PEDIATRIC TRAUMA

PEDIATRIC TRAUMA

Edited by

ROBERT J. TOULOUKIAN, M.D.

Professor of Surgery and Pediatrics
Chief, Pediatric Surgery
Yale University School of Medicine
Yale–New Haven Hospital
New Haven, Connecticut

SECOND EDITION
With **485** *illustrations*

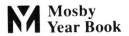

Mosby
Year Book

St. Louis   Baltimore   Boston   Chicago   London   Philadelphia   Sydney   Toronto

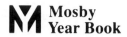

**Mosby
Year Book**

Dedicated to Publishing Excellence

Editor: Robert W. Reinhardt
Assistant Editor: Melba Steube
Project Manager: Patricia Tannian
Production Editor: John Casey
Book and Cover Design: Gail Morey Hudson

SECOND EDITION

Mosby–Year Book, Inc.
11830 Westline Industrial Drive, St. Louis, Missouri 63146

Library of Congress Cataloging in Publication Data

Pediatric trauma/edited by Robert J. Touloukian.—2nd ed.
    p.   cm.
  Includes bibliographical references.
  Includes index.
  ISBN 0-8016-5067-4
  1. Children—Wounds and injuries. I. Touloukian, Robert J.,
1936-
  [DNLM: 1. Wounds and Injuries—infancy & childhood. WO 700
  P3714]
  RD93.5. C4P43   1990
  617.1'0083—dc20
  DNLM/DLC
  for Library of Congress 90-6234
                CIP

GW/MV/MV 9 8 7 6 5 4 3 2 1

Contributors

BONNIE L. BEAVER, M.D.

Assistant Professor of Surgery and Pediatrics, University of Maryland School of Medicine and The Johns Hopkins University School of Medicine, Baltimore, Maryland

DEBORAH F. BILLMIRE, M.D.

Assistant Professor of Surgery and Pediatrics, St. Christopher's Hospital for Children, Philadelphia, Pennsylvania

MICHAEL R. CLEMMENS, M.D.

Assistant Professor of Pediatrics, University of Colorado School of Medicine; Director of Emergency Services, Children's Hospital of Denver, Denver, Colorado

DONALD R. COONEY, M.D.

Professor of Surgery and Pediatrics, University of Buffalo School of Medicine, State University of New York; Chairman of Pediatric Surgery and Surgeon-in-Chief, The Children's Hospital of Buffalo, Buffalo, New York

PETER DILLON, M.D.

Assistant Professor of Surgery, Division of Pediatric Surgery, Medical College of Virginia, Richmond, Virginia

MICHAEL A. DIPIETRO, M.D.

Associate Professor of Radiology, Section of Pediatric Radiology, University of Michigan Hospitals, Ann Arbor, Michigan

JOHN M. DRISCOLL, Jr., M.D.

Professor of Clinical Pediatrics, Columbia University College of Physicians and Surgeons; Director, Neonatal Intensive Care Unit, Columbia-Presbyterian Medical Center (Babies Hospital), New York, New York

CHARLES C. DUNCAN, M.D.

Associate Professor of Surgery (Neurosurgery), Yale University School of Medicine and Yale–New Haven Hospital, New Haven, Connecticut

MARTIN R. EICHELBERGER, M.D.

Professor of Surgery and Child Health and Development, George Washington University; Director, Emergency Trauma Services, Children's Hospital National Medical Center, Washington, D.C.

FREDERICK FINSETH, M.D.

Attending Plastic Surgeon, El Camino Hospital, Mountain View, California and Stanford University Hospital, Stanford, California

MARK GALLOWAY, M.D.

Assistant Clinical Professor of Orthopedics and Rehabilitation, Yale University School of Medicine and Yale–New Haven Hospital, New Haven, Connecticut

RICHARD H. GRANGER, M.D.

Professor, Child Study Center and Pediatrics, Yale University School of Medicine, New Haven, Connecticut

J. ALEX HALLER, Jr., M.D.

Robert Garrett Professor of Pediatric Surgery, Professor of Emergency Medicine, Professor of Pediatrics, The Johns Hopkins University School of Medicine; Children's Surgeon-in-Charge, The Johns Hopkins Hospital, Baltimore, Maryland

W. HARDY HENDREN, M.D.

Robert E. Gross Professor of Surgery, Harvard Medical School; Chief of Surgery, The Children's Hospital, Boston, Massachusetts

TERRY W. HENSLE, M.D.

Professor of Urology, Columbia University College of Physicians and Surgeons; Director, Pediatric Urology, Columbia-Presbyterian Medical Center (Babies Hospital), New York, New York

DENNIS J. HOELZER, M.D.

Chief, Pediatric Surgery, and Associate Chairman, Department of Surgery, The Medical Center of Delaware, Wilmington, Delaware; Clinical Associate Professor of Surgery, Jefferson Medical College, Philadelphia, Pennsylvania

MARC S. KELLER, M.D.

Associate Professor of Diagnostic Radiology and Pediatrics, Chief, Section of Pediatric Radiology, Yale University School of Medicine and Yale–New Haven Hospital, New Haven, Connecticut

MARGARET A. KENNA, M.D.

Associate Professor of Surgery (Otolaryngology and Pediatrics), Yale University School of Medicine; Attending Physician, Yale–New Haven Hospital, New Haven, Connecticut

GEORGE LISTER, M.D.

Professor of Pediatrics and Anesthesiology, Yale University School of Medicine, New Haven, Connecticut

J. KEVIN LYNCH, M.D.

Associate Clinical Professor of Orthopedics and Rehabilitation; Co-Director, Sports Medicine Center, Yale University School of Medicine and Yale–New Haven Hospital, New Haven, Connecticut

RICHARD I. MARKOWITZ, M.D.

Associate Professor of Diagnostic Radiology, University of Pennsylvania School of Medicine; Attending Radiologist, Children's Hospital of Philadelphia, Philadelphia, Pennsylvania

ALEKSANDRA MAZUREK, M.D.

Associate Clinical Professor of Anesthesiology, Northwestern University School of Medicine; Attending Anesthesiologist, Children's Memorial Hospital, Chicago, Illinois

LAURA R. MENT, M.D.

Professor of Neurology and Pediatrics, Yale University School of Medicine and Yale–New Haven Hospital, New Haven, Connecticut

THOMAS S. MORSE, M.D.

Professor of Surgery, University of Massachusetts Medical School, Worcester, Massachusetts

KURT D. NEWMAN, M.D.

Assistant Professor of Surgery and Child Health Development, George Washington University; Attending Surgeon, Children's Hospital National Medical Center, Washington, D.C.

JOHN A. OGDEN, M.D.

Chief of Staff, Shriners Hospital for Crippled Children, Tampa, Florida; Professor of Orthopedic Surgery and Rehabilitation, University of South Florida College of Medicine

JAMES A. O'NEILL, Jr., M.D.

C. Everett Koop Professor of Surgery, University of Pennsylvania School of Medicine; Surgeon-in-Chief, Children's Hospital of Philadelphia, Philadelphia, Pennsylvania

H. BIEMANN OTHERSEN, Jr., M.D.

Professor of Surgery and Pediatrics and Chief, Pediatric Surgery, Medical University of South Carolina, Charleston, South Carolina

DONALD H. PARKS, M.D.

Professor of Surgery and Chief, Division of Plastic and Reconstructive Surgery, University of Texas Health Science Center at Houston; Director, Hermann Burn Center, Houston, Texas

J. JULIO PÉREZ FONTÁN, M.D.

Assistant Professor of Pediatrics, Yale University School of Medicine, New Haven, Connecticut

CRAIG A. PETERS, M.D.

Research Fellow in Surgery, The Children's Hospital, Boston, Massachusetts

MAX L. RAMENOFSKY, M.D.

Professor of Pediatric Surgery, University of Pittsburgh School of Medicine

NANCY S. ROSENFIELD, M.D.

Associate Professor of Diagnostic Radiology and Pediatrics, Yale University School of Medicine and Yale–New Haven Hospital, New Haven, Connecticut

BARTON D. SCHMITT, M.D.

Professor of Pediatrics, University of Colorado School of Medicine; Director of Consultative Services, The Children's Hospital, Denver, Colorado

JOHN N. SCHULLINGER, M.D.

Professor of Clinical Surgery, Columbia University College of Physicians and Surgeons; Attending Surgeon, Columbia-Presbyterian Medical Center (Babies Hospital), New York, New York

MARVIN L. SEARS, M.D.

Professor and Chairman, Department of Ophthalmology and Visual Science, Yale University School of Medicine and Yale–New Haven Hospital, New Haven, Connecticut

JOHN H. SEASHORE, M.D.

Professor of Surgery and Pediatrics, Yale University School of Medicine; Attending Surgeon, Yale–New Haven Hospital, New Haven, Connecticut

RICHARD S. STAHL, M.D.

Associate Professor of Surgery (Plastic and Reconstructive), Yale University School of Medicine; Assistant Director (Surgery) Emergency Service; Attending Surgeon, Yale–New Haven Hospital, New Haven, Connecticut

ROBERT J. TOULOUKIAN, M.D.

Professor of Surgery and Pediatrics, Chief, Pediatric Surgery, Yale University School of Medicine and Yale–New Haven Hospital, New Haven, Connecticut

JOAN L. VENES, M.D.

Professor of Surgery and Pediatrics, Chief, Pediatric Neurosurgery, University of Michigan and Mott Children's Hospital, Ann Arbor, Michigan

TO OUR CHILDREN

Preface—FIRST EDITION

Although many books are available on all aspects of trauma, management of childhood trauma requires knowledge of the special ways children differ from adults. Each phase of the care of the injured child from the time of transport, resuscitation, clinical and roentgen diagnosis, anesthesia, and operative treatment to postoperative management requires knowledge of such differentiation. This information is the substance of *Pediatric Trauma*.

My aim has been to describe in comprehensive detail all important trauma problems encountered in infants and children, and I take particular pride in the list of outstanding contributors, many of whom are the leading authorities in their field. Part 1 emphasizes certain important general considerations such as the psychologic aspects of trauma, anesthesia and intensive care, the battered child syndrome, and birth injuries. Part 2 comprises more detailed discussions of all the important organ system injuries. These chapters deal with the essentials of diagnosis and management and highlight the mechanism and pathophysiology of injury, infection prevention and the use of antibiotics, and athletic injuries and their prevention.

I hope that *Pediatric Trauma* will appeal to the pediatrician, the family practitioner, and the emergency room physician, who are almost always called upon to initiate resuscitation and diagnostic procedures, as well as to the surgeon who must direct subsequent care of the severely injured child. More and more, the properly trained pediatrician must assume the role of the "team captain," particularly during the most important early phase of management, and be fully aware of how to work up and assess the injured child. Furthermore, many minor injuries, if appropriately treated by a primary physician, never require a surgeon. The importance of this book to both general and pediatric surgeons should be obvious. There are numerous illustrations and figures to help in preoperative decision making and in performing the operation itself. Extensive bibliographies following each chapter supplement those in existing works on the management of trauma.

R.J.T.

Preface

The past decade has been marked by a burgeoning interest in and dedication to the care of the injured child. The childhood injury fact sheet is well known. More children die from preventable injuries each year than from all childhood diseases combined. One child in four will suffer a preventable injury severe enough to require medical attention. The first edition of *Pediatric Trauma* focused on the many distinctions in transport, resuscitation, clinical and roentgen diagnosis, anesthesia, and opoperative treatment between the child and adult trauma patient. The text was patient-physician oriented and remains so, but during the 1980s the need for progress in developing trauma-specific hospital systems, education, prevention of injury and standards of care, and research and development has made pediatric trauma a valid medical specialty. National organizations such as the American Academy of Pediatrics, the American College of Emergency Physicians, the American College of Surgeons, and the American Pediatric Surgical Association have sections devoted to member education in pediatric trauma and to the provision and development of pediatric trauma care. There is increasing support for federal legislation that would strengthen state emergency medical services (EMS) and establish regional trauma systems. Parallel developments in diagnostic imaging, critical care, monitoring, prehospital transport capability, and surgical technology have revolutionized the care of the trauma patient.

With that background, the need for a revised edition of *Pediatric Trauma* was apparent, and the Editor is pleased that Mosby–Year Book, Inc. sought to make the second edition a reality. The format of the original version has been retained, but we take pride in adding six new chapters to make the second edition more comprehensive. Included now are chapters such as "Prehospital Resuscitation and Transport," "Metabolism and Nutrition in Severe Injury," "Respiratory Failure," "Maxillofacial Trauma," "Sports Injuries," and "Insect and Spider Bites."

As before, each author is a recognized authority in his or her field of interest. The intention is not only to make the second edition of *Pediatric Trauma* the standard reference for my colleagues in children's surgery, but also to please an expanded audience including general surgeons, emergency medicine physicians, and the pediatrician. Finally, the book is devoted to our children, prevention of injury when possible, and excellence in medical care to facilitate full recovery.

Robert J. Touloukian

Contents

PART I

GENERAL CONSIDERATIONS

1

Overview of Pediatric Trauma

J. Alex Haller, Jr. and Bonnie L. Beaver

So much has been written and said in the professional and lay press about the tragic loss of children from congenital heart disease, birth defects, and cancer that it is easy to overlook the fact that half of the children who die in the United States succumb from the immediate effects or aftereffects of major injuries.[10] Almost 50% of deaths occurring during childhood, from ages 1 through 14, in the United States are the result of major trauma, as compared with approximately one death in twelve from injuries in the total general population.[1,4] A similar situation exists in most industrialized nations. For example, in 1964 Stolowsky[29] reported that more than one third of childhood deaths in Germany resulted from major trauma. Although cardiovascular diseases, cancer, and pulmonary disease are the leading causes of death in the American population as a whole, trauma is the leading cause of death in children by a wide margin.[9,11]

The death of an otherwise normal child is always a great tragedy. On the other hand, crippling injuries to a child and the resulting need for rehabilitation may have an even greater effect on our health care system than the child's death per se. The expenditure of resources and personnel and the economic loss from termination of work potential when a child is seriously handicapped are relatively enormous when compared with similar costs resulting from adult injuries. This is true not only because of the long-term nature of such rehabilitation, but also because of the difficult problems of growth and development that must take place simultaneously in an immature child. These adjustments to severe disability and a child's image of himself as an incomplete individual may be overwhelming to the young patient unless highly trained professionals participate in the process of rehabilitation. It has been estimated that more than

100,000 children are seriously crippled in the United States each year by injuries and that another 2,000,000 may be temporarily incapacitated. As the number of children increases in our country, along with the general population increase, emergency medical services for immediate resuscitation and long-term rehabilitation will put further strains on our overburdened health care systems unless we can become innovative in preventing injuries and more aggressive toward providing better acute care management, both of which will decrease the need for long-term rehabilitation.

Since 1982 several guidelines for components of emergency medical systems for children have been suggested, and for the first time, specific standards of pediatric trauma care were formulated collaboratively. This "J Document" is a summation of the "Standards of Care for the Critically Injured Pediatric Patient." It was endorsed by the American Pediatric Surgical Association and the Committee on Trauma of the American College of Surgeons.[26,30] The American Academy of Pediatrics Provisional Committee on Emergency Medicine has been charged with the responsibility of developing national standards of emergency care for acute medical illnesses in children and are currently at work on such a landmark document.

We have had a functioning statewide system for the management of life-threatening injuries in children in Maryland for the past 13 years. In 1985 320 children were admitted to our regional Pediatric Trauma Center. The evolution, organization, and current status of the Maryland system are described as one example in this discussion. It is hoped that our experience may serve as a successful model that could be modified for use in other regions of this country and abroad.

Regional trauma centers have gradually evolved

in the United States to focus on the "disease of modern society," as trauma has been called by physicians working in the field of multiple-organ injuries. One of the earliest of these regional trauma centers was the Maryland Shock Trauma Unit under the direction of Dr. R.A. Cowley. It subsequently developed into a more complex statewide emergency system, now called the Maryland Institute of Emergency Medical Services Systems (MIEMSS). Similar trauma centers have been organized, with a very impressive impact on the management of trauma in the San Francisco area, Seattle, San Diego, and Denver, to mention but a few of the leading trauma centers in the United States. These units have been responsible for the development of standards of care based on solid clinical and laboratory research. In this way the acute care of patients has been improved, and to some extent, the long-term care and ultimate outcome have been enhanced. Regional trauma centers have not only improved the outcome of resuscitation in life-threatening injuries, but also, as a result of this focused attention, better systems of transportation from the scene of the accident to the appropriate center, as well as ongoing intensive care within the trauma institution, have been documented. This approach is still evolving; the concept is accepted, and the preliminary evidence clearly documents an improved level of care for this complicated disease called *trauma*.

MAIN CAUSATIVE FACTORS IN BLUNT INJURIES TO CHILDREN

In attempting to evaluate children with non-penetrating trauma, it is helpful to consider the kinds of forces that might be responsible for traumatic injuries. These can be arbitrarily identified as crushing, compressing, and decelerating forces. Crushing injuries are those in which the child's body is mashed against an unyielding surface, such as a loading platform or wall; a moving missile presses against the body. This is somewhat different from the compressing injury, in which there is usually a vector force of motion across the body, such as the passage of an automobile wheel over the child's body. This introduces an additional factor of movement and the tearing stress associated with it.

By far the most important group of forces is that associated with decelerating or accelerating injuries in which different organ systems are set in motion

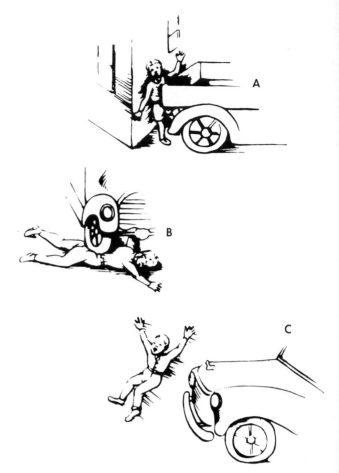

Fig. 1-1 **A,** Crushing, **B,** compressing, and **C,** decelerating forces are responsible for a variety of blunt abdominal injuries. (From Haller JA Jr: Clin Pediatr 5:476, 1966.)

depending on their masses. This results in differential ripping forces within the body. This may result in a tear, for example, at the stanchion points of the small intestine, Treitz's ligament, and the ileocecal area. Whiplash forces may be brought to bear and subsequently result in disruption or devascularization of the intestine with consequent perforation. Other forms of deceleration injuries may occur in the vascular system and in solid organs (Fig. 1-1).

BLUNT INJURIES IN CHILDREN

By far the commonest group of injuries that we see in the childhood age group is blunt as opposed to penetrating injuries. It has been estimated that at least 90% of life-threatening injuries in children occur as a result of blunt forces. Blunt trauma introduces a number of significant factors that complicate patient management. For example, blunt injuries are much more frequently associated with head injuries in children, and the evaluation of a semicomatose patient presents a communication problem, particularly the absence of important feedback from the patient in response to pertinent questions. In addition, blunt trauma is often associated with little evidence of external injury, yet the possibility of life-threatening internal injury may be present. It is this type of injury, a blunt injury, that emphasizes the need for highly experienced professionals working in emergency facilities to perform the initial evaluation and resuscitation of children. No injury is more complicated than one that is blunt. Despite this fact, often times patients are initially evaluated by the least experienced members of the emergency care team. This fact underlines the importance of reevaluating staffing policies in emergency rooms and considering the addition of full-time emergency medical staff with experience in blunt trauma who can supervise the training of younger health professionals and be available for important decisions commonly associated with the management of blunt injuries.[23]

Blunt Abdominal Injuries

Blunt abdominal trauma resulting in retroperitoneal injuries is especially difficult to evaluate. For example, compression injury to the pancreas may result in a hematoma in the body of the pancreas with leakage of activated pancreatic juices into the retroperitoneal space. Autodigestion may occur if this is not recognized, yet there may be very little evidence of this injury when the child is first evaluated. The retroperitoneal area is a relatively quiet area in terms of physical signs, and only later will evidences of peritoneal irritation become obvious. The same may be said for more extensive injuries to the pancreas, including transection, in which major hemorrhage may occur. The evidences for a specific cause of hypovolemic shock are not easily ascertained. The adjacent duodenum may be injured from the same compression force, with resultant retroperitoneal perforation or intramural hematoma, resulting in obstruction of the lumen. These must be considered in the differential diagnosis with any blunt injury to the abdomen. The solid organs (pancreas, liver, spleen and kidney) all may be injured from blunt trauma. Documentation of solid organ injury has been best

achieved by contrast-enhanced computed tomography (CT).[2,15-18,25]

Blunt injury to the kidney may result in transection of a portion of the parenchyma and laceration of the blood vessels and drainage system. The CT scan has greatly improved the ability to diagnose specific injuries, and, more and more frequently, no surgery is required. Extravasation of urine or contrast medium on the CT scan or intravenous pyelogram (IVP) is no longer an absolute indication for exploration because some of these injuries can heal. Furthermore, if the patient is stable, a more conservative approach is indicated. Occasional aortography may be indicated, especially if no contrast is secreted from a kidney. Partial resections rather than nephrectomy for major vascular injuries to the kidney are possible.[18] A massively expanding hematoma in the retroperitoneal area still represents a rare indication for exploration.

Blunt injuries to the liver may result in major fractures of the parenchyma with both hemorrhage and bile leakage; however, laparotomy may not be necessary, even with documentation of injury by CT scan. Techniques of hepatic artery ligation, intraoperative cholangiography, and finger fracture methods of resection have improved overall salvage of these potentially lethal injuries.[17,25]

The commonest solid organ to be injured is the spleen. Nonoperative management of splenic fracture or laceration is the primary goal of management. A child's spleen has a very important immunologic function, especially in his or her resistance to certain types of infections. It is the primary source of antibodies against encapsulated gram-positive organisms, such as pneumococcus and meningococcus, and gram-negative organisms such as *Haemophilus influenzae*. Much experience has been documented in nonoperative management.[6,8,19] Attempts to preserve the spleen are clearly indicated, and recent studies with splenorrhaphy support preservation even for critical splenic injuries. Rarely is splenectomy necessary. Certainly, following splenectomy, all children should be placed on prophylactic penicillin and receive vaccinations against pneumococcal and *Haemophilus* species to decrease the chances of overwhelming infections, which have now been very well documented following the seminal observations of surgeons in Indianapolis in 1952.[19,20]

Blunt injury to hollow viscera may result in compression perforation or perforation due to tearing of the mesentery and intestine. These may also be difficult injuries to diagnose initially because there may be very little evidence of peritoneal irritation, especially in a child with a head injury who is semicomatose from the concussion effects. Careful observation in the hospital for this type of injury is imperative so that insidiously developing peritonitis is not overlooked. After 24 to 36 hours of leakage from the intestine, clear-cut evidence of peritoneal irritation should be present, and with expeditious exploration and repair, purulent peritonitis, a much more serious complication than chemical peritonitis, can usually be prevented.

Peritoneal lavage should be reserved for those settings in which CT scanning is unavailable or other life-threatening injuries take precedence over abdominal CT assessment. For example, should the patient require urgent operative intervention for head injury, open lavage or laparotomy or both can be quickly performed in the OR area at the same time.[3,7,27]

PENETRATING INJURIES IN CHILDREN

Penetrating injuries do occur in childhood. In perhaps 10% of the abdominal injuries seen in major emergency rooms a penetrating force is involved. These are not as difficult to evaluate and manage because most penetrating injuries require an exploratory operative procedure. Various kinds of diagnostic studies that employ injection of contrast media have been used in children and adults, and they have their place in selected overall management. By and large, a penetrating injury is an indication for surgical exploration as soon as the patient has been totally evaluated and is hemodynamically stable.

THERMAL INJURIES

A major burn is one of the most serious diseases of childhood. The immediate mortality associated with an extensive burn is still quite high, and the associated morbidity of a major burn is often overwhelming in terms of commitment of professional personnel and the financial load on the family. The anguish of debridement followed by multiple skin grafting procedures adds to the severity of the injury to the child. In addition, long-term rehabilitation, cosmetic disfigurement, and emotional adjustments in an immature child add to the tragedy of this preventable injury.

VASCULAR INJURIES

Vascular injuries in children have become a significant problem, especially in regional referral centers. Penetrating trauma is responsible for most of these vascular injuries, but they may also result from blunt trauma. The commonest cause of vascular injuries in major diagnostic centers is the complication of an invasive diagnostic study, such as cardiac catheterization and arteriography.[22,28] This fact does not imply that these tests should not be carried out but serves to underline the potential hazard of such tests, particularly in young children, and to emphasize the importance of having skilled personnel and excellent facilities for these highly specialized studies. Of all penetrating injuries there has been a striking increase in the number of cases of lethal gunshot wounds in young children, resulting from increased availability of guns, largely handguns, in the home.

UNUSUAL RESPONSES OF A CHILD TO A MAJOR INJURY

A small child may respond differently from an older patient and adult to major injuries. For example, paralytic ileus following blunt abdominal trauma may be of greater consequence in children because abdominal distention in a young child may elevate the diaphragm and interfere more with limited pulmonary function. In a relative sense, therefore, paralytic ileus is of greater consequence in an infant or young child. The same may be said for blood losses in a small patient whose blood volume is less. For example, a closed fracture of the femur in a 10-year-old patient may be associated with 300 or 400 ml of blood lost into the soft tissues. The same amount of blood for a similar injury in an adult would be of little consequence; but in the child this may represent 10% to 25% of the total circulating blood volume and contribute to hypovolemic shock. Unless these relative differences are recognized, such blood losses may not be considered significant in the smaller patient. Major heat losses may occur in a young child who is unclothed in an air-conditioned emergency room for proper evaluation and who may remain there for several hours. A drop in core temperature of several degrees may interfere with normal enzyme function and other metabolic processes. These changes may add a further metabolic insult to a child's response to the stress of trauma.

Congenital abnormalities rarely complicate evaluation and management of adults with major injuries. They can cause serious complications in young children whose congenital anomalies may not have been detected and may not have interefered with reasonably normal function up to the time of injury. For example, a 5-year-old child with 50% second- and third-degree burns recently went into profound congestive heart failure during the resuscitative process of fluid and electrolyte replacement. He was then found to have an asymptomatic ventricular septal defect, but under the stresses of rapid fluid replacement, acute myocardial decompensation and heart failure occurred. Possible complications of unrecognized congenital abnormalities must be remembered in the total evaluation of a child treated for major trauma.

The rapidity with which metabolic and cardiovascular responses can occur serves to emphasize the importance of good monitoring systems to evaluate the responses of young children to emergency treatment. Whereas monitors are useful in adults, they are mandatory in a small patient because minor changes in response to treatment must be detected early to prevent more serious sequelae.

Head injuries are much more commonly associated with blunt trauma in children than in adults, and they complicate the overall evaluation of the child. Why head injuries occur so commonly is not always obvious. It may be that a child's head is relatively larger and therefore more exposed to trauma than that of the adult, or that the child's head is less well supported on the neck and shoulder girdle. Regardless of an exact explanation, head injuries are very frequently associated with blunt trauma in children. Aside from the errors in diagnosis, which may result from evaluating an obtunded child, the lethal effects of hypoxia, hypoperfusion, and progressive cerebral edema from blunt trauma are major causes of death from head injury. Although mass lesions such as subdural or epidural hematomas occur less frequently in children than in adults, they require aggressive operative treatment.

The emotional impact of an emergency room experience cannot be overemphasized. A child with a relatively minor injury is often triaged into a corner of a general adult emergency room while patients with life-threatening injuries are given their proper first priority. What a young child may see during a 2-hour stay in such an environment is often frightening and emotionally disturbing. Gunshot wounds, stab wounds, and drunken adults in various states of disarray represent horrible visual experiences to an immature child. Unless these are necessary components of the child's emergency room experience, perhaps better care can be administered in an environment designed and staffed for his or her age group. For many years we have recognized that children have special needs and that we need to design pediatric departments and children's units within our larger medical centers accordingly. The same approach is long overdue in emergency room areas. Whether we design separate but equal facilities for children alongside adult units, or whether we identify committed areas for children within adult emergency room environments, are individual decisions for each regional medical center. The important principle is to design and staff appropriate areas especially for children and their particular needs. These facilities must contain the best available quality care for the management of life-threatening and less serious injuries to children.

If a compromise in the organization of these facilities must be made, it would be far better to bring children with life-threatening injuries into an adult environment because the resuscitative efforts are much more important than sheltering children from potentially frightening environmental influences, especially since these children are often unconscious. However, it is also very important to designate special areas for evaluating children with minor injuries who are threatened by this environment. Obviously a child who is semicomatose or in shock is not likely to remember the environmental aspects of his resuscitative treatment, but a child with a cut finger, a stubbed toe, or a minor burn may more greatly feel the effects from emotional trauma than from the physical injury itself.

The identification of such specialized children's units within the total emergency facility offers a number of other significant possibilities for improving patient care. This would give surgeons and pediatricians in training the opportunity to work as partners in the care of children with major injuries and serious acute illnesses.

Identification of a captain of the trauma team is essential to prioritizing and directing appropriate management of multiple-organ injuries. Children, as well as adults, with complex injuries are at great risk of being separated by organ system for management by different surgical specialists. For example, the child with a head injury, a fractured femur, and hematuria may have a neurosurgeon, orthopedic surgeon, and urologist each demanding that a particular organ receive priority in management. Under these circumstances the pediatric trauma victim desperately needs a child advocate, one who can intelligently establish priorities in management and organize the team effort in resuscitation and continuing treatment. Of course, highly skilled surgical specialists must be immediately available to such emergency facilities for the care of children. These surgical specialists should have special expertise in the management of children's surgical problems and be familiar with some of the unique features of the care of children. A natural leader for such a team approach would be a general pediatric surgeon or, in his absence, a very experienced physician in pediatric emergency medicine.

Any consideration of the design of such dedicated outpatient emergency facilities must be combined with the development of inpatient facilities that are dedicated to the continuing care of injured children. These include an operating room that is always available for life-threatening emergencies requiring immediate surgery, including pediatric anesthesiologists as a part of the treatment team. Intensive care units designed for children and staffed for their care may also parallel intensive care facilities for adults, depending on inpatient organization in individual regional centers. A helicopter receiving area is necessary for expeditious transport from the scene of injury and for the transfer of newborn infants with life-threatening emergencies. These combined facilities can be expected to deliver high-quality care with special emphasis on the unusual needs of children. As a complex they would then represent a proper regional trauma center for children.

Discussed below is an outline for the continuum of care of the injured and ill child, in an organized Emergency Medical System for children.

COMMUNICATION

Recent experience in several medical centers has emphasized the importance of two-way radio communication between ambulance personnel at the scene of an emergency and medical personnel in a receiving hospital. This voice system makes it possible to notify a hospital that a child will be transported to their special facilities and enables the physician and emergency medical technician at the scene to discuss management. In this system, advice on special forms of treatment, such as management of flail chest, may be given directly to the emergency medical technician.

TRANSPORT SYSTEM

A transport system is an integral part of a regional trauma center concept. The support components of the system include *helicopter transport* on a radio-controlled basis, which is initiated through an *emergency medical relay center,* which functions as a communication link for the system. Transportation is arranged through the relay center for each case, and the appropriate specialty facility to which the patient should be taken is determined.

Transport of children from the emergency scene into the emergency room often requires special instrumentation including small airways and splints and miniaturized equipment. The use of this equipment must be included in the emergency medical technician training courses and should be a special part of the communication and transport system. Half of the preventable deaths associated with major trauma are estimated to occur between the scene of the accident and arrival in the emergency room. Only by better training and communication with improved transport can this inexcusable loss of life be prevented.

FIRST RESPONDERS AT THE TRAUMA SITE

The *emergency medical technicians* must receive specialized training in the care of infants and children from medical specialists such as neonatologists, pediatric emergency physicians, and pediatric surgeons and anesthesiologists. They are then certified to begin intravenous treatment of small infants and to intubate babies and young children if indicated. Their pediatric training must be a part of the ongoing training program for emergency medical technicians within the regional system.

PEDIATRIC TRAUMA CENTER

A resuscitation unit is a basic component of a regional pediatric trauma system. After communication from the scene of the life-threatening injury, the child is brought by appropriate transportation to the designated emergency room and is met by a team of pediatric resuscitation and pediatric surgery specialists who are trained in initial man-

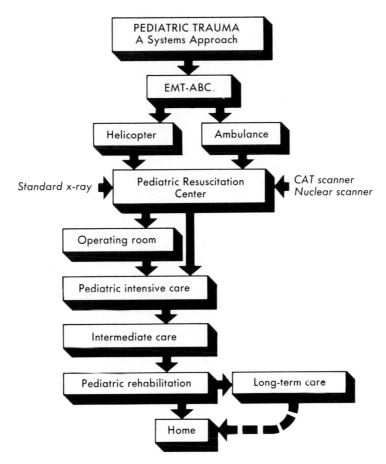

Fig. 1-2   Plan for a systematic approach to emergency medical services for children with major injuries.

agement of life-threatening injuries (Fig. 1-2).

The child should be managed in a resuscitation unit designed specifically for children, with miniature intubation equipment (including tracheostomy tubes) and other specialized equipment (including central venous pressure lines for children). The captain of the trauma resuscitation team should be either a senior resident in pediatric surgery or a staff pediatric surgeon working closely with well-trained emergency pediatric staff. Available on call within minutes must be key pediatric surgical specialists, such as pediatric neurosurgeons and pediatric orthopedic surgeons. X-ray equipment must be immediately available in the unit for both the initial diagnostic studies and subsequent special films, including computerized axial tomography. It is important to emphasize that all children with major injuries should be resuscitated by emergency pediatricians and pediatric surgeons, all of whom are part of an organized pediatric trauma team.

After initial stabilization, with appropriate diagnostic tests and specialty consultations, a child may go directly to the operating room or be admitted to a pediatric intensive care unit (PICU).

PEDIATRIC INTENSIVE CARE UNIT

Pediatric intensive care units should also be centralized. All patient stations should be equipped with multiple-channel monitoring equipment and ventilators and staffed for the immediate detection of cardiopulmonary arrest and for resuscitation and continuing posttrauma management. Other equipment may include a mass spectrometer, cardiac output computers, blood gas analyzers, ionized calcium analyzers and gamma cameras for determination of cardiac output and similar clinical research studies. A small designated on-site blood gas laboratory should provide immediate blood gas determination.

NEUROLOGY-NEUROSURGERY INTERMEDIATE CARE UNIT

A neurology-neurosurgery intermediate care unit for pediatric trauma is directed by a pediatric neurosurgeon and a pediatric neurologist who both have special interests in the care of the child with head injuries. This is a direct continuation of the intensive care of children with brain injuries, including continued monitoring of their neurologic recovery when they no longer require constant monitoring and the use of intracranial probes for pressure measurements. Within this unit, pediatric rehabilitation begins and the involvement of the pediatric behavioral medicine specialists becomes an increasingly important component of patient management. Children with long-term physical rehabilitation requirements need continued assessment and structured therapy conducted by specialists in physical medicine and rehabilitation. Eventually, these children will be transferred to a formal pediatric trauma rehabilitation unit.

Preliminary evidence from our experience strongly suggests that children with major head injuries that result in coma lasting longer than 24 hours have a higher recovery rate than reported in the literature. These data suggest that only 10% of the surviving children have an intellectual or motor residual and 88% of the survivors over 2 years of age have good recovery without measurable major motor or intellectual deficits. Although it remains to be seen whether these preliminary data will reflect continuing trends, they are certainly encouraging.[21]

PEDIATRIC TRAUMA REHABILITATION UNIT

One pediatric trauma rehabilitation unit, located in the John F. Kennedy Rehabilitation Institute, is an important new program that has been given a high priority within that institution. An eight-bed unit has been designed to allow for inpatient care and parent participation in ongoing subacute and intermediate rehabilitation programs and evaluation. This provides not only for better day-to-day patient care, but also an opportunity to study the emotional and physical responses to rehabilitation and to design new protocols for early rehabilitation. This provides another important component of an integrated program that has committed itself to intermediate and long-term management of children with residual neurologic and physical problems following major injuries. This unit has full-time pediatric supervision, and all of the physician members of the pediatric trauma group are an important part of the consultative staff and participate in frequent interdisciplinary discussions and presentations.

CHILDREN'S TRAUMA REGISTRY: LOCAL AND NATIONAL

Within such specialized facilities it then becomes possible to establish a statistical survey system, or trauma registry, in which each child with a major injury is documented within a protocol. These data are available for careful retrospective evaluation and computerization at the local, state, and national level. Frequent review of the results of treatment patterns of trauma will be invaluable in subsequent training of emergency medical personnel. By quality assurance review of available facilities for the treatment of children, one may focus on areas requiring change. Within the emergency department, these registries can be used for inservice education, review of patient care, and discussion of better patient management. An ongoing clinical pathologic conference remains the best form of teaching and best means of improving delivery of emergency care.[5,13,14]

Local

Our experience in pediatric trauma at The Johns Hopkins Hospital between July 1985 and June 1986 emphasizes the unique features of childhood injuries that have led to modification of our approach to diagnosis, resuscitation, and definitive management of injured children.

Between July 1, 1985 and June 30, 1986 the care of children treated at the Maryland Regional Pediatric Trauma Center was analyzed. Patients were evaluated and initially stabilized in the main emergency area by the pediatric/surgical trauma team. This team consisted of a senior pediatric surgical resident (sixth to seventh postgraduate year), a pediatric intensivist, a surgical resident (fourth postgraduate year), and a pediatric intern. Diagnostic studies were obtained in the emergency room and the adjacent CT area. Patients were then transferred to the PICU or pediatric surgical ward for definitive care. A trauma registry was used to record prospectively the demographic data, mechanism of injury, systems injured, types of injuries, vital signs, trauma scores (including Glasgow coma scores), and patient outcome.

Table 1-1   Mechanisms and types of injury

	Number of patients	Percentage
Blunt trauma		
Motor vehicle accidents (pedestrian)	130	41
Motor vehicle accidents (passenger)	37	12
Motor vehicle accidents (bicycle)	28	9
Falls	85	26
Other	28	9
Penetrating trauma		
Gunshot	4	1
Knife-stab injury	6	2
Other	2	0.5

Table 1-2   Organ systems

	Number of patients	Percentage
Type of system		
Central nervous	198	62
Maxillofacial	23	7
Skeletal	82	26
Abdominal	60	20
Chest	25	10
Soft tissue	55	17
Number of systems involved		
Single-system injury	222	69
Two-system injury	65	20
≥Three-system injury	33	10

Table 1-3   Complications

Type of complication	Number of patients
Septic	
Pneumonia	4
Central line	8
ICP/Bolt	3
Urinary tract	1
Wound/soft tissue	2
Delay or error in diagnosis	
Facial bone fracture	2
Extremity fracture	2

During the 12-month span, 320 patients were admitted to the hospital. All children were less than 15 years of age (mean age was 7.2 years). Of these 320 patients, 210 were males and 110 were females; 144 were black, 168 were white, and 8 were of other races. Helicopter transport accounted for 42% of patient transport, and 58% were transported by ambulance. Approximately 85% were admitted directly from the scene. The types of injury (blunt and penetrating) and the mechanisms of injury are depicted in Table 1-1.

The overwhelming majority of blunt trauma injuries were associated with pedestrian/motor vehicle accidents (42%). Falls were second in frequency (26%). The remaining 28 patients sustained other injuries, including burns (8), crush injuries associated with sports (10), abuse and assault (8), and near drowning events (2).

Although penetrating injuries were infrequent, the gunshot wounds included one head injury (fatal), one abdominal, and two soft tissue injuries. The knife stab wounds to the chest caused pneumothorax four times and two soft tissue injuries. Two other penetrating injuries were associated with falls. The breakdown of frequency of injury to organ systems was as follows: central nervous system (62%), skeletal (26%), abdominal (20%), soft tissue (17%), chest (10%), and maxillofacial (7%). Of these patients, 69% had a single-system injury, 20% had a two-system injury, and 10% had an injury to three or more systems (Table 1-2). There were 22 complications: 85% were septic and 20% were due to a delay or an error in diagnosis (Table 1-3).

The overall mortality was 3.4%, or 11 patients. All 11 patients had *closed head injuries* associated with their multisystem trauma. *All of the patients died as a result of their head injuries.* Seven children died after admission during their early hospital course in the PICU; the other four patients died in the emergency room.

National

As of October 1989, more than 11,900 pediatric trauma patients had been entered in the centralized Pediatric Trauma Registry of the National Institute on Disability and Rehabilitation Research. This reflected data contributed by 50 institutions.

The male-to-female ratio was 2:1. The age distribution was, for the most part, between 1 to 10 years of age (62%), with ages 11 to 15 years accounting for 23.5%. Eight-four percent of injuries were associated with blunt mechanisms of injury, 12.1% were caused by penetrating trauma, and others (drowning, crush injury, ingestion) accounted for 3.5%. The largest number of injuries were associated with motor vehicle encounters (40%), followed by falls (34%), firearm and stab injuries (5%), and miscellaneous (20%).

Organ systems injured, in decreasing frequency of occurrence, were closed head trauma, skeletal, superficial and deep soft tissue, thorax, abdomen, and spine. The overall mortality was 3.3%.[24]

DISCUSSION

Since 1963 a statewide network for the care of injured patients has served both urban and rural areas in Maryland. In 1972 the Regional Pediatric Trauma Center at The Johns Hopkins Hospital became an integral part of the Maryland Institute of Emergency Medical Systems Services. Our experience with all injured children under 15 years of age for the past 16 years has provided an opportunity to evaluate resuscitation and management strategies in the immediate postinjury period, as well as to initiate studies on injury control and prevention.

Several unique aspects of trauma in children have now been documented. The increased incidence of head injury in children with blunt trauma and the associated morbidity and mortality involving the central nervous system have mandated a more aggressive approach to the management of brain injury, including intracranial monitoring to facilitate control of cerebral edema. CT in the immediate postinjury period and sequential scanning has been invaluable in following the clinical courses of these patients. Indeed, no trauma center for children can function properly without the immediate availability of CT scanning and intracranial monitoring.

The management of blunt abdominal injury for the most part has become largely nonoperative. Abdominal CT has played a major role in assessing blunt abdominal injury. CT scanners have become our method of choice in all children who have altered neurologic states and whose physical examination is unreliable.

Both head and abdominal CT are conducted sequentially and have been used effectively after the initial assessment and stabilization. Close proximity of the radiologic suites to the main trauma room permits expedient evaluation.[2] The multidis-

ciplinary approach to the injured child is coordinated through a general pediatric surgeon who consults the neurosurgeon, orthopedic surgeon, and the pediatric anesthesiologist/intensivist.[12] For the child who is being managed nonoperatively, a team effort with constant monitoring is required in a PICU at least for the first 24 hours.

The rehabilitative pathway is just the beginning for many trauma patients, particularly those children who survive head injuries. An excellent quality of life may be anticipated, even in children with severe head trauma.[21] A plan for immediate and long-term rehabilitation for children with neurologic and orthopedic injuries should be formulated early in the intensive care phase of treatment. This requires early input from pediatric neurologists and pediatric physiatrists. With this systems approach of integrated prehospital treatment and transport, hospital resuscitation, intensive care, and rehabilitation of the injured child, optimal management of this "most fatal disease of modern society" can be attained. Trauma management and injury control are a challenge and an opportunity for all emergency physicians, especially pediatric surgeons throughout the world.

REFERENCES

1. Baker SP, O'Neill B, and Karpf RS: The injury fact book, Lexington, Mass, 1987, DC Heath and Co.
2. Beaver BL et al: The efficacy of computed tomography in evaluating abdominal injuries in children with major head trauma, J Pediatr Surg 22:1117, 1987.
3. Bivins BA, Jonei JZ, and Belin RP: Diagnostic peritoneal lavage in pediatric trauma, J Trauma 16:739, 1976.
4. Tabulations prepared by Children's Bureau, Welfare Administration, based on data of the National Center for Health Statistics, Public Health Service, Department of Health, Education and Welfare, Rockville, Md., 1980.
5. Colombani PM et al: One-year experience in a regional pediatric trauma center, J Pediatr Surg 20:8, 1985.
6. Douglas GJ and Simpson JS: The conservative management of splenic trauma, J Pediatr Surg 6:565, 1971.
7. Drew R, Perry JF, and Fischer RP: The expediency of peritoneal lavage for blunt trauma in children, Surg Gynecol Obstet 145:885, 1977.
8. Eraklis AJ and Filler RM: Splenectomy in childhood: a review of 1413 cases, J Pediatr Surg 7:382, 1972.
9. Gratz RR: Accidental injury in childhood: a literature review on pediatric trauma, J Trauma 19:551, 1979.
10. Haller JA: Newer concepts in emergency care of children with major injuries, Pediatrics 52:485, 1973.
11. Haller JA: Pediatric trauma, the No. 1 killer of children, JAMA 249:47, 1983.
12. Haller JA: Emergency medical services for children: what is the pediatric surgeon's role? Pediatrics 79:576, 1987.
13. Haller JA et al: Use of a trauma registry in the management

of children with life-threatening injuries, J Pediatr Surg 11:381, 1976.

14. Haller JA et al: Organization and function of a regional pediatric trauma center: does a system of management improve outcome? J Trauma 23:691, 1983.

15. Jones TK, Walsh JW, and Maull KI: Diagnostic imaging in blunt trauma of the abdomen, Surg Gynecol Obstet 157:389, 1983.

16. Karp MP et al: The role of computed tomography in the evaluation of blunt abdominal trauma in children, J Pediatr Surg 16:316, 1981.

17. Karp MP et al: The nonoperative management of pediatric hepatic trauma, J Pediatr Surg 18:512, 1983.

18. Karp MP et al: The impact of computed tomography scanning on the child with renal trauma, J Pediatr Surg 21:617, 1986.

19. King DR et al: Selective management of injured spleen, Surgery 90:677, 1982.

20. King H and Schumacker HB Jr: Splenic studies—I. Susceptibility to infection after splenectomy performed in infancy, Ann Surg 136:239, 1952.

21. Mahoney WJ et al: Long-term outcome of children with severe head trauma and prolonged coma, Pediatrics 71:756, 1983.

22. McCroskey BL, Moore EE, and Rutherford RB, editors: Vascular trauma, Surg Clin North Am 68:683, 1988.

23. Morse TS: Triage, technicians, and teaching in a children's emergency room, J Pediatr Surg 8:701, 1973.

24. Report of the National Institute on Disability and Rehabilitation Research Pediatric Trauma Registry, Boston, October 1989.

25. Oldham KT et al: Blunt liver injury in childhood: evolution of therapy and current perspective, Surgery 100:542, 1986.

26. Ramenofsky ML and Morse TS: Standards of care for the critically injured pediatric patient, J Trauma 22:921, 1982.

27. Root HD et al: Diagnostic peritoneal lavage, Surgery 57:633, 1965.

28. Shaker IJ et al: Special problems of vascular injuries in children, J Trauma 16:863, 1976.

29. Stolowski HJ: Blunt abdominal trauma and intestinal perforation in childhood, Chirurg 36:4, 1965.

30. Trauma Committee of the American Pediatric Surgical Association in conjunction with the Committee on Trauma of the American College of Surgeons: Appendix J to hospital resources document, Planning Pediatric Trauma Care, 1982.

2

Prehospital Resuscitation and Transport

Max L. Ramenofsky

Injury continues to be the number one cause of death in the pediatric age group.[6,13] As in the adult population, death from trauma in childhood follows a trimodal distribution.[14] The first peak occurs within seconds to minutes after the occurrence. Death during the first peak is "usually due to lacerations of the brain, brain stem, high spinal cord, heart, aorta, or other large vessels."[2] The second peak occurs within minutes to several hours after the incident and is usually the result of subdural and epidural hematomata, hemopneumothorax, ruptured spleen, major liver lacerations, pelvic fractures, or other injuries that result in major blood loss. The third peak occurs days to weeks after the injury and is most always due to multiple-organ system failures and sepsis. Although many fewer deaths occur in children than in adults during the third peak, as treatment modalities improve, more children will succumb during this period, although total mortality should fall.

Prehospital care directly affects the first two time periods and indirectly affects the third. A major influence on the first period is the result of effective injury-prevention methodologies. However, with appropriate identification of an accident and a rapid prehospital response to the scene of an injury, a small number of victims will be salvaged who would otherwise die on the scene before the rescue squad arrives.[11]

The second peak is affected by the care given by the prehospital personnel, the speed with which the patient is delivered to the pediatric trauma center, and the care given in the first hour following arrival in the center.[5]

The third peak of death is affected by all that has occurred up to the point of the patient's recovery.

A major problem in the prehospital care rendered the injured child is the pediatric education of the prehospital provider. Only 2% to 3% of the curricula of most paramedic training courses is in pediatrics. This deficiency has been noted by most of the Emergency Medical Services for Children grants given by the Maternal Child Health Division of the Department of Health and Human Services.[8] Consequently, most of the 12 recipients of these grants have implemented a pediatric training module for paramedics in their states. The majority of states, however, do not have such an expanded pediatric curriculum.

The pediatric trauma surgeon should expect to receive the injured child in the best possible condition. Should this not occur, it becomes the responsibility of the surgeon to provide continuing education programs for the prehospital care providers so that care can be improved. The purpose of this chapter is to describe the evaluation, care, packaging, and transport of an injured child.

PREHOSPITAL CARE
EMS/Trauma System

The concept of a trauma system is not new. Trauma systems were mandated by the US Congress in the 1970s via the EMS Systems Acts.[4] There are, however, only a few areas in the United States where fully functioning trauma systems are in place. These few areas provide the population that they serve a better than expected outcome from life-threatening traumatic events.[15]

A well-organized trauma system will have a number of mandatory components such as integrated, designated trauma centers, triage protocols, and adequate communication and transportation systems, including an aeromedical component.[8]

The purpose of trauma center designation and

verification is to allow significantly injured patients to be transported to a hospital that has committed itself to care of the injured without the imposition of unacceptable delays. This includes 24-hour/7-day in-house trauma teams and immediate access to all hospital equipment and facilities the injured patient may require. This obviously requires a major commitment from hospital administration, physicians, nursing, and other paramedical personnel. The degree of the commitment should be judged not by the hospital itself but by an unbiased group of trauma surgeons, nurses, and administrators from outside of the immediate area that the hospital serves. This verification group will generally use a set of standards for trauma center verification, such as those developed by the American College of Surgeons Committee on Trauma.[1]

Personnel

A statewide Emergency Medical Service System now exists in every state in the United States. Some are quite sophisticated, whereas many are only embryonic in the care they provide. There are three general training levels of rescue personnel in these systems. The Emergency Medical Technician I (EMT-I) is an individual who has been trained in basic life support (BLS). BLS is noninvasive life support, such as CPR. The second level of training is the EMT-intermediate. Such an individual has been trained in BLS and intravenous cardiac drug use. The highest level of training is the EMT-paramedic (EMT-P). Such an individual has been through hundreds of hours of didactic and clinical experience and can provide advanced life support (ALS), which includes invasive procedures, such as endotracheal intubation and chest tube insertion. Throughout this chapter the term "EMT" will be used to identify the EMT-P.

The personnel component of a rescue squad will vary regarding the skill level of the individuals composing that squad. A squad may be composed of all paramedics, but more often the majority will be EMT I–trained individuals. Thus, the care any given rescue squad can provide will depend on the makeup of the individual squad.

The specifics of care that a rescue squad can provide in the field are generally defined by the area's EMS system. For example, even though paramedics have been trained in the techniques of endotracheal intubation, the EMS system and medical control may not allow prehospital personnel to perform that procedure. It is helpful for the hospital-based trauma surgeon or physician to be aware of what the rescue squad can and cannot do.

Medical Control

Prehospital personnel function under the medical license of a physician who has been charged with the responsibility of overseeing what these individuals do. The physician component of an EMS system is referred to as medical control, of which there are two types, on-line and off-line. On-line medical control is provided by a physician at a base station who is in radio or telephone contact with the EMTs on the scene. The EMTs provide verbal descriptive reports to the physician, who then tells the EMT to carry out a given treatment.

Not infrequently, it is impossible to be in voice contact with medical control, and when that occurs, the EMT or paramedic functions via preapproved written protocols for the medical emergency at hand.

Off-line medical control is the quality-assurance mechanism of an EMS system. After a "run," a responsible physician must evaluate and critique the rescue squad. When errors are identified, a mechanism should be in place to correct these errors. Off-line medical control also refers to care given to certain subsets of patients, such as the child, the burn victim, and the spinal cord–injured patient. Although specialists for these types of patients may not be in direct voice contact with the EMTs, the prehospital care provider should have preapproved protocols by such specialists, or alternatively, medical control may be in contact with these specialists and relay orders to the EMTs in the field.

The Scene

The scene of an accident is not a familiar venue for the physician. It is perhaps the most hostile patient care environment imaginable. The EMT, by attitude and training, is in fact a more ideal care provider than a physician for an injured patient at the scene of the injury. The physician expects an organized, well-lighted, quiet, well-controlled environment in which to treat a patient. The EMT treats patients in a most uncontrolled environment. The patient may be entrapped, bleeding, and unable to maintain his or her airway. The outside, ambient temperature may be below freezing or it may be in excess of 100° F; it may be raining, snowing, hailing, in a house or building fire, in the midst of a hurricane or tornado; there may be a crowd milling about, a riot, upset parents or relatives, drunk and disorderly patients and/or bystanders, or there may have been a gunfight.[3] The scene can be in the center of an area of urban blight, within a poorly maintained tenement building, in the center of a large metropolitan area during the peak of rush hour, in an outlying affluent suburb, in a corn field, in the middle of a forest, or on a mountainside. The incident may be the result of a terrorist shooting or bombing. The EMT not only must provide immediate lifesaving care, but also must treat and triage multiple victims simultaneously, with a limited number of personnel having varying amounts of training, in addition to providing crowd control. Thus the job of the EMT is complex, unpredictable, occasionally dangerous and, at all times, hurried.

Initial Assessment and Primary Survey

The physician should expect to receive the patient in the best possible condition. The trauma surgeon should be aware of the routine practiced by the EMT.

The EMT is acutely aware that the time spent on the scene *must* be kept to a minimal.[9,11] After extraction of a patient from a vehicle, a fire, or any situation in which the EMT must use his or her nonmedical skills to gain access to the patient, it is reasonable to expect the time at the scene to be 10 minutes or less. If lifesaving care cannot be completed within 10 minutes, valuable time is being lost and the child is being treated in the most poorly equipped and lighted emergency room in town.[9]

Initial assessment and the primary survey are the ABCs of lifesaving care and are based on the principles of Advanced Trauma Life Support (ATLS) of the American College of Surgeons[2] and Pre-Hospital Trauma Life Support (PHTLS) of the National Association of Emergency Medical Technicians.

The ABCs are an easily remembered and practiced mnemonic: *A*—Airway assessment and management and cervical spine control; *B*—Breathing; *C*—Circulation; *D*—Disability or a rapid neurologic examination; and *E*—Exposure of the patient so that injuries can be seen, evaluated, and stabilized.

The ABCs are aimed at immediately identifying and treating life-threatening injuries such as airway obstruction, tension pneumothorax, pericardial tamponade, and hypovolemic shock. In fact, the ABCs were developed to treat the greatest threats to life in the order in which these threats kill. For example, an obstructed airway is more quickly fatal than a tension pneumothorax, which is more quickly fatal than shock.

The initial assessment of the injured child proceeds through the same steps as those used to assess an injured adult; however, a number of aspects of the ABCs require a different approach.

Airway

The approach to the child's airway requires knowledge of the child's anatomy. The position the airway occupies in the pharynx, the surrounding, potentially obstructing structures, the angle and softness of the vocal cords, the shortness of the trachea, and the position of the head relative to the neck when the child is lying supine are vital anatomic facts the EMT must know.

The first maneuver is to clear the airway by sweeping the finger into the pharynx and using suction to remove solid debris, blood clots, broken teeth, and so forth.

To open the airway the head is brought slightly forward relative to the neck, the so-called sniffing position. Once the airway has been opened by these physical maneuvers, it must be maintained. If an oral airway is used in the child, it is inserted along the curvature of the tongue rather than the 180-degree reverse insertion used in adults. An oral airway cannot be used in the child with an intact gag reflex. The nasopharyngeal airway can similarly be used in the child, but care must be used in its insertion because of the fragile nature of the nasal and pharyngeal mucous membranes.

Endotracheal intubation may be necessary for a variety of reasons. Attention must be paid to the size of the endotracheal tube. Cuffed endotracheal tubes are not used in children because of the softness of the airway and the potential damage even a low-pressure cuff can cause. Due to the ease with which the child's vocal cords can be damaged when an endotracheal tube is forced through the cords, it is best to select a tube that easily passes the cords. An air leak through the cords is the rule and can be compensated for by an increased flow rate rather than a tighter fitting tube.

It is usually impossible to rule out a cervical spinal cord injury in the field; thus the cervical spinal cord must be protected at all times during resuscitation. Early in-line immobilization of the cervical spine is warranted either by manual technique or the use of a cervical collar and cervical immobilizer device (CID). Spinal cord injury without radiographic abnormality (SCIWORA) occurs in the child and must be evaluated in the same way as in an adult.[7] Good presumptive evidence of a normal cervical spine includes the lack of localizing neurologic deficits and a lack of tenderness during neck examination. In the field, presumptive evidence is not adequate, and thus in-line cervical spinal immobilization is mandatory.

Breathing

Assessment of breathing in the injured child is no different from that of an adult but is often easier to evaluate because of the compliance of the chest wall. EMTs are taught that the optimal position to auscultate and evaluate breath sounds is in each axilla. They are also taught to evaluate the respiratory rate and the depth and equality of the respiratory effort.

Circulation

Evaluation of the circulatory status requires significant knowledge of cardiovascular physiology to prevent the delayed identification of occult bleeding and development of hypovolemic shock. Most EMTs are taught neither the subtle changes seen in the child that occur early in shock nor how to treat these changes.

The initial maneuver in assessing and treating the child's circulation is to arrest hemorrhage. This can most often be accomplished by applying direct pressure on a bleeding site. Tourniquets are not used to stop bleeding because of the damage caused distal to the application site of a tourniquet.

Controversy exists regarding the use of the pneumatic antishock garment (PASG). Most authorities feel its use is not warranted if the transport time will be short, that is, less than 20 minutes. However, the severely fractured diastatic pelvis with accompanying serious hemorrhage is one clear-cut indication for its use. EMTs are carefully taught the use of the PASG, specifically how to apply it. When it is used the leg compartments are inflated first and, if necessary, the abdominal compartment last. Once the PASG has been applied the trauma surgeon should know how to remove it. Each compartment is deflated in the reverse order of its inflation, with careful monitoring of pulse and blood pressure. Should significant deterioration be identified, the last deflated compartment is again expanded.

Volume resuscitation in the injured child is carried out in much the same way as it is in the adult. Once it has been determined that the child is suffering a volume deficit, large-bore intravenous lines should be rapidly inserted and a rapid infusion of crystalloid fluids started. Lactated Ringer's solution is generally used. The initial infusion volume should be based on replacing 25% of the child's blood volume. A reasonable estimate of that blood volume is 80 ml/kg. To replace 25% of the blood volume using a crystalloid solution, a total volume of 60 ml/kg may be necessary. A fluid bolus of 20 ml/kg should initially be infused; this may be repeated twice, for a total volume of 60 ml/kg. After the initial fluid bolus has been given, the patient's hemodynamic status should be *reassessed,* and if at that time more volume is indicated, it should be given.

Disability

The next priority in the primary survey is to evaluate the neurologic status of the patient. This is a rapid neurologic examination that evaluates the level of consciousness and the presence of abnormal pupillary findings. In addition to the pupillary evaluation the neurologic examination is carried out via the pneumonic AVPU: *A* describes an awake, alert child; *V* denotes a child who is responsive to verbal stimuli; *P* describes a child who is responsive to only painful stimuli; and *U* stands for an unresponsive child. Pupillary response is evaluated by the size and equality of the pupils. These two simple modalities provide a quick and accurate description of the child's CNS status.

Some authorities feel that the Glasgow coma score (GCS) is a more useful tool. However, some question the accuracy of the GCS when it is used to evaluate the nonverbal child.

Exposure

It is not appropriate to totally expose the child in the field. Not only is the removal of the child's clothing inappropriate in terms of temperature maintenance, but also the modesty and comfort of the child must be considered.

Reassessment

The ABCs must be completed before the EMT proceeds to the next step. In fact, it is not a particularly infrequent occurrence for the EMT not to be able to go beyond the ABCs because immediately life-threatening injuries have not or cannot be adequately controlled in the field. If one assumes for the moment that the ABCs have been carried out and the patient is stabilized, the next priority is to assess the results of their actions. Assessment and reassessment is a cornerstone of what an EMT does. Should it be found that the patient is again deteriorating, attention must once again be focused on the cause of that deterioration, and attempts should be made to arrest the process, albeit temporarily.

Secondary Survey

After the initial assessment, the primary survey, and continual reassessment, the EMT should undertake the secondary survey. In practice the secondary survey is often not conducted because of limited time; however, it should be performed.

The secondary survey is a rapid head-to-toe examination, the purpose of which is to identify other injuries that may ultimately jeopardize the child's outcome. It is during this phase of care that previously nonapparent fractures, penetrating injuries, and significant lacerations are often identified. For example, should a fracture be identified, the application of an appropriate splint will provide some degree of pain control and also a safe package for patient transport.

Packaging

Once the child's immediately life-threatening injuries have been temporarily treated, secure packaging for the transport is required. Most often the child will be securely attached to a long spineboard,

and not infrequently, to a short spineboard as well. The cervical collar should be stiff but allow access to the airway, should that become necessary. The CID is added to immobilize the head and neck with the rest of the body. Splints attached to the child are left in place, as are dressings. Once the child has been fully immobilized the entire litter is placed into the transporting vehicle.

PEDIATRIC TRAUMA SCORE

The development of the pediatric trauma score (PTS) has provided the prehospital/provider and the trauma surgeon with some options not previously available. The PTS, developed by Tepas et al.,[12] is a combination anatomic-physiologic score that has several distinct advantages over other clinical scoring systems. The score is an accurate predictor of severity of injury, is useful by itself as a triage tool, and provides a checklist similar to the initial assessment of ATLS, which quickly identifies life-threatening injuries, as well as less severe injuries that may not be life threatening but, if overlooked, add significantly to morbidity if not mortality (Fig. 2-1).

The PTS is the only scoring system developed with the special needs of the child in mind. All other trauma scoring systems fail to give appropriate consideration to the differing anatomic and physiologic aspects of the injured child.

The PTS is determined by evaluating each of six components (size, airway, central nervous system status, systolic blood pressure, open wounds, and

Severity	+2	+1	−1
Weight	>44 lbs.	22-44 lbs.	<22 lbs.
	(>20 kg)	(10-20 kg)	(<10 kg)
Airway	Normal	Oral or nasal airway	Invasive
			Intubation
			Cricothyroidotomy
Blood pressure	>90 mm Hg	50-90 mm Hg	<50 mm Hg
Level of consciousness	Awake	Obtunded	Comatose
	Alert	Any LOC*	
Open wound	None	Minor	Major or penetrating
Fractures	None	Single	Open or multiple
		Simple	
TOTALS			

*Any loss of consciousness

Fig. 2-1 Diagrammatic representation of the pediatric trauma score (PTS). One severity score is circled for each individual component, and the scores are totaled. The pediatric trauma score ranges from +12, indicating minor or no injury, to −6, indicating uniformly fatal injury.

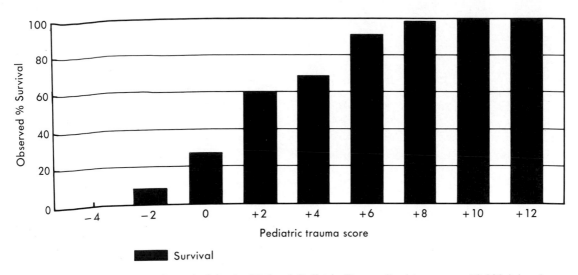

Fig. 2-2 Observed survival in the National Pediatric Trauma Registry among 10,098 injured children. There is uniform fatality for pediatric trauma scores of -3 or less and uniform survival for patients with pediatric trauma scores of $+10$ and greater.

fractures) at one of three severity levels ($+2$ = mild, $+1$ = moderate, and -1 = severe, potentially life threatening). When each component has been scored all of the individual scores are added, thus constituting the PTS. The PTS ranges from $+12$, indicating no or minimal injury, to -6, indicating fatal injury. Each individual PTS is associated with its own mortality rate and has been correlated with injury severity scores and mortality rate (Fig. 2-2).[12] The PTS accurately predicts significant injury and insignificant injury (predictive validity) and has a high interrater reliability among emergency medical technicians and physicians.[10]

SUMMARY

The Trauma/EMS system provides a rapid access system for traumatic and medical emergencies. The appropriate designation of trauma centers provides hospitals with commitment to rapid, state-of-the-art trauma care. EMTs generally provide prehospital care in such a system and should be expected to deliver the injured child to the trauma center in the best possible condition.

The resuscitation delivered in the field is described by the initial assessment or primary survey, reassessment, secondary survey, packaging, and transport.

It is the responsibility of the pediatric trauma surgeon to act as on-line and/or off-line medical control, the purpose of which is to provide quality assurance for the Trauma/EMS system.

REFERENCES

1. American College of Surgeons, Committee on Trauma: Hospital and prehospital resources for optimum care of the injured patient and appendices A-J, 1987, The College.
2. American College of Surgeons: Advanced trauma life-support program manual, 1989, The College.
3. Barlow B, Gandhi R, and Niermirska M: Ten years experience with pediatric gunshot wounds, J Pediatr Surg 17:927, 1982.
4. Emergency medical systems act of 1973, Public Law 93-154, Washington, DC, 1976, US Government Printing Office.
5. Luterman A, Ramenofsky ML, and Berryman C: Evaluation of prehospital emergency services (EMS): defining areas for improvement, J Trauma 22:702, 1983.
6. National Safety Council: Accident facts, 1988 edition, 1988, The Council.
7. Pang D and Wilberger JE: Spinal cord injury without radiographic abnormality, J Neurosurg 57:114, 1982.
8. Ramenofsky ML: Emergency medical services for children and pediatric trauma systems components, J Pediatr Surg 24:153, 1989.
9. Ramenofsky ML et al: EMS for pediatrics: optimium treatment or unnecessary delay, J Pediatr Surg 18:498, 1983.
10. Ramenofsky ML et al: The predictive validity of the pediatric trauma score, J Trauma 28:1038, 1988.
11. Ramenofsky ML et al: Maximum survival in pediatric trauma: the optimal system, J Trauma 24:818, 1984.
12. Tepas JJ et al: Pediatric trauma score as a predictor of injury severity in the injured child, J Pediatr Surg 22:14, 1987.
13. Tepas JJ et al: The national pediatric trauma registry, J Pediatr Surg 24:153, 1989.
14. Trunkey DD: Trauma, Sci Am 249:28, 1983.
15. West J and Trunkey D: Systems of trauma care: a study of two counties, Arch Surg 114:455, 1979.

3

Evaluation and Initial Management

Thomas S. Morse and Robert J. Touloukian

The emergency care of injured children calls for a systematic approach that has been mentally rehearsed until it has become automatic. The plan includes an understanding of airway management, control of hemorrhage, and the principles of resuscitation. Once the overall condition of the patient is stabilized, an assessment of the extent of injury can be undertaken and priorities in emergency treatment established. In this chapter, the evaluation and initial management of the entire patient are discussed. Various specific forms of injury are detailed in subsequent chapters.

AIRWAY

Life depends on ventilation and circulation. When a child cannot breathe adequately, the physician must correct this deficiency before turning attention to any other consideration. The first requirement is a patent airway.

Airway Obstruction

In unconscious children the tongue tends to fall backward and obstruct the airway. Obstruction is accentuated if the neck is either flexed or overextended and is minimized by placing the child's head in the "sniffing" position (Fig. 3-1). Foreign matter such as blood or vomited stomach contents can be quickly wiped or aspirated away. Foreign matter that cannot be removed readily may be expelled using the residual air in the child's lungs, as described by Heimlich. The heel of one hand is placed on the abdomen midway between the umbilicus and the xyphoid; a quick inward and upward thrust compresses the lungs by driving the liver and diaphragm upward. The maneuver may be repeated if necessary.

Oxygen should be supplied by the most readily

available means, usually first by mouth-to-mouth resuscitation. The exhaled air of an adult contains plenty of oxygen for this emergency purpose. A few puffs in a child's mouth with the nose pinched shut, or with the physician's mouth covering both the nose and mouth of an infant (Fig. 3-2), can be followed with air from a self-inflating bag until oxygen by mask and ventilating bag are available. A plastic oral airway, if the child will accept it, may be slipped into the mouth to hold the tongue forward.

Intubation

Only after the above simple measures have been applied should the use of an endotracheal tube be considered. In emergency situations, this tube should be passed through the mouth, to be replaced later, if necessary, by a nasotracheal tube. The size of the tube can be judged from the fact that the child's nostril is nearly always about the same size as the narrowest part of the airway through which

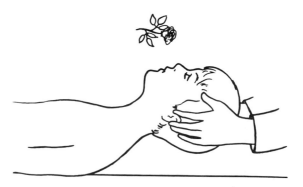

Fig. 3-1 "Sniffing" position to minimize upper airway obstruction. The neck is neither flexed or overextended. The head is lifted as if to help the child sniff an imaginary flower held above the face.

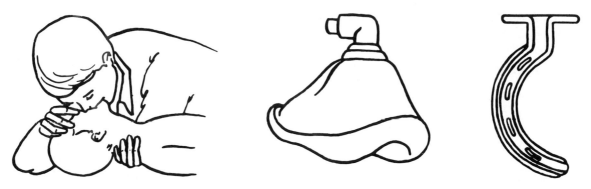

Fig. 3-2   Mouth-to-mouth resuscitation or administration of oxygen via a mask should precede intubation. An oral airway is useful if the child will accept it.

the tube is to be inserted (Fig. 3-3). Thus a tube that would fit comfortably in the nostril is of an appropriate size for emergency orotracheal intubation. Age-related guidelines for the size of the endotracheal tube and the appropriate orotracheal distance inserted to prevent main-stem bronchial intubation are found in Table 3-1. As the tube is inserted, an assistant places his or her finger over the trachea just above the suprasternal notch to feel the tip of the tube pass beneath the notch, indicating that the tube has been inserted to the proper depth. If it is passed too far, the tip of the tube may enter one main bronchus, obstructing the other, and only one lung will be ventilated. If the tube is properly placed, both sides of the chest rise equally with each inspiration, and breath sounds are heard equally over both lungs. A stethoscope placed over the stomach will identify misplacement of the tube in the esophagus. To prevent dislocation of the endotracheal tube, a Logan bow or Neckel's arch is invaluable (Fig. 3-4). Using a tincture of benzoin

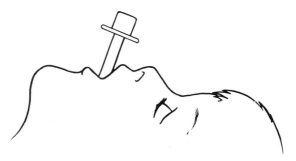

Fig. 3-3   Emergency intubation is performed via the mouth using a tube of the same diameter as the child's nostril.

Table 3-1   Guidelines for size of endotracheal tube

Age	Internal diameter (mm)	Orotracheal distance (cm)
Newborn-6 months	3.5*	11
6-12 months	4.0*	12
1.5 years	4.5*	13
2 years	4.5*	14
3-4 years	5.0*	16
5-6 years	5.5*	18
7-8 years	6.0*	20
9-11 years	6.5	22
12 years	7.0	24

*Uncuffed tube

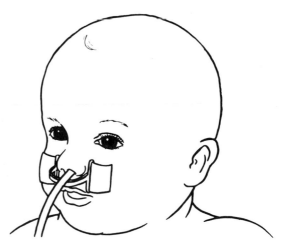

Fig. 3-4   After the emergency phase, the endotracheal tube may be removed and a new one passed transnasally. The Neckel's arch helps to fix the tube in place.

to ensure adhesion, the arch is taped to the cheeks and the tube taped to the arch.

VENTILATION

Mechanical ventilation with a volume ventilator may be substituted for hand ventilation by Ambu bag once the endotracheal tube is properly secured and chest movement monitored to determine that adequate excursions are achieved. Children of school age can be ventilated appropriately with about 20 inspirations per minute, but younger children require 30 per minute (Fig. 3-5). Tidal volume setting for a child weighing more than 5 kg should be set to deliver 10 to 15 ml/kg and 3 to 4 cm H_2O of positive end-expiratory pressure.

In the final analysis, mechanical ventilation must be monitored by arterial blood gas determination. The primary aim is to maintain the PaO_2 at 80 to 100 torr by controlling the inspiratory oxygen quotient, inspiratory pressure, and respiratory rate with the ventilator. If the arterial pH falls below 7.35 in the presence of an increasing base excess, hyperventilation and infusion of sodium bicarbonate are usually required to correct the metabolic acidosis. The formula for using $NaHCO_3$ (mEq/l) equals the body weight (kg) × base excess ×0.3. Half of the total calculated dose is given initially and the patient hyperventilated to reduce the $PaCO_2$ to 20 to 25 torr. The remainder of the $NaHCO_3$ infusion can be given to correct the serum pH further. Further details on ventilation management in respiratory failure are presented in Chapter 5.

CIRCULATION

Once the airway has been cleared and ventilation ensured, circulation becomes the prime consideration. The urgent problems are arrest of hemorrhage and recognition and treatment of shock. Less frequently encountered, but no less critical, are cardiac tamponade and cardiac arrest.

Control of Hemorrhage

Direct pressure over the bleeding point is usually the safest way to control bleeding. Simply elevating the bleeding part may greatly reduce the loss of blood. This is particularly true of the head. Children with massive bleeding from scalp wounds *should not* be made to lie flat but should be treated with the head elevated. Scalp wounds from which blood pours profusely usually overlie compound skull fractures with torn intracranial veins. Application of direct pressure to these veins is impossible, but blood loss will be minimal if the laceration in the vein is kept a few inches above the level of the heart. Spurting vessels may be clamped with hemostats only if the bleeding points are clearly visible. In most areas of the body, major arteries are closely accompanied by important nerves to which irreparable damage may be done by blind clamping.

Bleeding from extremity wounds may be controlled temporarily by tourniquets. Preferably, blood pressure cuffs should be used because these deliver measurable pressure over a broad area. The pressure must exceed the child's systolic blood pressure, or else blood will escape into the limb only to be prevented from returning to the body. A tourniquet that is too loose actually promotes blood loss and is worse than none at all. Damage to underlying nerves may be caused by narrow makeshift tourniquets twisted too tight. If used at all, tourniquets should be replaced within a few minutes by sterile pressure dressings over the wound because the ischemia produced by a tourniquet soon results in intolerable pain. There is always the danger that a tourniquet may be applied to an unconscious child and forgotten, resulting in loss of the extremity.

The application of the military antishock trouser (MAST) during the prehospital resuscitation of children in shock has largely replaced the use of tourniquets. The MAST garment has particular value in patients with unstable pelvic fractures and those with extensive intraabdominal injury. The advantages of the MAST garment are to reduce hemorrhage and sustain circulation to the heart, lungs, and brain. Filling of the upper extremity veins may also facilitate placement of an intravenous cannula for giving fluid volume.

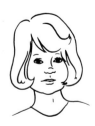

Fig. 3-5 Appropriate ventilatory rate is about 40/min for infants, 30/min for preschool children, and 20/min for school and teenage children.

SHOCK

Shock following injury is nearly always due to blood loss. Trauma to the central nervous system practically never causes shock, and circulatory collapse due to autonomic response to fear or pain is usually of such brief duration that it is no longer present when the child arrives in the emergency department. Myocardial insufficiency is very rare. Shock resulting from infection is usually a late complication and is seldom encountered in the emergency department.

Hemorrhagic Shock

Hemorrhagic shock is characterized by hypotension, tachycardia, cool, pale, or slightly cyanotic extremities, restlessness or obtunded sensorium, and oliguria. Hypotension results directly from the diminished blood volume. Tachycardia is a compensatory mechanism, as is increased peripheral vasoconstriction, which produces the cool, pale extremities. The central nervous system aberrations result from cerebral hypoxia due to inadequate perfusion of the brain. Oliguria results from reduced glomerular filtration secondary to hypotension and from renal cell hypoxia. Whenever oxygenation of the brain and kidneys is inadequate, the same is true of the myocardium. If myocardial hypoxia persists, hypovolemic shock is complicated by a cardiogenic component. Eventually all body cells, which at first were hungry for oxygen, become incapable of utilizing it, and death invariably follows.

Recognition of Shock

Familiarity with the normal blood volume of children is fundamental to rational initial management. A child's blood volume relates directly to his body weight and for practical purposes is 80 ml/kg regardless of age or size (Fig. 3-6).

The upper limits of normal for pulse rate are 160/min in infants, 140/min in preschool children, and 120/min in everyone else (Fig. 3-7). The normal systolic blood pressure in millimeters of mercury for children from 1 to 20 years of age is 80 plus twice the age in years. The normal diastolic pressure is two thirds the normal systolic pressure. Thus for a 5-year-old child, normal systolic pressure is $80 + 5 \times 2 = 90$ mm Hg, and normal diastolic pressure is $90 \times \frac{2}{3} = 60$ mm Hg.

Normal minimal urine output averages 2 ml/kg/hr in small children and 1.0 ml/kg/hr in older children and adults (Fig. 3-8).

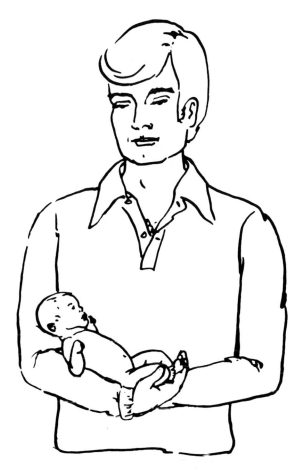

Fig. 3-6   For practical purposes the normal blood volume is 40 ml/lb, regardless of size or age.

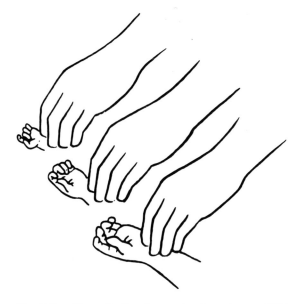

Fig. 3-7   Upper limits of normal pulse rates are 160/min for infants, 140/min for preschool children, and 120/min for everyone else.

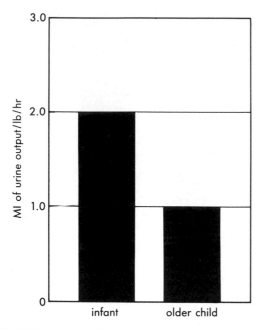

Fig. 3-8 Acceptable minimal urine output is 2 ml/lb/hr for infants and 1 ml/lb/hr for older children.

The accompanying table (Table 3-2) is a helpful guide to the first signs of circulatory compromise based on heart rate and blood pressure in the pediatric age group.

Initial Management of Shock

A previously healthy child who is in shock after an injury has lost at least one fourth and usually not more than one half of normal blood volume. Most children seen in the emergency department in hemorrhagic shock have lost between 20 and 40 ml/kg of blood. The Advanced Trauma Life Support Classification of Hemorrhage recommended by the American College of Surgeons is useful in defining the severity of hemorrhage (see box below) and can be used to estimate crystalloid and blood volume fluid replacement.

Vascular access

Saphenous and antecubital vein cutdown and percutaneous insertion have been the traditional favored sites for venous access in the acutely injured patient. Prompt cannulation may be difficult because of vasoconstriction and movement, particu-

For practical purposes, an injured child is in shock if tachycardia and cool, pale extremities accompany a drop in systolic pressure. The first preventable error is failure to recognize the *presence* of shock. An even more common mistake is failure to recognize the *development* of shock after initial evaluation has been completed. The only way to be sure that these mistakes are never made is to assume that shock is present or will develop in every significantly injured child and to insist on frequent determination and accurate recording of the pulse rate and blood pressure. The alterations in heart rate and systolic blood pressure that occur following hemorrhage are related not only to the extent of blood loss but also the age of the patient.

Table 3-2 Heart rate and systolic blood pressure alterations as initial signs of hemorrhagic shock

Age	Heart rate	Systolic blood pressure
1 year	160	50
1-2 years	150	60
Preschool	140	70
School age	130	80
Adolescent	120	90

AMERICAN COLLEGE OF SURGEONS: ADVANCED TRAUMA LIFE SUPPORT CLASSIFICATION OF HEMORRHAGE

Class I hemorrhage	Up to 15% blood loss (10 ml/kg), minimal tachycardia, no measurable change in blood pressure, pulse pressure, respiratory rate, or capillary refill time (CRT)
Class II hemorrhage	15% to 30% blood loss (10-20 ml/kg), tachycardia, tachypnea, decreased pulse pressure (decreased diastolic pressure), increased CRT, decreased urine output
Class III hemorrhage	30% to 40% blood loss (20-30 ml/kg), overt shock, tachycardia, hypotension, tachypnea, depressed level of consciousness, oliguria
Class IV hemorrhage	40% blood loss (30 ml/kg), profound hypotension, tachycardia, tachypnea, anuria, profound depression of consciousness, cold pale skin

Table 3-3 Catheter size (gauge) guidelines for vascular access

	Peripheral	Central	Seldinger technique (femoral, jugular, subclavian)
Infants	22-24	18-22	20-22 (3-4 Fr)
Toddlers, preschool	20-22	16-20	16-20 (4-6 Fr)
School age	16-20	10-16	6+ Fr

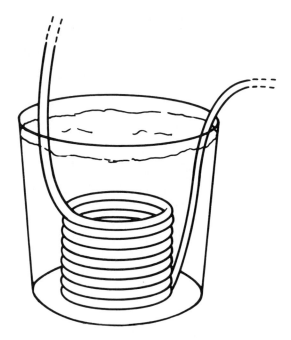

Fig. 3-9 Simple coil of tubing inserted in water at body temperature safely warms blood for rapid infusion.

larly in a small child. Under these circumstances, alternatives include using a smaller gauge plastic cannula than required to begin fluid resuscitation, performing a saphenous vein cutdown at the groin, or inserting a percutaneous catheter in the external jugular vein. The use of an upper extremity catheter is preferred, particularly when the question of intraabdominal injury is raised. Percutaneous subclavian insertion has become extremely popular in adult patients, but this exposes the uncooperative child to the risks of vessel injury or pneumothorax. For those reasons, we have been quite selective in its use for children, limiting central venous placement until after initial resuscitation has been completed. Guidelines recommended for catheter size in various age groups are found in Table 3-3.

Crystalloid

Once adequate intravenous access is established, a bolus of Ringer's lactate or similar crystalloid fluid is rapidly infused. Patients sustaining hemorrhage of 10% to as high as 30% of estimated blood volume may be resuscitated with crystalloid at the rate of 3 ml for every 1 ml blood lost and may never require a blood transfusion. The response to this initial bolus of electrolyte solution determines further management. If the blood pressure returns to normal, Ringer's lactate solution at a maintenance rate of 1500 ml/m^2/24 hours is continued, and the pulse rate and blood pressure are measured at frequent intervals. If these remain normal, one can be confident that blood loss is not continuing and that blood transfusion will not be needed.

If the pulse rate remains elevated and the child is still hypotensive, a second bolus of Ringer's lactate solution equal to 30 ml/kg of body weight is given as rapidly as the first. The need for this second bolus implies that blood transfusion will be needed because dilution of the patient's remaining

blood will have reduced its oxygen-carrying capacity.

Blood

Blood should be transfused after the child has been given an amount of Ringer's lactate solution equal to one half of the total blood volume. The freshest whole blood available is preferable to packed red blood cells for preserving coagulation function. Because it should be given rapidly in boluses, the blood should be warmed to body temperature with the use of a blood warming coil (Fig. 3-9). Each bolus should bear a definite relationship to the normal blood volume. The first bolus is usually 20 ml/kg. Subsequent volumes of blood administered are based on magnitude of blood loss. The American College of Surgeons guide to therapy based on hemorrhage classification is useful for estimating the volume of blood and crystalloid required (Table 3-4).

Central venous pressure

In our experience there is no danger of overloading the circulation of a child in hemorrhagic shock until sufficient Ringer's lactate solution and blood have been administered. A central venous catheter is of no value in the *initial* management

Table 3-4 Fluid therapy based on hemorrhage classification

ACS class	Blood loss (ml/kg)	Crystalloid therapy (ml/kg)	Blood (PRBC) (ml/kg)
I	10	30	—
II	10-20	30-60	—
III	20-30	20+ (may repeat)	20
IV	30	20+ (may repeat)	20+

of hypovolemic shock, and attempting to insert one before giving the child 30 to 60 ml/kg of Ringer's lactate solution and 20 ml/kg of blood is generally a waste of valuable time. After these fluids have been given, many children become normotensive and stable and do not need a central venous monitor. Those who have not been resuscitated completely by the above measures are candidates for insertion of a percutaneous internal jugular venous line, which can be very valuable in their further management.

Urinary catheter

Tissue perfusion is adequate when the sensorium is lucid, the skin warm and pink, and the rate of urine output normal. The most reliable and easily documented of these parameters is the hourly urine output. If the patient is rapidly and easily stabilized, a urinary catheter is superfluous, but when the indications for a central venous catheter are present, an indwelling Foley catheter also should be inserted. Both catheters carry a risk of introducing infection; both should be inserted with calm care and precision *after* the initial steps described previously have been taken, and both should be removed as soon as they are no longer needed.

Hematocrit

The hematocrit is of little value in the initial management of children in hemorrhagic shock, but it is extremely helpful in the hours that follow. It reflects changes more slowly than do the vital signs, central venous pressure, and rate of urine output. Its greatest usefulness is as an indicator of gradual blood loss. Changes in serial hematocrits are more valuable than any single determination.

OCCULT BLEEDING

Children who require more than 20 ml/kg of whole blood in addition to 40 ml/kg of Ringer's lactate solution often are still bleeding. It is much easier to detect continuous bleeding if blood is replaced rapidly in boluses than if it is infused at a constant rate. Vital signs, hematocrit, and rate of urine output are recorded before and immediately after each bolus is administered. Changes in these pretransfusion and posttransfusion values reflect primarily the influence of the rapid intravenous intake. During the subsequent period of maintenance fluid administration, changes in hematocrit, pulse rate, blood pressure, and rate of urine output quickly reflect a decreasing blood volume due to ongoing hemorrhage. If continuous blood loss and replacement are allowed to proceed simultaneously, recognition of ongoing blood loss may require a much longer observation period.

Fractures of the pelvis or major long bones may be associated with a loss of more than one fourth of the total blood volume, and bleeding from fractures may continue for many hours after injury. Provided vital signs, hematocrit, and rate of urine output are followed with a high index of suspicion, the physician will not be caught unaware when occult bleeding causes shock. A more dangerous error is to assume that, because major fractures are present, *they* are responsible for all the loss of blood. This erroneous assumption may lead to failure to recognize potentially lethal lesions, such as rupture of the liver or spleen.

Significant occult bleeding is usually intraabdominal and is manifested by abdominal tenderness. In simple injuries the diagnosis of intraabdominal bleeding is not difficult, but in more complicated injuries many factors may make a clinical diagnosis unreliable or impossible. The most common complication factor is a head injury. Since tenderness is the most important clinical feature of intraabdominal bleeding, head injuries that obtund the sensorium deprive the clinician of his or her most valuable observation. Pelvic or rib fractures may produce pain when the abdomen is pressed, and one cannot be sure whether the patient is reacting to motion of the fracture or whether abdominal tenderness is being elicited. Renal injuries produce tenderness and hematuria. The coexistence of rupture of the liver or spleen is easily missed if all the tenderness is mistakenly attributed to a renal injury. These combined injuries are common. Of 44 children with injuries of the left kidney, 11 (25%) also had a ruptured spleen. An abdominal CAT scan has proven invaluable in assessing for visceral injury in the multiple-trauma patient.

Abdominal Paracentesis

Paracentesis is neither indicated in perfectly lucid children without abdominal findings nor when the diagnosis of an intraabdominal injury requiring operation has been based on clinical grounds, including diagnostic imaging. We use paracentesis liberally in patients with head injuries who are difficult to examine or uncooperative or when an abdominal CAT scan cannot be obtained. Paracentesis is performed with a 17-gauge Angiocath*; we have not found peritoneal dialysis catheters necessary. The finding of gross blood that does not clot indicates an intraabdominal injury. If blood does not return, 20 ml/kg of saline is infused. This corresponds to about 1.5 to 1.8 liters in the adult and nearly always ensures a return via the catheter. An RBC count of over 100,000/cu mm or an inability to read newsprint through a test tube full of the effluent is taken as significant.

CARDIAC TAMPONADE

Cardiac tamponade is a rare cause of circulatory insufficiency that results from accumulation of blood within the pericardium. It is caused by a penetrating wound of the heart, and usually a wound of entrance can be identified. The condition is characterized by a very weak rapid pulse and a narrow pulse pressure. Because the heart cannot expand normally, the central venous pressure is high, as suggested by the finding of distended neck veins.

---

*Deseret Company, Salt Lake City, Utah.

The emergency treatment of cardiac tamponade consists in removing some of the liquid portion of the extravasated blood by inserting a large caliber needle into the pericardial sack. The needle is inserted at the xyphoid and aimed at the middle of the left scapula, 45 degrees upward and 45 degrees laterally from the point of entrance (Fig. 3-10). Removal of as little as 10 to 20 ml of blood may greatly improve the child's condition, at least temporarily, but aspiration is usually not adequate definitive treatment because aspiration does not close the rent in the myocardium and because much of the blood in the pericardial sac is clotted. Emergency pericardiotomy with evacuation of the clots and repair of the myocardial wound is usually indicated.

CARDIAC ARREST

Cardiac arrest in the emergency department usually portends to a fatal outcome for an injured child. If there is incontrovertible evidence that the heart has been stopped for 10 minutes or more, resuscitation should not be attempted. Unless one can be certain of this, attempts at salvage are justifiable and occasionally may succeed.

The first step is to ensure adequate ventilation. It does no good to circulate anoxic blood. Myocardial compression at a rate of five compressions for each pulmonary insufflation is appropriate at all ages. The child should be placed supine on a firm surface, such as a chest board, and the heart compressed with the heel of the hand over the middle of the sternum (Fig. 3-11). In the case of infants the physician may stand at the head and slip both hands behind the scapulae, compressing the heart with his or her thumbs over the middle of the ster-

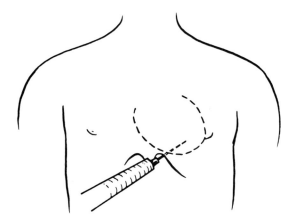

Fig. 3-10 Emergency treatment of cardiac tamponade. The needle is aimed 45 degrees upward and 45 degrees laterally from the point of entrance at the xyphoid.

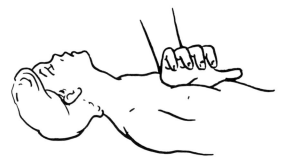

Fig. 3-11 Cardiac massage. The heel of the hand is on the middle of the sternum.

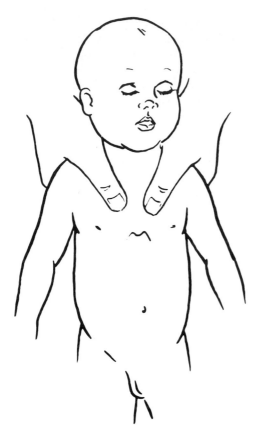

Fig. 3-12 Cardiac massage in an infant. The physician stands at the head and slips both hands behind the scapulae, compressing the heart with thumbs over the middle of the sternum.

num (Fig. 3-12). Care must be taken to avoid pressing on the xyphoid, since this results in inefficient compression of the heart and may injure the liver.

If the blood volume is normal, each compression should result in a readily palpable pulse in the temporal, radial, or femoral artery. With adequate ventilation and with cardiac massage producing a palpable pulse, the emergency is under control. An assistant should cannulate a large vein and inject 2 ml/kg of undiluted sodium bicarbonate followed by 2 ml of 1:10,000 adrenalin. Perfusion of the myocardium with oxygenated blood may be all that is needed to initiate a normal heart beat. Oxygenation and perfusion should be continued for a full 5 minutes. If a normal beat has not been restored, the electrocardiogram should be checked.

If the electrocardiogram shows asystole, 1 ml of 10% calcium chloride should be diluted with 10 ml of saline and injected intravenously. Ventilation

and massage are continued for 2 minutes, and then the doses of sodium bicarbonate, adrenalin, and calcium chloride are repeated.

If the electrocardiogram shows fibrillation, calcium chloride is omitted. The dose of bicarbonate is repeated and preparations are made to defibrillate the heart. Ventilation and compression must be continued up to the moment of massage because the fibrillating heart does not pump blood and because anoxic heart muscle cannot be defibrillated. The heart should be shocked once with 150 Wsec. Compression is withheld for 20 seconds, but ventilation is resumed at once. If fibrillation persists, massage is resumed. After about 2 minutes, the dose of bicarbonate is repeated and the heart shocked with a higher current. If a regular beat returns but remains weak, the circulation may be supported by an intravenous drip of 2 mg of isoproterenol (Isuprel) (usually 10 ampules) in 500 ml of Ringer's lactate solution. If fibrillation persists or recurs repeatedly, 5 ml of 1% procaine hydrochloride may be injected intravenously.

Nearly all cases of cardiac arrest in savable injured children are due to correctable respiratory failure. If the primary cause of arrest is exsanguination the prognosis is almost hopeless. Clinically the child in profound hemorrhagic shock and the child in cardiac arrest due to exsanguination look remarkably similar. An electrocardiogram is essential to making a rational decision concerning how and whether to attempt resuscitation. Many children in profound hemorrhagic shock can be salvaged if treated promptly and vigorously, provided their heart has not stopped beating before resuscitation is begun.

FURTHER EVALUATION

The evaluation and management of every injured child must begin in the same way and must proceed to this point in the same orderly fashion if life is not to be lost by squandering the few precious moments during which it can be saved by restoring ventilation and circulation. Beyond this point the order in which the regions of the body are evaluated and treated will vary with the nature of the injury. These body regions are discussed below in a sequence that roughly parallels the descending order of urgency with which the usual injuries of childhood must be managed.

The importance of complete evaluation and accurate documentation cannot be overemphasized.

Many preventable deaths have occurred because obvious injuries were assumed to be the only injuries. Serious wounds of the head and extremities are readily apparent, while equally serious injuries within the thorax and especially within the abdomen often have been overlooked.

THORAX

Urgent thoracic injuries produce airway obstruction, tension pneumothorax, hemothorax, sucking wounds, flail chest, or cardiac tamponade. More subtle and insidious are mediastinal contamination due to esophageal rupture and progressive pulmonary insufficiency due to aspiration of gastric contents or pulmonary contusion. The major goals of management are the following:

1. To intercept exsanguination and life-threatening infection by prompt recognition and surgical closure of rents in the heart, major vessels, and esophagus
2. To rid the pleural cavities, mediastinum, and pericardium rapidly of space-occupying air, blood, or fluid
3. To reexpand collapsed lungs as quickly and completely as possible, closing tears in the trachea and major bronchi when necessary
4. To guard against reaccumulation of air, blood, or fluid and recurrence of pulmonary collapse

Airway Obstruction

Blood may be present in the tracheobronchial tree from pulmonary contusion, from bronchial or tracheal injury, or from aspiration from the nose or mouth. Repeated gentle suction via an endotracheal tube is usually adequate. Aspiration of stomach contents produces not only obstruction but also a severe chemical pneumonitis. If the material removed by suction resembles stomach content or is acid, bronchoscopy usually should be performed to achieve as complete removal as possible. Systemic antibiotics and hydrocortisone, 100 mg, intravenously every 8 hours for six doses are indicated if aspiration of gastric contents is suspected. Insertion of a nasogastric tube is usually indicated, as discussed below. The tube should be aspirated while the tip is in the midesophagus on the way to the stomach. The finding of a small amount of acid material at this point implies regurgitation of gastric contents, and the child should be treated as if aspiration of gastric contents had occurred (Fig. 3-13).

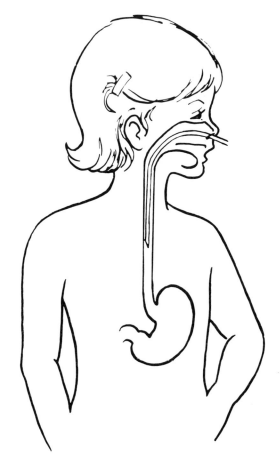

Fig. 3-13   Aspiration of the nasogastric tube with the tip in the midesophagus. If the aspirate is acid, pulmonary complications resulting from aspiration of stomach contents can be anticipated.

Tension Pneumothorax

Tension pneumothorax is a very common cause of embarrassed ventilation in injured children. One hemithorax is hyperresonant with diminished distant breath sounds. The trachea and mediastinum are shifted toward the opposite side. If pneumothorax is suspected a needle on a syringe should be inserted into the chest in the midaxillary line. In our experience this simple emergency maneuver never has done harm, often has helped a hypoxic child, and occasionally has been lifesaving.

Needle aspiration should not be considered definitive treatment for traumatic pneumothorax. Even if the amount of air in the chest is minimal an indwelling chest tube should be inserted and connected to underwater seal. If complete reexpansion does not result, gentle suction should be applied. If air escapes so rapidly that suction cannot keep the lung expanded, a tear in a major bronchus or the trachea should be assumed to be present and emergency bronchoscopy and thoracotomy performed. If saliva or gastric contents emerge from the chest tube, an emergency contrast esophagram is indicated, followed by operative closure of the esophagus and mediastinal drainage.

Hemothorax

Significant hemothorax produces dullness and diminished or absent breath sounds and a shift of the mediastinal structures to the opposite side. Management depends on the amount of blood in the chest and the rapidity with which it accumulates. A large chest tube is inserted in the midaxillary line and the amount of blood initially removed is recorded. Hourly blood loss up to 4 ml/kg, particularly if the rate is slowing, usually indicates a wound that will stop bleeding and heal without operation. If the loss exceeds 30 ml/kg in the first 8 hours, and particularly if the loss accelerates, early operation is indicated. As a rule, if bleeding into the chest is sufficient to cause hemorrhagic shock, operation is urgently needed.

Hemopneumothorax

Usually the finding of both blood and free air in the pleural cavity indicates a laceration of the pulmonary parenchyma. Most of these lacerations heal spontaneously. If one chest tube is not adequate to remove both air and blood, a second chest tube should be inserted.

Roentgenography

The roentgenographic findings produced by the injuries just discussed are described in the chapter on thoracic trauma. No significant injury can be managed properly without roentgenographic documentation. Roentgenograms supplement but do not substitute for careful examination and sound clinical judgment. In dealing with some thoracic injuries, particularly tension pneumothorax, the physician must be prepared to initiate emergency treatment before stopping to obtain a chest x-ray.

ABDOMEN

The usual abdominal injuries are rupture of the spleen, liver, or intestine. Less common are injuries of the pancreas or major vessels. Often more than one organ is injured. Rupture of the spleen or liver produces bleeding; rupture of the bowel produces peritonitis.

Tenderness

Blood or intestinal content in the peritoneum produces abdominal tenderness. It is absolutely essential that the physician determine whether an injured child's abdomen is tender. A calm, unhurried reassuring manner and gentle palpation with warm hands are invaluable. Often, despite commendable efforts to be gentle and reassuring, the physician finds a tense, frightened child unable to relax sufficiently for accurate evaluation. A subcutaneous injection of secobarbital (Seconal), 4 mg/kg, allows the child to become drowsy and relaxed but does not mask true tenderness. The virtue of a nonnarcotic sedative for a screaming 2-year-old child is obvious to all, but the value of barbiturates in the examination of apparently stoic older children is not generally appreciated. We use Seconal as described, regardless of age, if we have any doubt as to the presence or absence of abdominal tenderness.

Decisions made on the basis of frequently repeated examinations are much more reliable than those made after a single evaluation. Many children whose abdomens appear rigid and very tender initially soon lose all evidence of discomfort. Others, particularly those with slow blood loss or small perforations of the intestine, appear essentially asymptomatic on first evaluation but develop increasing evidence of tenderness in the ensuing hours. The abdomen should be examined repeatedly.

Distension

Two differences between children and adults bear on the evaluation of abdominal distension. The first is that changes in abdominal girth caused by intraabdominal bleeding are easier to detect in a small abdomen than in a larger one. The addition of a moderate amount of blood to an abdomen with a girth of 14 inches causes a much greater percentage increase in girth than the addition of the same amount to an abdomen with a girth of 40 inches. We measure and record repeatedly the girth of every child suspected of intraabdominal injury. A simple ink mark on the abdomen ensures that the girth is repeatedly measured at the same level.

Gastric Dilatation

The second difference between children and adults is the increased frequency with which children develop acute gastric dilatation. The left upper quadrant of the abdomen is tympanitic. In extreme cases the abdomen is distended and respiration is embarrassed. A nasogastric tube should be inserted and left in place for several hours because the child requires time to settle down and stop swallowing extra amounts of air. As described previously, the tube should be aspirated when the tip is in the midesophagus so that respiratory complications of aspirated gastric contents can be anticipated.

Paracentesis

The primary purpose of paracentesis is to detect the presence of blood in the peritoneal cavity. Its use is discussed in the section on occult bleeding. Withdrawal of fluid resembling bowel content is nearly always indicative of traumatic perforation of the stomach or intestine. In our experience penetration of intestine by the paracentesis needle has not occurred. We are very careful not to tap the abdomen near a surgical scar to which a loop of intestine might be adherent.

Amylase

The serum amylase level is elevated in many children with insignificant abdominal injuries. In these children the elevation usually does not exceed twice the normal value and returns to normal within a week. Rapid rise of serum amylase to levels more than four or five times normal signifies either an injury to the pancreas or a perforation of the duodenum or jejunum through which intestinal content rich in amylase escapes into the peritoneal cavity. Usually these children have clear evidence of peritoneal irritation demanding abdominal exploration, and the amylase level in these instances is not helpful in making the clinical decision. Occasionally it has been helpful in evaluating an unconscious child. Certainly the finding of an elevated amylase level should not deter the clinician from an operation that appears indicated on clinical grounds. The assumption that the amylase level is elevated because of an isolated pancreatic injury that will heal without operation cannot be justified.

Perhaps the most important contribution of the serum amylase level is in the early detection of the child who is developing a pancreatic pseudocyst. We obtain baseline levels on all children with suspected abdominal injuries and follow those with an elevated serum amylase level until it returns to normal. Children whose amylase levels do not return to normal within 10 days are prime candidates for late complications of pancreatic injury.

If pure blood returns on abdominal paracentesis we do not test it for amylase, but any fluid resembling bowel content, urine, or blood mixed with either of these is routinely tested for amylase content.

Penetrating Wounds

In general, children with penetrating wounds of the abdomen are not subjected to laparotomy unless the abdomen is tender. This nonoperative policy demands appropriate local care to the abdominal wall wound and repeated observation for detection of developing signs of intraabdominal injury. Many stab wounds meet stringent criteria for nonoperative management. Most gunshot wounds require exploration because of obvious abdominal pain, tenderness, or loss of blood.

Roentgenologic Findings

Roentgenologic findings will be discussed in detail in the chapter dealing with abdominal injuries. Abdominal radiographs are essential to the management of all children with significant abdominal injury. They should be obtained as soon as the child has been evaluated and respiration and circulation stabilized. Usually the nasogastric tube, central venous pressure line, and Foley catheter, if indicated, should be inserted before the x-ray films are taken. Paracentesis usually should be performed after the abdominal films have been viewed. Free air in the peritoneal cavity is best seen on the upright chest roentgenogram.

HEAD

The usual mistakes in the care of children with head injuries are failure to support ventilation and circulation and failure to detect additional injuries in other regions of the body. Brain injuries do not cause shock. If shock is present, additional injuries are invariably present.

The usual injuries are cerebral concussion and contusion, for which operation is not indicated, and expanding hematomas, compound skull fractures, and significantly depressed skull fractures, which do require operation. The objectives of the neurologic evaluation are to detect hematomas requiring operation and to detect deterioration of brain function requiring intensification of nonoperative management. In essence, one is looking for the appearance of localized neurologic defects, changes in vital signs, and deterioration in the level of consciousness.

Once ventilation and circulation are restored or are being supported, heroic speed is seldom needed except to stop bleeding or to decompress a rapidly expanding hematoma.

Bleeding

Bleeding from the scalp can be controlled by pressure, hemostats, or rapid suturing. If the blood is escaping rapidly from inside the skull via a compound fracture, the head should be elevated even if the child is in shock. Exsanguination can occur in minutes from a large tear in a dural sinus unless the opening in the vein is kept above the level of the heart.

Expanding Hematoma

Many epidural hematomas are immediately fatal. Savable children have initial loss of consciousness, then a period of consciousness and head pain followed by rapid deterioration with hemiparesis, unconsciousness, and a single dilated pupil. Subdural hematomas may be clinically indistinguishable from epidural hematomas but usually are more indolent.

If a rapidly expanding hematoma is suspected, burr holes made in the emergency room carry far less risk than helpless inactivity. A short vertical incision is made above and in front of the ear on the side of the dilated pupil. The skull is drilled with a twist drill. If blood does not emerge, a small incision is made in the dura. If no blood is released, the procedure is repeated on the opposite side.

By partially relieving the rapidly increasing intracranial pressure the emergency burr hole may be lifesaving but is seldom appropriate definitive treatment. Formal emergency craniotomy is required to control the bleeding and to evacuate clotted blood.

Evaluation

Evaluation of a head-injured child is remarkably simple. The three important parameters are the level of consciousness, vital signs, and localized neurologic deficits.

Level of consciousness

Any intelligent observer, regardless of inexperience, can place a patient in one of the following six categories:

1. Alert, oriented, able to move all extremities appropriately
2. Slow but correct answers to questions asked once, correct response to clear commands given once
3. Responsive only to repeated questions or to commands repeated and reinforced by painful stimuli
4. Unresponsive to voice, purposeful response to painful stimuli
5. Unresponsive to voice, withdrawal only from pain
6. Totally unresponsive

These categories do not depend on such words as "comatose" or "stuporous," which may mean different things to different observers.

Vital signs

Slowing of the pulse and respiration and a rising blood pressure suggest increasing intracranial pressure. Frequent, accurately recorded determinations are essential.

Localized neurologic deficits

Localized neurologic deficits, that is, weakness or asymmetry of motion, position, or muscle tone, imply a localized lesion that may be surgically remediable. They should be described as accurately as possible. The finding of one pupil that is dilating or deviated outward and downward suggests a localized hematoma.

Observations relating to the state of consciousness, vital signs, and localized neurologic deficits form a baseline from which the trend of the patient's course can be charted. Children who are at least somewhat responsive, who show no localizing neurologic signs, and whose level of consciousness remains the same or gradually improves usually recover without operation. Unresponsive children, those whose level of consciousness deteriorates, or those who show progression of a neurologic deficit may be candidates for operation or may require more intensive medical care, for example, hypothermia.

Management

Most children with brain injury do not have hematomas requiring operation. Treatment is aimed at supporting vital functions, minimizing brain swelling, treating convulsions, and preventing infection and other complications such as bowel and bladder distention, pressure to insensitive body areas, malnutrition, and contractures.

Brain swelling

Nearly all head injuries result in some degree of brain swelling. If the child is responsive enough to handle secretions, the head should be raised about 20 degrees. If unresponsive but not in need of endotracheal intubation, the child should be kept on his or her side with the body level and the head slightly below the axis of the spine. Meticulous attention to ventilation is perhaps the most important aspect of care, since accumulation of carbon dioxide in the serum seriously aggravates intracranial pressure. As the pressure within the skull rises, circulation is impaired and transport of oxygen to the brain decreases.

Dexamethasone, 5 to 10 mg intravenously followed by 3 to 5 mg every 6 hours, appears to be helpful in the early management of cerebral edema. Mannitol and urea effectively shrink brain tissue but should be avoided early because they may act so rapidly and aggravate intracranial hemorrhage.

Fluid administration must be adequate to resuscitate the child from shock, but thereafter a rate of 1000 ml/m^2/day is appropriate for the first few days.

Hypothermia, producing a subnormal body temperature, is not an appropriate emergency measure, but fever threatens the brain by increasing the need for oxygen at a time when perfusion is impaired by brain swelling. Temperature should be carefully monitored and fever vigorously treated.

Convulsions

Convulsions are not only a symptom of brain dysfunction but also are capable of producing further brain damage. They should be vigorously treated with intravenous sodium amytal. The child may require as much as 5 mg/lb of sodium amytal. In addition, diphenylhydantoin (Dilantin) 2 mg/lb intramuscularly, is given at once, followed by 1 ml/lb every 6 hours. Phenobarbital and other long-acting agents are avoided in the early treatment of convulsions because of their depressive effect.

Roentgenography

Millions of medically unnecessary skull x-ray films are taken each year. The essential quesiton usually is not whether the skull is fractured but whether the contents have been injured. Emergency radiography of the skull is very rarely indicated, and radiographs obtained in the emergency department with portable equipment are often of such

poor quality as to be useless. The most reliable imaging study is a CT scan with bone windows. The indications for obtaining a CT scan are summarized in the chapter on head injury.

Skull Fractures

Linear skull fractures are very common and usually insignificant. Those crossing the path of the middle meningeal artery may be accompanied by epidural hemorrhage. Fractures of the facial bones may produce asymmetry and malocclusion requiring early elective correction. Hematomas around the eyes and mastoid processes and bleeding from nose or ears suggest the presence of a basilar skull fracture.

Compound skull fractures, including basilar skull fractures, are treated with sulfadiazine. The initial dose is 60 mg/lb intravenously. This ancient drug is preferred because it passes the blood-brain barrier more readily than do antibiotics.

Depressed skull fractures may require operative elevation. Usually those in which the fragment is depressed less than the thickness of the adjacent skull do not require operative treatment.

NECK

Spinal cord damage due to motion of a broken neck is a disastrous complication. All children who complain of neck pain and all with head injuries should be suspected of cervical spine fracture. They should be moved only with manual traction, with the neck slightly extended.

Each spinous process should be palpated. Displacement or pain on palpation is characteristic of vertebral fracture. Conscious children should be checked for pain in the neck or for pain or paresthesias in the extremities. Arm and leg movement is checked for power and symmetry. Unconscious children usually will withdraw all four extremities from painful stimuli, indicating that sensory and motor pathways are intact.

Spinal cord injuries should always be considered reversible, and emergency neurosurgic consultation should be obtained immediately. If weakness suggests spinal cord injury, dexamethasone, 5 to 10 mg intravenously, is appropriate emergency treatment.

A nasogastric tube and a Foley catheter should be inserted before dilatation of the stomach or bladder occurs. Anesthetic areas must be protected from pressure injury. An ounce of prevention is worth tons of cure.

Penetrating wounds of the neck should be explored under general endotracheal anesthesia in an operating room. The probing of neck wounds in the emergency department is fraught with danger to vital structures and may initiate life-threatening hemorrhage.

GENITOURINARY SYSTEM
Kidney

Renal injuries are characterized by flank pain and tenderness and by the presence of red blood cells in the urine. In unconscious children hematuria may be the only clue. Since the amount of blood in the urine does not correlate well with the severity of injury, all children with any red blood cells at all in the urine should be suspected of harboring a renal injury. If the child cannot void after a reasonable time, a Foley catheter should be gently and carefully inserted into the bladder so that the presence or absence of hematuria can be determined.

High-dose intravenous pyelography, using 1 ml of contrast material per pound of body weight, should be obtained as soon after initial stabilization as possible. Pyelograms obtained soon after injury yield much better visualization than those obtained a few hours later because as the renal parenchyma swells within the unyielding renal capsule the collecting system becomes compressed and can contain less opacified urine.

Renal contusions, with or without perirenal hematoma, account for about 75% of renal injuries. They require no treatment. Renal lacerations permitting the escape of opacified urine into the perirenal space are best treated by early elective debridement, repair, and drainage. Vascular injuries are uncommon but require emergency management if the kidney is to be salvaged. These are characterized by absence of visualization on intravenous pyelography. Retrograde pyelography, arteriography, or radioisotope renal scanning, if conducted on an emergency basis, may clarify the diagnosis in time for emergency operation to permit salvage of the kidney.

An isolated renal injury may permit enough blood loss to produce shock but not enough to cause exsanguination. About 40% of renal injuries are accompanied by injuries to other organs. Rupture of the spleen is seen in about 25% of the children

with injuries of the left kidney. Because of the frequency of associated intraabdominal injuries, the presence of abdominal pain and tenderness accompanied by hematuria is an indication for paracentesis.

Ureter

Ureteral injuries are very seldom seen in children. Most are due to penetrating injuries and are characterized by extravasation of urine along the course of the ureter. They usually are found in conjunction with other injuries requiring emergency surgery.

Bladder

Rupture of the bladder frequently accompanies pelvic fractures that are characterized by pain when the greater trochanters are compressed. A distended bladder may be ruptured in the absence of pelvic fracture. Lower abdominal pain and tenderness are associated with urine containing red blood cells.

A cystogram may be obtained either by filling the bladder with contrast material via a catheter or by clamping the catheter and allowing the bladder to fill with opacified urine following intravenous pyelography. In either case, the distended bladder may obscure minor degrees of extravasation, and a film should be exposed after the bladder has been emptied. Bladder rupture is treated by operative repair and suprapubic cystostomy.

Urethra

Urethral injuries are more common in boys than in girls. They are easily overlooked on initial evaluation. The hallmarks are perineal swelling and the presence of a drop of blood at the urethral meatus. Retrograde urethrography, using contrast material injected via the tip of the penis, will demonstrate the point of disruption. Passage of a catheter should not be attempted if urethral injury is suspected because it may transform an incomplete urethral tear to a complete disruption. The bladder can be decompressed via a suprapubic polyethylene catheter.

EXTREMITIES

The urgent problem in the extremities are uncontrolled bleeding and injuries that compromise the blood supply of the hands or feet. Bleeding is controlled by direct pressure when possible in preference to the use of tourniquets. Impaired blood supply is characterized by cool, pale, or slightly cyanotic extremities with absent pulses. Loss of tissue viability is preceded by loss of sensation in the affected part. Sensory loss demands emergency evaluation, often including arteriography.

Compound fractures, dislocations, and other fractures that are accompanied by impaired blood flow require early treatment. Other extremity injuries can be dealt with after more critical injuries have been managed. Suspected fractures should be splinted before moving the patient and should be evaluated with appropriate x-ray studies.

Arterial lacerations in the leg or forearm may be ligated, but if they are multiple, an attempt should be made to repair at least one artery. Arterial lacerations proximal to the bifurcation of the popliteal or brachial artery should be repaired.

Nerve injuries produce areas of sensory loss and loss of one of the following motor functions:

1. Axillary—abduct arm
2. Brachioradialis—flex biceps
3. Ulnar—spread fingers
4. Median—touch thumb to little finger
5. Radial—extend wrist and fingers
6. Femoral—flex hip
7. Sciatic—flex foot
8. Peroneal—extend foot

AFTER INITIAL EVALUATION

The initial evaluation usually is conducted without benefit of a detailed account of how the accident occurred and with little knowledge of the past medical or surgical history of the child. Once respiration and circulation have been ensured and the major regions of the body assessed, this information can be obtained in a thorough and unhurried interview. Often the mechanism of wounding suggests injuries that may have been overlooked, prompting reevaluation of specific areas.

As soon as the physician can reasonably do so, he or she should give the parents a summary of the findings and prognosis. A serious injury to their child is a frightening experience for all parents, even if some cannot vocalize this fear. Although they often do not express guilt, and may not even be aware of it, their anxiety is always compounded by feelings of guilt, for they know, at least subconsciously, that if they had exercised their responsibility as parents more effectively their child would not have been injured. The physician who understands these simple facts and deals effectively with the fears and guilt of parents will be rewarded with their lasting gratitude.

BIBLIOGRAPHY

Betts J: Shock resuscitation in the pediatric trauma patient in critical care of the pediatric surgical patient, Postgraduate course, American College of Surgeons, San Francisco, 1987.

Committee on Trauma, American College of Surgeons: Early care of the injured patient, Philadelphia, 1982, WB Saunders Co.

Committee on Trauma, American College of Surgeons: Advanced trauma life support course, Chicago, American College of Surgeons, 1984.

Eichelberger M and Randolph J: Pediatric trauma: an algorithm for diagnosis and therapy, J Trauma 23:91, 1983.

Haller JA: Pediatric trauma, JAMA 249:47, 1983.

Lucking S and Pollack M: Shock following generalized hypoxic-ischemic injury in previously healthy infants and children, J Pediatr 108:354, 1986.

O'Neill JA: Special pediatric emergencies. In Bostwick JA, editor: Emergency care, Philadelphia, 1981, WB Saunders Co.

Rutherford RB and Buerk CA: The pathophysiology of trauma and shock. In Zuidema GD, Rutherford RB, and Ballinger WF, editors: The management of trauma, Philadelphia, 1979, WB Saunders Co.

Shires GT: Crystalloid resuscitation in shock. In Najarian JS and Delaney JD, editors: Emergency surgery, Chicago, 1982, Year Book Medical Publishers.

Trunkey DD: Toward optimal trauma care, Bull Am Coll Surg 69:2, 1984.

4

Metabolism and Nutrition in Severe Injury

John H. Seashore

Trauma is a systemic disease. The specific injuries and their correction tend to dominate our attention, but the more generalized effects must not be overlooked. Hemodynamic and cardiopulmonary consequences of injury are often apparent in the emergency room and for several days thereafter. Resuscitation and initial management are discussed elsewhere in this book. Less well recognized are the metabolic effects of injury. Trauma is the most severe metabolic stress that humans can suffer, and an understanding of the biochemical changes following trauma is essential to proper management. Appropriate and timely nutritional support may be critical to recovery of function or even survival in the severely injured patient. This chapter reviews the metabolic effects of trauma and provides guidelines for nutritional support.

METABOLIC CONSEQUENCES OF INJURY

Dr. Francis Moore's book *Metabolic Care of the Surgical Patient,* first published in 1952, is still a classic.[27] His ideas have been modified and better defined by subsequent clinical research, but the basic principles remain valid. He defined four phases of recovery from injury. The first, or *injury phase,* is characterized by pain, immobility, ileus, hemodynamic instability, retention of sodium and water, and catabolism evidenced by a marked increase in nitrogen excretion and fat oxidation. The cardinal elements of patient care in this phase are hemodynamic and cardiopulmonary resuscitation and good surgical technique including repair and/ or debridement and drainage of wounds to promote clean, nonseptic healing.

The second phase, or *turning point,* begins a few days after injury in uncomplicated cases. It is characterized by clinical signs of recovery, diuresis,

and beginning wound healing. The patient is still catabolic, but nitrogen excretion is much lower. This phase may last for a few days to a few weeks, depending on the severity of injury. Adequate nutrition is critical to limit the rate and extent of catabolism.

The third phase, *increasing muscular strength,* begins as clinical recovery appears to be complete. The patient is anabolic and in positive nitrogen balance as the lost lean body mass is resynthesized. A diet high in quality and quantity is essential at this time. Duration depends on the severity of injury and the patient's ability to ambulate and exercise. Muscle mass and strength increase slowly, if at all, in patients who are bedridden or immobilized.

The fourth phase, *fat restoration,* lasts weeks to months and is characterized by positive energy balance. Obviously, good nutrition is necessary in this phase as well.

The metabolic events of simple short-term fasting are shown in Fig. 4-1. Most of the organs derive their energy from fatty acids. However, fatty acids do not cross the blood-brain barrier, so the central nervous system requires glucose for fuel. This must be supplied by gluconeogenesis from amino acids mobilized mainly from skeletal muscle. Following major injury, however, there is a change in the hormonal milieu (Fig. 4-2). There is significant hypersecretion of catecholamines, corticosteroids, and glucagon, probably mediated by lymphokines or other messengers liberated by the injured parts.[1] These hormones have many and varied effects, but all three are catabolic with respect to the major metabolic substrates—glucose, protein, and fat.[45]

Glucose is the major substrate for the brain and probably for healing wounds as well. Blood glucose concentration is significantly elevated following trauma, partly from glycogenolysis but more

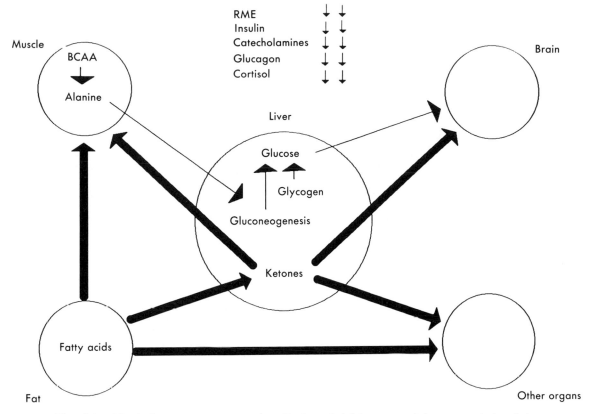

Fig. 4-1   Metabolic response to starvation. During a brief fast most of the organs derive their energy from oxidation of fatty acids, either directly or after conversion to ketone bodies in the liver. There is, however, a substantial breakdown of muscle proteins, especially branched-chain amino acids (BCAA), which are converted to glucose by gluconeogenesis to provide fuel for the central nervous system. Metabolic expenditure and hormone secretion are low.

importantly from an increased rate of gluconeogenesis from amino acids derived from catabolism of muscle protein.[23] This increased rate of gluconeogenesis is not suppressible by exogenous administration of glucose, except in excessive quantities.[16,24] Although the serum concentration of insulin, the primary anabolic hormone, is also increased, it is low relative to blood glucose, and there is evidence of insulin resistance at the cellular level and a decreased half-life of insulin.[6,25] The net effect of these changes is a marked increase in glucose flow through the system, depletion of glycogen stores, wasting of skeletal muscle, and an increased but inefficient utilization of glucose as a fuel.

Hypersecretion of the three counterregulatory hormones significantly increases the rate of protein catabolism, primarily in skeletal muscle. The branch chain amino acids (BCAA) valine, leucine,

and isoleucine appear to play a key role. They are preferentially, but only partially, catabolized in muscle, then converted to alanine, which is transported to the liver where it serves as the primary substrate for gluconeogenesis.[17] It has generally been assumed that protein synthesis is suppressed during the acute injury phase, but studies have shown that, under some circumstances, protein synthesis is increased, particularly in the liver.[4,40] However, this increase is not enough to offset the increased rate of catabolism, so the net effect is negative nitrogen balance and depletion of the lean body mass.

The effects of trauma on fat metabolism have been a subject of controversy; some authors argue that fat is not well utilized,[13,21] whereas others claim that fat is a preferential fuel.[20,30,44] The weight of current evidence is that fat oxidation is normal in injured patients unless mitochondrial function is

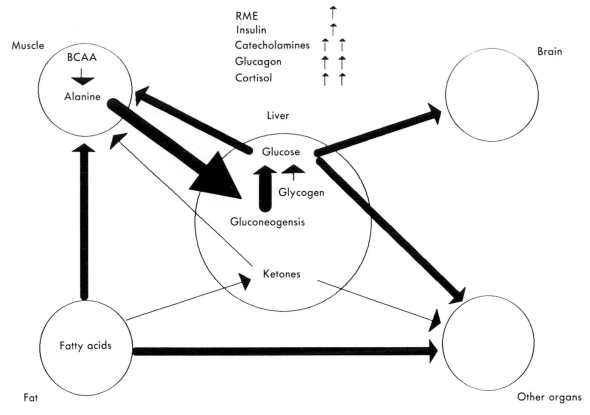

Fig. 4-2 Metabolic response to injury. Following injury there is an increase in metabolic rate and secretion of cortisol, glucogen, and catecholamines that significantly increases glucose production from protein. Insulin secretion is also increased, but there is relative insulin resistance, leading to poor utilization and hyperglycemia, often called the "diabetes of injury." Increased insulin also inhibits ketosis, but fatty acids continue to be oxidized by most organs.

impaired by shock or sepsis.[18] Exogenously administered lipids are metabolized normally in most traumatized patients. However, as noted above, the serum concentration of insulin is increased following trauma. Insulin has a potent antilipolytic effect, so it is likely that endogenous fatty acids are not made available to the periphery as readily as they are in the nonstressed starving patient with low insulin concentration. One of the major mechanisms of adaptation to starvation in the nonstressed individual is a 100-fold increase in the serum concentration of ketone bodies (Fig. 4-3).[10] At this level, ketone bodies can cross the blood-brain barrier and replace glucose as the primary fuel for central nervous system metabolism.[29] This mechanism significantly decreases the need for gluconeogenesis and spares an equivalent amount of protein.[33] However, the ketosis normally seen in starvation does not occur in severely injured patients.[37]

The antilipolytic and antiketotic effects of insulin and the gluconeogenic effect of the counterregulatory hormones tend to increase protein breakdown.

Paralleling the increased breakdown of protein and excretion of nitrogen is an increase in metabolic rate following trauma. Cuthbertson[12] first made both of these observations more than 50 years ago while studying patients with long bone fractures. Spencer and co-workers[38] developed a method of indirect calorimetry using a sealed canopy to measure oxygen consumption and carbon dioxide production. Energy expenditure can be calculated from these data using standard formulas. Gas exchange data are collected several times a day for up to an hour each time to ensure a reliable estimate of total daily energy expenditure. The original studies by Kinney et al.[20] showed a 10% to 20% increase in metabolic rate following skeletal trauma, a 15% to

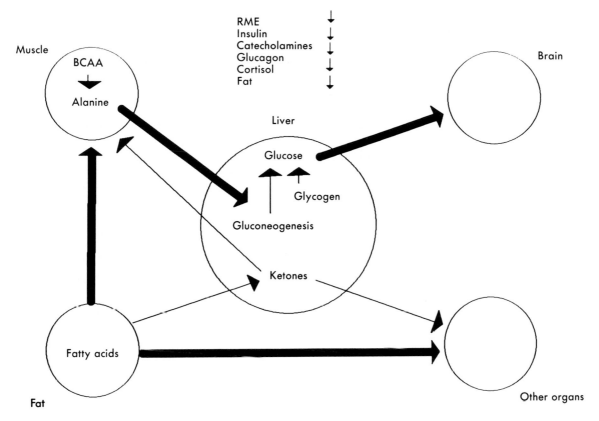

Fig. 4-3   Metabolic adaptation to prolonged starvation. During prolonged starvation metabolic rate and hormone secretions are low. The most important metabolic change is a marked increase in production of ketone bodies that at high concentration cross the blood-brain barrier and become the primary fuel for the central nervous system. This has a powerful protein-sparing effect.

50% increase from peritonitis, and a 40% to 100% increase from major burns. Wilmore[43] published a nomogram in 1977 that incorporated these and other data and included an estimate of a 30% to 50% increase in energy expenditure in patients with multiple trauma. All of these estimates are lower than the 200% to 300% increase in metabolic rate suggested by previous authors based on the degree of weight loss commonly observed following injury.

Wilmore's nomogram has been widely used as the basis for determining energy requirements in injured and septic patients. More recent studies have found lesser increases in metabolic rate. Askanazi et al.[3] reported a mean increase in metabolic rate of 14.2% in a group of injured and/or septic adults. Winthrop et al.[45] studied a group of injured children and found a mean increase of 14% in metabolic rate and a direct correlation between meta-

bolic rate and injury severity score. These differences may be explained in part by differences in methodology and the assumptions made in calculating energy expenditure from gas exchange data. There is clearly a need for better methods to determine the metabolic cost of injury. There is, however, a definite trend in current practice toward using lower estimates of the energy requirements of injured patients. This is in part due to recognition of the ill effects of excessive caloric administration, including fat and glycogen deposition in the liver, and lipogenesis without further synthesis of lean body tissue. Excessive glucose administration leads to increased carbon dioxide production, the excretion of which may be detrimental to patients whose ventilatory function is impaired.

Malnutrition develops slowly in the nonstressed, starving individual because of the adaptation described previously and a gradual decline in metabolic rate. The severely injured patient, however, is unable to adapt by ketosis and a fat dominated fuel economy and also has a significantly increased metabolic rate.[11,43] Therefore it is not surprising that malnutrition occurs rapidly. Even a healthy, well-nourished adult can develop life-threatening malnutrition in as few as 10 to 15 days after a very severe injury. Children have a higher basal metabolic rate than adults and relatively lower endogenous caloric reserves. In a young child, even 4 or 5 days of starvation after injury may lead to significant nutritional deficits.[34]

CONSEQUENCES OF MALNUTRITION

Many studies have demonstrated a close association between malnutrition and increased morbidity and mortality. Weight loss, decreased albumin and other serum proteins, impaired cell-mediated immunity, and more complex nutritional assessment indices all correlate very well with clinical outcome. Malnutrition cannot be measured by any single parameter, and the degree of malnutrition can only be estimated. Furthermore, it is almost impossible to separate the underlying disease and malnutrition as risk factors in clinical studies in humans. Therefore it is difficult to prove a cause-and-effect relationship between malnutrition and outcome, but the overwhelming weight of evidence is that malnutrition prolongs illness, predisposes to complications, and increases mortality.

Prevalence studies indicate that one third to one half of all hospitalized patients have one or more abnormal nutritional parameters.[5,8,26,41] Obviously, not all of these patients suffer increased morbidity simply because their serum albumin or triceps skin fold thickness is a little low. The question of how much evidence of malnutrition is acceptable and when malnutrition becomes a risk factor is not easily answered. For example, a 5% to 10% loss of body weight in most adults is probably not significant, but if it occurs rapidly as a result of a hypermetabolic condition such as trauma, it may be serious. Children, however, are normally expected to be growing, so any weight loss should be regarded as evidence of malnutrition.

Muscle wasting and loss of lean body mass make the patient weak and bedridden. Eventually the chest muscles become so wasted that the patient cannot cough and clear secretions. Bronchopneumonia supervenes and is one of the most common causes of death in malnourished individuals. Visceral proteins, as measured indirectly by albumin, transferrin, and other serum proteins are depleted, since catabolism exceeds synthesis. This implies a decreased turnover of hormones, enzymes, and other metabolically active proteins, which leads to organ dysfunction. Immune function is also impaired, notably by a loss of cell-mediated immunity and a decrease in secretory IgA. The malnourished patient is more susceptible to infection and is less able to localize and destroy organisms or repair tissue damaged by infection. The combination of sepsis and malnutrition is probably the primary cause of multiple-organ failure, which is the most common cause of death in patients hospitalized for more than 2 weeks.[39]

INDICATIONS FOR NUTRITIONAL SUPPORT

Nutrition is of secondary importance during the injury phase for the reasons discussed earlier. Intravenous solutions containing 5% dextrose should be provided to take advantage of the protein-sparing effect of carbohydrate, particularly in patients with relatively minor trauma.

The second phase, beginning 3 to 5 days after uncomplicated injury, is also the turning point for nutrition. The vast majority of injured patients are recovering at this time and are ready to resume eating. The primary nutritional task for the clinician is to monitor intake to ensure that the intake of calories and protein is adequate to meet the increased needs of healing.

Some patients are unable to eat at this point, however, and it is imperative that the clinician identify them and begin some sort of nutritional support. Patients who have sustained multiple severe injuries, particularly if abdominal viscera are involved, cannot be fed normally. Children who are comatose following closed head injury obviously cannot be fed by mouth and often have a prolonged ileus as well. Similarly, patients who require mechanical ventilation cannot eat, and the narcotics and paralyzing agents administered to keep them from fighting the ventilator usually cause gut dysfunction. Septic complications further increase the metabolic rate and impair both the ability and desire to eat. The septic, traumatized patient almost always needs aggressive nutritional support.

The most severely injured patients, who are clearly not going to be eating for some time, should receive complete nutritional support, usually by central total parenteral nutrition (TPN), starting by the fourth or fifth day after injury. In other patients it may not be clear whether long-term support will be needed or recovery will proceed rapidly. This is the time to begin enteral feedings slowly through a nasogastric tube or a jejunostomy catheter, anticipating that it will take several days to achieve full intake. Peripheral TPN with lipid may be appropriate at least to hold the line until the time course of recovery is apparent.

By 7 to 10 days after injury, most patients should be in the third phase of recovery. They should be anabolic and in positive balance for nitrogen and energy. If the patient is not eating an adequate diet by this time, nutritional support is indicated to provide complete nutritional requirements either enterally or by central TPN.

ESTIMATION OF ENERGY REQUIREMENTS

The energy requirements of children vary widely with age, sex, and nature of illness, so it is essential to have some method to calculate appropriate caloric intake. The basal energy expenditure (BEE) formula of Harris and Benedict is a regression equation based on age, sex, height, and weight.[7] The BEE is widely used but is fairly cumbersome. The Recommended Dietary Allowances give a range of nutrient intake for children of different ages but is based on normal, healthy, active, growing children and is not as applicable to hospitalized patients.[28] Many hospitals use metabolic carts to measure oxygen consumption and carbon dioxide production and calculate energy expenditure. These measurements are carried out for a relatively short period (an hour or so) and therefore may not accurately predict metabolic rate over a 24-hour day. We prefer to use a simple formula that calculates basal metabolic rate as the following:

$$55 - (2 \times \text{age in years}) \text{ kcals/kg/day}$$

This formula correlates well with measured basal metabolic rate (BMR) in children between the tenth and ninetieth percentiles of weight for age.[34] To account for cold stress, minimal activity, and specific dynamic action (the metabolic cost of oxidizing nutrients), 20% of BMR is added to estimate the resting metabolic expenditure (RME).[43] As shown in Table 4-1, additional increments are added for trauma, sepsis, activity, and growth. Excessive caloric intake can certainly be harmful, but

Table 4-1 Energy requirements in children

	Percent of BMR	kcals/ kg/day
Basal metabolic rate (55 − 2 × age in years)		————
Resting metabolic expenditure	20	————
Activity	0-25	————
Sepsis	13%/1° C	————
Simple trauma	10-15	————
Multiple trauma	20-40	————
Burns	50-100	————
Growth/anabolism	50	————
TOTAL		————

we believe it is better to err slightly on the side of too many calories rather than too few. We generally add 10% of BMR for single-organ injuries and 20% to 30% for multiple injuries. Burns may entail substantially higher energy intake. The figure of 13% per degree centigrade of fever is well documented in adults, though not in children.[43] Since patients rarely have sustained temperature elevation above 39° C, addition of 15% to 20% of BMR is usually about right.

Muscular activity increases energy expenditure. Indirect calorimetry in patients who are ambulatory about the hospital ward shows about a 20% increase in oxygen consumption.[22] Patients who are on ventilators and receiving paralyzing agents obviously are not active. A child who is immobilized in traction for leg or pelvic injuries may initially have very little activity, but as recovery progresses and a trapeze is added to the bed to encourage upper body activity, energy expenditure will increase.

Growth and/or regrowth of lost body mass is a primary goal during recovery from injury in children. Any positive energy and nitrogen balance should lead to accretion of lean body mass. However, addition of 50% of BMR is advisable to ensure steady and measurable weight gain.

This formula for estimating energy requirements obviously has its limitations and is only broadly based on the available evidence. Nonetheless, it is a simple and useful way to initiate nutritional therapy. Further adjustments can be made as dictated by the patient's clinical course.

TECHNIQUES OF NUTRITIONAL SUPPORT
Enteral Nutrition

Enteral feeding is cheaper, safer, and metabolically more effective than parenteral nutrition and should always be considered first. The most common route is through an indwelling nasogastric tube. It is important that the large nasogastric tube used initially for gastric decompression be replaced with a small (8Fr) silicone or polyurethane tube for feeding. The smaller, softer tubes are much less likely to cause nasopharyngeal and esophageal irritation or reflux, vomiting, and aspiration. Gastric retention and diarrhea are the two major reasons for failure of tube feedings. In some patients these problems indicate that the gut is not able to tolerate enteral feedings, and parenteral nutrition is necessary. In many cases, however, they are the result of poor technique. Enteral feedings are always given as a continuous 24-hour infusion in acutely ill patients; bolus feedings are much more likely to cause gastric retention.[9] Feedings are initiated slowly (at about one quarter the eventual desired rate) using a formula that is diluted to about one half the osmolality of serum, or 150 mOsm/kg. Small, frequent increments of both strength and concentration over 48 to 72 hours are less likely to cause problems than large increases. Standard commercially available formulas (for example, Ensure and Isocal) are inexpensive, nutritionally complete, lactose-free, and isotonic and work well in most patients. However, if the small bowel mucosa has been damaged by injury, illness, or malnutrition, absorption of fat and complex carbohydrates and proteins may be impaired. A trial of an "elemental" diet containing little or no fat, disaccharides or monosaccharides, and protein hydrolysates or amino acids (for example, Criticare, Vivonex, and Vital) may work. Since these formulas are hypertonic, feedings must be advanced even more slowly. Diarrhea is the primary symptom both of malabsorption and of excessive osmolality, so it can be difficult to decide the best dietary manipulation if diarrhea is a problem. Trial and error is often the only recourse. One simple bedside test that can be helpful is testing for reducing substances in the stool. A positive test indicates carbohydrate malabsorption, and a formula containing simpler carbohydrates can be tried.

The ileus that follows abdominal injury, laparotomy, or both is usually most profound and long-lasting in the stomach and colon, whereas small bowel motility may be relatively normal. The technique of needle catheter jejunostomy was described in 1973 and is used extensively in adults.[14] Numerous studies have shown that intrajejunal feedings are well tolerated in many patients even as early as 12 to 24 hours after operation, thus obviating the need for parenteral nutrition.[15,31] Needle catheter jejunostomy has been used successfully in children as well and should be considered in children who require laparotomy for major abdominal trauma.[2] In young children, however, the bowel wall is too thin to allow safe submucosal tunnelling of the catheter through a needle; a standard Witzel jejunostomy must be performed. The incidence of leak and other complications following Witzel jejunostomy is much higher, and in our experience this method is rarely indicated.

A more recent innovation is a double-lumen gastrostomy tube through which a silicone rubber catheter is passed and manipulated into the proximal jejunum. This allows simultaneous gastric decompression and jejunal feeding and prevents the risk of direct jejunostomy.

If initial attempts at enteral feeding are unsuccessful, the child should receive parenteral nutrition. However, enteral feeding should be retried periodically. It is to be expected that well over half of all children who require nutritional support will eventually tolerate gastrointestinal feeding.

Parenteral Nutrition

The protein-sparing effect of carbohydrate has already been mentioned. Intravenous solutions containing 5% dextrose should always be provided to children who are NPO. The addition of 2% to 4% amino acids, vitamins, and minerals provides some nutritional benefit but increases the cost about 50-fold. Nitrogen equilibrium or positive balance can be achieved only if the *total* energy and protein requirements of the patient are provided. The maximal concentration of intravenous fluids that peripheral veins will tolerate is about 900 mOsm/kg. Appropriate solutions of dextrose and amino acids for peripheral vein infusion in children are shown in Fig. 4-4. Osmolality ranges from 800 to 914 mOsm/kg and they provide 0.33 to 0.45 kcals/ml. It is rarely possible to give a large enough volume

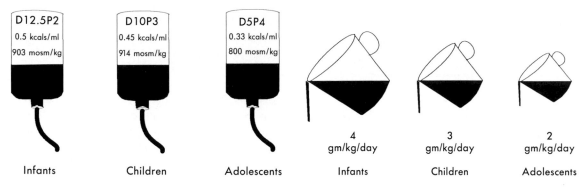

Fig. 4-4   Standard peripheral TPN solutions for children in different age groups.

Fig. 4-5   Recommended doses of fat emulsion for infants, children, and adolescents.

of these solutions to meet energy requirements. The only way to achieve this goal is to include intravenous fat emulsion in the prescription. Twenty percent lipid emulsions provide 2 kcals/ml and are isotonic and nonirritating to peripheral veins. Soybean and safflower oil emulsions are very stable, are similar to normal chylomicrons, and are very safe when administered in the recommended doses (Fig. 4-5). The fat overload syndrome, which results from inadequate clearing of the emulsion from the serum (leading to destabilization, formation of large fat globules, and fat emboli), is very rare with current fat emulsions. As noted earlier, fat is a major fuel in injured patients, and exogenous fat is metabolized effectively. The only absolute contraindications to fat administration are the very rare allergic reactions, known hyperlipidemia, and documented intolerance of fat emulsion. The latter can be monitored by periodic measurement of serum lipid concentration by nephelometry (normal <100 mg/dl) and serum triglyceride concentration (should be less than two times the upper limit of normal during infusion of lipid).

Peripheral TPN with fat is a more important part of the nutritional armamentarium for children than it is for adults, since the water requirements and fluid tolerance of children are much higher, even relative to energy requirements. Maintenance fluid requirements of children are as follows:

Weight	Requirement
<10 kg	100 ml/kg
10-20 kg	1000 ml + 50 ml/kg over 10 kg
>20 kg	1500 ml + 20 ml/kg over 20 kg

The potential value of peripheral TPN in a hypothetical child with moderate injury (for example,

blunt abdominal trauma with mesenteric hematoma and prolonged ileus) is illustrated in the box below. Fluid requirements are calculated as previously shown and minimal energy requirements from the formula in Table 4-1, assuming 10% increments for trauma and activity but nothing for growth. If the maximal dose of fat is used and fluids are administered at maintenance rates, caloric intake is inadequate. However, if the fluid intake is increased to 1.5 × maintenance, caloric intake approximates the estimated requirement. In general, peripheral TPN is effective only if (1) the maximum dose of fat is used; (2) the rate of fluid administration is well above maintenance requirements; and (3) the patient actually receives the volume of TPN that is ordered. The latter is often a problem if the patient has only one intravenous line

---

PERIPHERAL TPN—MODERATE TRAUMA

30 kg, 8-year-old male with blunt abdominal trauma, mesenteric hematoma, and prolonged ileus

Fluid requirements		1700 ml/day
Energy requirements		59 kcals/kg/day
		1770 kcals/day
D10P3	1250 ml	560 kcals
20% fat	450 ml	900 kcals
	1700 ml	1460 kcals
D10P3	2050 ml	920 kcals
20% fat	450 ml	900 kcals
	2500 ml	1820 kcals

Table 4-2 Central TPN solutions*

	Concentration per liter		
	Infants	Children	Adolescents
Calories	760	970	1020
Amino acids	20 g	30 g	40 g
Dextrose	200 g	250 g	250 g
Sodium	25 mEq	35 mEq	35 mEq
Potassium	25 mEq	36 mEq	30 mEq
Chloride	33 mEq	48 mEq	35 mEq
Calcium	16 mEq	12 mEq	4.6 mEq
Magnesium	7.2 mEq	4.0 mEq	5.0 mEq
Phosphorus	8 mM	8 mM	15 mM
Acetate	32 mEq	55 mEq	68 meq
Zinc	2.5 mg	4 mg	†
Copper	200 mcg	400 mcg	†
Manganese	50 mcg	100 mcg	†
Chromium	2 mcg	4 mcg	†

*Recommended fat- and water-soluble vitamins added daily.
†Trace elements added only for long-term TPN.

that is also used to give antibiotics or other medications or if the IV infiltrates frequently.[35] Thrombophlebitis and skin sloughs are other problems associated with peripheral TPN.

Central TPN is indicated for children who need *hyper*alimentation and prolonged nutritional support or those with limited peripheral venous access. The composition of standard central TPN solutions for children of different ages is shown in Table 4-2. It is generally possible to achieve adequate nutrient intake using rates of administration that are equal to or slightly above maintenance fluid requirements. There is some evidence that traumatized patients need a higher protein intake than nontraumatized patients. Therefore we often use 4% protein for children and occasionally use 5% protein for adolescents.

Percutaneous subclavian catheterization is the best method for central venous access in most children. Jugular or facial vein cutdown is a good alternative. A stiff central venous catheter is often inserted during initial resuscitation of injured children. These are usually contaminated and should not be used for TPN. In older children we change this catheter over a wire or insert a new one before instituting central TPN. In young children Silastic catheters are by far the best choice because of their pliability and low tissue reactivity. The incidence of venous perforation and thrombotic complications is much higher with other catheter materials. In all age groups, the Broviac catheter is more

secure and possibly less prone to infection than conventional central catheters and is particularly suited to children who will need long-term (more than 10 days) nutritional support.

Bacteremia is the most common complication of central TPN, occurring in about 20% of children. The most common organism is coagulase-negative staphylococcus, often resistant to oxacillin. Use of central venous catheters for multiple purposes (for example, TPN, medications, blood sampling) is widely practiced despite considerable controversy in the literature about risk factors for bacteremia. Our own experience (unpublished data) suggests that the risk of bacteremia is higher with TPN than with other uses and highest when TPN is combined with other uses. If at all possible we prefer to use catheters for TPN only. If the patient has a double-lumen catheter, one port is reserved for TPN. Meticulous catheter care and dressing changes by properly trained nurses are essential. It has been shown repeatedly that the incidence of bacteremia is lower when catheter care is supervised by a nutrition support team.[32]

Children who develop fever and clinical signs of sepsis while receiving central TPN are thoroughly evaluated for sources of infection. Broad spectrum antibiotic therapy, including vancomycin, is instituted pending results of blood culture and sensitivity testing. Several studies, as well as our own experience, have demonstrated that 50% to 75% of bacteremias can be treated with appropriate antibiotics without having to remove the catheter.[19,36] However, the catheter is removed if the patient has overwhelming sepsis, persistent unexplained fever (more than 48 hours), positive blood culture while receiving antibiotics to which the organism is sensitive, or fungal sepsis. The risk of death or secondary infectious complications is very low if these principles are followed.

SUMMARY

Knowledge of the metabolic and nutritional consequences of trauma is essential in the management of injured children. The vast majority of children resume eating within a few days and recover uneventfully. Multiple or severe injuries, particularly of the head or abdomen, prolonged ileus, mechanical ventilation, and septic complications are indications for aggressive nutritional support that may be lifesaving. The period from the fifth to the tenth day after injury is the critical time to establish adequate nutritional intake by whatever means possible. Enteral feeding is always preferable to parenteral nutrition and is frequently possible. Use of age-appropriate TPN solutions, careful monitoring and meticulous catheter care, all supervised by a nutrition support team, will minimize the risk of complications.

REFERENCES

1. Alberti KGMM et al: Relative role of various hormones in mediating the metabolic response to injury, J Parenteral Enteral Nutr 4:141, 1980.
2. Andrassy RJ et al: The role and safety of early postoperative feeding in the pediatric surgical patient, J Pediatr Surg 14:381, 1979.
3. Askanazi J et al: Influence of total parenteral nutrition on fuel utilization in injury and sepsis, Ann Surg 191:40, 1980.
4. Birkhahn RH et al: Whole-body protein metabolism due to trauma in man as estimated by 1-[15N]alanine, Am J Physiol 241:E64, 1981.
5. Bistrian BR et al: Prevalence of malnutrition in general medical patients, JAMA 235:1567, 1976.
6. Black PR et al: Mechanisms of insulin resistance following injury, Ann Surg 196:420, 1982.
7. Blackburn GL et al: Nutritional and metabolic assessment of the hospitalized patient, J Parenteral Enteral Nutr 1:11, 1977.
8. Bollet AJ and Owens S: Evaluation of nutritional status of selected hospitalized patients, Am J Clin Nutr 26:931, 1973.
9. Bury KD and Jambunathan G: Effects of elemental diets on gastric emptying and gastric secretion in man, Am J Surg 127:59, 1974.
10. Cahill GF Jr: Ketosis, JPEN 5:281, 1981.
11. Cahill GF Jr and Aoki TT: How metabolism affects clinical problems, Res Staff Physician 32:96 1973.
12. Cuthbertson DP: Observations on the disturbance of metabolism produced by injury to the limbs, Q J Med 2:233, 1932.
13. Das JB, Joshi ID, and Philippart AI: Depression of glucose utilization by intralipid in the posttraumatic period: an experimental study, J Pediatr Surg 15:739, 1980.
14. Delaney HM, Carnevale NJ, and Garvey JW: Jejunostomy by a needle catheter technique, Surgery 73:786, 1973.
15. Dunn EL, Moore EE, and Bohus RW: Immediate postoperative feeding following massive abdominal trauma— the catheter jejunostomy, J Parenteral Enteral Nutr 4:393, 1980.
16. Elwyn DH et al: Influence of increasing carbohydrate intake on glucose kinetics in injured patients, Ann Surg 190:117, 1979.
17. Felig P: The glucose-alanine cycle, Metabolism 22:179, 1973.
18. Giovannini I et al: Respiratory quotient and patterns of substrate utilization in human sepsis and trauma, J Parenteral Enteral Nutr 7:226, 1983.
19. King DR et al: Broviac catheter sepsis: the natural history of an iatrogenic infection, J Pediatr Surg 20:728, 1985.
20. Kinney JM et al: Tissue fuel and weight loss after injury, J Clin Pathol 4:65, 1970.
21. Liddell MJ et al: The role of stress hormones in the catabolic metabolism of shock, Surg Gynecol Obstet 149:822, 1979.
22. Long CL, Kopp K, and Kinney JM: Energy demands during ambulation in surgical convalescence, Surg Forum 20:93, 1969.
23. Long CL et al: Carbohydrate metabolism in man: effect of elective operations and major injury, J Appl Physiol 31:110, 1971.
24. Long CL et al: Gluconeogenic response during glucose infusions in patients following skeletal trauma or during sepsis, J Parenteral Enteral Nutr 2:619, 1978.
25. Meguid MM, Aun F, and Soeldner JS: Temporal characteristics of insulin: glucose ratio after varying degrees of stress and trauma in man, J Surg Res 25:389, 1978.
26. Merritt RJ and Suskind RM: Nutritional survey of hospitalized pediatric patients, Am J Clin Nutr 32:1320, 1979.
27. Moore FD: Metabolic care of the surgical patient, Philadelphia, 1959, WB Saunders Co.
28. National Academy of Sciences: Recommended dietary allowances, ed 9, Washington, DC, 1980, US Government Printing Office.
29. Owen OE et al: Brain metabolism during fasting, J Clin Invest 46:1589, 1967.
30. Robin AP et al: Plasma clearance of fat emulsion in trauma and sepsis: use of a three-stage lipid clearance test, J Parenteral Enteral Nutr 4:505, 1980.
31. Ryan JA Jr and Page CP: Intrajejunal feeding: development and current status, J Parenteral Enteral Nutr 8:187, 1984.
32. Ryan JA Jr et al: Catheter complications in total parenteral nutrition: a prospective study of 200 consecutive patients, N Engl J Med 290:757, 1974.
33. Saudek CD and Felig P: The metabolic events of starvation, Am J Med 60:117, 1976.
34. Seashore JH: Nutritional support of children in the intensive care unit, Yale J Biol Med 57:111, 1984.
35. Seashore JH and Hoffman M: Use and abuse of peripheral parenteral nutrition in children, Nutr Support Serv 3:8, 1983.
36. Shapiro ED et al: Broviac catheter-related bacteremia in oncology patients, Am J Dis Child 136:679, 1982.
37. Smith R et al: Initial effect of injury on ketone bodies and other blood metabolites, Lancet 1·1, 1975.
38. Spencer JL et al: A system for continuous measurement of gas exchange and respiratory functions, J Appl Physiol 33:523, 1972.
39. Steffee WP: Malnutrition in hospitalized patients, JAMA 244:2630, 1980.
40. Stein TP et al: Changes in protein synthesis after trauma: importance of nutrition, Am J Physiol 233:E348, 1977.
41. Weinsier RL et al: Hospital malnutrition: a prospective evaluation of general medical patients during the course of hospitalization, Am J Clin Nutr 32:418, 1979.
42. Wilmore DW: Hormonal responses and their effect on metabolism, Surg Clin North Am 56:999, 1976.
43. Wilmore DW: The metabolic management of the critically ill, New York, 1977, Plenum Publishing Corp.
44. Wilmore DW and Aulick LH: Systemic responses to injury and the healing wound, J Parenteral Enteral Nutr 4:147, 1980.
45. Winthrop AL et al: Injury severity, whole body protein turnover, and energy expenditure in pediatric trauma, J Pediatr Surg 22:534, 1987.

5

Respiratory Failure

J. Julio Pérez Fontán and George Lister

Respiratory failure is often viewed as an aberration in gas exchange and is frequently described in terms of the concentration or partial pressure of oxygen (P_{O_2}) or carbon dioxide (P_{CO_2}) in the blood. This approach has been particularly convenient because it is easy to measure blood gas tensions even in very small children. Unfortunately, blood gas tensions alone may be easily subject to misinterpretation because they are often maintained near normal levels with oxygen supplementation of inspired air. In addition to impaired blood gas exchange, traumatic injury to the lungs or chest wall invariably causes disruption of mechanical function. Furthermore, it is fatigue (from the excessive work of breathing) rather than hypoxemia that frequently precipitates a respiratory arrest in the traumatized child. Therefore any review of the pathophysiology and management of respiratory failure caused by trauma in the child must consider the disturbances in both mechanical and gas exchange function. In this chapter we will first discuss the general principles of respiratory gas exchange and mechanical function because these are essential background for an understanding of pathologic conditions. In the process we will highlight some of the features unique to the child that influence the response to trauma and accidents that injure or tax the respiratory system. We will next describe the general approach to the recognition and management of respiratory failure of the child. Finally, we will consider the pathogenesis of some specific injuries that are common causes of respiratory failure in children.

BLOOD GAS EXCHANGE
Normal Carbon Dioxide and Oxygen Exchange

To understand how to detect and quantify disturbances in the blood gas exchange, we will first examine the factors that determine arterial oxygen and carbon dioxide tensions under normal conditions. If we first consider gas exchange for the entire respiratory system, the tidal volume (V_T), or the volume of gas moving in or out of the lungs per breath, is composed of alveolar (V_A) and dead space (V_D) volumes: $V_T = V_A + V_D$. The alveolar volume is the portion of tidal volume that provides fresh gas for uptake of oxygen and removal of carbon dioxide. The (physiologic) dead space is the volume of gas that enters the lung with each breath but does not participate in gas exchange. These volumes can also be multiplied by the respiratory rate, or frequency (f), to obtain the respective minute expired ($\dot{V}_E$), alveolar ($\dot{V}_A$), and dead space ($\dot{V}_D$) ventilations:

$$V_T f = (V_A + V_D) f = \dot{V}_E = \dot{V}_A + \dot{V}_D \quad (1)$$

Arterial P_{CO_2}

If we now briefly view gas exchange for a single alveolar-capillary unit, the difference of volume of carbon dioxide or oxygen entering and leaving an alveolus per unit of time is the rate of carbon dioxide production or oxygen uptake for that alveolus. The ratio of these gas exchange rates is the respiratory quotient. Because the inspired carbon dioxide is usually zero, the rate of carbon dioxide production ($\dot{V}_{CO_2}$) or elimination can be simply related to the local alveolar ventilation or carbon dioxide concentration (F_{ACO_2}) as follows:

$$\quad (2)$$

[volume of CO_2 out–in]: $\quad (\dot{V}_A F_{ACO_2}) - 0 = \dot{V}_{CO_2}$

Rearranging terms,

$$F_{ACO_2} = \dot{V}_{CO_2}/\dot{V}_A \quad (3)$$

From this it follows that alveolar P_{CO_2} (which is proportional to F_{ACO_2}) will be directly related to the carbon dioxide production and inversely proportional to alveolar ventilation.

46

Simultaneous with the movement of gas in and out of the alveolus, blood flows through the pulmonary capillaries, providing a large surface for gas exchange. The driving force for the exchange of carbon dioxide and oxygen is the difference in pressures of these gases between venous blood and alveolar gas. Normally there is enough time for blood to reside at the blood-gas interface to allow complete equilibration of both oxygen and carbon dioxide. In this manner the Po_2 and Pco_2 of pulmonary capillary blood at equilibrium are equivalent to the Po_2 and Pco_2 of the alveolar gas.

If we now again consider gas exchange for the whole lung, the pulmonary venous and arterial Pco_2 and Po_2 are a function of the (volume-weighted) average of the capillary carbon dioxide and oxygen concentrations from the millions of alveolar-capillary gas exchange units. Therefore the arterial Pco_2 ($Paco_2$) can be related to overall carbon dioxide production and to alveolar or tidal ventilation as follows[87]:

$$Paco_2 \, \epsilon \, \dot{V}co_2 / \dot{V}_A \, \epsilon \, \dot{V}co_2 / (V_T - V_D) \, f \qquad (4)$$

In the normal subject, most of tidal ventilation is used for gas exchange (that is, dead space is usually one third of tidal volume). Therefore increases in minute ventilation are usually an efficient way of decreasing or maintaining arterial Pco_2 in response to increased carbon dioxide production, as might occur with fever or excessive catabolism after severe trauma or burns. However, when injuries increase dead space, ventilation becomes relatively inefficient and there are two immediate consequences: (1) the arterial Pco_2 may rise unless minute ventilation can be increased substantially, and (2) the work of breathing will increase at least in proportion to minute ventilation (and often much higher because the pathologic process interferes with efficiency of mechanical function).

Arterial Po_2

The arterial Po_2 at equilibrium is also a function of several variables: the Po_2 of gas entering the alveolus, the Po_2 of blood entering the capillaries, the capacity of blood to carry oxygen (hemoglobin oxygen capacity), and the respective gas ($\dot{V}A$) and capillary blood ($\dot{Q}c$) flows. For a given hemoglobin concentration and mixed venous and inspired Po_2, the greater the gas flow is in relation to the blood flow (high $\dot{V}A/\dot{Q}c$), the closer the equilibrium Po_2 will be to that of inspired gas and the higher will be the alveolar and capillary Po_2. Conversely, when

gas flow is low in relationship to perfusion (low $\dot{V}A/\dot{Q}c$), the equilibrium reached is closer to the mixed venous Po_2.

In the normal lung the average $\dot{V}A/\dot{Q}c$ is in the range of 0.8 to 1.0. However, neither ventilation nor perfusion is uniform throughout the lung. This leads to regional differences in ventilation-to-perfusion relationships, such that $\dot{V}A/\dot{Q}c$ is lowest in the dependent portions of the lung. This heterogeneity of $\dot{V}A/\dot{Q}c$ gives rise to regional differences in the alveolar and pulmonary capillary Po_2 and, when accentuated, can cause arterial hypoxemia. In the normal lung, however, regional decreases in alveolar Po_2 also cause vasoconstriction of local arterioles (hypoxic pulmonary vasoconstriction), thereby reducing blood flow to poorly ventilated alveoli (that is, reducing $\dot{V}A/\dot{Q}c$ heterogeneity) and minimizing the potential for hypoxemia. It is very important to recognize that areas with a low capillary Po_2 do more to decrease the arterial oxygen concentration and Po_2 than areas with a high capillary Po_2 do to raise it. This is caused by the shape of the oxygen-hemoglobin equilibrium curve in the range of 80 to 120 torr, where increases in Po_2 barely increase blood oxygen concentration, but comparable decreases in Po_2 decrease oxygen concentration measurably.

Without detailed knowledge of the ventilation and perfusion in all areas of the lung, it would be difficult to predict what the (volume-weighted) mean pulmonary capillary or pulmonary venous Po_2 ought to be in a given child. However, we can derive an ideal alveolar (PAo_2) or pulmonary capillary oxygen tension that permits an estimation of the highest arterial Po_2 that could be expected if gas exchange (that is, $\dot{V}A/\dot{Q}c$ ratios) were homogeneous. If we view the lungs as a single alveolus, we can calculate the following ideal alveolar oxygen tension:

$$(5)*$$
$$PAo_2 = PIo_2 - Paco_2/R + [(1-R) \, FIo_2 \, Paco_2]/R$$

or simplified

$$PAo_2 = PIo_2 - Paco_2/R \qquad (6)$$

where R is the respiratory exchange ratio of carbon dioxide and oxygen, which is usually estimated to be 0.8 for the whole lung. The inspired Po_2 (PIo_2) is calculated as ($PB - PH_2O$) FIo_2, where PB is the barometric pressure and PH_2O is the water vapor

---

*See footnote on p. 48.

pressure at body temperature (47 mm Hg at 37° C).

Under normal conditions, while breathing room air, the predicted alveolar P_{O_2} is usually within 5 mm Hg of the measured arterial P_{O_2} (the difference is somewhat larger in very young patients). The small alveolar-arterial P_{O_2} difference is caused by normal shunt pathways that carry 3% to 5% of the venous return. Because the alveolar-arterial P_{O_2} difference is easily calculated at the bedside, it provides a simple means for detecting derangements in oxygen exchange.

Pathogenesis of Arterial Hypoxemia
Causes of alveolar-arterial P_{O_2} difference

In the presence of pulmonary disease arterial blood will invariably have a P_{O_2} that is much lower than that predicted from ideal alveolar gas (that is, there is a large alveolar-arterial P_{O_2} difference, or AaD_{O_2}). An increased AaD_{O_2} can be caused by one of a combination of impairments of gas exchange as outlined below.[83]

True intrapulmonary shunt ($\dot{V}_A/\dot{Q}c = 0$). When the systemic venous blood perfuses nonventilated areas, there is no increase in the oxygen content of this blood on passage through the capillary bed. Shunt may be caused by conditions such as atelectasis or alveolar consolidation.

Ventilation-perfusion mismatch. In alveoli with low ventilation to perfusion, there may be an insufficient amount of oxygen entering the alveoli per unit of time to saturate the hemoglobin of mixed venous blood entering the capillaries at the same time. This will cause a low pulmonary venous P_{O_2} that, as discussed earlier, will not be offset by areas

with a high ventilation to perfusion ratio. Ventilation-perfusion mismatch is common in the young child (especially when supine) in whom airway closure may occur during expiration. The resultant decrease in local alveolar ventilation may be the primary cause for the lower arterial P_{O_2} of the infant as compared with that of the child and adult.[53] Ventilation-perfusion mismatch occurs with pathologic processes, such as interstitial edema, that reduce, but do not eliminate, air entry into an alveolus. When 100% oxygen is breathed, there will be more oxygen available for uptake by systemic venous blood in regions with low ventilation to perfusion, and the AaD_{O_2} owing to this problem will be eliminated.

Diffusion impairment. Equilibrium of oxygen pressure may not be reached because the diffusion of oxygen into blood is impeded. Whether this is a significant problem for children is unclear, but when present the AaD_{O_2} caused by diffusion impairment will be eliminated with oxygen breathing.

Response to hypoxemia

Shunt and ventilation-perfusion mismatch are hallmarks of respiratory failure, as commonly occurs with traumatic injuries to the respiratory system. Decreases in arterial P_{O_2} and hemoglobin oxygen saturation stimulate the chemoreceptors to increase ventilatory drive. The increase in alveolar ventilation then causes arterial P_{CO_2} to decrease and alveolar and arterial P_{O_2} to rise slightly (equation 6). The manner in which ventilation is increased is dictated primarily by the mechanical state of the lungs (see subsequent discussion), but the overall response is usually arterial hypoxemia combined with hypocapnia. Thus a low arterial P_{CO_2} should be anticipated as a response to hypoxemia, and when not present one should suspect that the child has fatigue or a depressed ventilatory drive and global hypoventilation (for example, from head trauma or medications).

Quantitation of hypoxemia in terms of shunt

Although calculation of an AaD_{O_2} is a convenient way to detect aberrations in pulmonary gas exchange, the magnitude of this difference may also be affected by numerous factors, including inspired oxygen concentration or cardiac output.[73] Therefore venous admixture is often quantified as the fraction of total cardiac output shunted *right-to-left*. The shunt fraction ($\dot{Q}sh/\dot{Q}t$) is an estimate of total cardiac output that bypasses areas for gas

---

*(Refers to p. 47) The alveolar P_{O_2} (P_{AO_2}) may be derived from the equations for alveolar gas exchange and R, the respiratory exchange ratio, which is equivalent to $\dot{V}_{CO_2}/\dot{V}_{O_2}$. In conceptual terms the alveolar P_{O_2} should be the pressure of O_2 in the alveolar gas after equilibrium between gas and blood has been reached. Since total alveolar gas pressure must remain constant during gas exchange, the oxygen removed from inspired gas must be replaced with either CO_2 or additional fresh gas (some of which contains O_2) entering the alveolus. The partial pressure of the oxygen taken up is P_{aCO_2}/R because CO_2 is exchanged for O_2 in a ratio of R. To keep total pressure constant, the additional gas entering from the atmosphere must have a total pressure equal to the difference between the pressure of gas removed (P_{aCO_2}/R) and that replaced by gas exchange (P_{aCO_2}) and of this a fraction (F_{IO_2}) contains oxygen. Therefore the O_2 pressure in the alveolus at equilibrium (P_{aO_2}) must be $P_{IO_2} - P_{aCO_2}/R + (P_{aCO_2}/R - P_{aCO_2}) F_{IO_2}$ or $P_{IO_2} - P_{aCO_2}/R + (1-R)/R$ $F_{IO_2} P_{aCO_2}$.

exchange. It is calculated as if venous return were divided into two compartments, one with perfect gas exchange ($\dot{Q}v$) and one with no gas exchange at all ($\dot{Q}sh$). Shunt fraction therefore includes components that can be described as "true shunt" ($\dot{V}_A/\dot{Q}c = 0$, where $\dot{Q}c$ represents pulmonary capillary blood flow, intracardiac shunt) and those that cause "shunt-like" effects ($\dot{V}_A/\dot{Q}c$ mismatch) but where some gas exchange still takes place. (Note that the term "shunt" is often used for two purposes, which can be a source of confusion.) The shunt equation is a practical means of describing a degree of gas exchange abnormality and for tracking changes consequent to therapy. As derived in the legend of Fig. 5-1, the shunt fraction [$\dot{Q}sh/\dot{Q}t = (Cc'O_2 - CaO_2)/(Cc'O_2 - C\bar{v}O_2)$] can be calculated from knowledge of mixed venous ($C\bar{v}O_2$) and arterial oxygen (CaO_2) contents and the pulmonary capillary oxygen content ($Cc'O_2$), computed from the alveolar gas equation and the hemoglobin concentration. The figure specifically demonstrates that the arterial oxygen content and PO_2 vary with factors other than intrapulmonary pathology: they depend on inspired oxygen fraction, hemoglobin concentration, cardiac output, and oxygen consumption, as well as the net right-to-left shunt. Remembering this important point can help to prevent misinterpreting the cause of a change in arterial PO_2, and it provides the basis for treatment of hypoxemia (see "Management of Respiratory Failure"). It is also important to recognize that shunt fraction, like the $AaDO_2$, can vary with oxygen breathing.[85] The contribution to shunt fraction of $\dot{V}_A/\dot{Q}c$ mismatch (and diffusion impairment, when present) will decrease as inspired oxygen concentration increases. Therefore the change in shunt when inspired oxygen concentration is increased may be helpful to elucidate the cause for the hypoxemia (Table 5-1); although in practice there is usually a variety of causes, so one can only determine which cause or causes dominate.

RESPIRATORY MECHANICS

Almost all forms of respiratory failure occurring after trauma are associated with mechanical dysfunction of the respiratory system. Certainly, compensation for respiratory failure always requires an increase in the mechanical activity of the muscles that participate regularly in respiration, especially the diaphragm. Accordingly the following paragraphs attempt to provide some basic understanding of respiratory mechanics and to familiarize the reader with the unique mechanical features of the child's respiratory system.

The respiratory system can be simplified as consisting of a mechanical pump (the chest wall and lungs) controlled by a neural generator (the respiratory center in the brain stem). The generator is in turn regulated by the input of sensors located in

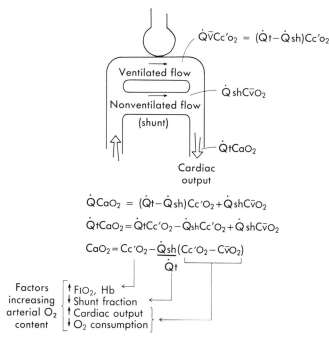

Fig. 5-1 Factors increasing arterial oxygen content in the presence of intrapulmonary or intracardiac *right-to-left* shunts. Two pathways are shown for mixed systemic venous blood: one via well-ventilated alveoli in the lung and the other via an intracardiac or an intrapulmonary *right-to-left* shunt. The sum of the flow of oxygen through these pathways is equivalent to the oxygen transported in the aorta: $\dot{Q}tCaO_2 = (\dot{Q}t - \dot{Q}sh) Cc'O_2 + \dot{Q}shC\bar{v}O_2$. Rearranging, $\dot{Q}tCaO_2 = \dot{Q}tCc'O_2 - \dot{Q}sh (Cc'O_2 - C\bar{v}O_2)$ Therefore, $CaO_2 = Cc'O_2 - (\dot{Q}sh/\dot{Q}t) /(Cc'O_2 - C\bar{v}O_2)$. This leads to a formulation of the factors that can influence arterial oxygen content: an increase in pulmonary capillary oxygen content, a decrease in the shunt fraction, or a decrease in the difference between pulmonary capillary and mixed venous oxygen contents. The equation for arterial oxygen content can also be rearranged to produce the standard shunt equation that is used to calculate the fraction of net *right-to-left shunt:* $(\dot{Q}sh/\dot{Q}t) = (Cc'O_2 - CaO_2)/(Cc'O_2 - C\bar{v}O_2)$. $\dot{Q}t$, Systemic blood flow or cardiac output; $\dot{Q}sh$, shunt blood flow; $C\bar{v}O_2$, CaO_2, $Cc'O_2$, oxygen contents in mixed systemic venous, arterial, and pulmonary capillary blood, respectively.

Table 5-1   Intrapulmonary causes of hypoxemia and response to oxygen breathing

Physiologic disturbance	Effect on AaDo$_2$	Effect on calculated shunt fraction	Effect of 100% O$_2$
True shunt	Increases	Increases	No change in calculated shunt; Po$_2$ increases (change depends on initial Po$_2$)
Ventilation-perfusion mismatch	Increases	Increases	Calculated shunt decreases; Po$_2$ increases to normal
Diffusion impairment	Increases	Increases	Calculated shunt decreases; Po$_2$ increases to normal
Global hypoventilation	No change	No change	No change in calculated shunt; Po$_2$ increases to normal

the central nervous system (chemoreceptors) and in the pump itself (stretch receptors). Disturbances in the control of respiration can occur after head trauma and after a sustained compensatory effort (the so-called central respiratory fatigue). However, as is the case with complicated mechanical systems, the moving parts of the respiratory system are the most likely to malfunction.

Similar to any other system that performs external work, the function of the respiratory pump must be analyzed in terms of energy requirements. These requirements depend on both the amount and the efficiency of the work performed by the pump. Assuming no change in temperature, the amount of work performed by the pump in each cycle depends on the volume change experienced by the lungs and the pressure generated by the respiratory muscles to produce this volume change. The efficiency of the pump is highly variable and depends on the passive condition of the chest wall and lungs and the functional condition of the respiratory muscles. We will examine first the mechanical factors that define the work performed by the respiratory system and analyze later the factors that affect the pump's efficiency.

Mechanical Factors of Respiratory Work

The work performed by the respiratory system can be defined by the integral of volume changes with respect to pressure. Volume changes are relatively fixed by the need of a certain minute alveolar ventilation to maintain arterial Pco$_2$ within acceptable limits (equation *4*). The pressure required to generate the volume changes, on the other hand, can vary widely. Increases in this pressure will inevitably result in a greater work load for the respiratory muscles.

The volume-pressure relationship of the thorax results from the combined volume-pressure relationships of the lungs and chest wall. (The latter is understood here in a wide sense and includes the rib cage and the abdomen.) From a mechanical point of view, we say that the chest wall and the lungs are *in series* because changes in the volume of the lungs (dVL), chest wall (dVw), and thorax (dVTH) are identical:

$$dV_{TH} = dV_L = dV_W \qquad (7)$$

This identity stems from the fact that the pleural space, which forms the boundary between the lungs and chest wall, normally does not change volume during respiration.

Unlike volume, the pressures needed to inflate the lungs (PL, usually known as transpulmonary pressure), chest wall (Pw), and thorax (PTH) are different from each other. Each of these pressures can be defined as the pressure difference across the specific component:

$$P_L = P_M - P_{pl} \qquad (8)$$

$$P_W = P_{pl} - P_B \qquad (9)$$

$$P_{TH} = P_M - P_B \qquad (10)$$

where *P*M represents the pressure measured at the mouth, *P*pl the pleural pressure, and *P*B the atmospheric pressure (which is conventionally taken as the zero reference). These pressures depend not only on the volume of inflation but also on whether that volume is held constant (static conditions) or changes continuously (dynamic conditions). We will examine the volume-pressure relationships of lungs, chest wall, and thorax first under static and then under dynamic conditions.

Static volume-pressure relationships: elastic recoil and compliance

When thoracic volume is held constant, there is no gas flow in the airways. Having no frictional or other flow-related pressure losses in the airways, alveolar (P_A) and mouth pressure become identical (provided that the glottis is open). Under the conditions of this static equilibrium, the pressure differences measured across lungs, chest wall, and thorax at a specific volume must equal their respective elastic recoils ($PelL$, $Pelw$, and $PelTH$):

$$PelL = P_A - Ppl \qquad (11)$$

$$Pelw = Ppl - P_B \qquad (12)$$

$$PelTH = P_A - P_B \qquad (13)$$

The elastic recoil pressure of the thorax is the sum of those of the lungs and chest wall. This can be derived by subtracting $PelL$ (equation *11*) and $Pelw$ (equation *12*) from $PelTH$ (equation *13*):

$$PelTH = PelL + Pelw \qquad (14)$$

In this expression, *Pel*TH represents not only the sum of the elastic recoils of the lungs and chest wall, but also the total pressure that the respiratory muscles need to generate to maintain a given thoracic volume.

The volume-pressure relationships (Fig. 5-2) of the lungs, chest wall, and thorax differ considerably.[1] The relaxation volume (the volume at which elastic recoil pressure is zero) of the lungs is much lower than that of the chest wall. This arrangement has two important consequences. First, the relaxation volume of the thorax occupies a position intermediate between that of the lungs and that of the chest wall. Under most circumstances this volume is the same as the functional residual capacity (FRC), the volume contained in the lungs at the end of a tidal expiration. Second, the opposing forces generated by the lungs (to relax at a lower volume) and chest wall (to relax at a higher volume) generate a negative pressure at their boundary, the pleural surface. If a communication is open between the atmosphere and the pleural space, this negative pressure will draw gas into the pleural space until the lungs and chest wall reach their relaxation volumes.

If we wished to characterize the relationship between volume and pressure changes, a reasonable approach would be to determine the ratio of these changes, dV/dP. This ratio defines the compliance of the thorax, lungs, or chest wall, depending on

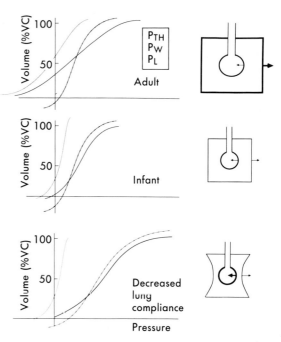

Fig. 5-2 *Left,* Static volume-pressure relationships of the thorax, lungs, and chest wall in the adult, the normal infant, and the infant with decreased lung compliance. Volume in the ordinates is shown as a percentage of the vital capacity. Pressure in the abscissa indicates the pressures across the thorax (P_{TH}), lungs (P_L), and chest wall (P_W). (The relaxation volume of the thorax is similar to the functional residual capacity under most circumstances.) *Right,* Idealized representations of the chest wall and lungs at the relaxation volume of the thorax. The arrows represent the recoil forces of chest wall and lungs. Because these forces are at equilibrium, the length of the arrows is the same. In the adult the importance of the chest wall recoil in determining thoracic relaxation volume is emphasized with a thicker arrow. In the infant the recoil of the lungs is relatively unopposed by that of the chest wall, resulting in a lower thoracic relaxation volume (and functional residual capacity). In the infant with decreased pulmonary compliance the high recoil of the lungs *(thick arrow)* results in an even lower thoracic relaxation volume. In addition, because of its high compliance, the chest wall undergoes deformation, which limits lung expansion.

whether we use dP_{TH}, dP_L, or dP_W in the denominator. Unfortunately, as shown in Fig. 5-2, dV/dP is not constant, and the volume-pressure relationship cannot therefore be described by a single compliance value for the entire range of thoracic volume. Compliance decreases both at high and low thoracic volumes. At intermediate volumes, however, compliance is maximal and relatively constant. For this range of volumes, which is where normal respiration takes place, we can safely consider:

$$Pel = V/C \qquad (15)$$

In this equation, which is valid for the thorax, lungs, or chest wall, *Pel* represents the pressure generated by elastic recoil of any of these structures after undergoing a volume change V, if its compliance were C.

The static volume-pressure relationships of the lungs and chest wall vary with size and age as the lungs and, especially, the chest wall mature. The chest wall of the infant is extremely compliant in comparison to that of the adult and older child.[38,86] This feature has several consequences. First, due to the series arrangement of lungs and chest wall, the contribution of the chest wall to the overall volume-pressure behavior of the thorax is very small in the infant. Consequently the volume-pressure relationship of the thorax approaches that of the lungs alone (Fig. 5-2). Second, the decreased recoil of the chest wall results in a lower relaxation volume of the thorax. Newborns and small infants are capable of maintaining their functional residual capacity above this low relaxation volume by various mechanisms directed at breaking expiratory flow.[35,70,75] Unfortunately, these mechanisms may not be effective when lung compliance is reduced, when neurologic control is impaired (for example, during anesthesia), or when the infant's trachea is intubated. Under these circumstances, the functional residual capacity may decrease to volumes incompatible with alveolar stability, resulting in alveolar closure and increased shunt fraction. Finally, negative pleural pressures created in the course of respiratory efforts result in greater deformation of the chest wall (Fig. 5-2). This deformation, which is expressed as visible retractions of the rib cage, greatly reduces the overall efficiency of the pump[41] and decreases the ability to compensate under conditions of respiratory compromise.

Dynamic volume-pressure relationships: resistance and airway obstruction

Until now we have considered only the pressure changes generated by the elastic properties of the lungs and chest wall during thoracic volume changes. The analysis of the volume-pressure relationships of the thorax becomes more compli-

cated if we also consider the pressure changes produced by the movement of gas inside the airways (and to some extent also by the movement of the tissue itself) during thoracic inflation and deflation. Although the gas contained in the airways has low viscosity and density, it moves at relatively high velocity and undergoes quick accelerations and decelerations during the respiratory cycle. As a result, frictional and convective (accelerative) pressure losses are generated. The addition of these pressure losses increases the total pressure, and therefore the work, needed to inspire to a given thoracic volume. Under most circumstances, resistive pressure losses are only relevant during inspiration because expiration is passive and requires no expenditure of energy by the respiratory muscles to overcome resistance.

Resistive pressure losses depend on gas flow in the airways. If we assume that the relationship between resistive pressure losses (Pres) and flow ($\dot{V}$) is linear, we can write the following:

$$Pres = R\,\dot{V} \qquad (16)$$

where *R* represents the resistance of the thorax, lungs, or chest wall. Unfortunately, this expression, which is often used to calculate thoracic and pulmonary resistances, is an oversimplification because R is not really constant. If flow is high enough, as commonly occurs during rapid breathing, turbulence ensues and R starts to depend on flow. In addition, the airway caliber, and thus the airway resistance, depend on both lung volume and the phase of the respiratory cycle. This principle is essential for understanding and recognizing airway obstruction in children and deserves some special attention.

Airways are collapsible tubes rather than rigid pipes; their caliber is determined by the airway's intrinsic compliance and the pressure across the airway wall. This pressure, the airway transmural pressure, is the difference between the pressure of the gas column inside the airway and the pressure of the tissue surrounding the airway. The pressure inside any airway is relatively easy to predict. During inspiration the action of the respiratory muscles generates an increasingly negative pleural pressure. Pleural pressure is applied in part to overcome elastic recoil and expand the lungs and in part to create negative alveolar pressures that will cause gas to flow from the mouth (where pressure is zero) into the alveolar spaces. During expiration the direction of gas flow reverses. Reversal of flow is facilitated by lung recoil, which now makes alveolar pressure positive with respect to the pressure at the mouth. The pressure outside the airways varies depending on whether the airways are intrathoracic or extrathoracic. The outside pressure of extrathoracic airways is essentially equal to the atmospheric pressure (zero) and constant during the respiratory cycle. The outside pressure of intrathoracic airways is similar to pleural pressure, and thus it is a function of lung volume.

From the previous discussion it is evident that inspiration and expiration will have different effects on the transmural pressure and caliber of the airways depending on whether the airways are intrathoracic or extrathoracic. During inspiration extrathoracic airways will narrow because their inside pressure will decrease without change in their outside pressure. Intrathoracic airways, on the other hand, will expand because their outside pressure (pleural pressure) will decrease more than their inside pressure. During expiration the changes will be reversed. The extrathoracic airway will expand as the inside pressure becomes positive with respect to the outside pressure, and the intrathoracic airway will narrow as the inside pressure decreases with respect to pleural pressure. The narrowing of the intrathoracic airways during expiration is contingent on airway pressure decreasing enough downstream from the alveoli so that the inside pressure will at some point become equal to pleural pressure. At this *equal pressure point*,[64] the inside pressure will be lower than alveolar pressure in a magnitude equivalent to the elastic recoil of the lungs (which is the difference between alveolar and pleural pressure, as we have previously seen). Since lung elastic recoil depends on lung volume, the equal pressure point moves toward the mouth (and possibly outside the chest) at high lung volumes and toward the periphery of the lung at low lung volumes. Accordingly, intrathoracic airway resistance increases at the end of expiration, when lung volumes are low.

Airway obstruction causes an exaggeration of these normal changes in airway caliber (Fig. 5-3). With extrathoracic airway obstruction (for example, subglottic edema after intubation), airway pressures have to be more negative during inspiration to overcome the resistance of the obstruction. Therefore the extrathoracic airway will tend to collapse, producing a typical turbulent noise that is recognized clinically as inspiratory stridor. The obstruction is unchanged or somewhat relieved dur-

ing expiration because the pressure inside the airway becomes more positive with respect to the atmospheric pressure surrounding it. When the obstruction is intrathoracic, as with bronchospasm or impaction of the bronchi with mucus or aspirated material, the airway caliber increases during inspiration permitting relatively free entry of gas into the distal air spaces. During expiration, however, the obstruction causes the airway pressure to decrease abruptly downstream (towards the mouth) from the obstruction point. The equal pressure point moves to the lung periphery, and airway diameter decreases even at high lung volumes. This additional decrease in airway diameter may limit expiratory flow,[102] making the rate of lung deflation independent of the patient's expiratory effort. Expiration is thus characteristically prolonged, especially at low lung volumes. In addition, the reduced airway diameter promotes turbulence, which is responsible for an audible wheezing noise. It is important to remember that, although expiratory prolongation and wheezing are traditionally associated with small airways disease, they can also be present with obstruction of the intrathoracic trachea and major bronchi.

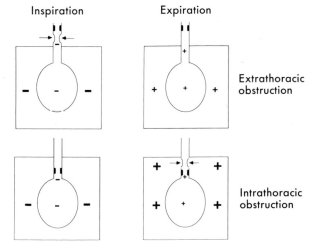

Fig. 5-3 Effect of the phase of the respiratory cycle on the dimensions of the airways during extrathoracic and intrathoracic airway obstruction. Extrathoracic airway obstruction worsens during inspiration because the negative pressure inside the airway is unopposed by the atmospheric pressure outside the airway. Intrathoracic airway obstruction worsens during expiration because the positive pressures outside the airways (pleural pressure) exceed the pressure inside the airways downstream from the obstruction point.

Compliance, resistance, and the work of breathing

As we have discussed, the pressure across the thorax or, in other words, the pressure that the respiratory muscles have to generate to produce a respiratory excursion, is the sum of two components. The first component is the pressure needed to overcome the elastic recoil of the lungs and chest wall (PelTH) and depends on thoracic volume. The second component is the pressure used to overcome airway and tissue resistance (PresTH), and depends on gas flow. These two components are summarized in the following equation of motion of the respiratory system.[61]

$$\text{PTH} = \text{PelTH} + \text{PresTH} = \text{V}/\text{CTH} + \text{RTH} \: \dot{\text{V}} \: (17)$$

where CTH and RTH are the thoracic compliance and resistance, respectively. As long as thoracic volume changes and gas flow are unchanged, decreases in thoracic compliance (restrictive respiratory disease) or increases in thoracic resistance (obstructive disease) will increase PTH, thereby increasing the work load of the respiratory muscles.

Restriction of thoracic expansion by a reduced pulmonary or chest wall compliance is the most common mechanism of respiratory pump failure in children after trauma. Lung compliance can decrease because the parenchymal substance of the lungs is infiltrated with blood or edema fluid. Lung compliance also decreases when the number or volume of ventilated alveoli is diminished, as when an area of the lung becomes atelectatic or an entire lung is compressed by a tension pneumothorax. In both examples a greater airway pressure is needed to overdistend the remaining alveolar units to the same final lung volume. Chest wall compliance is less frequently reduced in traumatized children. This reduction almost always involves abdominal distention and increased intraabdominal pressure. On rare instances, infiltration of the chest wall by hemorrhage or edema may decrease chest wall compliance enough to restrict respiration.

Whether originating in the lungs or the chest wall, a decreased thoracic compliance has two mechanical consequences. First, as previously stated, the work of breathing increases. Second, the relaxation volume of the thorax, and thus the functional residual capacity, decreases. This decrease in lung volume, which further reduces compliance and increases the work of breathing, may be more pronounced in infants whose thoracic relaxation volume is already low. At low lung volumes the

alveoli are particularly unstable and tend to collapse, increasing venous admixture. A deep inspiration (that is, a sigh) may reverse this tendency and improve oxygenation by recruiting collapsed alveoli, which remain open for a certain period, improving lung compliance.[63] This effect of the volume history of the lung on pulmonary compliance is important to explain some of the benefits of intermittent positive pressure inflation of the lungs (see "Institution of Ventilatory Support"). Unfortunately the improvement of alveolar stability induced by a deep inflation is usually short-lived in patients with restrictive respiratory disease who require repeated inflations to maintain lung volume.

Airway obstruction is relatively common after trauma in children. The short neck of the infant and young child may protect against direct upper airway injuries, which are relatively rare at early ages. On the other hand, the small diameter and high compliance of the developing intrathoracic airways predispose to airway obstruction. The airways of the infant and small child have a reduced diameter and a high resistance. This high resistance causes no problem under normal conditions because airway flow is low. Small decreases in airway diameter, however, produce a disproportionate increase in airway resistance, which is exponentially (at least to the fourth power) related to changes in diameter. Resistive work increases in the same exponential fashion, leading rapidly to respiratory failure. As an example, subglottic edema after trauma during endotracheal intubation is much more likely to cause respiratory failure in the infant than in the older child or the adult. The same increase in mucosal thickness will almost completely obstruct the airway of the infant, whereas it will still leave a large opening in the larynx of the older child and adult. Developing airways are also characteristically more compliant than mature airways.[13,94] Accordingly, similar decreases in their transmural pressure will cause a large reduction in diameter. The infant's larynx, for example, will collapse easily during inspiration when there is subglottic obstruction. Similarly the intrathoracic airways of the infant are more likely to become obliterated during expiration when the bronchi are obstructed by mucus or bronchospasm.

Factors Affecting Respiratory Efficiency

To maintain a normal arterial P_{CO_2}, the respiratory system must maintain a certain minute alveolar ventilation. Therefore when the work load of the respiratory muscles increases in the course of an illness, the system is faced with two alternatives for compensation. The first and most simple is to increase the output of the respiratory muscles even at the cost of a greater energy expenditure. The second alternative is to improve the efficiency of respiration, adapting the respiratory pattern to the conditions imposed by the illness. Patients with respiratory failure usually take both alternatives. The respiratory effort of these patients increases visibly. In addition, their breathing pattern usually exhibits characteristics typical of the mechanical derangement of their respiratory system.[31,59] Children with decreased thoracic compliance will breathe rapidly and shallowly because, with this pattern, less work per unit of time is needed to maintain the same minute alveolar ventilation. The tachypneic response to restrictive respiratory disease is amplified in the infant, who already has a high respiratory rate and a low total thorax compliance. Children with increased thoracic resistance will breathe more deeply and slowly because less work per unit of time is required with this pattern.

The configuration of the chest wall and the power of the respiratory muscles essential for the compensatory effort are frequently impaired in the course of respiratory failure. The respiratory muscles are capable of developing their maximal force only if they are stretched to an optimal length. This length is achieved for a certain chest wall configuration. The diaphragm reaches its optimal length at low lung volumes, when it adopts the shape of a dome-capped cylinder (Fig. 5-3).[26] This geometric design has two advantages. First, diaphragmatic contraction shortens the sides of the cylinder, which then functions like a piston acting on the lungs.[18] Second, the sides of the diaphragmatic cylinder are apposed to the internal surface of the rib cage.[62] The area of apposition of diaphragm and chest wall is exposed to intraabdominal pressure, which increases as the diaphragm descends during inspiration, pushing the rib cage forward and laterally to increase lung volume further (Fig. 5-4).

Both thoracic hyperexpansion and abdominal distention spread out the insertions of the diaphragm (Fig. 5-4). Under these conditions the stretched diaphragmatic fibers start their contraction at a suboptimal length, which limits their ability to generate force. In addition, the diaphragm loses its cylindrical shape and its area of apposition, resulting in a much smaller change in lung volume

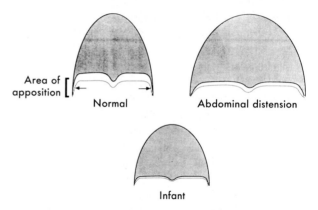

Fig. 5-4 Schema of the shape of the diaphragm in a normal adult or older child, in the adult or older child with abdominal distention, and in the normal infant. The developed diaphragm has the shape of a dome-capped cylinder whose walls are apposed to the rib cage. The abdominal pressure acts on the area of apposition (*arrows*), increasing the excursion of the rib cage at the end of inspiration (*broken line*). Abdominal distention obliterates the area of apposition and flattens the diaphragmatic dome, decreasing tidal volume. The horizontal insertions of the diaphragm have a similar effect in the normal infant.

for the same energy expenditure. Thoracic hyperexpansion is not rare after trauma in patients who develop intrathoracic airway obstruction or extrapulmonary collections of gas or liquid inside the chest. Abdominal distention, which is even more common in the traumatized child, has the additional disadvantage of increasing the intraabdominal pressure, which opposes diaphragmatic descent and increases the mechanical demands on the diaphragmatic muscle.

For a diaphragmatic contraction to produce a maximal volume expansion, the rib cage must undergo expansion in all its points. If an area of the rib cage moves in an expiratory direction, the tidal volume of the lungs decreases. Because the diaphragm still has to do work to produce this expiratory deformation of the chest wall, the system becomes less efficient. This paradoxic movement of the rib cage occurs in patients with extensive rib fractures that weaken the frame of the rib cage (flail chest). As pleural pressure becomes negative during inspiration, the weakened area becomes depressed, causing a net loss in the tidal volume of the lungs. The abdominal wall can also experience a paradoxic inward movement during parts of inspiration when the contractility of the diaphragm diminishes due to muscle fatigue. This abdominal paradox also decreases the tidal volume of the lungs and is an important sign of respiratory muscle fatigue.

The arrangement of the chest wall in children, and particularly in small infants, has some apparent disadvantages that may make them more vulnerable to respiratory failure. The lower portion of their rib cage has large anteroposterior and lateral diameters that, similar to abdominal distention, make the costal insertions of the diaphragm horizontal and decrease the area of apposition.[96] In addition, the infant's rib cage and, to a lesser extent, the child's rib cage are very compliant.[38,86] Although such compliance represents a mechanical advantage to withstand trauma, it also favors distortion and paradoxic inspiratory movement of the rib cage. Paradoxic movement is also favored by the low tone of the rib cage muscles,[42] whose contribution to respiration consists mainly of contracting simultaneously with the diaphragm to stiffen the rib cage and minimize distortion during inspiration.

It is important to recognize that the efficiency of respiration is also affected by the functional state of the respiratory muscles. Sustained intense activity of these muscles is likely to result in decreased contractility and muscle fatigue. In the context of this discussion, respiratory muscle fatigue will be defined as the inability of the muscle to generate enough force to maintain an adequate minute alveolar ventilation.[90] Respiratory muscle fatigue may be a response to a variety of physiologic alterations. The most common is the imbalance between the energy demands of the muscle's contractile machinery and the substrates available to satisfy those demands. Whether the imbalance is due to circulatory shock[8] or to the inadequate coupling of the excitation-contraction processes inside the muscle cell, the final result is always a decrease in the force generated by the muscle, even if its energy consumption is increased. The respiratory muscles, particularly the diaphragm, contain a high proportion of high-oxidative, slow-twitch fibers, which are resistant to development of fatigue. In contrast with the adult, the diaphragm of the infant contains a greater proportion of low-oxidative, fast-twitch fibers, which are fatigue-susceptible.[49]

RECOGNITION OF RESPIRATORY FAILURE

The child's limited capability of respiratory compensation makes the early recognition of any re-

spiratory embarrassment essential. Ideally, respiratory failure should be anticipated rather than recognized so that the appropriate measures can be taken before gas exchange is severely altered. Early intervention will prevent the effects of hypoxemia and hypercarbia on the already taxed central nervous and circulatory systems of the traumatized patient.

During physical evaluation the examiner should avoid disturbing the patient's mechanisms of respiratory compensation. Often, patients in respiratory failure will not tolerate well the supine position because the weight of the abdominal organs interferes with diaphragmatic function. The agitation induced by separating a child from his mother may increase the work of breathing and precipitate respiratory failure, particularly in the presence of airway obstruction.

The evaluation of a child after trauma should include first a quick assessment of the adequacy of ventilation, particularly in those patients who have sustained head, chest, or abdominal injuries or have signs of circulatory impairment. This assessment includes the presence and vigor of the respiratory effort, respiratory rate, extent of the chest excursions, and existence of signs of airway obstruction. A child with grossly inadequate respiratory efforts or complete airway obstruction will not survive unless ventilation of the lungs is restored immediately.

The alterations of gas exchange characteristic of respiratory failure can be difficult to detect by physical examination. Cyanosis is influenced by perfusion and is therefore an unreliable sign of hypoxemia, even when lighting conditions are optimal.[22] Hypoventilation or hypercarbia are equally difficult to detect by physical examination.[65] If severe enough, hypoxemia and hypercarbia impair the function of the central nervous and circulatory systems. Confusion, lethargy, or even combativeness are thus common signs of respiratory failure and are due to brain hypoxia. Similarly, tachycardia is a frequent response to hypoxemia and hypercarbia.

A first inspection of the child in respiratory failure will almost always demonstrate abnormalities of the breathing pattern. If the failure is the result of dysfunction of the central nervous system, the child's breathing rate may be abnormally low or the breathing rhythm periodic. If, on the other hand, the failure is the result of a mechanical derangement, the breathing pattern will denote compensatory changes, which often provide important clues about the nature of the mechanical derangement itself.[31,59] Tachypnea, or a pattern of rapid, shallow respirations, is the normal response to decreases in the compliance of the thorax. Very deep, slow respirations accompanied by accentuated effort suggest airway obstruction. Inspiration is typically prolonged in extrathoracic airway obstruction, whereas expiration is prolonged in intrathoracic airway obstruction. The increased effort of the respiratory muscles results in distortions of the chest wall, particularly at the level of the costal insertions of the diaphragm (subcostal retractions) and the intercostal spaces (intercostal retractions). These distortions are particularly noticeable in infants, owing to the high compliance of their chest wall.[38,86] As failure progresses and more compensation becomes necessary, incorporation of accessory muscles to the breathing effort and the greater amplitude of the contractions of the regular respiratory muscles give an impression of air hunger, as if the patient's attention were solely concentrated in breathing.

Inspiratory stridor is usually the result of extrathoracic airway obstruction, whereas abnormal expiratory noises result from intrathoracic airway obstruction. Grunting usually represents an attempt to increase functional residual capacity by stopping gas flow through the glottis at the end of expiration, thus creating a positive end-expiratory pressure in the airways.

Auscultation of the chest provides information about the entry and distribution of gas in the lungs. Breath sounds will often be decreased in intensity if gas entry is poor. However, the small size of the infant's chest facilitates the transmission of tracheal sounds to the thoracic surface, limiting the ability to judge the volume of gas that actually enters the lung periphery. Gross asymmetries between the two lungs are always abnormal, and in the traumatized child, they often indicate abnormal accumulations of gas or liquid in the pleural space. The absence of these asymmetries, however, does not rule out such accumulations in the infant or small child because breath sounds can be easily transmitted from the trachea or the contralateral side. Crackles and rales suggest the presence of liquid or atelectasis in the peripheral air spaces.

MANAGEMENT OF RESPIRATORY FAILURE

The goal of therapy in the child with respiratory failure is to restore and maintain adequate gas exchange at the minimal energy cost and with minimal complications. Often this goal can be achieved by interventions that improve the efficiency of the respiratory pump, but on occasions the entire function of the pump must be substituted and ventilation be supported artificially.

Of the two gas exchange aberrations that occur during respiratory failure, hypoxemia is by far the most dangerous for the patient. Usually it is also the easiest to correct. Initial administration of supplemental oxygen is a safe precaution in all patients with any substantial trauma, even if there is no apparent hypoxemia. Oxygen can be administered with face masks, face tents, or nasal cannulae while the patient is being evaluated. Oxygen hoods are a convenient way of delivering oxygen to small infants, who may not tolerate face masks. Unfortunately, hoods are bulky and have little place in the initial treatment of the patient in the emergency room, where a mask, a face tent, or even a high flow of humidified oxygen directed at the mouth and nose may be more appropriate. The initial measures directed at increasing inspired oxygen concentration, however, may be insufficient to improve tissue oxygenation in the child with very severe trauma. It is then imperative to provide additional ventilatory support.

Institution of Ventilatory Support

The indications for ventilatory support in the traumatized child are often a matter of clinical judgment. As such, they are based on multiple factors and influenced by the experience of the clinician making the judgment. There is, however, one absolute indication: the presence of decompensated respiratory failure, independent of whether this is due to an abnormal respiratory drive, unsurmountable mechanical dysfunction, or respiratory muscle fatigue. In any of these circumstances the adequacy of gas exchange in the lungs, and ultimately the respiratory function of the peripheral tissues, are threatened and need to be secured.

Other indications of ventilatory support may be less clear and need to take into account factors such as the availability of skills and equipment. In an attempt to systematize these indications, we will consider three categories of patients. The first category includes those with compensated but progressive respiratory dysfunction that is anticipated to result in decompensated respiratory failure. An example of this category is the child who develops clinical signs of the adult respiratory distress syndrome (ARDS) soon after trauma. ARDS is a progressive disorder (see later discussion), and it is likely that the patient's respiratory function will worsen to follow a prolonged course. Similarly a child with severe abdominal injuries is likely to develop abdominal distension and impaired diaphragmatic function and should therefore be considered for ventilatory support. The second category comprises children with moderate respiratory impairment but who have a limited capability of respiratory compensation (for example, a child in shock). Shock limits the compensatory response of the respiratory muscles and can induce respiratory failure by decreasing respiratory muscle blood flow.[8] Mechanical support of the respiratory function will not only prevent the often fatal development of muscle fatigue but will also facilitate the redistribution of cardiac output to other underperfused vital organs and reduce tissue hypoxia. Newborns and small infants with any severe respiratory or nonrespiratory injury should be considered in this second category because of their limited respiratory reserve. Finally, the third category includes children with potential for respiratory failure that, if materialized, would severely threaten the function of vital organs. An example of this category is the child with head trauma and intracranial hypertension, for whom hypoxemia and hypercarbia would result in further increases in intracranial pressure and brain injury.

Mechanical Ventilation

Once the decision is made to provide assisted ventilation, a secure airway access becomes necessary. This is usually accomplished by intubation of the trachea, a procedure that is discussed in detail elsewhere. It is important to note here, however, that endotracheal intubation is not devoid of risks. These risks need to be evaluated carefully before making the decision to initiate mechanical ventilation. This evaluation is particularly pertinent in children with unstable cardiovascular function or head and neck injuries and when the personnel performing the intubation are not fully experienced.

Types of mechanical ventilators

Several types of mechanical ventilators can be used in children. Lung deflation is passive with all these ventilators. Inflation is produced by a pneumatic mechanism regulated to generate a certain tidal volume. Depending on the regulatory mechanism, the ventilators can be pressure cycled, time

cycled, or volume cycled. Pressure-cycled ventilators have fallen in disuse and do not merit much discussion. Time-cycled ventilators are widely used for newborns and infants. Lung inflation with these ventilators is controlled by a timing mechanism that opens and closes an expiratory valve. Closure of the valve diverts a constant inspiratory flow circulating in the ventilatory circuit to the patient's lungs, whereas opening the valve permits both the constant flow of the ventilator and the gas contained in the lungs to exit to the atmosphere. A pop-off safety valve limits the inspiratory pressure developed in the airway. When used as described, time-cycled ventilators deliver a rather consistent tidal volume, whose magnitude depends on the duration of the inspiratory time and the constant flow in the ventilator. Time-cycled ventilators, however, are often used as pressure-limited, time-cycled ventilators by establishing a relatively low-inspiratory pressure limit, which renders tidal volume and alveolar ventilation dependent on thoracic compliance and resistance, similar to the pressure-cycled ventilators. With volume-cycled ventilators, lung inflation ceases only when a certain tidal volume has been delivered to the ventilator circuit. These ventilators, which provide the most consistent tidal volume, are equipped with a safety valve that can effectively limit airway pressure.

Principles of ventilatory management

All types of mechanical ventilators are designed for a single purpose: to provide adequate alveolar ventilation with minimal barotrauma. From a functional point of view, mechanical ventilation is usually initiated with two additional goals: preservation of lung volume and replacement of respiratory muscle function. Certain principles of ventilator management are common to all ventilators. Since alveolar ventilation is proportional to both ventilatory rate and tidal volume (equation *4*), reciprocal adjustments of these ventilatory variables will usually achieve the desired level of alveolar ventilation and CO_2 removal. Finer adjustments in ventilatory support, which affect oxygenation and CO_2 removal, should be directed at correcting specific physiologic abnormalities. Frequently, these abnormalities involve changes in the relaxation volume of the thorax and the functional residual capacity.

When lung or chest wall compliance is decreased, the relaxation volume of the thorax is reset at a lower value and the patient breathes at a lower functional residual capacity. As lung volume decreases, the alveolar structures become unstable and some alveoli collapse. Alveolar collapse reduces lung compliance further, increasing the work of breathing if the patient breathes spontaneously, or decreasing tidal volume (or increasing airway pressure) if the patient is already mechanically ventilated. In addition, collapsed alveoli may continue to be perfused and act as shunt units, increasing shunt fraction and causing hypoxemia (Fig. 5-5). These abnormalities can be reversed, at least in part, if the thorax is distended by applying positive airway pressure. Several approaches can be used. Increasing tidal volume will distend some of the collapsed alveoli, improving alveolar ventilation and reducing venous admixture. Intermittent lung distention with a large tidal volume will improve alveolar stability and reduce the overall number of collapsed alveoli, but as the thorax is allowed to reach its relaxation volume at the end of expiration, some alveoli may still collapse. The addition of positive end-expiratory pressure (PEEP) circumvents this problem. PEEP raises the functional residual capacity above the relaxation volume of the thorax[32,48,50] and provides more stable alveolar recruitment (Fig. 5-5). Consequently, thoracic compliance and alveolar ventilation increase and shunt fraction decreases.[30,52,95]

Both increases in tidal volume and PEEP result in a greater average thoracic volume. With conventional modes of ventilation, this average volume is reflected by the mean distending pressure applied to the airways, which is known as the mean airway pressure. Mean airway pressure is easily computed electronically and correlates well with oxygenation in restrictive lung disease. In addition to increasing tidal volume and PEEP, mean airway pressure can be increased by lengthening inspiration or by modifying inspiratory pressure waveform to make it approach a square shape.

Increases in intrathoracic airway resistance are less common than restrictive respiratory disease in traumatized children. Intrathoracic airway obstruction causes expiratory retardation with gas trapping. The patient's functional residual capacity is thus greater than the relaxation volume of the thorax. To allow for the complete emptying of the lungs after each inflation the longest expiratory time compatible with adequate ventilation should be used. A long expiratory time requires a relatively low ventilatory rate. Applying low inspiratory flows appears to promote a more homogeneous

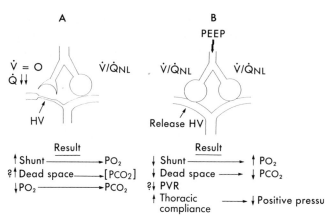

Fig. 5-5 Idealized schema of the effects of PEEP in restrictive lung disease. **A,** Atelectatic areas with a decreased ventilation-perfusion ratio $(\dot{V}/\dot{Q})$ increase the shunt fraction and dead space, causing hypoxemia and hypercarbia. These are partially offset by the arteriolar vasoconstriction *(HV)* induced by alveolar hypoxia and by the hyperventilatory response to hypoxemia. **B,** Reexpansion of the atelectasis following the application of PEEP normalizes the ventilation perfusion ratio $(\dot{V}/\dot{Q}_{NL})$, reducing the shunt fraction and dead space and improving the hypoxemia and hypercarbia. In addition, the release of hypoxic vasoconstriction by lung expansion may reduce pulmonary vascular resistance *(PVR)* and the afterload to the right ventricle. Finally, recruitment of collapsed alveoli improves thoracic compliance and decreases ventilatory pressures.

distribution of gas in the lungs.[9] In patients with airway obstruction, PEEP may increase lung overdistention and is not recommended as a first approach.

Modes of ventilatory support

The aforementioned principles can be applied in various modes of ventilatory support. Ventilation is *controlled* when the ventilator delivers a predetermined rate, independent of the patient's respiratory effort. For efficiency and safety, controlled ventilation requires that the patient's spontaneous respirations are suppressed or kept to a minimal. Ventilation is *assisted* when the ventilator cycles are triggered by the patient's own effort. Most ventilators will still deliver a preset minimal number of breaths even if there is no triggering effort. By allowing the patient to determine minute ventilation, assisted ventilation decreases respiratory work and facilitates adaptation to the ventilator. Unfortunately, many children and infants develop respiratory alkalosis and gas trapping during periods of agitation, especially if the triggering airway pressure is set low. Intermittent mandatory ventilation (IMV) and its more recent modification in which ventilation is synchronized (SIMV), were introduced as *weaning* modes. During IMV the patient breathes spontaneously from a constant flow through a pressurized circuit. The ventilator delivers a preset minimal number of breaths, which contribute a variable portion of the patient's minute ventilation. Through the effect of lung volume history on lung compliance, ventilator breaths improve mechanical function in the spontaneous breaths that follow each ventilator breath, further reducing the work of breathing. SIMV differs from IMV only in that the ventilator can be triggered (assisted) by the patient's effort. Either of these modes can be used with or without PEEP. In practice, controlled ventilation is usually provided with an IMV circuit so that the patient may obtain gas flow when taking an occasional spontaneous breath. Continuous positive airway pressure (CPAP) provides a consistent distending pressure by allowing the patient to breathe from a pressurized circuit that contains a constant flow. The increase in functional residual capacity produced by the application of CPAP often increases lung compliance and decreases work of breathing enough to obviate the need for mechanical ventilation.

Complications of ventilatory support

The most common complications of mechanical ventilation arise from the application of positive pressure to the airways. Positive pressure ventilation increases the intrathoracic pressure surrounding the vascular structures contained in the chest.[89] As a consequence, venous return to the heart decreases, and blood pools in the venous compartment outside the thorax. In addition, the right ventricle may have to empty against the increased impedance opposed by compressed alveolar vessels. Increased respiratory variability of cardiac output, decreased cardiac output, and right ventricular failure are common complications of positive pressure ventilation.[27,46,100] These complications negate one primary objective of ventilatory support by limiting the convective transport of oxygen by the arterial blood. Frequently, increased administration of fluid and inotropic support are necessary to restore oxygen delivery to the tissues.

Perivascular and pleural pressure are very similar. Both undergo regional variations within the chest. Also, both depend on alveolar pressure and the volume-pressure characteristics of the lungs and chest wall. When lung compliance is reduced (and lung elastic recoil is increased), high alveolar pressures are not transmitted to the pleural and perivascular spaces.[76] Accordingly, patients with severe restrictive lung disease tolerate positive pressure better than those with a more normal lung compliance. When chest wall compliance is reduced, on the other hand, the same alveolar pressure will result in greater pleural and perivascular pressures (equation *12*). Patients with a restrictive chest wall (for instance, due to abdominal distention) are thus more prone to experience decreases in cardiac output during positive pressure ventilation because of the need for high alveolar pressures to distend the chest and the ready transmission of these pressures to the perivascular space.

Patients with decreased lung compliance require high transpulmonary pressures to distend their lungs. These high pressures place rather strenuous stresses on the walls of airways and alveoli, which can rupture, allowing gas to leak into the pulmonary interstitium. Interstitial gas dissects along the lung septations, becoming visible on chest radiographs as interstitial emphysema.[47] On rare occasions, gas can penetrate pulmonary veins, resulting in fatal arterial air embolism.[39] More frequently, extraalveolar gas reaches the pleural surface of the lung and enters the pleural space (pneumothorax) or the mediastinum (pneumomediastinum). The malignancy of these gas collections is related to their impedance of venous return and severe reduction of cardiac output. From the mediastinum, pressurized gas can follow cleavage planes to enter the perivascular sheaths of the great vessels, the pericardial sac (pneumopericardium), the retroperitoneum and peritoneum (pneumoperitoneum), and the subcutaneous tissue of the neck, face, trunk, and extremities.[54] Compression of the heart, intrathoracic vessels, and lungs by extraalveolar gas demands immediate evacuation.

Prolonged administration of high oxygen concentrations during mechanical ventilation is known to result in both epithelial and endothelial injuries in the lungs. Although immature lungs appear to be somewhat more resistant to oxidant lung injury than mature lungs,[36] it is probably wise to decrease the fractional concentration of O_2 in the inspired gas as soon as possible, even if this requires an increase in the distending pressures applied to the lung.

Strategies to Improve Oxygenation

Following the initiation of mechanical ventilation, many patients continue to have refractory hypoxemia. Furthermore the cardiac output of these patients may be decreased, owing to the effect of positive pressure ventilation on the circulation. The net result is a critically reduced oxygen transport (cardiac output × arterial oxygen concentration) and tissue hypoxia. It may therefore be necessary to use other strategies to augment oxygenation to preserve vital organ functions. The following is a brief discussion of these strategies and the potential hazards of trying to manipulate oxygen transport.

Inspired O₂ concentration (FIo₂)

Increasing inspired oxygen concentration is usually the easiest and most accessible means for the immediate improvement of arterial oxygenation. The increase in pulmonary capillary oxygen content in the ventilated and perfused lung regions predictably leads to an increase in oxygen content

in both arterial and mixed venous blood. Accordingly, even with severe hypoxemia and a large shunt, raising inspired oxygen concentration increases arterial oxygen content and saturation. However, the exact level of arterial P_{O_2} that will be attained cannot be accurately predicted for a number of reasons.[85] First, the change in P_{O_2} may not be dramatic if the initial arterial P_{O_2} is low. Because of the shape of the oxygen-hemoglobin equilibrium dissociation curve, large increases in oxygen saturation may result in only small increases in P_{O_2} (Fig. 5-6). Second, raising inspired oxygen may actually decrease the shunt fraction by diminishing the venous admixture from areas of low ventilation to perfusion or areas with diffusion impairment (Table 5-1). Finally, in some patients, shunt fraction can also increase by raising inspired oxygen, owing to resorption atelectasis or abolition of hypoxic pulmonary vasoconstriction. Regardless of this lack of predictability, arterial P_{O_2} and oxygen content invariably increase when inspired oxygen concentration is raised, and the short-term risks are minimal. There does not seem to be immediate toxicity to the lungs from short-term use of oxygen (24 hours), and only in the premature newborn infant is there much risk of injury to retinal vessels.

Shunt fraction

As has been discussed, positive pressure ventilation with PEEP is the primary therapy employed to decrease intrapulmonary shunt fraction in a patient with respiratory failure. Positive pressure breathing usually increases lung volume, improves ventilation to perfusion matching, and may expand nonventilated areas, thereby decreasing shunt fraction and dead space while improving lung compliance. Although this usually results in an increased arterial oxygen content, positive pressure ventilation can also have an adverse influence on perfusion and gas exchange, which negates some of its effects on tissue oxygenation. PEEP can increase dead space, lung water, and epithelial permeability and decrease cardiac output.[2] Therefore an optimal level of positive pressure or PEEP has often been suggested, at which oxygen transport (cardiac output × arterial oxygen content) is maximal. This optimal level may not necessarily be where shunt fraction has returned to normal or is minimal.[95] Others have suggested using the lowest level of PEEP that permits adequate oxygenation

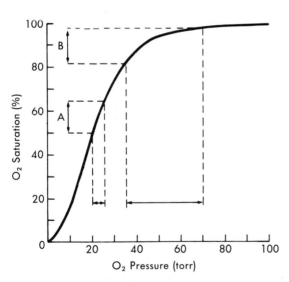

Fig. 5-6 Changes in hemoglobin oxygen saturation and P_{O_2} that can be anticipated when inspired oxygen is increased from 21% to 100% and right-to-left shunt fraction is constant. When the initial shunt is large the P_{O_2} is very low; the change in oxygen saturation (A) is about 15%, but the P_{O_2} change is minimal. In contrast, when the initial P_{O_2} is higher, there is still a 15% increase in O₂ saturation (B), but the change in P_{O_2} is much larger.

with an inspired oxygen concentration less than 70%.[2] Another important strategy that has been used to reduce shunt, particularly when there is pulmonary edema, is the administration of diuretics.[4,5] Furosemide, in particular, seems to improve pulmonary blood flow distribution and thereby decrease shunt. However, as with PEEP, these drugs have the risk of diminishing cardiac output and must be used with caution.

Hemoglobin concentration

Increasing hemoglobin concentration will raise the content of oxygen throughout the circulation even if arterial P_{O_2} is not changed because of the augmentation in oxygen-carrying capacity. However, an increase in hematocrit also increases the viscosity of the blood and can reduce cardiac output. Therefore there seems to be an optimal level of hemoglobin concentration for which oxygen transport is maximized.[71] This optimal level is rarely known for a given patient and may vary with age or clinical condition, but in most experimental studies it is in the range of 35% to 45%.[23,33]

Cardiac output

An increase in cardiac output will raise mixed venous P_{O_2} and oxygen concentration (that is, the shunted blood) and increase arterial oxygenation by this mechanism.[84] Augmentation of systemic blood flow can be effected by a variety of means and may not only have the benefit of increasing oxygen supply to the tissues but also the delivery of other nutrients. Unfortunately each of the means for augmenting cardiac output can also compromise oxygen transport, and therefore these means need to be used with precaution. Blood volume expansion, used to raise end diastolic filling of the ventricle, has the risk of enhancing pulmonary edema. Some authors have strongly recommended that patients with ARDS be maintained at as low a filling pressure as tolerable.[104] Catecholamines may stimulate cardiac contractility and heart rate, thereby augmenting cardiac output. However, they also raise metabolic demands[45,93] and, in some cases, they may only yield a marginal improvement in the relation between tissue oxygen supply and demand.[20] Catecholamines are indicated when ventricular function is depressed, but it is less certain whether they are of any benefit when ventricular function is normal. Vasodilators may also improve cardiac output by reducing afterload on the right or left ventricle. However, vasodilators may disrupt

pulmonary vasoregulation (as can catecholamines) and increase shunt fraction.[21] Finally, some authors have reported that increasing cardiac output in patients with hypoxemic respiratory failure increases perfusion to nonventilated lung and raises shunt fraction.[25] Regardless of these risks, in the child with life-threatening hypoxemia, augmentation of cardiac output should be considered an integral part of the management.

Oxygen consumption

Reduction of metabolic demands can reduce the extraction of oxygen from the tissues, thereby raising mixed venous oxygen content and consequently arterial oxygen content. This provides some of the rationale for the use of sedation in patients with respiratory failure. Although such therapy may be beneficial for a variety of important reasons, when metabolic demands are diminished, cardiac output often decreases in proportion, and there may be no net improvement in oxygenation.[84] Other techniques, such as the induction of hypothermia to reduce metabolic demands, have not proven to be very effective and may have adverse effects.[17]

Although manipulation of each of the above mentioned factors is part of the standard management of patients with severe hypoxemia due to respiratory failure, the treatments need to be used with caution and as part of an empirical trial in each patient. It is very difficult to predict a priori whether they will be effective. It is most prudent to decide which factors, if any, should be manipulated first based on the condition of the patient, the urgency for additional therapy, and one's best estimate of outcome. Furthermore, it is unclear what level of arterial oxygenation is acceptable to support aerobic function. The arterial P_{O_2} taken alone is a poor predictor of tissue oxygenation and must be used in conjunction with other determinants of oxygen transport, especially cardiac output and hemoglobin concentration. Finally, the traditional concept of maintaining arterial P_{O_2} as high as 80 to 100 mm Hg, even at the expense of high inspired oxygen concentrations and high mean airway pressures, may need reexamination. A much lower arterial P_{O_2} may be tolerated with less toxicity from therapy.

Decreasing and Discontinuing Ventilatory Support

Ventilatory support should be decreased only when the reasons for its initiation are no longer present. Discontinuation of mechanical ventilation always requires a rigorous evaluation of each aspect of respiratory function: control, airway protective reflexes, pump function, and gas exchange. Often, the patient's ventilatory requirements will decrease rapidly, and there will be little question about the opportunity of discontinuing support. At times, however, *weaning* a patient from mechanical ventilation is a long and complicated process, the analysis of which goes beyond the scope of this chapter. Ventilatory modes such as IMV and SIMV are useful to decrease ventilatory support progressively and allow conditioning of the patient's respiratory muscles. In addition, pressure-supported spontaneous breaths or sprinting (periods of spontaneous respiration) have been used widely in adults to facilitate weaning. Whatever mode is used, it is important to observe the patient while he or she is breathing to ensure that the pattern is coordinated and effective. This is a particularly important issue in the child who has received ventilatory support for a long time. Unfortunately the decision to discontinue support in these patients must often be based on subjective clinical criteria, although bedside measurements of mechanical function may be helpful (see "Monitoring").

Adjuncts to Ventilatory Support

Nutritional support has become an essential part of the treatment of respiratory failure in recent years.[15] Its importance is supported by the demonstration of profound abnormalities in both respiratory control and respiratory muscle function in critically ill adults and children.[7,82] The hypercatabolic state that inevitably follows trauma and surgery further emphasizes the need for adequate nutritional intake. Fever and increased work of breathing increase the nutritional demands of traumatized patients. Enteral or parenteral (whenever the enteral route is unavailable) alimentation should be begun as soon as possible with the aim of maintaining a caloric intake sufficient to prevent loss of muscle mass. Caloric needs are difficult to estimate in critically ill children. However, simple bedside determinations of the nitrogen balance or oxygen consumption may be of help in estimating these needs.[11,16,44]

Adequate sedation is particularly important in mechanically ventilated children. The objective of this sedation is to eliminate agitation and anguish. Excessive movement may jeopardize certain surgical interventions and cause damage to the intubated larynx and trachea. Agitated breathing and crying efforts interfere with ventilator therapy. However, appropriate use of sedation should always start by evaluating the reasons for the state of agitation and trying to rectify them. Hypoxemia and hypercarbia are frequent causes of restlessness and should always be considered. Pain and discomfort are a common reason for agitation, and therefore analgesics are frequently given along with sedatives. The combination of a benzodiazepine and a narcotic is usually effective in achieving both sedation and analgesia. The half-lives of both drugs are prolonged in infants and young children. Therefore it is important to assess carefully the respiratory drive of those receiving these medications before discontinuing ventilatory support.

Muscle paralysis induced by nondepolarizing agents (for example, pancuronium) is used on occasion to suppress spontaneous movement and respiration and facilitate mechanical ventilation. This therapy has several disadvantages, including the inability to assess the state of sedation, the development of peripheral edema, and the elimination of spontaneous respiratory efforts that can be lifesaving if the ventilator malfunctions. We usually limit its use to patients with extremely severe mechanical dysfunction who can benefit from the small increase in chest wall compliance. The use of these agents to restrain patients is inappropriate if the same objective can be accomplished with sedatives and gentle physical measures.

RESPIRATORY MONITORING

Appropriate monitoring of patients who have or are at risk of developing respiratory failure is essential to detect the effects of therapy or to help prevent sudden deterioration. Monitoring of the respiratory system includes three general areas: (1) assessment of blood gas exchange, (2) assessment of mechanical function, and (3) assessment of the physical signs of respiratory distress.

Blood gas exchange (Table 5-2) is most directly evaluated from measurement of arterial Po_2, Pco_2 and pH in concert with knowledge of the inspired oxygen concentration of the patient. As mentioned earlier the difference between the alveolar and the arterial Po_2 ($AaDo_2$) provides a guide to pulmonary gas exchange, although this difference is sensitive to other variables. For years, direct measurement of blood gas tensions in arterial blood was the mainstay of monitoring of gas exchange because the

Table 5-2   Blood gas exchange monitoring in common use for children

Sample source/site	Measurement	Comments/precautions
Invasive monitoring		
Arterial blood	P_{O_2}	Usually need at least 0.2 mL; estimate of Hb_{O_2} saturation; erroneous estimate of Hb_{O_2} saturation when carbon monoxide in blood or altered Hb_{O_2} affinity
	Hb_{O_2} saturation	Need at least 0.1 mL; not very sensitive to changes in blood gas exchange when $> 95\%$
	P_{CO_2}	Usually need at least 0.2 mL
Mixed venous blood	P_{O_2}	Not a reliable estimate of arterial P_{O_2}; insensitive to changes in blood gas exchange; useful as guide to cardiac output
	P_{CO_2}	Somewhat sensitive to blood gas exchange; when cardiac output is normal, about 5-6 mm higher than arterial P_{CO_2}; sensitive to changes in perfusion
Capillary blood (heel, toe, finger)	P_{O_2}	Erroneous and unpredictable estimate of arterial P_{O_2} when extremity perfusion reduced
	P_{CO_2}	Erroneous estimate of arterial P_{CO_2} when extremity perfusion reduced
Noninvasive monitoring		
Skin surface	P_{O_2}	Erroneous and unpredictable estimate of arterial P_{O_2} when perfusion skin reduced; most useful in small infants; easily dislodged with motion
	P_{CO_2}	Erroneous estimate of arterial P_{CO_2} when skin perfusion reduced; most useful in small infants; easily dislodged with motion
Peripheral artery (pulse oximetry)	Hb_{O_2}	Difficult to obtain when there is motion, very poor perfusion, arrhythmias; error increases with severe hypoxemia; insensitive to carbon monoxide
Expired gas	End-tidal P_{CO_2}	May underestimate arterial P_{CO_2} when there is heterogeneous emptying of alveoli (e.g. bronchopulmonary dysplasia or wheezing), large alveolar dead space (e.g. high PEEP), or very fast respiratory rates

technology had been developed and it was relatively easy to obtain samples from direct puncture of the vessel or withdrawal from an indwelling catheter. Although removal of blood can be a problem in a small child, this approach to monitoring gas exchange is still the most widely used and available in the United States. Approximately 15 years ago skin surface electrodes were developed. These electrodes estimate capillary P_{O_2} and P_{CO_2} as these blood gases diffuse through the skin, which has been warmed to enhance local blood flow.[43] Skin surface P_{O_2} and P_{CO_2} have been particularly useful for the small infant with relatively thin skin. Unfortunately such measurements are considerably less useful when perfusion is poor or when there is much motion of the electrode.[78] These problems restrict the use of skin surface electrodes in most children with trauma. More recently, measurement of hemoglobin oxygen saturation by pulse oximetry have provided a major advance for monitoring oxygenation in children.[105] With this technique, light of two wavelengths is passed through tissue with a pulsating artery and the amount of light transmitted is detected. The absorbance of light differs for oxyhemoglobin and deoxyhemoglobin, so the photodetector can determine the relative proportions of each. Although the pulse may be difficult to obtain when there is considerable motion, a light beam automatically searches for a pulse so that, as soon as the motion stops, monitoring can continue. Finally, arterial carbon dioxide tension can be approximated by measurement of alveolar carbon dioxide tension at the end of a tidal breath. This method is most commonly used in intubated patients, although nasopharyngeal catheters that withdraw gas at a slow rate may be used for some nonintubated patients. Despite its utility, there are some important sources of error that can cause the end-tidal P_{CO_2} to underestimate arterial P_{CO_2} by an unpredictable amount. Although each of the above mentioned noninvasive approaches has its own unique problems, there is usually a combination of monitoring that can be devised to minimize blood sampling and provide a frequent and reasonably accurate estimate of gas exchange for a given patient.

Monitoring of mechanical functioning of the lungs for pediatric patients is considerably less sophisticated than assessment of gas exchange. This is a result of two major obstacles: the ability of the patient to cooperate and the lack of a leak-free system either in the unintubated or intubated patient. In adult patients, measurements of mechanical functions, particularly forced vital capacity, inspiratory force, and lung compliance, have provided useful information about the need for mechanical ventilation or the change in function during the period of ventilatory support. Forced vital capacity is particularly important because it provides some estimate of whether the subject can generate intermittent sighs needed to maintain lung volume. In general, a vital capacity of at least 15 ml/kg is necessary for a patient to sustain spontaneous breathing.[34] Because a forced vital capacity is a voluntary maneuver, its validity depends on patient cooperation. Some investigators have tried using the volume attained with crying as a crude approximation of vital capacity in infants, but this is not particularly helpful in very sick patients. The maximal inspiratory force or pressure is obtained following the occlusion of the airway during expiration and does not require cooperation. It provides some estimate of the strength of the inspiratory muscles and usually needs to be more negative than -20 cm H_2O.[34] However, if lung compliance is very poor, more muscle strength may be necessary to sustain respiration. Total respiratory system compliance can be measured in intubated patients in whom there are no air leaks. From knowledge of the exhaled volume, the end expiratory pressure, and the airway pressure when it is stable following cessation of flow (usually within 1 second) the static compliance can be calculated. Although normal values vary as a function of age and size, changes in thoracic compliance may provide considerable inference about the evolution of underlying parenchymal lung disease during an acute respiratory illness.

Finally, there is no substitute for frequent observation and examination for signs of respiratory distress. Respiratory rates should be measured often or continuously in all patients with respiratory failure or who are at risk for it. Because a decrease in lung compliance is almost an invariable consequence of injury to the respiratory system, an increase in respiratory rate is usually an early warning sign of impending respiratory failure. The presence of retractions, nasal flaring, and use of accessory muscles are also reliable signs of respiratory distress and are much less subject to interobserver variability than the quality of the breath sounds of auscultation. Therefore these are particularly useful signs when multiple observers are examining a child over a sustained period.

SPECIFIC INJURIES TO THE RESPIRATORY SYSTEM
Adult Respiratory Distress Syndrome

It is now well recognized that the lungs may develop a characteristic response to a variety of insults, some of which directly injure the lungs (for example, contusion and aspiration) and others that seem to damage the lungs more indirectly (for example, circulatory shock).[88] An increase in capillary permeability initially causes pulmonary edema and subsequently leads to impaired gas exchange and lung compliance. In addition, a cascade of events damages the vascular endothelium because of the release of proteases and lipolytic substances into the circulation. This entity of edema from increased permeability, or "low pressure" pulmonary edema, was first called "shock lung" and is now known as ARDS. The syndrome occurs in children[91] as well as adults, and although the impairments in gas exchange and mechanics are analogous to those of idiopathic respiratory distress syndrome of the neonate, the etiology is different. The exact trigger for the alteration in endothelial permeability is unknown, but ARDS can be provoked by injury from the airway side (for example, pneumonia) or from the vascular side (for example, sepsis). The list of problems that can evolve into ARDS is very long and continues to expand. Each of the clinical entities discussed in subsequent sections is well recognized as an injury that frequently progresses to ARDS.

The inciting event may be clearly defined and precede the onset of ARDS by as much as 48 to 72 hours, although more commonly the latent period between injury and respiratory distress is less than 24 hours.[80] Following the period with minimal or no apparent evidence of lung injury, there is rapid development of diffuse bilateral lung disease and physical signs of respiratory distress including tachypnea, cyanosis, retractions (in the younger child), and dyspnea.[81] In addition, the radiograph of the chest shows diffuse disease characterized by interstitial edema and alveolar infiltration and consolidation (Fig. 5-7). The edema and infiltration may be homogeneous or heterogeneous, but they are widespread. Many factors, including the posture of the patient and the nature of the specific injury, influence the radiographic distribution of the densities.

In practice, the diagnosis of ARDS in children is made from a cluster of findings. These include the physical and radiographic signs mentioned previously with no evidence of high left atrial filling pressure. The latter criterion may be satisfied indirectly by the size of the atrium demonstrated with a radiograph or by echocardiogram, or directly

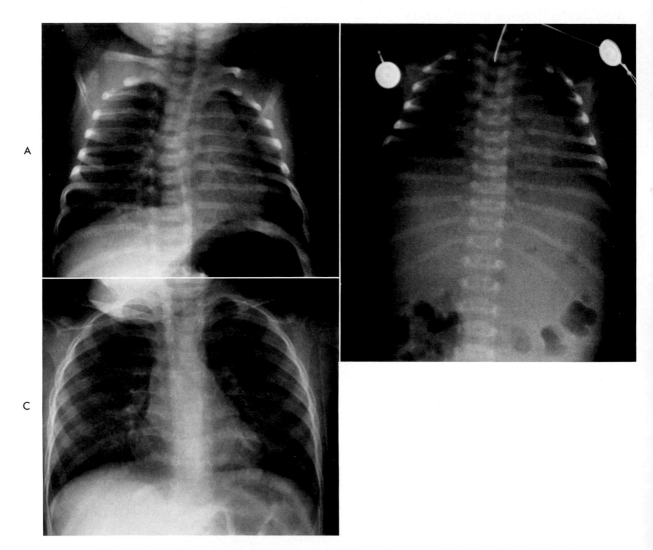

Fig. 5-7 **A,** Chest radiograph of a 3-week-old infant who was accidentally suffocated. At admission, she was in no respiratory distress, and the chest radiograph showed minimal atelectasis. **B,** Within 72 hours, she developed severe respiratory difficulty and bilaterally consolidated lungs, consistent with ARDS. She required mechanical ventilation with high-inspiratory and end-expiratory pressures. Despite this, her lung volumes remained reduced, and she maintained a large $AaDo_2$ for more than 2 weeks. **C,** Eighteen months later, she was asymptomatic, and her chest radiograph was almost normal.

from wedge pressure measurements (not commonly available in children). The hypoxemia is usually severe (that is, necessitating at least 40% inspired oxygen), and it should be clear that this represents a recent change.

The pathology is characterized by atelectasis, consolidation, hemorrhage, congestion, and inflammation with infiltration of leukocytes.[14,88] The fluid that produces the alveolar exudate has a high protein concentration (approximately equivalent to that of plasma) and is rich in polymorphonuclear leukocytes as well as oxidants and proteases.

Although a host of substances have been implicated as participants in the lung injury, no single mediator or single pathway has been identified as necessary and sufficient for the genesis of ARDS.[14,91] It is very likely that once an injury starts multiple triggers set off various pathways to produce lung damage. In addition, once treatment for the respiratory distress is initiated, injury is propagated further by the high oxygen concentrations and high pressure necessary to sustain gas exchange. It is generally accepted that neutrophils become activated (in the circulation or after migration to the lung) and generate toxic oxygen metabolites (free radicals and peroxide), producing tissue damage.[58,97] However, ARDS has been demonstrated in patients and in experimental animals with neutropenia.[55] Thus other inflammatory cells, such as macrophages and platelets, are thought to be important, although their role as essential components of the lung injury remains speculative. In addition, it is attractive to postulate that humoral mechanisms are important in initiating the lung damage. Complement and arachidonic acid metabolites are the two categories of substances with the strongest presumptive evidence for a central role. Complement activation can provoke lung injury in certain experimental models of ARDS, but the mechanistic link in humans is lacking.[40] Similarly, by-products of both the cyclooxygenase and lipoxygenase pathways can mimic many of the features of ARDS experimentally, and it is clear that they are involved in propogating the lung damage.[91] What is less clear is their specific place in initiating the cascade of ARDS. Finally, there is also much interest in the importance of the cytokine cachectin (tumor necrosis factor) in the precipitation of ARDS in patients with sepsis and shock.[98] Current concepts in lung injury with ARDS have been reviewed elsewhere, and the interested reader is referred here for more detailed information.[101]

Once ARDS develops, treatment is aimed at preventing life-threatening hypoxemia and attempting to minimize the extrapulmonary effects of mechanical ventilation.[57] Although there is nothing unique about the management of ARDS, a few key issues merit some clarification. First, a number of incidents have been identified in adult populations as having a high risk for the development of ARDS.[80] These include sepsis, aspiration of gastric contents, multiple transfusions, and shock. It is also clear that the presence of more than one of these conditions raises the likelihood of the development of ARDS even further. Next, in a group of patients identified at high risk for the development of ARDS, neither the early application of PEEP[79] nor the administration of corticosteroids[12] alter the likelihood of developing ARDS or its outcome. To date, no particular therapies have been identified that, when applied before the florid manifestations of ARDS, influence the incidence or the outcome. High-frequency ventilation and extracorporeal membrane oxygenation[106] have been tested in experimental trials with no compelling evidence for their benefit after the development of ARDS. Recently, there has been renewed interest in extracorporeal carbon dioxide removal, but conclusive data are not available.[37] Accordingly, the major aim of treatment for ARDS is to sustain gas exchange while the lungs have an opportunity to heal following the injury. Although this sounds simple, the high levels of positive pressure breathing and oxygen promote continued injury to the lung in the process of "treatment." Therefore the eventual respiratory disturbance includes a mixture of the initial insult and the damage from therapy. Furthermore, numerous complications arise from the need for prolonged respiratory support, invasive monitoring, altered nutrition, and the generally debilitated state. The most important problem, and one which is a common cause of death, is infection. Although there are no large series in pediatric patients, the mortality in adults with ARDS is in the range of 50% to 75%.[14] Despite the severe derangement in gas exchange, it seems to be less common for hypoxemia to be a cause of death than infection.

Patients who recover from ARDS usually have had a prolonged period of mechanical ventilation and require an extensive hospital stay, during which time they need supplemental oxygen and frequently require physical rehabilitation. Despite this, in follow-up studies of adult patients there is surprisingly little residual lung disease within a year.[3] The commonest abnormalities that have been found include a decrease in diffusion capacity and the presence of reactive airways disease. Such follow-up data are not available in children, but from our experience the recovery often seems dramatic, and there may be little or no evidence of respiratory compromise within a few years. Part of this remarkable recovery may be a consequence of ongoing lung growth that occurs up to about 8 years of age (Fig. 5-7).

Fat Embolism

Fat embolism may occur following fractures of long bones, particularly the femur and humerus. It results in a lung injury requiring a clinical course similar to that of ARDS. Whereas the triad of neurologic dysfunction, petechiae, and hypoxemia is characteristic of fat embolism, the diagnosis is often made by exclusion of other causes for these findings. There is no specific diagnostic test, although the diagnosis is dubious if fat globules are not found in the urine.[69] The pulmonary injury seems to follow the release of triglycerides in the bone marrow and their conversion to free fatty acids by circulating lipoprotein lipase. This usually takes 1 to 2 days to become manifest. Although fat embolism is always considered a potential problem following long bone fractures, its occurrence is exceedingly rare in pediatrics.[72] We have not had a patient with fat embolism in over 10 years at our institution.

Water Submersion

Drowning is the second most common cause of accidental death in children, and near-drowning is probably every bit as important as the cause of long-term disability from cerebral anoxia.[77] As might be expected, submersion is particularly common in the toddler and preschool child. Although much has been written regarding the differences in electrolyte disturbances and lung injury between fresh water and salt water submersion,[66] most of this information comes from experimental studies with tracheal installation of fluid.[68] Aspiration of fluid is certainly a cause of respiratory distress after submersion injury, but asphyxia is the major cause for mortality and morbidity in these patients.

When a patient becomes submersed in water, there is usually some aspiration of fluid. The development of laryngospasm seems to prevent massive aspiration except under some unusual circumstances (such as neurologic impairment before entering the water). The patient may swallow water in panic. Eventually, as hypoxia progresses, the larynx relaxes in many patients, and more water is aspirated into the lungs.[51] Most patients, however, aspirate very little water (less than 22 ml/kg).[67] There is minimal differences between submersion in fresh water, sea water, and chlorinated water even though there are some distinct alterations in blood volume and serum electrolytes that may be present experimentally. These differences do not last very long and are rarely apparent in the patient who has been resuscitated.

Respiratory disease may occur because of alveolar collapse, pulmonary edema, and exudate following aspiration of water and stomach contents. Despite the potential severity of the pulmonary changes and their importance in the production of hypoxemia, these problems often resolve with positive pressure ventilation, unless there is a complication of respiratory support. This is particularly true for children who are submerged in relatively clean water. However, if the submersion takes place in stagnant or contaminated water, overwhelming pneumonia, often with unusual organisms, may become a life-threatening problem (Fig. 5-8).

With the improved techniques in respiratory support, it has become apparent that the major influence and outcome from submersion is now primarily a function of the rapidity with which resuscitation ensues. A number of authors have found that patients who rapidly regain respiratory function and neurologic activity have an excellent prognosis, whereas patients who require cardiorespiratory support and are comatose following resuscitative efforts have a uniformly poor outlook.[67,74] Aggressive management of intracranial hypertension has not seemed to affect outcome once cerebral anoxia has occurred.[17]

Although the data in warm water submersion are relatively clear with regard to outcome, for patients who are submerged in cold water it is very unpredictable who will survive and with what sequelae (Figs. 5-9 and 5-10). There are numerous reports of prolonged (greater than 15 minutes) submersion in ice water, with apparent full recovery of neurologic and respiratory function following resuscitation.[77] However, if there is no cardiac activity, it may be virtually impossible to obtain circulation and warming of the body core even with the use of warm intravenous fluids or lavage of the gas-

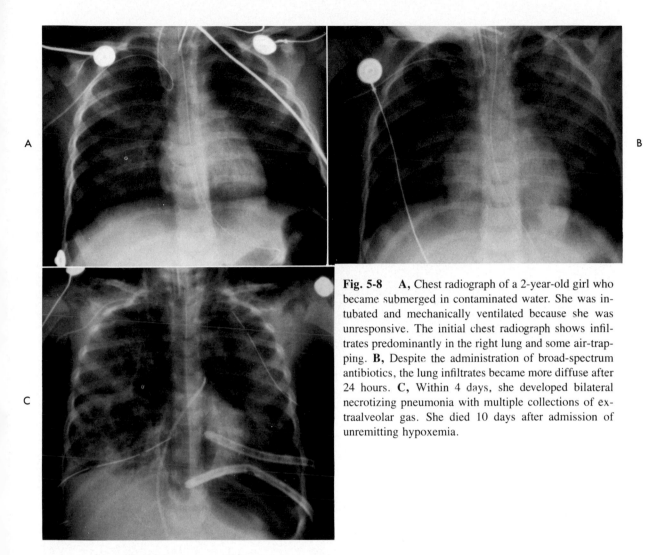

Fig. 5-8   A, Chest radiograph of a 2-year-old girl who became submerged in contaminated water. She was intubated and mechanically ventilated because she was unresponsive. The initial chest radiograph shows infiltrates predominantly in the right lung and some air-trapping. **B,** Despite the administration of broad-spectrum antibiotics, the lung infiltrates became more diffuse after 24 hours. **C,** Within 4 days, she developed bilateral necrotizing pneumonia with multiple collections of extraalveolar gas. She died 10 days after admission of unremitting hypoxemia.

trointestinal tract. At our own institution we have had siblings survive following 50 minutes of ice water submersion and cardiac arrest, but we used cardiopulmonary bypass to accomplish rewarming.[92] We are particularly aggressive in attempting to restore body temperature and perfusion in patients with cold water submersion even if they have no apparent cardiac or respiratory activity on presentation to the emergency room. As with patients with submersion in warm water, the respiratory disease is usually not the overwhelming problem, although severe respiratory distress can occur. In summary, the respiratory complications of submersion range from minimal disability, which may not even merit admission to the hospital, to adult respiratory distress syndrome and its complications. For the most part the respiratory management is not unique and is merely support of respiratory function and prevention of hypoxemia.

Inhalational Injury

Inhalation of noxious gases can result in severe pulmonary injury. The most common form of inhalational injury occurs in fire victims, and it involves three major mechanisms: thermal injury, chemical injury, and carbon monoxide (CO) poisoning.

Thermal injury is usually restricted to the upper airway, where most of the heat is exchanged. This injury often results in life-threatening airway ob-

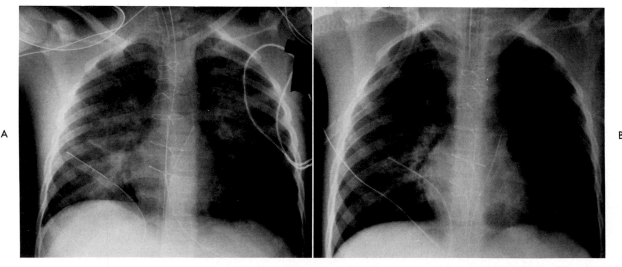

Fig. 5-9   Radiographs of a 6-year-old girl whose family vehicle slid off the road into an icy river. She was submerged for at least 50 minutes and brought to the hospital in cardiac standstill. **A,** Chest radiograph showed pulmonary consolidations, primarily on the right side, immediately after rewarming by cardiopulmonary bypass. **B,** Within 72 hours she developed severe pulmonary edema and bilateral lung consolidation, requiring vigorous ventilatory support. She improved gradually and was discharged 49 days later with no respiratory dysfunction.

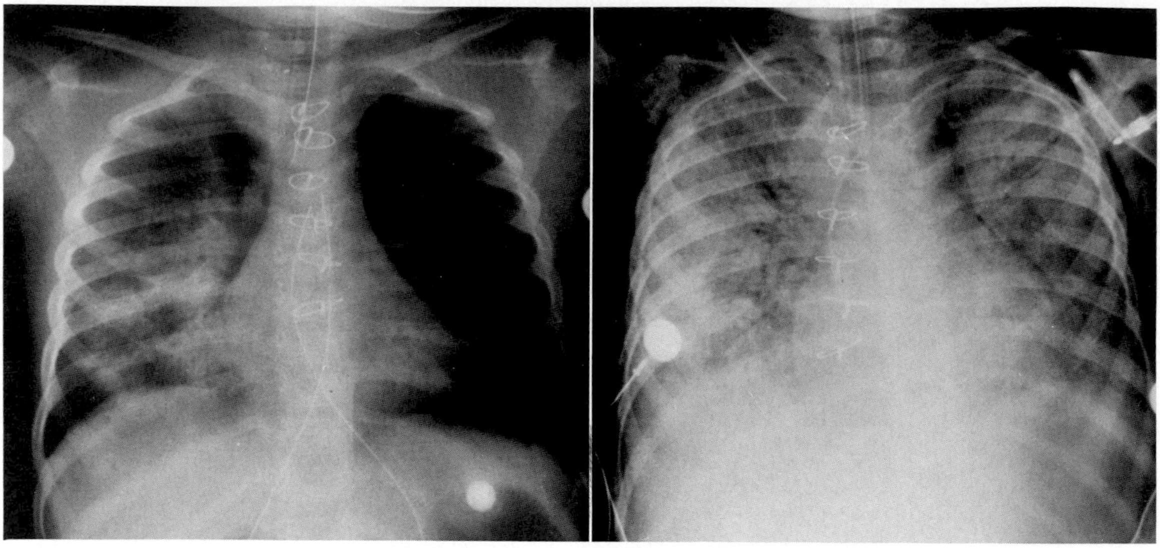

Fig. 5-10   This 12-year-old sibling of the girl shown in Fig. 5-9 was rescued at the same time as his sister and also brought to the hospital pulseless. **A,** Chest radiograph demonstrated bilateral infiltrates immediately after rewarming by cardiopulmonary bypass. **B,** However, 2 days later, most of the infiltrates had cleared. He was extubated shortly after this radiograph was obtained and discharged within 1 week. These siblings who sustained a similar insult illustrate the unpredictability of the respiratory complications of cold water submersion.

struction, which typically develops in an insidious manner. Airway thermal injury should be strongly suspected when there are burns in the nose, lips, or oral cavity. The presence of these signs with or without stridor in a child rescued from a fire is almost always an indication for tracheal intubation. Particularly if stridor is present, the airway should be intubated under the most controlled circumstances, if possible under inhalational anesthesia in the operating room. Thermally induced parenchymal injury is rarer, but can be present, especially with steam inhalation. Steam has a much greater specific heat than air and therefore delivers a greater amount of heat to the lung periphery.

Smoke or soot in itself is not acutely damaging to the lung parenchyma and airways. Unfortunately, combustion of most household and construction materials liberates organic acids, aldehydes, and other substances capable of producing a lung injury. This injury usually involves the airways as well as the lung epithelium and endothelium. Consistently, patients develop symptoms of small airway obstruction (wheezing and expiratory prolongation) and a low-pressure pulmonary edema, similar to that observed in ARDS. The clinical examination is therefore characterized by hypoxemia, decreased pulmonary compliance, and radiologic signs of edema and atelectasis. Treatment of this chemical injury is mainly supportive and includes bronchodilators, judicious use of fluid restriction and diuretics, and ventilatory support when necessary.

Carbon monoxide poisoning is very common in children who are victims of household fires because they are frequently the last to be rescued.[56] It should always be assumed present in such patients to prevent delays in the treatment while awaiting confirmation. Carbon monoxide binds hemoglobin with an affinity 240 times greater than oxygen.[103] It also binds preferentially to the intracellular heme cytochromes, thereby impeding both oxygen transport and its utilization in the respiratory chain. The injury produced by carbon monoxide is therefore a hypoxic injury, the consequences of which depend on the magnitude of the tissue hypoxia and the ability of each specific tissue to tolerate it. The high metabolic demands of children, particularly in a situation of panic, limits tissue tolerance.

The brain is the organ most vulnerable to carbon monoxide—induced tissue hypoxia. If this hypoxia is severe enough, irreparable brain damage may occur before treatment can be started. There is a correlation between the carbon monoxide saturation of hemoglobin and the severity of the outcome. Carbon monoxide saturations greater than 30% are life threatening and demand immediate treatment. Although lower saturations are better tolerated, they should not be considered a guarantee against severe hypoxic damage, particularly if some time has elapsed since the inhalation and the measurement of the carbon monoxide saturation.

Children with carbon monoxide inhalation develop hypoxemia without cyanosis. Their arterial Po_2 will reach normal values for the inspired oxygen concentrations. Pulse oximetry does not detect this hypoxemia because this monitoring method determines the ratio of oxygen-saturated hemoglobin to hemoglobin oxygen-binding capacity, both of which are reduced. Signs of tissue hypoxia are usually present. Central nervous system dysfunction ranging from confusion to coma is prominent. Cardiac hypoxia can be detected as changes in the repolarization in the electrocardiogram. Lactic acidosis, a sign of increased anaerobic metabolism, is common and indicates insufficient delivery of oxygen to the tissues. Although these clinical signs are important, determination of carboxyhemoglobin is the only reliable diagnostic test to detect and quantify carbon monoxide intoxication.

Treatment of carbon monoxide poisoning requires immediate administration of 100% oxygen.[107] This not only improves oxygen delivery to the tissues by increasing the volume of oxygen dissolved in the arterial blood, but also enhances carbon monoxide dissociation from hemoglobin by a competitive mechanism. Mechanical ventilation is indicated if the patient is in coma or has other injuries that may interfere with adequate ventilation for carbon monoxide removal. Administration of 100% oxygen reduces the half-life of carbon monoxide dissociation to one fourth of the time. Oxygen administration should be continued until carbon monoxide saturations are below 5% and there is minimal impairment of oxygen transport and utilization. Carbon monoxide dissociation can be further enhanced with hyperbaric oxygen administration. Although this therapeutic modality is not widely available and severely restricts access to the patient, it represents a viable alternative in children with severe carbon monoxide intoxication.

Aspiration Pneumonia

Aspiration pneumonia is a common complication of trauma in children. Its frequency along with its devastating mortality (probably greater than 30%) emphasize the importance of prevention and early diagnosis. Gastric material is aspirated into the airways only when the airway-protective mechanisms are not intact. This occurs under two circumstances in traumatized children. First, when the patient's sensorium is depressed, laryngeal and coughing reflexes are inefficient, and vomiting will inevitably be followed by aspiration, especially if the patient is breathing spontaneously. Second, intrusion of the airway by endotracheal intubation or tracheostomy impairs the patient's ability to occlude the laryngeal entrance, even if the sensorium is not depressed. This latter consideration is particularly important in children with abdominal distension, who are prone to vomit during resuscitation.

The severity of the pulmonary injury depends greatly on the volume and quality of the aspirate. Traditionally, the acid pH of the stomach contents has been associated with a more severe disruption of the pulmonary structure. Unfortunately, even when the aspirate is not acid, hypoxemia and hypoventilation will result from the aspiration of a significant volume of fluid. Aspiration of gastric material causes a nonspecific injury affecting both the airways and the alveolar epithelium and endothelium. Frequently, the clinical presentation is not distinguishable from that of ARDS, which in itself is a common complication of aspiration pneumonia. The infiltrates seen on chest radiograph tend to be heterogeneous with a preference for the right lung, but they can also be confluent and bilateral. The clinical course varies. In those who survive, the infiltrates may take several weeks to resolve.

In many traumatized children, aspiration pneumonia is preventable. All traumatized patients should be treated as if they had a full stomach. Coma with inability to cough or gag is an indication for intubation. Whenever possible, a cuffed endotracheal tube should be used. This is an impossibility in infants for whom cuffed endotracheal tubes are not commonly manufactured (sizes < 4 mm ID). A nasogastric or orogastric tube should be inserted early in the treatment of traumatized children for evacuation of gastric contents. The act of intubation in itself represents a major opportunity for aspiration and should be performed by the most experienced personnel with adequate suction available.

The treatment of aspiration pneumonia is mostly supportive. Mechanical ventilation and oxygen ad-

ministration are frequently necessary. Vigorous suction is recommended immediately after the episode, but unfortunately liquids diffuse rapidly into the periphery of the lungs. Corticosteroids have been used to diminish the inflammatory response in the lungs, but they have provided no proven benefits in study trials.[19] Broad-spectrum antibiotics are often given because infection is a common complication of aspiration, but this practice is not strongly supported by experimental proof. Anaerobes are the most common organisms recovered.[10] Microbiologic examination of the sputum correlates poorly with the causal organisms in patients developing bacterial pneumonitis.[6] Recent studies suggest that the acidity of the gastric pH may actually limit bacterial growth and contamination.[29] The frequent administration of antacids in patients with trauma may eliminate this protection, making bacterial pneumonitis more common.

Chest Wall Injuries

Children are rarely exposed to injuries that cause penetration of the chest wall. When present, these injuries usually involve various intrathoracic structures and require immediate surgical treatment. Chest wall damage caused by blunt trauma is also rare in children. The presence of multiple skeletal fractures without other obvious chest wall damage should also raise suspicion of child abuse. In this case, the fractures are frequently at various stages of repair. The highly compliant chest wall of the child can sustain a high degree of deformation without fracturing the skeletal structure. Therefore puncture or laceration of the lungs by rib fragments is uncommon. Similarly rare are multiple rib fractures resulting in instability and inward paradoxic motion of the chest wall during inspiration (flail chest). Management of children with multiple fresh fractures requires mechanical ventilation with positive pressure, usually for several days.[24] Analgesics are necessary to facilitate spontaneous breathing.

Diaphragmatic rupture can occur during both thoracic and abdominal blunt trauma. It is more frequent on the left side, where the supporting effect of the liver is missing, and should be suspected when the elevation of a hemidiaphragm persists, frequently after draining the associated pneumohemothorax. The negative pressure of the pleural space pulls the stomach and other abdominal viscera into the chest cavity. Therefore this injury, which requires immediate surgical repair, can often be confirmed by introducing a cannula into the stomach and demonstrating the displaced stomach radiographically.

Pulmonary Contusion

Pulmonary contusions are relatively frequent and should be investigated in children with blunt chest trauma. They are characterized by nonspecific radiologic findings of pulmonary edema, hemorrhage, and atelectasis in the vicinity of the traumatized area. Hemoptysis and gas leaks are seen on occasions. When extensive, pulmonary contusion can alter the mechanical properties of the lung and cause substantial right-to-left shunt and hypoxemia. The treatment is entirely supportive. Local infection is a relatively common complication. Antibiotics are recommended if the patient develops fever or a purulent sputum, usually several days after the injury.

Tracheobronchial Tears and Gas Leaks

Tracheobronchial tears are common after both penetrating and nonpenetrating injuries to the chest and neck. Their most common consequence is the passage of airway gas into the tissue surrounding the airways and its eventual migration into the pleural or the mediastinal space. From there, gas can reach a number of other spaces and tissues, as described with the complications of mechanical ventilation. The presence of extraalveolar gas should alert the clinician about the possibility of a tracheobronchial tear (Fig. 5-11). Diagnosis often requires bronchoscopic visualization of the tear. Surgical repair may be necessary, especially when the tear involves the trachea or the major bronchi. In mechanically ventilated patients, the fistulous pathway created by the tear may offer less impedance to gas flow than the lungs themselves. If so, a large portion of the minute ventilation is directed to this pathway, sometimes limiting alveolar ventilation severely. Although high-frequency ventilation may increase the impedance of the fistula with respect to that of the lung and decrease fistula flow, this technique is still controversial in patients with large tracheobronchial tears.[28,99]

Accumulations of gas in the pleural space are poorly tolerated when pleural pressure increases enough to interfere with both ipsilateral and contralateral pulmonary expansion and venous return to the heart (tension pneumothorax). Respiratory

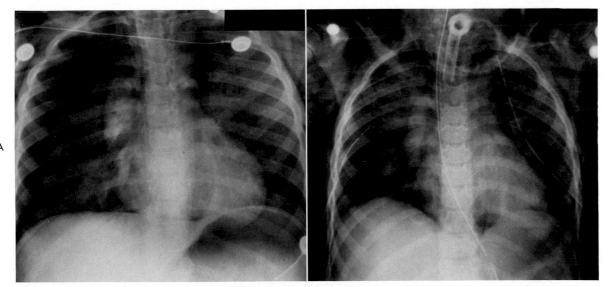

A   B

Fig. 5-11   This 8-year-old boy hit his neck on the handle bars of his bicycle and developed respiratory difficulty. **A,** On arrival to the emergency room, he had substantial subcutaneous emphysema in the neck and face. Chest radiograph showed a pneumomediastinum and a right pneumothorax. **B,** A tracheostomy was performed emergently and chest tubes were inserted. He recovered rapidly, and his tracheostomy was decannulated before discharge from the hospital.

and circulatory failure develop rapidly under these circumstances. Lung compression decreases the size and number of alveolar units available for ventilation. Consequently the effective compliance of the lungs and thorax is reduced and the work of breathing increased. In addition, the extraalveolar gas contained in the pleura pushes the diaphragm down into the abdomen, limiting its efficiency to respond to the increased working load. The cardiovascular compromise dictates emergency treatment. Vascular compression decreases the transmural pressure of the atria, reducing ventricular filling and cardiac output. Children with tension pneumothorax present with tachycardia, markedly decreased pulse pressure, and hypotension. Pneumomediastinum is better tolerated because there is a more limited space for gas accumulation and the pressure builds up rapidly, forcing the gas into other areas (soft tissues of the neck and retroperitoneum). However, penetration of gas into the pericardial sac may result in cardiac tamponade and require immediate evacuation.

REFERENCES

1. Agostoni E and Mead J: Statics of the respiratory system. In Fenn WO and Rahn H, editors: Handbook of Physiology, vol 1, Respiration, Washington, DC, 1964, American Physiological Society.
2. Albert RK: Least PEEP: primum non nocere, Chest 87:2, 1985.
3. Alberts WM, Priest GR, and Moser KM: The outlook for survivors of ARDS, Chest 84:272, 1983.
4. Ali J, Chernicki W, and Wood LDH: Effect of furosemide in canine low-pressure pulmonary edema, J Clin Invest 64:1494, 1979.
5. Ali J and Wood LDH: Pulmonary vascular effects of furosemide on gas exchange in pulmonary edema, J Appl Physiol 57:160, 1984.
6. Andrews CP et al: Diagnosis of nosocomial bacterial pneumonia in acute, diffuse lung injury, Chest 80:254, 1981.
7. Askanazi J et al: Nutrition and the respiratory system, Crit Care Med 10:163, 1982.
8. Aubier M, Trippenbach T, and Roussos C: Respiratory muscle fatigue during cardiogenic shock, J Appl Physiol 51:499, 1981.
9. Bake B et al: Effect of inspiratory flow rate on regional distribution of inspired gas, J Appl Physiol 37:8, 1974.
10. Bartlett JG, Gorbach SL, and Finegold SM: The bacteriology of aspiration pneumonia, Am J Med 56:202, 1974.
11. Benotti P and Blackburn GL: Protein and caloric or macronutrient metabolic management of the critically ill patient, Crit Care Med 7:12:520, 1979.
12. Bernard GR et al: High-dose corticosteroids in patients with the adult respiratory distress syndrome, N Engl J Med 317:1565, 1987.
13. Bhutani VK, Rubenstein D, and Shaffer TH: Pressure-induced deformation in immature airways, Pediatr Res 15:829, 1981.
14. Biondi JW et al: The adult respiratory distress syndrome, Yale J Biol Med 59:575, 1986.
15. Blackburn GL, Maini BS, and Pierce EC: Nutrition in the critically ill patient, Anesthesiology 17:181, 1977.
16. Blackburn GL et al: Nutritional and metabolic assessment of the hospitalized patient, JPEN 1:11, 1977.
17. Bohn DJ et al: Influence of hypothermia, barbiturate therapy, and intracranial pressure monitoring on morbidity and mortality after near-drowning, Crit Care Med 14:529, 1986.
18. Braun NMT, Arora NS, and Rochester DF: Force-length relationship of the normal human diaphragm, J Appl Physiol 53:405, 1982.
19. Bynum LJ and Pierce AK: Pulmonary aspiration of gastric contents, Am Rev Respir Dis 114:1129, 1976.
20. Cain SM: Peripheral oxygen uptake and delivery in health and disease, Clin Chest Med 4:2, 1983.
21. Colley PS and Cheney FW: Sodium nitroprusside increases Qs/Qt in dogs with regional atelectasis, Anesthesiology 47:338, 1977.
22. Comroe JH and Botelho S: The unreliability of cyanosis in the recognition of arterial anoxemia, Am J Med Sci 214:1, 1947.
23. Crowell JW and Smith EE: Determinants of the optimal hematocrit, J Appl Physiol 22:501, 1967.
24. Cullen P et al: Treatment of flail chest: use of intermittent mandatory ventilation and positive end-expiratory pressure, Arch Surg 110:1099, 1975.
25. Dantzker DR, Lynch JP, and Weg JG: Depression of cardiac output is a mechanism of shunt reduction in the therapy of acute respiratory failure, Chest 77:636, 1980.
26. De Troyer A and Loring SH: Action of the respiratory muscles. In Macklem PT and Mead J, editors: Handbook of physiology, vol 3, Respiration, Bethesda, Md, 1986, American Physiological Society.
27. Dorinsky PM and Whitcomb ME: The effect of PEEP on cardiac output, Chest 84:210, 1983.
28. Drazen JM, Kamm RD, and Slutsky AS: High-frequency ventilation, Physiol Rev 64:505, 1984.
29. Driks MR et al: Nosocomial pneumonia in intubated patients given sucralfate as compared with antacids or histamine type 2 blockers, N Engl J Med 317:1376, 1987.
30. Dueck R, Wagner PD, and West JB: Effects of positive end-expiratory pressure on gas exchange in dogs with normal and edematous lungs, Anesthesiology 47:359, 1977.
31. von Euler C, Herrero F, and Wexler I: Control mechanisms determining rate and depth of respiratory movements, Respir Physiol 10:93, 1970.
32. Falke KJ et al: Ventilation with end-expiratory pressure in acute lung disease, J Clin Invest 51:2315, 1972.
33. Fan FC, Chen RYZ, and Schuessler GB: Effects of hematocrit variations on regional hemodynamics and oxygen transport in the dog, Am J Physiol 238:H545, 1980.
34. Feeley TW and Hedley-Whyte J: Current concepts: weaning from controlled ventilation and supplemental oxygen, N Engl J Med 292:903, 1975.
35. Fisher JT et al: Respiration in newborns: development of the control of breathing, Am Rev Resp Dis 125:650, 1982.
36. Frank L, Bucher JR, and Roberts RJ: Oxygen toxicity in

neonatal and adult animals of various species, J Appl Physiol 45:699, 1978.

37. Gattinoni L et al: Low-frequency positive-pressure ventilation with extracorporeal CO_2 removal in severe acute respiratory failure, JAMA 256:881, 1986.

38. Gerhardt T and Bancalari E: Chest wall compliance in full-term and premature infants, Acta Pediatr Scand 69:359, 1980.

39. Gregory GA and Tooley WH: Gas embolism in hyaline-membrane disease, N Engl J Med 282:1141, 1970.

40. Hammerschmidt DE et al: Association of complement activation and elevated plasma-C5alpha with adult respiratory distress syndrome, Lancet I:947, 1980.

41. Heldt GP and McIlroy MB: Distortion of chest wall and work of diaphragm in preterm infants, J Appl Physiol 62:164, 1987.

42. Henderson-Smart DJ and Read DJC: Reduced lung volume during behavior active sleep in the newborn, J Appl Physiol 46:1081, 1979.

43. Huch R, Lubbers DW, and Huch A: Quanitative continuous measurement of partial oxygen pressure on the skin of adults and newborn babies, Pflugers Arch 337:185, 1972.

44. Hunker FD et al: Metabolic and nutritional evaluation of patients supported with mechanical ventilation, Crit Care Med 8:628, 1980.

45. Jackson LK, Key BM, and Cain SM: Total and hindlimb O_2 uptake and blood flow in hypoxic dogs given dopamine, Crit Care Med 10:327, 1982.

46. Jardin F et al: Influence of positive end-expiratory pressure on left ventricular performance, N Engl J Med 304:387, 1981.

47. Joannides M and Tsoulos GD: The etiology of interstitial and mediastinal emphysema, Arch Surg 21:333, 1930.

48. Katz JA et al: Time course and mechanisms of lung-volume increase with PEEP in acute pulmonary failure, Anesthesiology 54:9, 1981.

49. Keens TG et al: Developmental pattern of muscle fiber types in human ventilatory muscles, J Appl Physiol 44:909, 1978.

50. Kumar A et al: Continuous positive-pressure ventilation in acute respiratory failure, N Engl J Med 283:1430, 1970.

51. Lougheed DW: Physiological studies in experimental asphyxia and drowning, Can Med Assoc J 40:423, 1939.

52. Malo J, Ali J, and Wood LDH: How does positive end-expiratory pressure reduce intrapulmonary shunt in canine pulmonary edema? J Appl Physiol 57:1002, 1984.

53. Mansell A, Bryan C, and Levison H: Airway closure in children, J Appl Physiol 33:711, 1972.

54. Marchand P: The anatomy and applied anatomy of the mediastinal fascia, Thorax 6:359, 1951.

55. Maunder RJ et al: Occurrence of the adult respiratory distress syndrome in neutropenic patients, Am Rev Respir Dis 133:313, 1986.

56. McBay AJ: Carbon monoxide poisoning, N Engl J Med 272:252, 1965.

57. McCaffree DR: Adult respiratory distress syndrome. In Dantzker DR, editor: Cardiopulmonary critical care, Orlando, Fla, 1986, Grune & Stratton, Inc.

58. McGuire WW et al: Studies on the pathogenesis of the adult respiratory distress syndrome, J Clin Invest 69:543, 1982.

59. McIlroy MB et al: The effect of added elastic and non-elastic resistances on the pattern of breathing in normal subjects, Clin Sci 15:337, 1956.

60. Mead J: Control of respiratory frequency, J Appl Physiol 15:325, 1960.

61. Mead J: Mechanical properties of lungs, Physiol Rev 41:281, 1961.

62. Mead J: Functional signifance of the area of apposition of diaphragm to rib cage, Am Rev Respir Dis 119:31, 1979.

63. Mead J and Collier C: Relation of volume history of lungs to respiratory mechanics is anesthetized dogs, J Appl Physiol 14:669, 1959.

64. Mead J et al: Significance of the relationship between lung recoil and maximum expiratory flow, J Appl Physiol 22:95, 1967.

65. Mithoefer JC et al: The clinical estimation of alveolar ventilation, Am Rev Resp Dis 98:868, 1968.

66. Modell JH and Davis JH: Electrolyte changes in human drowning victims, Anesthesiology 30:414, 1969.

67. Modell JH, Graves SA, and Kuck EJ: Near-drowning: correlation of level of consciousness and survival, Can Anaesth Soc J 27:211, 1980.

68. Modell JH et al: Physiologic effects of near-drowning with chlorinated fresh water, distilled water, and isotonic saline, Anesthesiology 27:33, 1966.

69. Moylan JA and Evenson MA: Diagnosis and treatment of fat embolism, Ann Rev Med 28:85, 1977.

70. Muller N et al: Diaphragmatic muscle fatigue in the newborn, J Appl Physiol 46:688, 1979.

71. Murray JF, Gold P, and JB Lamar: The circulatory effects of hematocrit variations in normovolemic and hypervolemic dogs, J Clin Invest 42:1150, 1963.

72. Nichols DG and Rogers MC: Adult respiratory distress syndrome. In Rogers MC, editor: Textbook of pediatric intensive care, Baltimore, Md, 1987, Williams & Wilkins.

73. Nunn JF: Applied respiratory physiology, London, 1977, Butterworths.

74. Oakes DD et al: Prognosis and management of victims of near-drowning, J Trauma 22:544, 1982.

75. Olinsky A, Bryan MH, and Bryan AC: Influence of lung inflation on respiratory control in neonates, J Appl Physiol 36:426, 1974.

76. O'Quinn RJ et al: Transmission of airway pressure to pleural space during lung edema and chest wall restriction, J Appl Physiol 59:1171, 1985.

77. Orlowski JP: Drowning, near-drowning, and ice-water submersions, Ped Clin North Am 34:75, 1987.

78. Peabody JL et al: Transcutaneous oxygen tension in sick infants, Am Rev Respir Dis 118:83, 1978.

79. Pepe PE, Hudson LC, and Carrico J: Early application of positive end-expiratory pressure in patients at risk for the adult respiratory distress syndrome, N Engl J Med 311:281, 1984.

80. Pepe PE et al: Clinical predictors of the adult respiratory distress syndrome, Am J Surg 144:124, 1982.

81. Petty TL and Newman JH: Adult respiratory distress syndrome, West J Med 128:399, 1978.

82. Pollack MM, Wiley JS, and Holbrook PR: Early nutritional depletion in critically ill children, Crit Care Med 9:580, 1981.

83. Pontoppidan H, Geffin B, and Lowenstein E: Acute respiratory failure in the adult, N Engl J Med 287:690, 1972.

84. Prys-Roberts C, Kelman GR, and Greenbaum R: The influence of circulatory factors on arterial oxygenation during anaesthesia in man, Anaesthesia 22:257, 1967.

85. Quan SF et al: Changes in venous admixture with alterations of inspired oxygen concentration, Anesthesiology 52:477, 1980.

86. Richard CC and Bachman L: Lung and chest wall compliance in apneic paralyzed infants, J Clin Invest 40:273, 1961.

87. Riley RC and Cournand A: Ideal alveolar air and the analysis of ventilation-perfusion relationships in the lungs, J Appl Physiol 1:825, 1949.

88. Rinaldo JE and Rogers RM: Adult respiratory distress syndrome: changing concepts of lung injury and repair, N Engl J Med 306:900, 1982.

89. Robotham JL and Scharf SM: Effects of positive and negative pressure ventilation on cardiac performance, Clin Chest Med 4:161, 1983.

90. Roussos C and Macklem PT: Inspiratory muscle fatigue. In Macklem PT and Mead J, editors: Handbook of physiology, vol 3, Respiration, Bethesda Md, 1986, American Physiological Society.

91. Royall JA and Levin DL: Adult respiratory distress syndrome in pediatric patients. I. Clinical aspects, pathophysiology, pathology, and mechanisms of lung injury, J Pediatr 112:169, 1988.

92. Saltiel A et al: Resuscitation of cold water immersion victims with cardiopulmonary bypass, J Crit Care 4:54, 1989.

93. Schmitt M et al: Catecholamines and oxygen uptake in dog skeletal muscle in situ, Pflugers Arch 345:145, 1973.

94. Shaffer TH and Bhutani VK: Alterations in bulk modulus of trachea during development, Respiration 39:344, 1980.

95. Suter PM, Fairley HB, and Isenberg MD: Optimum end-expiratory airway pressure in patients with acute pulmonary failure, N Engl J Med 292:284, 1975.

96. Takahashi E and Atsumi H: Age differences in thoracic form as indicated by thoracic index, Hum Biol 27:65, 1955.

97. Tate RM and Repine JE: Neutrophils and the adult respiratory distress syndrome, Am Rev Respir Dis 128:552, 1983.

98. Tracey KJ, Lowery SF, and Cerami A: Cachetin/TNF-a in septic shock and septic adult respiratory distress syndrome, Am Rev Respir Dis 138:1377, 1988.

99. Turnbull DD, Howland CG, and Beattie EJ: High-frequency jet ventilation in major airway or pulmonary disruption, Ann Thorac Surg 32:468, 1980.

100. Weisman IM, Rinaldo JE, and Rogers RM: Positive end-expiratory pressure in adult respiratory failure, N Engl J Med 307:1381, 1982.

101. Wiedemann HP, Matthey MA, and Matthey RA: Acute lung injury, Crit Care Clin 2:377, 1986.

102. Wilson TA, Rodarte JR, and Butler JP: Wave-speed and viscous flow limitation. In Macklem PT and Mead J, editors: Handbook of physiology, vol 3, Respiration, Bethesda, Md, 1986, American Physiological Society.

103. Winter PM and Miller JN: Carbon monoxide poisoning, JAMA 236:1502, 1976.

104. Wood LDH and Prewitt RM: Cardiovascular management in acute hypoxemic respiratory failure, Am J Cardiol 47:963, 1981.

105. Yoshiya I, Shimada Y, and Tanaka K: Spectrophotometric monitoring of arterial oxygen saturation in the fingertip, Med Biol Eng Comput 18:27, 1980.

106. Zapol WM et al: Extracorporeal membrane oxygenation in severe acute respiratory failure, JAMA 242:2193, 1979.

107. Zimmerman SS and Truxal B: Carbon monoxide poisoning, Pediatrics 68:215, 1981.

6

Anesthesia for the Trauma Patient

Aleksandra Mazurek

If you plan for a year, sow a seed; if you plan for years ahead, plant a tree nursery; if you plan for centuries ahead, concentrate on your children.

CHINESE PROVERB

The anesthesiologist's early involvement in the care of critically ill children transported to a tertiary care medical center is essential for improved survival. Fuller[27] found that 31% of patients required further airway intervention, and Macnab[47] concluded that the "incidence of avoidable secondary insults was four times higher when *pediatric trained transport personnel* were *not* utilized." Analysis of 10 years experience with mobile intensive care units in Creteil, France indicated a 30% increase in 24-hour survival of polytraumatized patients[32] when trained and experienced teams were involved in the transport.[26]

To act effectively, the role of every member of the team awaiting arrival of the patient has to be assigned and rehearsed.[26,48,63] The prearranged plan must be followed with reasonable flexibility allowing for particular circumstances.[74] Weibley and Holbrook[87] designed an easy to remember and execute algorithm of priorities:

A—Airway
B—Breathing
C—Circulation
D—Drainage (pneumothorax, hemothorax)
E—Elevation of the head
F—Fluid resuscitation

These priorities must be coordinated under naturally chaotic and stressful circumstances, when events are happening in a simultaneous rather than sequential order. Although the surgeon plays the leading role in determining diagnostic and thera-

peutic priorities, the anesthesiologist or intensivist may fulfill this task in the surgeon's absence.

The patient *has to be completely undressed* for the initial assessment. This ought to be done quickly, with no consideration given to the cost of clothing, while moving the patient as little as possible.[31] Subcutaneous emphysema or bone fractures are evident on surface inspection. The presence of crepitus indicates a violation of airway continuity and calls for aggressive investigation and cautious application of positive airway pressure until the situation is controlled by the insertion of a chest tube and other appropriate measures.

The role of the anesthesiologist on the team is initially focused on airway evaluation and management of oxygenation and ventilation.[29,50] Patients with multiple injuries should receive 100% O_2 as soon as possible. The most severe sequelae of trauma result from hypoxic brain injury.[88] Every child with multiple head injuries has to be approached as if there is a spine injury present or until it is ruled out. When it is unclear whether the patient has a cervical spine injury, the neck is immobilized with a cervical collar or manually before instituting artificial airway and ventilation. Although a cross-table radiograph of the cervical spine is expeditious and sufficient to establish the diagnosis,[74,82] a limited CT scan or three-view cervical spine series[68] is necessary when improved definition is required.

Basic respiratory monitoring and initial airway assessment (lasting no longer than 1 minute) should establish the presence or absence of facial or neck injuries. The assessment of skin color takes place together with the evaluation of the spontaneous respiratory pattern. Important parameters of airway function and pathology to note are the following:

1. Stridor
2. Nasal flaring
3. Use of accessory muscles
4. Chest excursion
5. Presence and symmetry of breath sounds
6. Presence of neck ecchymosis
7. Absence of thyroid cartilage prominence (Adam's apple)
8. Hemoptysis

AIRWAY MANAGEMENT

Appropriate airway management may be classified by both the nature of the injury and the likelihood of an intrinsic airway injury. The three common categories of airway management are the following:

1. *Care of a normal airway* in a traumatized child with peripheral organs injury requiring artificial airway (for example, exsanguinated victim of traumatic amputation)
2. *Normal airway management* in a child *with head injury* in addition to other organ injuries
3. *Care of a traumatized airway* in the presence or absence of other injuries

The care of the normal airway in a injured child is similar to ordinary operating room patient management and requires limited assistance. Awake intubation is considered the first and the easiest option.[7] Most youngsters, however, are frightened and uncooperative and are capable of putting on a spectacular fight against bona fide attempts, thereby turning an otherwise well-controlled situation into a sorry mess in which damage sometimes is difficult to undo and results in iatrogenic airway trauma, loss of intravenous access, and other possible complications. Usually, intubation without pharmacologic assistance (sedation and muscle relaxant) can be accomplished in the awake neonate or moribund child who does not express any spontaneous activity. Otherwise the technique applied is dictated by the presence or absence of foreseeable difficulty or head injury.

Awake intubation should be preceded by applying an ECG, sphygmomanometer, and pulse oximeter and inserting an intravenous line. Initially the face should be wiped dry and clean and ven-

tilation and oxygenation assessed and continued via mask and bag with 100% O_2 always bearing in mind the likelihood of cervical spine injury in which clinical immobilization is imperative. Danger of aspiration is often enhanced by unskilled or difficult bagging and stomach inflation. Proper position of the child's head, jaw thrust, and insertion of an oral airway with gentle institution of PEEP (about 5 cm H_2O) can correct a vast majority of problems. Application of cricoid pressure may take place during mask ventilation, thus reducing the danger of aspiration of stomach contents. Due to parasympathetic dominance in the pediatric autonomic system, atropine (20 ug/kg) is routinely administered intravenously to prevent bradycardia resulting from vagal airway stimulation.[33,76] The awake intubation of a neonate or infant requires considerable skills. The patient's head and shoulders have to be well immobilized. A moderate shoulder roll may help position the airway, and the procedure ought to be performed smoothly without undue delay. The administration of an intravenous hypnotic agent alone, like thiopental, for intubation is not popular because of inconsistency in the achieved depth of anesthesia and complications varying from hypotension to laryngospasm. However, etomidate (0.3 mg/kg) preceded by diazepam (0.2 mg/kg) was found by Ronchi and co-workers[66] to be very safe and satisfactory agents when used for this purpose in children, despite data indicating etomidate's disastrous influence on mortality in ICU trauma patients[43] (caused by adrenocortical suppression) when administered for long-term sedation.

Modification of the intubation technique when *increased intracranial pressure* is present calls for skillful manual cervical immobilization, administration of high O_2 concentration, hyperventilation, and intravenous administration of thiopental (5 mg/kg) and xylocaine (1.5 mg/kg) followed by a nondepolarizing muscle relaxant like pancuronium (Pavulon) (0.15 mg/kg) or vecuronium (0.28 mg/kg), all preceded by atropine (0.02 mg/kg) and followed by hyperventilation (see box on p. 79). The above plan is suitable only for the stable patient without cardiovascular or respiratory derangements. Real life seldom follows such a course. I have found succinylcholine to be my muscle relaxant of choice even in the presence of increased intracranial pressure when a full stomach, vomiting, or anatomic airway abnormality may modify the induction technique. The short duration of suc-

---

TRAUMA ROOM PROTOCOL

Children's Memorial Hospital
Chicago, Illinois

Operating room 8 has been designated the on-call emergency trauma room and is to be set up daily by the on-call resident as follows:

1. **Suction tubing with Yankauer suction tip attached**
   a. 8-, 10-, 14-, 18-gauge French catheters also to be opened and placed next to suction apparatus (e.g. on side of ECG machine)

2. **Breathing circuit**
   a. Humidifier in line filled with sterile water
   b. Ventilator tubing attached, with 1.0 liter reservoir bag; 0.5 liter and 2.0 liter reservoir bags in blue drawer under anesthesia machine
   c. Nos. 1, 2, and 3 trays containing neonatal, children's, and adolescent airway equipment
   d. Large adult mask, Ohio newborn and infant masks, and no. 2 straight blade on anesthesia cart

3. **Endotracheal tubes (ETTs)**
   a. One each of 2.5-6.0 uncuffed ETTs
   b. One each of 5.0-7.5 cuffed ETTs, with 5 cc syringe for cuff inflation
   c. Place ETTs in blue drawer under anesthesia machine
   d. One pediatric and one adult stylet placed on anesthesia machine
   e. ½-inch and 1-inch rolls of tape placed on anesthesia machine
   f. Additional laryngoscope handle

4. **Monitors**
   a. Infant pulse oximeter probe attached to cable
   b. Blood pressure gauge out on anesthesia machine
   c. Cable for esophageal temperature probe plugged into temperature machine
   d. ECG electrodes set up with ECG pads attached
   e. Arterial line tubing and stopcock in room

5. **Medications**
   a. Halothane and isoflurane vaporizers filled
   b. Drawn up:
      - Succinylcholine in 1 cc and 10 cc syringes
      - Pavulon in 1 cc and 5 cc syringes
      - Sodium thiopental in 1 cc and 10 cc syringes
      - Atropine in two 1 cc syringes
      - Epinephrine in one 1 cc syringe
   c. In room: In addition to "code" drugs in anesthesia cart:
      - Heparin—one vial
      - Bicarbonate—four amps
      - Ca Cl$_2$—two amps
   d. One infusion pump in room, with tubing placed on back of anesthesia cart

6. **Intravenous lines**
   a. One normal saline attached through blood warmer for reconstitution with PRBCs
   b. One dextrose (5%), Ringer's lactate

7. **Portable anesthesia cart for the following:**
   a. Supplement room 8 setup
   b. Facilitate setting up rooms other than room 8 at night or on weekends
   c. Help with major resuscitation in any room

---

cinylcholine action offers a definite advantage in case of failed intubation.[13,77] Noteworthy is the dose-related speed of onset of Pavulon's action.[18] Pavulon administered in high doses (0.15 to 0.2 mg/kg) results in acceptable intubation conditions within 60 seconds; however, the price to pay for this benefit is a prolonged duration of action.

Cricoid pressure is used whenever possible. According to Salem[71] it is also effective in the pres-

ence of a nasogastric tube. There are situations when Sellick's maneuver renders the intubation impossible because the infant's laryngeal cartilage is soft and may be occluded by vigorously applied pressure.* The anesthesiologist should keep this in mind when there is clear visualization of the vocal cords in the presence of a normal airway and un-

---

*References 7, 37, 69, 70, 72, 73.

EMERGENCY CART CONTENTS
Code Committee Recommendations

Children's Memorial Hospital
Chicago, Illinois

Top of cart

Suction bottle with 6-foot plastic tubing and Yankauer suction tip

Dextrose 50% in water—50 ml

Naloxone (Narcan) 0.4 mg/ml

Atropine 1 mg/ml

Phenytoin 100 mg

Propranolol Hcl (Inderal) 1 mg/ml

Isoproterenol (Isuprel) 1:5000-5 ml

Dopamine Hcl 200 mg (40 mg/ml)

Calcium gluconate 10%/10 ml

Sodium chloride (normal) 10 ml

Diphenhydramine 50 mg/1 cc

Dexamethasone 4 mg/ml

Bretylium tosylate (Bretylol) 10 ml

Povidone-iodine (Betadine) solution

Lidocaine 1% 20 ml

Four epinephrine 1:10,000-10 ml

Three lidocaine 1%—5 ml

Six sodium bicarbonate 8.4%—10 ml/10 mEq + 50 mEq

　Tuberculin syringe without heparine

Ten 2 × 2 gauze pads

Two tongue blades

One adhesive tape (1-inch wide)

Five alcohol sponges

Two scalpels (disposable) size no. 11

Two stopcocks with extension tubes

Two 2-inch, 14-gauge, 18-gauge, 20-gauge, "B-D" intravenous catheters

Four 1-inch, 22-gauge QUICK catheters

Two ⅝-inch, 24-gauge QUICK catheters

Two 20-gauge × 3½-inch intracardiac needles

Five 20-gauge × 1-inch, 18-gauge × 1-inch, 22-gauge × 1-inch hypodermic needles

Two 19-inch, 21-inch, 23-inch butterfly infusion sets

Disposable syringes: Two 20 cc without needles
　　　　　　　　　　Two 12 cc, 20 gauge × 1½-inch
　　　　　　　　　　Two 3 cc, 22 gauge × 1½-inch
　　　　　　　　　　One 33 cc catheter tip

Five Tuberculin syringes with 100 units of heparin (for arterial blood gas only)

Arrest flow sheet

Twenty labels (self-stick type for syringes)

Blood tubes (Vacutainer) one red (with gel), one red, one lavender, one gray

Drawer 1

Endotracheal tubes
　Uncuffed: 2.5 mm, 3.0 mm, 3.5 mm, 4.0 mm, 4.5 mm, 5.0 mm (two of each)
　Cuffed: 5.0 mm, 5.5 mm, 6.0 mm, 6.5 mm, 7.0 mm, 7.5 mm, 8.0 mm, 8.5 mm (two of each)

Two laryngoscope handles

Laryngoscope blades:
　Premature: No. 0, infant; no. 1, child; no. 2 (straight) (1 of each)
　Adult: no. 3 (straight); MacIntosh: no. 2 (curved), no. 3 (curved)

Laryngoscope bulbs: Large, small (two of each)

Two size C batteries

Tin-Co-Ben 4 fl. oz.

Several assorted safety pins

Forceps: Magill
　　　　　Kelly clamp

Triamcinolone acetonide cream 0.1%

Stylettes: Adult, child

Adhesive tape (1-inch wide)

Child Ohio Trimar mask

Newborn Ohio Trimar mask

Premature Ohio Trimar mask

Oral airways: Size 00, 0, 1, 2, 3, 5 (two of each)

Suction catheters: French 6 gauge, 8 gauge, 10 gauge, 14 gauge

Nasogastric tubes: Levin French 18 gauge

Anderson tubes: French 10 gauge

Adult Hope bag

Small Hope bag

0.5 liter Rusch bag

1.0 liter Rusch bag

Oxygen Flowmeter with 14 feet of oxygen tubing

Sterile gloves, size 8

Sterile gloves, size 6½

Yankauer suction tip

Metrisets

EMERGENCY CART CONTENTS, cont'd
Code Committee Recommendations

Children's Memorial Hospital
Chicago, Illinois

Drawer 2

Masks: Large Ohio Trimar mask, Medium Ohio
Trimar mask
Small Ohio Trimar mask (one of each)

Drawer 3

Intravenous solutions:
Normal serum albumin (human 5% solution 250 ml)
5% dextrose in 0.2% saline 500 cc
Normal saline 500 cc
Ringer's lactate 500 cc
Mannitol 20% 500 cc
Sterile normal saline 1000 ml (irrigating solution)
Blood pump kit

Bottom shelf

Suction machine (in the "on" position)
Adult Hope bag
Child Hope bag
Cut down tray

Side of cart

"E" Cylinder with 14 feet of oxygen tubing connected to 0.5 Rusch bag
Cardiac massage board

Tied to cart

Several tourniquets

---

expected resistance is experienced when passing an appropriate or smaller size endotracheal tube. Releasing the pressure may open the air passages.

For every emergency intubation there should be a full selection of uncut cuffed and uncuffed endotracheal tubes (see boxes on pp. 80 and 81). A stylet is used for all such intubations. In certain cases it is wise to exchange an oral endotracheal tube to the nasal route because of the greater stability achieved in this location. The child's cricoid cartilage corresponds in size to the anterior and posterior nostril. Therefore the larynx usually accepts the same size nasal tube as that of an oral one. A large air leak around an oral endotracheal tube requires the use of a larger nasotracheal tube. Nasal intubation should be avoided in the presence of basal skull fractures and injuries that are in close proximity to nasal air passages and sinuses. The tube change may be carried out at the end of surgery under controlled circumstances or when expedient and need not be the top priority when establishing vascular access or monitoring lines. For advance selection of an endotracheal tube appropriate for the treated child we use the following formula:

$$\frac{age}{4} + 4 = \text{endotracheal tube size}$$

Tubes one size larger and smaller are also made available. If circumstances allow it, the tube placement is verified by chest radiogram and the tube secured with benzoin, waterproof tape, a safety pin, foam pad, and umbilical clamp (Fig. 6-1).

Blind nasal intubation and retrograde intubation may be performed in exceptional cases. Details of this technique and its indications are available.[7,42]

Fiberoptic intubation can be carried out under sedation and local anesthesia in older children and teenagers.[4,60,61] In the younger population a more controlled situation is achieved with deep halothane anesthesia and spontaneous ventilation and can be continued with a muscle relaxant, hyperventilation, hyperoxygenation, and continuous monitoring of O_2 saturation. Ordinarily, fiberoptic intubation is limited to children older than 1 year of age, since the commonly available smallest fiberoptic bronchoscope with directed tip has an outside diameter of 3.5 mm and accepts the minimal #4.0 inner diameter endotracheal tube without the 15 mm connector (Fig. 6-2). Presently, Olympus is offering a custom-made ultrathin bronchoscope[39] (PF 27 [outer diameter 2.7 mm]) with directed tip, the very high cost and questionable durability of which make it an uncertain investment. Insertion

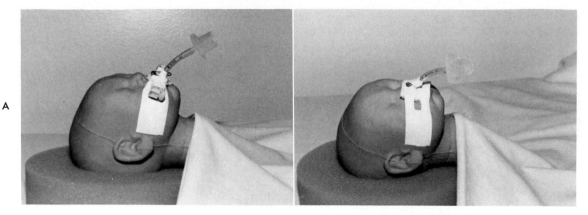

A   B

Fig. 6-1   Oral (**A**) and nasal (**B**) tubes secured with waterproof tape, safety pin, foam pad, and umbilical clamp.

of small tubes in infants can be accomplished with the help of a flexible guide wire introduced into the fiberoptic bronchoscope's working channel and passed into the trachea under endoscopic guidance. The endotracheal tube is then threaded over the wire. This technique requires special skills.[24, 83]

The presence of face and neck injury implies upper airway trauma. Complaints of neck pain, hoarse voice, or aphonia without airway impairment require a CT scan or endoscopy before a decision regarding definitive airway management can be made.

Severe airway impairment due to face and neck injury demands rapid decision making as to the practicality of attempting intubation or establishing

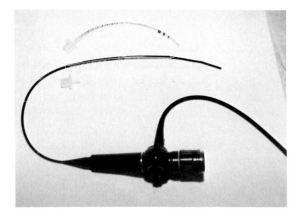

Fig. 6-2   Fiberoptic bronchoscope Olympus BF type 3C10 with size 4.0 inner diameter endotracheal tube threaded on; connector separated and 4.5 inner diameter endotracheal tube.

an alternative airway by needle or surgical cricothyroidotomy or emergency tracheotomy.[10,57]

Cricothyroidotomy is not favored by most otolaryngologists[30,85] because of (1) the small size of the cricothyroid membrane, (2) technical difficulties encountered, and (3) potential damage of important laryngeal structures in the process of airway insertion, all of which may eventuate in difficult or unsuccessful laryngeal reconstruction. Optimal conditions for performing tracheotomy are in the operating theater, with the patient intubated for total airway control. Only in rare circumstances is "slash" tracheotomy the preferred procedure.[30]

STABILIZATION OF THE CHILD

Once the safety of the patient's airway has been ensured, the anesthesiologist can leave further care to the respiratory technician and continue resuscitation with appropriate drug administration and attempt to restore cardiac function (Table 6-1). Temperature determination and monitoring are important for the effective management of hypothermia, which is an ominous predictor of survival.[36] In Jurkovich's study[36] no *adult* patient survived whose core temperature fell below 32° C. Anecdotal and scientific data indicate vast differences in physiologic responses to hypothermia between the pediatric and adult population, in some part because the ventricular fibrillation threshold is thought to be lower in children than in adults at 27° to 30° C. Data collected by Rosen and Rosen[67] confirm that belief. In infants and small children the ratio of body surface area to body weight is

Table 6-1   Code committee recommendations for resuscitation medications*

Children's Memorial Hospital
Chicago, Illinois

Essential life support medications

Medication	Initial dose (amount)	Initial dose (volume)	Subsequent dose
Atropine	0.01 mg/kg intravenous or intratracheal (min 0.1 mg; max 0.6 mg)	0.01 mg/kg intravenous or intratracheal	Total vagolytic dose: Child—1 mg; Adolescent—2 mg
Calcium gluconate	30 mg/kg intravenous (max 1g)	0.3 ml/kg intravenous	
Epinephrine	10 mcg/kg intravenous or intratracheal	0.1 ml/kg (1:10,000)	20 mcg/kg
Glucose	1 g/kg intravenous	2 ml/kg intravenous (50%)	
Lidocaine	1 mg/kg intravenous or intratracheal	0.1 ml/kg intravenous or intratracheal 1% solution	1 mg/kg to a maximal of 3 mg/kg
Sodium bicarbonate	1 mEq/kg intravenous	1 ml/kg intravenous	½ initial dose; than per blood gases

Useful life support medications

Medication	Initial dose (amount)	Initial dose (volume)	Subsequent dose
Diphenhydramine (Benadryl)	1 mg/kg intravenous	0.02 ml/kg intravenous	
Bretylium	5 mg/kg intravenous	0.1 ml/kg intravenous	10 mg/kg
Dexamethasone	1 mg/kg intravenous	0.25 ml/kg intravenous	
Furosemide	1 mg/kg intravenous	0.1 ml/kg intravenous	2 mg/kg
Mannitol	0.25 g/kg intravenous	1.25 ml/kg intravenous	
Naloxone	0.1 mg/kg intravenous	0.025 ml/kg intravenous	0.02 mg/kg

Infusion guidelines—initial dose

Medication	Amount/volume	Rate and corresponding dose
Dopamine/dobutamine	60 mg in 100 ml D5 0.2 NaCl	(patient's weight in kg) ml per hour = 10 mcg/kg/min
Isoproterenol/epinephrine	1 mg in 100 ml D5 0.2 NaCl	(patient's weight in kg) ml per hour = 0.167 mcg/kg/min
Lidocaine	100 mg in 100 ml D5 0.2 NaCl	(patient's weight in kg) ml per hour = 17 mcg/kg/min

Defibrillation current

For V. Fib.	2 watt-sec/kg	4 watt-sec/kg
For V. Tach/SVT	1-2 watt-sec/kg	Increase as needed

*Actual doses may vary depending on the patient's condition.

higher than that of the adults, making them more vulnerable to environmental heat losses. The same factor is responsible for rapid cooling during immersion in cold water, leading to initiation of "the diving reflex," which may eventually be responsible for successful resuscitation of near-drowning victims who survive several minutes of submersion. Hypothermic patients require active but gentle rewarming and should be not pronounced dead until their temperature reaches a normal level.[92] Radiant heat lamps, warm water, warm humidified air, and even extracorporeal circulation can be used. The process should be stopped when the core temperature reaches 33° to prevent overshoot.[81]

The anesthesiologist is responsible for ensuring that blood samples were sent to the laboratory for complete blood count, electrolytes, blood urea nitrogen, creatinine, and arterial blood gas analysis and that a reasonable amount of blood was ordered to be typed and crossmatched. The availability and readiness of the operating room ought to be checked, anesthetic equipment set up, and a sufficient amount of resuscitation fluid accessible.

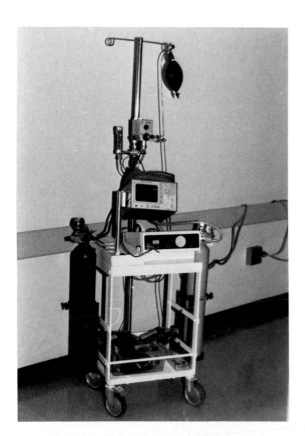

Fig. 6-3 Trolley for in-hospital transport.

The move to the operating room is undertaken with oxygen, monitors, emergency ventilation equipment, and fluids and drugs, as well as sufficient personnel to ensure safe and rapid transport. To minimize the risk of hemodynamic instability during transport,[14] we use a custom-made trolley fitted with oxygen and air, monitors and airway equipment (Fig. 6-3).

INTRAOPERATIVE MANAGEMENT

A significant number of patients undergoing emergency surgery will be intubated[74,90] before arrival at the hospital or in the emergency room, and a small number of patients (1% at Children's Memorial Hospital in Chicago) come to the operating room directly from the transport vehicle. Unfortunately the patient's condition is grave, blood is unavailable, the history is incomplete, and family members are not present to give their consent for surgery. Nonetheless, "In an emergency there is legally no need for consent," and "no physician has ever been sued successfully following treatment of a minor patient without parental consent when the treatment was necessary."[34]

Upon arrival to the OR the position and stabilization of the tube should be verified by auscultation, chest x-ray films, or both. Capnography or qualitative capnometry (the Biochem 515 CO_2 respiration monitor) serves as another way to confirm endotracheal placement of the ET tube.[65] The chest radiograph is the best diagnostic test to detect a possible pneumothorax.

Essential and standard monitoring equipment include an electrocardiograph, manual or automatic blood pressure cuff, temperature probe, SaO_2, Foley catheter, arterial line catheter, urine output, and central venous pressure.[5] Where available, capnography significantly contributes to the patient's safety and management. There certainly are instances when persistent attempts to insert an arterial line in the presence of profound hypotension would be a waste of time,[58] particularly if hypotension can be resolved by prompt surgical intervention. However, in a stable patient a reasonable amount of time can be spent obtaining additional vascular access. A saphenous vein cut down in the groin prepared into the abdominal operating field will ensure quick access for intravenous catheterization, and insertion of a double-lumen catheter allows fluid administration and simultaneous CVP monitoring.

A Swan-Ganz catheter seldom has application in acutely injured children, although it is used in further management of a variety of trauma complications and in the measurement of cardiac output by thermodilution.[48,55] It would be unjust to ignore the current development of the noninvasive pulse Doppler method in cardiac output determination,[2,3,35,93] with the aid of transesophageal or suprasternal probes, as well as the prospect of continuous monitoring of cardiac output via impedence measurement.[1,93] Both are attractive alternatives that have already delivered values correlating well with other methods.

INDUCTION OF ANESTHESIA

We treat all injured children as patients with a full stomach, regardless of their last food intake or the time elapsed between injury and operation. Stress, pain, and analgesic agents alter gastrointestinal motility, rendering NPO status unreliable. Preoperative intubation of the conscious patient *without* CNS injury is performed by rapid sequence induction as follows:

1. Awake patient
2. In rapid sequence
   a. Preoxygenation
   b. Intravenous administration of atropine, ketamine, or thiopental followed by succinylcholine
   c. Cricoid pressure application (concomitantly with injection of intravenous drugs), which is not released until correct placement of the tube is confirmed
   d. Rapid insertion of the endotracheal tube (with a stylet); correct placement is confirmed by presence of bilateral breath sounds auscultated in apical, maxillary, and epigastric areas

In the unstable patient who has lost a significant volume of blood (greater than 25% of estimated blood volume) ketamine 1 to 2 mg/kg intravenously is the preferred induction agent.[8,9,91] A decision in favor of thiopental ought to be weighed carefully and the dose appropriately adjusted to 1 to 2 mg/kg.

One volume of *fluid and blood administration* constitutes the major part of intraoperative management and may be modified by preexisting health problems, such as congenital heart disease, and current injuries, including head trauma or large vessel injury. The exact quantitation is usually aided by extensive monitoring and approximate calculation of estimated blood volume (EBV),[45] which can be summarized for each pediatric age group as follows:

Neonate—85 cc/kg
Infant—80 cc/kg
Child—75 cc/kg
Adolescent—65 cc/kg

The patient's body weight (often its approximation) serves as a guide in the administration of hourly fluid maintenance and in the calculation of 10 to 20 cc/kg boluses over 5- to 10-minute periods.[28]

If blood is not immediately available the advantage of colloids over crystalloids is debatable at best,[21,38,54,62] and the former can be administered only in limited quantities because of interference with blood crossmatching.[53] Nevertheless, colloids enhance the resuscitation effort for 24 to 36 hours because of their intravascular stability. Crystalloids administered in form of balanced salt solution (Ringer's lactate) offers only 2 to 3 hours of replacement support when infused at a 3:1 ratio to estimated blood loss. Crystalloids also carry a well-advertised price advantage. Regardless of the choice, all intravenous fluid should be *warmed*. Within the last few years our attention has been focused on the significance of the blood/brain glucose level versus the severity of neurologic sequelae on CNS hypoxia.[19,75] Therefore it is important to moderate glucose administration and monitor the glucose blood level, particularly in the presence of a CNS insult.[41,52,80]

Dealing with blood and blood products in the emergency situation, as in routine practice, calls for adherence to disease control measures recommended in the care of all patients,[64] despite the small risk of the hepatitis or AIDS virus.[53] Even in a pediatric hospital the HIV-positive material is more likely to come from blood donated by adults rather than from the patient population.[86] Nonetheless, universal protective measures must be carried out.

ANESTHETIC MANAGEMENT

Anesthetic management of these dramatically ill patients principally lays in *quantity* rather than *quality* of administered drugs. Some papers on the subject are so intensely focused on resuscitation issues that there is no mention of anesthetic drugs.[9] David L. Brown[38] points out that "We may need to consider ourselves, not inappropriately, resuscitologists rather than anesthesiologists."

In our goal of providing patient comfort through administration of hypnotic and analgesic agents, we should not lose sight of patient safety or be intimidated by the high rate of intraoperative recall in trauma victims, which Bogetz and Katz[12] report as 43% among trauma patients who had to be intubated while in shock or hypotensive.

Volatile anesthetics should not play a primary role in the administration of general anesthesia because of their myocardiodepressant properties and vasodilatatory action, but they should be used with caution as adjunctive agents to complement intravenous narcotics. Nitrous oxide has no cardiovascular advantage to offer and may expand a pneumothorax or pneumoperitoneum and also limit delivered FIO_2.[89] Most data concerning anesthetic agents are derived and extrapolated from adult or animal studies.[59] The most reliable information comes from research regarding sick infants and children, usually with congenital heart diseases. Very little is known of the hypovolemic child's response to medication.

Morphine (0.05 to 0.3 mg/kg) causes undesirable hemodynamic changes due to its histamine release and bradycardiac effects and is not the medication of choice for hypovolemic patients.[46]

Fentanyl, with its brevity of action and maintenance of cardiovascular parameters, offers the most versatile application in doses ranging from 5 to 100 ug/kg.[40]

Sufentanyl (0.2 to 10 ug/kg) like fentanyl is a synthetic opioid producing minimal hemodynamic changes easily counteracted by administration of atropine or pancuronium. It is a more rapid onset of action and a shorter elimination half-time than its predecessor.[20,56]

Alfentanil (2 to 50 ug/kg) is new to pediatric anesthetic practice and known to cause bradycardia and a hypotensive response when administered as a bolus. It has the shortest duration of action of the three synthetic drugs and offers little advantage in management of very sick, unstable patients. However, Alfentanil can serve as a useful supplement to inhalation anesthesia in minor trauma surgery in which there is no large fluid volume deficit.[79,84]

Scopolamine (7 ug/kg) given every 4 hours is a recommended amnestic agent.[59]

Benzodiazepines (Valium 0.1 mg/kg; Midazolam 0.08 to 0.1 mg/kg; lorazepam 0.1 mg/kg) may be used to produce intraoperative amnesia.

Intraoperative complications are a constant threat to all severely injured patients. Even the most extensive preoperative evaluation does not preclude the new development of a subdural hematoma, pneumohemothorax, air or fat embolism, or cardiac tamponade. The anesthesiologist has to be aware of this possibility constantly, particularly in the presence of persistent intraoperative hypotension.[11,90] A helpful tool to differentiate intraoperative hypotension is to remember the following mnemonic *HATCH*[23]:

H—Hemodynamics
A—Acid base
T—Temperature
C—Coagulation
H—Help

ANESTHESIA FOR MINOR TRAUMA

Children with complex fractures, lacerations, or eye injuries requiring urgent surgical treatment may incur a more significant risk with anesthesia than that imposed by the potential sequelae of the injury. Prompt suturing of a facial laceration or reduction of an open fracture is necessary, and delaying the procedure until the next morning will not significantly diminish the anesthetic risk. These patients generally are prepared for surgery according to the following rules that are applied to elective cases: preoperative interview with the parents and the patient, history and physical examination, appropriate premedication with sedation and analgesia, and acquisition of basic laboratory data. A complete blood count before a small procedure is not essential in a healthy patient who has no history of blood loss. Indeed, in certain situations, such as the presence of an open eye injury,[8] undue crying may have undesirable effects. The decision to delete the test or postpone its execution will depend on the anesthesiologist's attitude and expertise.

In exceptional cases in which even the stress of starting an intravenous line may cause irreparable damage, inhalation induction may be warranted, with cricoid pressure application. Open eye injury also calls for anesthetic management modification by substituting short-acting Succinylcholine with large doses of nondepolarizing muscle relaxants, such as Atracurium (0.5 to 0.6 mg/kg).[13,44,49] After induction is accomplished, the maintenance and course of anesthesia do not differ much from administering anesthesia to a healthy patient. Routine suctioning of the stomach after intubation does not ensure complete emptying of gastric contents, and awake extubation with the patient's eyes open or grimacing is mandatory.

During the last quarter of the century we have watched regional anesthesia regain its rightful place in anesthetic practice and advance into wide new avenues of continuous postoperative pain control and intrathecal narcotic administration.[6,16,17,22,25] Application of the new techniques for infants and children has met with growing interest only during the last 15 years. At present, regional anesthesia in pediatric practice has a recognized place in management of high-risk infants,[78] but most notably in postoperative pain relief. It is frequently used in conjunction with light general anesthesia, applied either at the beginning or end of the procedure.[51]

There is no literature addressing the practicality of regional techniques in acutely injured children. The anesthesiologist's skill and training, the predictable lack of cooperation from children in general, which may be further aggravated by stressful circumstances of injury, and the reports of paresthesias that cannot be relied upon are important considerations. The latter obstacle may be overcome by expert use of a block-aid monitor, which according to Wright[94] is an essential tool.

Candidates for nerve blocks ought to be selected carefully. Mature adolescents and some children are capable of assisting in the decision-making process. I recall a certain 8-year old who fell from an apple tree breaking both his forearms. The fear of parental wrath was such that he would have done anything to undo his mischief and therefore allowed bilateral placement of perivascular axillary blocks without hesitation.[95] More commonly, regional techniques in pediatric population are finding applications in perioperative pain control as continuous epidural local anesthetic injection, intercostal blocks, and infiltration blocks.[15]

ACKNOWLEDGMENT

My sincere appreciation to Allen I. Goldberg, M.D. for the opportunity, Marleta Reynolds, M.D., Lauren Holinger, M.D., and my boss, Frank L. Seleny, M.D. for their friendly assistance, and to Ms. Pat Peano for her invincible typing.

REFERENCES

1. Alverson DC: Noninvasive measurement of cardiac output in the newborn, J Perinat Med 3:16, 1984.
2. Alverson DC: Neonatal cardiac output measurement using pulsed Doppler ultrasound, Clin Perinatol 12:1, 1985.
3. Alverson DC et al: Noninvasive pulsed Doppler determination of cardiac output in neonates and children, J Pediatr 101:46, 1982.
4. Andrieu-Guitrancourt J et al: Utilisation du fibroscope dans les intubations difficiles chez le jeune enfant, Ann Otolaryngol Chir Cervicofac 101:481, 1984.
5. Barash PG: Controversies in cardiac monitoring, 1987 review course lectures, 1987, International Anesthesia Research Society.
6. Berde CB and Sethna NF: Regional anesthetic approaches to postoperative pain in children and adolescents, Intensive Care Med 13:460, 1987.
7. Berry FA: Anesthetic management of difficult and routine pediatric patients, Edinburgh, 1986, Churchill Livingstone, Inc.
8. Berry FA: Anesthesia for emergency pediatric surgery. In Donegan JH, editor: Manual of anesthesia for emergency surgery, Edinburgh, 1987, Churchill Livingstone, Inc.
9. Berry FA: Anesthetic management of the pediatric trauma patient, 1987 ASA annual refresher course lectures, Park Ridge, Ill, 1987, American Society of Anesthesiologists.
10. Bluestone CD and Stool SE: Pediatric otolaryngology, Philadelphia, 1983, WB Saunders Co.
11. Bodin L, Rouby JJ, and Viars P: Frequency of myocardial contusion after blunt chest trauma as evaluated by tallium 201 scintigraphy, Anesthesiology, 63:A123, 1985.
12. Bogetz MS and Katz JA: Recall of surgery for major trauma, Anesthesiology, 61:6, 1984.
13. Bonneru MC et al: Vecuronium or suxamethonium for rapid serivence intubation: which is better? Br J Anaesth 59:1240, 1987.
14. Braman SS et al: Complications of intrahospital transport in critically ill patients, Ann Intern Med 107:469, 1987.
15. Bridenbaugh PO: Regional analgesia for the trauma patient, 1987 ASA annual refresher course lectures, Park Ridge, Ill, 1987, American Society of Anesthesiologists.
16. Brodman LM: Regional anaesthesia in pediatric practice, Can Anaesth Soc J 34:543, 1987.
17. Brodman LM et al: The safety of caudal analgesia in children: experience with 2000 consecutive cases, Ninth World Congress of Anesthesiologists, Washington, DC, 1988, Park Ridge, Ill, 1988, American Society of Anesthesiologists.
18. Brown EM, Krishnaprasad D and Smiler BG: Pancuronium for rapid induction technique for tracheal intubation, Can Anaesth Soc J 26:489, 1979.
19. D'Alecy LG et al: Dextrose containing intravenous fluid impairs outcome and increases death after 8 minutes of cardiac arrest and resuscitation in dogs, Surgery 100:505, 1986.
20. Davis PJ et al: Pharmacodynamics of high-dose sufentanil in infants and children undergoing cardiac surgery, Anesth Analg 66:203, 1987.
21. Dodge C: What to transfuse: blood, blood components, colloid, or crystalloid? 1987 ASA annual refresher course lectures, Park Ridge, Ill, 1987, American Society of Anesthesiologists.
22. Eather K: Regional anesthesia for infants and children, Int Anesthesiol Clin 12:19, 1975.
23. Fairley HB: Perioperative management of thoracoabdominal trauma, First Annual Trauma Anesthesia and Critical Care Symposium, Washington, DC, May 1988, Park Ridge, Ill, 1988, American Society of Anesthesiologists.
24. Ford RWJ: Adaptation of the fiberoptic laryngoscope for tracheal intubation with small diameter tubes, Can Anaesth Soc J 28:479, 1981.
25. Francis M and Walbergh E: Caudal catheters in pediatric

patients: experience with 136 cases. Ninth World Congress of Anesthesiologists, Washington, DC, 1988, Park Ridge, Ill, 1988, American Society of Anesthesiologists.

26. Frutiger A: Emergency transport of trauma victims in a mountain area. In Vincent JL, editor: Update in intensive care and emergency medicine, New York, 1986, Springer-Verlag.

27. Fuller J, Frewen TS and Lee R: The anaesthetist's role in stabilization of the critically ill child, Can Anaesth Soc J 34:S55, 1987.

28. Furman EB: Pediatric fluid management during anesthesia, 1987 ASA annual refresher course lectures, Park Ridge, Ill, 1987, American Society of Anesthesiologists.

29. Grande CM, Stene JK, and Barton CR: The emerging concept of the trauma anesthesiologist, Md State Med J 37:512, 1988.

30. Handler SD: Trauma to the larynx and upper trachea, Int Anesthesiol Clin 26:39, 1988.

31. Harris BH: Management of multiple trauma, Pediatr Clin North Am 32:175, 1985.

32. Havre C, Gillard M and Huguenard P: Early medical care and mortality in polytrauma, J Trauma 27:1279, 1987.

33. Hendrix PH, and Govaerts MGM: Pediatric premedication: atropine or not, Acta Anaesthesiol Belg 31:195, 1980.

34. Hirsch HL: Informed consent: an anesthesiologist imperative, Practice Management Anesthesiol 1:1-4, 1988.

35. Imai M: Changes of hemodynamics during induction and tracheal intubation in children by ultrasonic Doppler method (Ultracom), Ninth World Congress of Anesthesiologists, Washington, DC, 1988, Washington, DC, 1988, World Federation of Societies of Anesthesiologists.

36. Jurkovich, GJ et al: Hypothermia in trauma victims: an ominous predictor of survival, Trauma 27:1019, 1987.

37. Kempen PM: Cricoid pressure, awake intubation, or both? Anesthesiology 64:831, 1986.

38. Kirby RR and Brown DL, editors: Anesthesia for trauma, Int Anesthesiol Clin 25:1, 1987.

39. Kleemann PP and Jantzen TP: Experience with the ultrathin fiberscope in the management of difficult airways in infants, Ninth World Congress of Anesthesiologists, Washington, DC, 1988, Washington, DC, 1988, World Federation of Societies of Anesthesiologists.

40. Koren G et al: Pediatric fentanyl dosing based on pharmacokinetics during cardiac surgery, Anesth Analg 63:577, 1984.

41. Lanier WL et al: Effects of IV dextrose and head position on neurologic outcome after complete cerebral ischemia, Anesthesiology 63:A110, 1985.

42. Latto IP and Rosen M: Difficulties in tracheal intubation, London, 1985, Baillière Tindall.

43. Ledingham I and Watt I: Influence of sedation on mortality in critically ill multiple trauma patients, Lancet I:1270, 1983.

44. Lennon RL, Olson RA, and Gronert GA: Atracurium or vecuronium for rapid sequence endotracheal intubation, Anesthesiology 64:510, 1986.

45. Levin FH and Horn BJ; The pediatric anesthesia handbook, ed 3, New Hyde Park, NY, 1985, Medical Examination Publishing Co.

46. Lynn AM and Slattery JT: Morphine pharmacokinetics in early infancy, Anesthesiology 66:136, 1987.

47. Macnab A et al: Optimal interhospital transport of polytraumatized children, Int Care Med 13:450, 1987.

48. Marcus RE: Trauma in children, Rockville, Md, 1986, Aspen Publishers, Inc.

49. Martin C et al: Vecuronium or suxamethonium for rapid sequence intubation: which is better? Br J Anaesth 59:1240, 1987.

50. Mayer TA: Emergency management of pediatric trauma, Philadelphia, 1985, WB Saunders Co.

51. McGown RG: Caudal analgesia in children (500 cases for procedures below the diaphragm), Anesthesia 37:806, 1982.

52. Michenfelder JD: Intelligence reports in anesthesia 5:13, 1988.

53. Miller RD: Current controversies in transfusion therapy. 1987 Review Course Lectures, 1987, International Anesthesia Research Society.

54. Millikan JS et al: Rapid volume replacement for hypovolemic shock: a comparison of techniques and equipment, J Trauma 24:428, 1984.

55. Moodie DS et al: Measurement of postoperative cardiac output by thermodilution in pediatric and adult patients, J Thorac Cardiovasc Surg 78:736, 1979.

56. Moore RA et al: Hemodynamic and anesthetic effects of sufentanil as the sole anesthetic for pediatric cardiovascular surgery, Anesthesiology 62:725, 1985.

57. Myers EN, Stool SE and Johnson TJ: Tracheotomy, Edinburgh, 1985, Churchill Livingstone.

58. Nelson LD: Monitoring in hemodynamics in trauma and acute illness, Anesthesiology 29:1, 1987.

59. Nicolson S: IV drugs in pediatric anesthesia—Narcotics. 1987 ASA annual refresher course lectures, Park Ridge, Ill, 1987, American Society of Anesthesiologists.

60. Ovassapian A et al: Difficult pediatric intubation—an indication for fiberoptic bronchoscope, Anesthesiology 56:412, 1982.

61. Patil VU, Stehling LC and Zauder HL: Fiberoptic endoscopy in anesthesia, Chicago, 1983, Year Book Medical Publishers.

62. Pavlin E: Fluid administration in the traumatized patient. First Annual Trauma Anesthesia and Critical Care Symposium, Washington, DC, May 1988.

63. Rayburn RL: Ventilatory therapy, anesthesia, and respiratory support. In Mayer TA, editor: Emergency management of pediatric trauma, Philadelphia, 1985, WB Saunders Co.

64. Recommendations for prevention of HIV transmission in health care settings, JAMA 258:1293, 1987.

65. Rodarte A: Perioperative management of pediatric trauma. First Annual Trauma Anesthesia and Critical Care Symposium, Washington, DC, May 1988.

66. Ronchi L et al: Etomidate for intubation of critically ill children, Int Care Med 13:449, 1987.

67. Rosen K and Rosen D: Occurrence of hypothermic ventricular fibrillation in children. Meeting of American Academy of Pediatrics, Elk Grove, Ill, Spring 1988.

68. Ross SE et al: Clearing the cervical spine: initial radiologic evaluation, J Trauma 27:1055, 1987.

69. Salem MR, Sellick BA, and Elam JO: The historical background of cricoid pressure in anesthesia and resuscitation, Anesth Analg 53:230, 1974.

70. Salem MR et al: Efficacy of cricoid pressure in preventing gastric inflation during bagmask ventilation in pediatric patients, Anesthesiology 40:96, 1974.

71. Salem MR et al: Cricoid compression is effective in oblit-

erating the esophageal lumen in the presence of nasogastric tube, Anesthesiology, 63:443, 1985.

72. Salem MR et al: In reply, Anesthesiology 64:832, 1986.

73. Sellick BA: The prevention of regurgitation during induction of anesthesia, First European Congress of Anesthesiology 89:1, 1962.

74. Shatney CH: Management of traumatic shock. In Vincent JL, editor: Update in intensive care and emergency medicine, New York, 1985, Springer-Verlag.

75. Sieber FE et al: Glucose: a reevaluation of its intraoperative use, Anesthesiology 67:72, 1987.

76. Smith RM: Anesthesia for infants and children, ed 5, St Louis 1989, The CV Mosby Co.

77. Sosis MB: Succinylcholine—relaxant for the 1990s? Anesthesiology 2:2, 1988.

78. Spear RM, Deshpande JK, and Maxwell LG: Caudal anesthesia in awake high-risk infant. Meeting of American Academy of Pediatrics, New York, Spring 1988.

79. Stanski DR: Pharmacokinetics and pharmacodynamics of Alfenta, Educational lecture series, Piscataway, NJ, 1987, Janssen Pharmaceutica, Inc.

80. Steward DJ, Da Silva CA, and Flegel T: Elevated blood glucose levels may increase the danger of neurologic deficit following profoundly hypothermic cardiac arrest, Anesthesiology 68:653, 1988.

81. Stoddart JC: Trauma and the anaesthetist, London, 1984, Baillière Tindall.

82. Storrs BB, and Walker ML: Spinal cord injuries, In Mayer T, editor: Emergency management of pediatric trauma, Philadelphia, 1985, WB Saunders Co.

83. Stiles CM: A flexible fiberoptic bronchoscope for endotracheal intubation in infants, Anesth Analg 53:1017, 1974.

84. Sudan NK, Michaels I, and Barash PG: Continuous narcotic infusions for pediatric patients: a reality? Anesth Analg 63:279, 1984.

85. Tucker GF: Personal communication, 1985.

86. Ward JW et al: Transmission of human immunodeficiency virus (HIV) by blood transfusions screened as negative for HIV antibody, N Engl J Med 318:473, 1988.

87. Weibley RE and Holbrook PR: Airway management in the traumatized child, Topics in Emergency Medicine, Oct 1982, Aspen Publishers, Inc.

88. Weiskopf RB: Anesthesia for major trauma, 1987 Review Course Lectures, International Anesthesia Research Society, 1987.

89. Weiskopf RB and Bogetz MS: Cardiovascular action of nitrous oxide of halothane in hypovolemic swine, Anesthesiology 63:503, 1985.

90. Weiskopf RB and Fairley HB: Anesthesia. In Trunkey DD and Lewis FR, editors: Current therapy of trauma, Philadelphia, 1986, BC Decker, Inc.

91. Weiskopf RB et al: Cardiovascular and metabolic sequelae of inducing anesthesia with ketamine or thiopental in hypovolemic swine, Ancsthesiology, 60:214, 1984.

92. White JD: Hypothermia. In Vincent JL, editor: Update in intensive care and emergency medicine, New York, 1985, Springer-Verlag.

93. Wong DG et al: Noninvasive cardiac output: two measurement methods compared with thermodilution and the importance of measured heart rate and ejection time, Anesth Analg 67:S262, 1988.

94. Wright B: A new use for block-aid monitor, Anesthesiology 30:236, 1969.

95. Zawadzki A: Personal communication, 1976.

7

Psychologic Aspects of Physical Trauma

Richard H. Granger

In almost all the industrialized countries of the world accidental injury is the major cause of morbidity and mortality in children and young adults. According to the national Health Interview Survey more than one third of children and youth in the United States incur at least one injury per year that requires medical attention or puts them out of action for at least a day, and each year there are about 22,000 injury-related deaths in those 0 to 19 years of age.[41] In a New Zealand birth cohort one in two children saw a physician at least once before the age of four for an accident-related injury, and one in five had two or more such occurrences. Approximately 9% of all these accidents resulted in hospital admission.[4] In a British birth cohort (all the children born in 1 week of April 1970) 43.9% had at least one accident between birth and 5 years of age, and 12% had two or more.[9]

Given these facts it is extraordinary that until recent years the psychologic aspects of physical trauma in children were largely neglected. The pediatric medical and surgical literature before that time, and even the specialized literature dealing exclusively with the developmental and psychologic aspects of child health, contains few mentions of the subject. The understanding of physical phenomena preceded and greatly outstripped the insight into psychologic phenomena. Therefore practical improvements in management of the physical aspects of care were numerous and sophisticated; those in management of the psychologic aspects were almost nonexistent. One might assume from this that not much was known about the effects of illness, accident, and their concomitants on children, but this was not the case. There was an extensive systematic literature on children's body image, reaction to illness (if not to accident, but often indistinguishable to the child), reaction to hospitalization and various surgical procedures (both

major factors in serious physical trauma), and the differences in these images and reaction based on age. Even 15 years ago this knowledge alone was sufficient to allow us to understand much about children's reactions to physical trauma of various kinds at various ages.

Now, however, there is enough additional direct evidence from observations and studies in the trauma field itself to confirm the accuracy and applicability of the more general information. This evidence, which has been systematically accumulated by pediatricians, pediatric surgeons, child psychiatrists, psychologists, epidemiologists and others, is now adequate to furnish guidelines for the management of injured children and to help redesign trauma services so that they will meet all the needs of such children. Furthermore, the evidence is now clear that such enhanced services will help shorten convalescence and improve physical, as well as psychological, outcomes. Before discussing specifics, however, it will help to examine some basic principles of psychologic development in children and how these relate to children's feelings about bodily dysfunction.

BARRIERS

Ravenscroft[94] states that "A child or adolescent suffering physical trauma is simultaneously plunged into acute emotional and social crisis. Patient and family go through several predictable phases—shock, denial and panic, protest and regression, oppositionalism, mourning, and readjustment." This fact is often not acknowledged in clinical settings. Significant and powerful factors interfere with the willingness and ability of adults to consider the psychologic pain of traumatized children. When children are injured the immediate concern of all is, as it should be, the quick and

90

thorough restoration of physical intactness and function. Under these circumstances psychologic considerations often seem secondary. The greater the injury and the more life threatening the insult are, the more this seems to be so. Among the tensions and pressures of trying to save lives and repair physical damage, psychologic prescriptions are often seen as a burden interfering with the smooth flow of services aimed at organic repair. In the emergency room and in the acute, immediate post-injury phase of treatment, psychologic issues must certainly take a back seat to those services. But the evidence is now compelling that, far from being a burden, good psychologic management quickens and enhances organic repair. Medical and surgical management of physical trauma can no longer be considered adequate or competent care when it does not incorporate knowledge of the psychosocial precursors and the psychologic sequelae of injury.

One factor that interferes is the manner in which most adults—parents and health professionals alike—deal with their own feelings and psychologic reactions. When children are injured, whether or not parental neglect or abuse is involved, parents feel guilty, ashamed, and defensive. At such times it is easier for them to focus on the physical realities of the injury than to consider the child's *feelings* of guilt, fear, and shame. The parents cannot contemplate the child's psychologic problems, so like their own, without increasing their own guilt and despair. Concentrating on the physical realities and ignoring the psychologic ones help parents maintain distance from the suffering of their children.

Similarly, health professionals often find themselves with an unacknowledged, but barely suppressed, anger directed toward the parents for having allowed the child to become so badly damaged. Whether they understand it or not, health professionals have trouble dealing with the conflicting emotions aroused in them by severely traumatized children. This is particularly so when close attention must be given to important decisions and actions involving survival or nonsurvival, intactness or permanent mutilation. Like the parents, the physicians and nurses also seek to distance themselves, especially when they must perform procedures (often repetitive ones) that they know are painful and distressing for the child.

So all the adults involved enter into a conspiracy of silence. Although they are aware of the child's suffering, it is more convenient for all of them to bury that awareness. In the face of considerable evidence to the contrary they choose to believe that the child has only a surface understanding of the trauma and its likely consequences. In this way the adults can refuse to face the fact that the injury and its sequelae have potent inner developmental and psychologic meanings for the child. The conspiracy does everyone a disservice. It prevents the adults from expressing their concerns, thereby making their pain easier to handle. In preventing adults from recognizing and accepting the child's priorities and needs, it makes impossible the planning for those procedures and services that would *really meet* developmental and psychologic priorities and needs.

There is no simple single formula for predicting or discussing the psychologic aspects of trauma in a given child. The importance of individualizing management is even greater in the developmental and psychologic areas than it is in the physical. No one would question that management considerations for adults must include many factors: the nature, location, severity, and symbolic importance of the injury; the patient's age and degree of understanding of the injury; the patient's relationship to family and friends; the patient's capacity to develop a trusting relationship with his or her caretakers; the preexisting mental health of the patient; and many others. These are developmental issues that are equally important in childhood, in which they are complicated by the fact that both the child's capacity for understanding and the symbolic importance of different injuries vary greatly with age and developmental level.

Beginning with an understanding of the developmental dynamics of the effects of illness and hospitalization, we can lay a sound foundation for a clearer understanding of the effects of trauma.

ILLNESS AND HOSPITALIZATION
Historical Overview

Reviewing some of the pioneer observations and recommendations in child illness and hospitalization is both inspiring and discouraging. It is inspiring because the observations were made by clinicians who saw clearly, described fully and accurately what they saw, and put their full recommendations at the service of the whole child. It is discouraging because reading these early observations makes painfully clear how little we have done to use this knowledge to improve the care and services for children.

As early as 1936 Beverly[8] wrote, "When studying emotional reactions of children in medical clinics, one is impressed with the frequency with which fears are related to medicine. By 'medical fears' we mean those stimulated by illness or therapeutic procedures including hospitalization." In 1938 Huschka and Ogden[51] advanced these observations and offered recommendations for minimizing emotional trauma in an outpatient clinic setting.

Jackson[52] in 1942 summarized these recommendations as follows:

honesty in acquainting the child with true facts about the procedure he is about to experience, whether painful or not; taking time to encourage patient's voluntary cooperation with minimizing of restraint; decreasing waiting time before a known uncomfortable test or treatment procedure, and immediate release of patient afterwards to congenial surroundings and normal play interests.

She draws attention to careless comments by nurses and physicians in front of children, the effect of separation from parents, the physician's error of mistaking the child's silence on a subject as an indication either of its unimportance or of the child's failure to understand it. All these contribute to the child's confusion and discomfort. Then she says, "All of these items might appeal to many as ordinary common sense, but their importance is often belittled and overlooked in practice—in ignorance of the predisposition to exaggerated fears which is characteristic of the age and the stage of development of the pre-school child." That these same points and recommendations are still appearing regularly in the literature as exhortations 45 years later indicates well how often they continue to be "belittled and overlooked."

Senn[107] and Langford[65] amplified these comments in discussions of psychologic healing during convalescence from physical illness or injury. Senn pointed out that the nature of disease itself was but one of four major factors that determined the child's emotional response to illness. The other three were psychological: "the physical, intellectual, and psychological status of the individual at the onset of his illness, . . . the meaning of the illness to the patient, . . . the interpersonal relationship of patient and nurse and patient and physician."[107] In relation to the nature of the disease itself he stated the following:

One which strikes with suddenness, demanding immediate change of setting without benefit of psychologic preparation, such as in a disease warranting immediate hospitalization and operation, stimulates feelings of uncertainty, confusion, fear and anxiety; these frequently result in emotional shock which persists for a long time in the period of recovery."

How well that statement describes the chain of events in physical trauma.

Agreeing with this, Langford[65] reports that "physical illness in a child, no matter how trivial, has its own unique meaning for the child and his parents and may be a focus out of which emerge emotional disturbances of far-reaching significance." For young children the most common meaning is that sickness is a punishment for their badness, and the most common reaction is regression to a more dependent state. Both Langford and Senn stress the need for attention to psychologic matters during convalescence equal to that given during the acute period of illness or injury.

In 1952 Anna Freud[34] provided the first theoretic framework for understanding the psychologic effects of illness on young children. Jessner[54] confirmed Freud's earlier observations with particular emphasis on the school-age child. It is important to note that although some of the work of Freud, Jessner, and others was derived retrospectively during psychotherapy or psychoanalytic treatment of adults, much of it was the result of direct, painstaking observations made in the children's wards and clinics of many hospitals. However, most of it was also naturalistic; it took advantage of what actually happened in those settings but made no effort to structure the settings or the selection processes to answer specific, preformulated research questions. Prugh et al[92] described the first large-scale, systematic, prospective study of the psychologic effects of hospitalization.

The information from all these studies still provides the basis of our knowledge today. It has been confirmed but little changed by subsequent years or newer studies. It can be best understood, however, in the context of some major, relevant developmental issues and landmarks. In this context it is important to note first that illness need not always be detrimental to developmental progress. Parmelee[85] points out that "Illnesses of a *minor* [emphasis added] nature, such as colds and GI upsets, are frequent events in the lives of all children . . . are generally not life threatening . . . (and) like other life perturbations, can expand children's personal and social experiences in ways beneficial to their behavioral development." He then goes on to make a plea for more studies to look at this side of illness in childhood.

Developmental Issues

Two types of developmental issues affect the reactions of individual children to illness, hospitalization, surgery, and physical trauma. Zuckerman and Duby[126] recommend a developmental approach to injury prevention that "emphasizes that children have different cognitive, perceptual, motor and language competencies" and they recommend attention to temperamental, motivational, and developmental capabilities and styles. This recommendation stresses the first type of developmental issue, which might be called longitudinal or historical considerations or issues. These deal primarily with such questions as how well the child has mastered, and been helped to master, previous developmental tasks and experiences. The ability of the child to master any new situation depends to a great extent on the success with which he or she has mastered previous challenges and the degree of personal intactness that has been reached at the moment of trauma. Children are proud of their increasing control of bodily functions and skills, feelings, and their environment. Although they may occasionally backslide a little on their own to experiment with the feeling of being more babyish, they fear and mistrust outside influences that make them regress. The loss, under stress, of recently acquired skills or controls adds greatly to their anxiety about the experience.

The second type of developmental issue might be called cross-sectional issues or developmental crises. These consist of recently arisen or long-standing unresolved problems in the child's life at the time of injury. If such problems exist, the psychologic impact of the trauma is likely to be greater and more difficult to master.

Longitudinal issues

Biologic endowment and prenatal and perinatal environment. Biologic endowment and prenatal and perinatal environment encompass genetic heritage, intrauterine influences (for example, nutritional and toxic), and the effects of the processes of labor, delivery, and newborn life. Awareness of and knowledge about these factors have been expanding at an enormous rate in recent years through work in such fields as obstetrics, pediatrics, genetics, developmental psychology, and so forth.

The Competent Infant[118] presents a wide selection of papers in all these fields.

What becomes clear from all this work is the incredible variability of newborn infants in their ability to interact with their environments, both physical and interpersonal. These differences are not always easy for clinicians to detect, but work in recent years, especially that of Brazelton,[14] has presented clinicians with useful tools for assessing newborns and young infants in a more detailed way than has ever been possible before.

Taken as a whole, the innate capacities and vulnerabilities of the individual child provide a life-long matrix for the child's ability to meet stresses and to deal with them constructively. Vulnerabilities may be ameliorated by good parents and other helpful influences, but they continue to be a determining factor.

Parent-child attachment. Numerous studies, such as those of Spitz[115] and Provence and Lipton,[91] have shown the critical importance of the early relationship between the infant and one or more nurturing adults. The relationship provides the substrate for cognitive development as well as for the more obvious areas of social and emotional development. Inadequate early attachment, stimulation, or both is a major factor in the subsequent inability of children or adults to meet stress with full resources.

Separation experiences. In the first months of life infants perceive themselves as extensions of nurturing adults rather than as separate individuals. About 8 months of age they begin to realize that they are separate and therefore separable, and they begin to fear that any separation may become permanent. The process of resolving this fear and learning that separations do not necessarily mean permanent loss of a loved one takes many months and careful attention by the parents. If it is handled well it is an important learning and maturing experience for the children. If it is not handled well, in a way that permits solution of the challenge, it recurs as a problem around every new type or example of separation. This is, of course, a major problem in relation to hospitalization. Illnesses or injuries that occur during the periods when anxiety about separation is at its height incur larger psychologic risks.

Language development. The development of language (facility of expression and a reasonable vocabulary) presents the child with the ability to communicate inner feelings and experiences if given the opportunity and encouraged to do so. The failure of adequate language development is a sensitive barometer of serious developmental difficulties and imposes a major barrier to helping the child deal with stressful situations.

Oedipal period. The Oedipal period is a more theoretic developmental concept than the others. Difficult to recognize clinically at the time it occurs, it has been described most completely retrospectively in psychotherapy. Nevertheless, there clearly are anxieties in children of both sexes emanating from their genital differences. These seem greatest in the 4- to 6-year-old child and are often extrapolated to include concerns about the intactness of, or injuries to, other parts of the body as well. How this developmental challenge is mastered is another important component of the way in which the child is able to deal with illness and bodily harm, particularly physical injury.

Cross-sectional issues

Injury during a normal developmental challenge. As discussed previously, physical trauma may create special difficulties for the child if it occurs when a major developmental challenge is undergoing resolution. If an accident occurs while the child is being toilet trained, for example, or immediately thereafter, the child is quite likely to become untrained, to regress to a period before any control was established. If the problem can be handled with special attention to the child's needs of the moment, the episode may be used by the child to enhance maturation. Poorly handled, however, the problem may interfere with the resolution both of the injury and of the normal developmental challenge being faced.

Separation crises. A number of family events (for example, divorce, illness, hospitalization or death of a parent or other close relative, the onset of schooling, or moving to a new house) may reactivate earlier separation anxieties, so the child has to work the issue through again. The effect of all this will be to increase anxiety about illness or hospitalization, but this can be helped by skillful, sympathetic handling. One of the more devastating effects of the parents' psychologic withdrawal when the child suffers serious illness or injury is that the withdrawal may be felt by the child as a loss as real and painful as that caused by physical separation.

Peer and sibling relationships. A new baby in the family, an inability to relate to peers or siblings, or other social maladjustments makes it more difficult for the child to use interpersonal relationships as a tool with which to work through crisis situations and stress.

Theoretical Considerations
Illness

In discussing the psychologic effects of illness in young children Freud[34] points out the most critical and most commonly overlooked fact: "The child is unable to distinguish between feelings of suffering caused by the disease inside the body and suffering imposed on him from outside for the sake of curing the disease. He has to submit uncomprehendingly, helplessly and passively to both sets of experiences." She then identifies the following factors, other than separation, that enter into the child's reaction to illness:

1. Parents almost inevitably change their patterns of child care when the child is sick. However they do this the change, the inconsistency, may be bewildering to the child who has grown accustomed to one way of being handled.

2. Adults view nursing care as "being treated like a baby" and are upset by it. Children are no less upset, particularly those who only recently have escaped from the reality of having been a baby. The feeling plays directly into their fears of not having really secured control, and they may truly regress in behavior and in patterns of training, especially those most recently established.

3. "Children defend their freedom of movement . . . to the utmost." When partial or total restraint is necessary, aggression is dammed up and may break through in young children as "restlessness, heightened irritability, the use of bad language, etc." In older children there may be a depressive or apathetic reaction.

4. Disruption of the integrity of the child's body—surgery, injury, casting, instrumentation—is viewed by boys as an attack or a mutilation and arouses fantasies of varying depth and severity, depending on the age and psychologic developmental stage of the child.

5. The reaction to pain varies from child to child as it does in adults, but the difference seems to be not physiologic but rather "the degree to which the pain is charged with psychic meaning. Pain augmented by anxiety, even if slight in itself, represents a major event in

the child's life and is remembered for a long time afterward, the memory being frequently accompanied by phobic defenses against its possible return."

6. The process of illness or injury requires the child to pay more than normal attention to his or her body and its needs. Energy that might otherwise be devoted to other, more constructive activities is turned inward and may cause the child to withdraw from normal, everyday activities. Or, unable to supply their own energy needs in this way, children may demand extra attention from the caretaking parent, as though they might attract energy to meet their inner needs.

7. Finally, children who have been parented well as infants—those whose bodily and psychologic needs were met with regularity and sensitivity— tend to feel secure about their bodies and bodily needs and therefore pay only casual attention to measures of hygiene and health. On the other hand, parentless children—those from institutions or neglecting homes for whom adequate attachment never took place in infancy—tend to have much more bodily concern, or overconcern, in a way that is reminiscent of adult hypochondriacs.

In summary, the child's reaction to illness derives from three diverse components—the pathophysiologic elements of the disease, the child's relationship to parents and other caretakers, and the child's reactions to his or her own inner life and body needs and to past and present developmental challenges. To attempt to treat one part of this triad without considering the others is to risk an outcome that is psychologically crippling to the child, in one way or another.

Hospitalization

Working from this theoretic framework Prugh and his associates[92] took advantage of the introduction of new nursing and visiting programs on the wards of Children's Hospital in Boston. They sought to discover which children reacted in which ways to the hospital experience and whether the newly designed services could modify those reactions for the better. They set up a reasonably controlled experiment with two groups of 100 children each, admitted for acute illness, and matched as closely as possible for age, sex, diagnosis, and degree of psychologic adjustment before hospital-

ization. The control group (hospitalized before the changeover of services) experienced the traditional ward management practices of limited visiting and no ward play groups or educational programs. The experimental group was exposed to the new ward program—liberal visiting, play groups, teachers, but stopping short of rooming-in for patients.

The results were supportive of the theoretic constructs. All children in both groups showed at least minimal reactions to hospitalization. However, in the control group 92% had significant reactions (36% severe), and in the experimental group only 68% had significant reactions (only 14% severe). These differences were highly significant ($p < 0.01$). The greatest number of severe reactions was in the developmentally more vulnerable younger children 2 to 5 years of age, with the control group showing almost twice as much difficulty as the experimental group (43% to 23%). In the 6- to 12-year-old group 27% of the controls had severe reactions, whereas none in the experimental group had them.

The children who had the fewest and mildest reactions in the hospital were those whose histories revealed the greatest adaptive capacity and the soundest developmental patterns before entering. Specifically, those children did best who had the most satisfying relationships with their parents and whose parents, in turn, showed the greatest ability to take advantage of the new ward program. Neither type of illness nor length of stay seemed to correlate in any age group with severity of reactions. Furthermore, 70% of the admissions were unplanned, which makes the data more applicable to the issues of children admitted for physical trauma.

The posthospitalization data are admittedly somewhat less reliable. Nevertheless, they essentially confirm the in-hospital observations: the experimental groups showed fewer and milder continuing reactions at all ages. Most of those children who continued to show reactions more than 3 months out of hospital were those who had shown the poorest adjustment in the hospital. In addition, 6 months after hospitalization there was a continuing drop in the persistence of severe reactions, with the control groups still showing more difficulty. The new, more humane hospital program clearly was helpful to all the children and their parents, although more so to the more competent children and parents who were better able to take advantage of it.

In examining the nature of the children's reactions Prugh says, "The most common manifestation of disturbance in adaptation at any age level or in either group was that of overt anxiety." How this was manifested differed in each age group. For those children 2 to 4 years of age separation anxiety was the major problem. The reactions were the same in both groups but less frequent and less severe in the experimental group. Crying, fearful behavior, and regression in feeding and toileting were among the symptoms shown. In the 4 to 6 year olds of the control group overt anxiety was still primary but was demonstrated differently. Phobic reactions and obsessive fears were more common, and somatic symptoms (urinary frequency or urgency, vomiting, diarrhea, dizziness, and so forth) were maximal in this age group. As predicted by Anna Freud's exegesis, this age group had particular trouble accepting the dependent needs fostered by nursing care and increased mothering. In general the experimental group showed the same trends but worked through their feelings through aggressive behavior and angry language in play and school situations.

In the 6- to 10-year-old children anxiety was more clearly related to their previous adjustment patterns and less so to specific acute stresses. Their aggression and acting out were under better control than that in the younger children, but they showed some hyperactivity. Conversion symptoms replaced psychosomatic reactions. Denial became a common way of dealing with threatened loss of control, and fantasies of mutilation and death became more evident. Again the experimental group showed fewer and less severe reactions and seemed better able to use the features of the new program to help work through their feelings.

This study clearly indicates that the major variable in children's reactions in hospitalization is their degree of adjustment before entry and particularly their satisfactory and supportive interactions with their parents. Jackson et al.[53] make the same point in their study of children's response to anesthesia and surgery.

The program described by Prugh has long been instituted in most, although not all, major pediatric centers in the country, and most of them have been further enhanced by rooming-in arrangements for parents and by more sophisticated knowledge of, and attention to, the psychologic processes of children. When such programs and processes are instituted in an intelligent and whole-hearted manner, they can, as Solnit[113] suggested in 1960, "create an environment in which certain children for a short time can deal with their physical and emotional needs better than at home. . . . The hospitalization, worked out as a helpful experience for both the child and the mother, has furthered the solution of these problems and promoted the healthy development of the child." Unfortunately, these principles and practices have yet to be applied systematically in a large percentage of the settings in which acutely, severely ill children are hospitalized.

According to Roskies et al.,[98]

Anyone concerned with the psychological trauma that can result from the hospitalization of a young child should, theoretically, be particularly sensitive to the hazards of *emergency* hospitalization . . . [which] contains not only the usual stresses (separation, unfamiliar surroundings, restricted mobility, and so forth) in an intensified fashion, but might also be expected to engender a host of other factors known to be harmful such as lack of preparation and a high anxiety level in parents.*

They go on to point out that

Children who enter via emergency experience a greater trauma, not only because they are sicker and therefore subjected to more painful procedures, but also because they receive less support from the adults around them and, at the same time, are deprived of the techniques that a child this age (8 months to 4 years) would usually use to master anxiety.

Thus the difference between regular and emergency admissions becomes quantitative as well as qualitative with the multiple stresses having a multiplicative effect.

These stresses and limitations are heightened by the frightening environment of the pediatric intensive care unit (PICU), with its high-tech equipment, buzzers, beepers, and flashing lights and with the tension inherent in the presence of numbers of severely ill or damaged children and manifested in the behaviors of the parents and professional personnel. In two related studies Cataldo et al.[19] assessed the state of the patients in such a unit and found that "one third of the patients were conscious and alert but markedly nonengaged with their environment." In the second study they used a hospital staff member to enlist those alert patients in individual activities: "the activity intervention was found to increase attention and engagement

---

*References 38, 39, 57, 89, 97, 121.

and positive affect, and to decrease inappropriate behavior." They suggest "that behavioral assessment procedures can provide an empirical basis for redesigning PICU routines affecting children's psychosocial status, and, thus, complement current procedures designed to provide quality medical care." Certainly it is time some such humane basis was applied to the design of such units for the benefit of the professional staff and the parents as well as the patients.

Surgery

In 1941 Pearson[86] commented, "Surgeons are well aware that operative procedures are associated with surgical shock. . . . Operative procedures are associated also with psychic shock in all children. . . . Physical shock shows its effects immediately. Emotional shock may not express itself openly for some time." A number of psychiatrists and psychoanalysts, among them Deutsch,[27] Jessner and Kaplan,[56] and Levy,[71] working with both adults and children have confirmed that, as Deutsch puts its, "operations performed in childhood leave indelible traces on the psychic life of the individual."

For many years the most common operation performed on children, tonsillectomy has been used as a paradigm of surgical intervention, and its psychologic side effects have been studied by a great many observers. These studies range from the observations of a single child (Robertson[96] of her own daughter) to carefully planned studies of large numbers of children.[55] Robertson's carefully kept diary shows how much can be learned from a single case by a skilled observer and offers evidence that a well-planned and well-handled hospitalization can, in fact, be a strengthening and maturing experience. However, the postscript shows that even so, new events in the child's life can reactivate many of the anxieties originally brought out by the surgical experience.

Jessner et al.[55] found the four main foci of anxiety in their children were separation and the strangeness of the hospital, the anticipation of anesthesia, the operation itself, and the fear of needles. The degree to which each of these was important shifted with age. Separation was most important for children under 5 years of age and decreased thereafter, whereas the fears around the surgery itself, and particularly the anesthesia, increased with age. As in Prugh's study, the only important correlation with serious psychologic re-

actions was the existence of previous neurotic tendencies in the children and their families.

Hoch[49] goes beyond this to point out that "A distinction must be made, however, between elective and emergency surgical procedures. When surgery can be anticipated, there is time to develop coping defense reactions. . . . Traumatic reactions of all kinds are vastly increased in emergencies because there was not enough time for defensive activity to take place." As a possible solution to at least part of this, Edwinson et al.[31] describe a program designed to prepare children psychologically to undergo acute appendectomy. The program, which reduced anxiety (and apparently the level of premedication needed) in the study group, had three main components. In the first a nurse described to the child all parts of the procedure he or she would actually see (not including the actual surgery); second, the actual instruments and items to be used were demonstrated on a doll; and, finally, the child was shown actual photographs of another child undergoing the procedure.

Trauma
Burns

No form of traumatic injury in children has been explored more fully in relation to its psychologic roots and sequelae than burns. Our country has the largest number of fires in the world, and approximately 3000 children a year die of burns. Beyond this "it has been estimated that for each child who dies of a burn, 10 to 15 are burned severely enough to require some degree of medical treatment.[15] Severe burns present as complicated a management problem as any other form of physical injury. Shock, pain, electrolyte imbalance, immobilization, immediate surgical intervention (perhaps for tracheotomy) are all likely to occur. Beyond the initial treatment is a long, tortuous course of continuing procedures, many of them painful. The final result is often disfigurement and limitation of motion secondary to scarring. These events alone would undoubtedly produce severe psychologic after effects, but the course of burned children is further complicated by the evidence that many of them are already psychologically scarred or vulnerable at the time the burn occurs.

Long and Cope[72] were the first to report a high incidence of emotinal maladjustment among burned children and/or a high likelihood that they come from broken homes or families in which one or both parents are mentally ill. Benians[5] and Bernstein et al.[7] agree with this and add the fact that burned children are more likely to come from chaotic families mired in poverty and in crowded and decrepit homes. Seligman et al.[106] following severely burned children in an intensive care unit, point out a common background of preexisting family and individual emotional problems, especially "acting out, aggressive, self-destructive behavior," and state that the injury seemed more related to these problems than to casual accident. The same authors[105] also point out that a number of the parents of burned children had themselves suffered early parental loss. Wright and Fulwiler,[124] comparing the mothers of burned children with a control group, report that those mothers have a low self-perception and a low estimate of their own abilities as mothers.

Galdston,[37] examining the natural history of burns in 100 children, reveals that two thirds of them were burned in their own homes, and most of the rest of them in their own immediate neighborhood. Although 75% of the children were burned by their own actions, 10% were burned deliberately by the actions of adults. Almost all the burns were caused by agents or objects commonly available in the home and represented a combination of the child's curiosity and impetuosity with a lapse of parental attention, which was due either to gross neglect—children left unattended or with immature caretakers—or to parental distraction secondary to overburdening or depression.

These factors, added to the fact that fires often claim more than one victim at a time, lead to the presence of extensive guilt feelings on the part of both children and parents. When the child has been the cause of the fire, the parents may well turn their own guilt feelings into anger reflected back on the burned child. Bernstein et al.[7] suggest an immediate role for the psychiatrist on the burn team as an "agent of clear communication for the staff and family . . . assess(ing) parental reactions . . . and help(ing) them to cope with it." Morse[81] goes further to suggest that it is important to "inform severely burned children that the same fire which caused their injury took the life of a parent or sibling." He recommends that this be done as soon as possible, within a few hours, opening up the subject to help the child air feelings that are better not repressed. Parents need to be helped to understand why this should be done and to participate in the telling.

A number of authors[7,37,43,72] point out that on admission, when the physical care problems are emergent, the psychologic problems are not. The shock, of destruction of skin and nerve endings and of the diversion of psychic energy into physiologic stabilization, results in the child feeling relatively little pain or discomfort at first. The dressings cover damaged areas, and neither patient nor parents are aware of the extent of the damage done. The patient is described by Long and Cope as "reasonable, cooperative, grateful." Soon, however, pain begins and is made worse by any movement, by the removal of dressings, by baths, debridement, and other treatments. The child is now "irritable, whining, uncooperative, aggressive"[72] or screaming and panicking with every dressing change.[73] The removal of the dressings reveals the extent of tissue destruction. This may make some parents so anxious that it is better to limit their visiting for a time, especially around the time of treatment procedures.

There is little doubt that pain, especially from the treatment, is the overriding problem. Generally viewed by the child as punishment for the burn episode itself or for previous misdeeds, it is so all pervasive that it saps the child's energy. Unable to understand the pain and procedures or to communicate the depth of it, the child slips into loneliness and isolation. The fact that the pain is made worse by treatments increases the tension between patient and staff. The child feels betrayed by the parental lack of foresight or actual neglect and can often get less support than usual from the parents' presence.

Such "severely burned children use all their energy—psychic and physical—to survive. In general they are not able to deal with emotional situations or conflicts. They are fortunate (perhaps?) if they have in their coping armamentarium mechanisms of denial, withdrawal, and splitting of the ego, which have gained our respect as survival mechanisms."[105] Regression, that most constant accompaniment of severe illness, is marked in these patients and universally noted. Solnit and Priel[114] state, "Regressive reactions usually are in the service of recovery," and Loomis[73] notes, "Regression into an extremely dependent position seemed to be protective against the more severe disturbance of withdrawal of interest from the outside world and . . . should be permitted." Both agree as to the utility of regression in facilitating both physical and psychologic healing. As the child begins to improve he or she can be helped to deal with the regression by being encouraged to participate in his or her own care and support.[37,114]

Any question that pain is the major cause of difficulty for both patient and staff is dispelled by Nover's study[83] of a 5-year-old boy with a myelomeningocele and paraplegia with no sensation below the waist. Partly because of that defect the child suffered a moderately severe burn on the left lower extremity. However, because of his sensory defect he felt no pain and showed none of the behavioral symptoms described above. He ignored the area of the burn, showed little regression, developed no cycle of anger or aggressive behavior, and was continually cooperative with dressing changes, debridements, and other procedures.

Stoddard[117] uses "The treatment of children aged 1-18 who experienced physical pain from an acute burn and the emotional pain of disfigurement (as) a prototype for treatment of pain and understanding its impact on the child's emotional life." He discusses (with case examples) the way in which children of different ages experience pain and suffering, and he then makes recommendations for age-appropriate treatment in the burn unit.

However, pain is not the only problem. As the child begins baths and debridements he sees himself and reveals to others the extent of skin destroyed. He watches pieces of skin float away. The sight and smell are both painful stimuli, and procedures that bring them about should not be done near mealtimes, since they will interfere with the child's appetite. Children misinterpret procedures, and these are rarely explained by the staff in terms the child can understand. Shorkey and Taylor[110] describe the use of positive reinforcement to help children distinguish between painful treatment procedures (for example, debridement) and pleasurable activities (for example, feeding).

Children develop both positive and negative attachments to nurses and doctors. These feelings are intensified and threatened when staff members rotate off service and new relationships must be formed. Particularly for young children, the need to travel to bath or physical therapy areas with different staff members increases separation anxiety and strains their ability to relate positively to staff members. Especially at high risk in this regard were those children "who could not develop basic trust in other individuals because of a poor experience with their mothers initially."[7] Loomis describes the use of foster grandparents on the ward to help such children relate to a nurturing figure.

In particular these mother substitutes are encouraged to hold and to love the children and to help their mobility by wheeling them around, by feeding them, by reading to them, and by tolerating their aggression and their regression.[73] An important issue for school-age children is the long period away from school that decreases their proficiency and increases their fear of returning to a situation in which they will be far behind. A good school program on the wards can be extremely helpful in planning remediation for the child.

Loomis,[73] Bernstein,[7] and Solnit[114] each discuss the need for the child psychiatrist to be a part of the regular burn treatment team. Bernstein notes,

The psychiatrist can give the burned child a sense of continued relationship with a person who does not cause him pain, does not even wear a white uniform, and who will get him some of the things he needs. The child can also get information and retranslations of what he has been told in a supportive and informative manner.

There is also good evidence that the psychiatrist can help other members of the team—house staff, nurses, even ward cleaning help—deal with their own reactions to caring for burned children.[93]

Following hospitalization there is need for continuing attention to the psychologic effects of burns. Herndon and his associates[47] followed the 12 survivors of "21 children admitted with greater than 80% total body surface area burn . . . One third of the children had excessive fear, regression, and neurotic and somatic complaints, but all of them showed remarkable energy in adapting to their disabilities." They point out that these patients seem to be doing better than one might expect, but that the long-term effects cannot really be known until the children reach adult life and that the final outcomes will depend on a number of intense intervention and reparative programs including long-term psychotherapy. Byrne et al.[18] reviewed the records of 145 of 337 children admitted to a regional burn unit in Canada to examine the factors that might improve the long-term outcomes for such children. Almost all the factors that enhanced social competence in the children were those that might be derived from well-functioning families involved with their communities and their own family members in positive activities.

Society in general and most individuals are intolerant of disfigurement, particularly around the face. Postburn disfigurement consists of discoloration, distortion of structures, and immobility secondary to scarring. Intolerance to people who look different causes many people to shun the disfigured. There is also evidence that many school systems refuse to take back children who have been significantly disfigured by burn injuries. Inasmuch as burns tend to occur along with social and family disorganization, the child and his or her family may have few strengths with which to cope with these sequelae. In a second study, Love and co-workers[74] looked at 42 adults who had been burned in childhood and found that "lower adjustment correlated with visible disfigurement and less peer support rather than with the severity of burn." One result of this long-term problem is the tendency of burn-disfigured patients to become lost to follow-up, to become, in fact, lost in society. Such behavior is, of course, crippling and needs vigorous attention both before and after the children leave the hospital.[6]

Head injury

As early as 1902 Still[116] suggested that injury to the brain in childhood might predispose to the development of a psychiatric disorder. In the years since that time a great many studies have examined the relationship between head trauma and cognitive and psychologic problems as both precursors and sequelae of each other. The center point of the argument has gone back and forth.

The first studies looked primarily at the effect of injury on cognitive abilities. In the early 1930s, when surgery on the brain was still quite problematic, two investigators[87,109] looked at the treatment of subdural hematomas in children both by subdural taps and by craniotomy. They found that the latter led to high mortality but a lower incidence of mental retardation in the survivors and that the former showed the reverse effect. In a more recent study of the same problem Gutierrez and Raimondi[40] achieved similar results, but none of the survivors in either group had an IQ over 98. More recently, Slater and Bassett[111] looked at short-term outcomes of closed head injury (CHI) in adolescents. They compared a group of 33 such patients injured in motor vehicle accidents with 11 orthopedically injured and 35 noninjured adolescents and reported the following:

Immediately after injury patients with CHI performed poorer than their counterparts on measures of intelligence, cognitive flexibility, memory (particularly verbal recall), and verbal fluency. Thus the findings indicate that adolescents who sustain CHI experience pervasive

cognitive deficits immediately after injury that potentially interfere with reentry into their home, school and peer activities.

In the 1950s and 1960s studies first focused a great deal of attention on what was known as the posttraumatic syndrome in children and how it differed from the same syndrome in adults. In 1961 Dillon and Leopold[28] pointed out that adults with concussions have primarily somatic symptoms—headache and vertigo—with irritability as the only common psychologic symptom. Children, on the other hand, have headache to a lesser degree and for a shorter time than adults, but, as least in this study, 47 of the 50 children studied had marked psychologic symptoms of which the most common were anxiety symptoms, sleep disturbances, withdrawn behavior, enuresis and hyperkinesis. Rowbotham et al.[99] Bochner,[13] and Peterson[88] all reported similar findings, although the latter indicated that accident proneness in restless, hyperactive children might be an etiologic selection factor rather than a sequela.

In 1969 in a report on the first 105 cases of a prospective, longitudinal study, Black et al.[12] confirmed that the posttraumatic syndrome in children was different from that in adults. Noting that 22% of their group had developed behavioral symptoms and that "the injury itself . . . appeared to be responsible for the development of or aggravation of symptoms," they state the following:

Although the majority of children remained symptomatically unchanged there was a considerable increase in the incidence of various symptoms or negative behavioral traits. These features may be regarded as characteristic of a "posttraumatic syndrome" subsequent to head injury in children. The four most common problems (designated as "major symptoms") were anger control problems, hyperkinesis, impaired attention, and headache. The following four traits (designated as "minor symptoms") occurred less frequently: discipline problems, hypokinesis, eating problems and sleep disturbances. One or more of the eight symptoms occurred in a given child. Headache was the single most common complaint, but it was usually mild or negligible in degree. Some of the other complaints, notably anger control problems, discipline problems and hyperkinesis constituted serious disturbances.

The picture is further complicated, however, by other groups of studies that examined more carefully the sequelae of head injury in relation to preexisting problems. Dillon and Leopold,[28] for example, noted that many of the children with head injuries came from underprivileged backgrounds. Two extensive Scandinavian studies[48, 100] came to the conclusions that head injuries were more likely to occur in children who already had cognitive or psychologic defects and that such children were more likely to suffer psychologic and behavioral symptoms as a result of head injury. They also suggest that disorganization in the home environment and emotional problems in the parents may also play both an etiologic and prognostic role. In 1958 Harrington and Letemandia[44] reported on a complicated comparison of two groups of children with head injuries. One group consisted of children seen in a psychiatric clinic and found to have a history of head injury. The other group consisted of children who had been admitted to a children's surgical ward with head injury. Although the latter group had the more severe head injuries, they had considerably less psychiatric difficulty. The authors conclude that "many of the chronic symptoms seen were not attributable to the head injuries alone, but were products of other factors, such as the family background, pretraumatic personality and intelligence, and might well have manifested themselves in many cases without head injury."

British psychiatrist Michael Rutter and his associates[101] in 1960 surveyed children 5 to 15 years of age on the Isle of Wight and found that psychiatric disturbances appeared five times more often in children who were brain injured or epileptic than in normal children and three times more often than in children with physical disorders that did not involve the central nervous system. Shaffer,[108] reviewing this and other studies in 1973, concluded much of the same as Still[116] did 71 years earlier: "Children suffering with brain injury or epilepsy run an appreciable increased risk of developing a psychiatric disorder." He then goes on to point out that the reasons for this are not clear and that there is not necessarily a specific connection between the type and severity of injury and the type of psychologic sequela.

Ten years later Rutter looked more extensively at this question but in inner-city London. Attempting to look at the role of head injury in actually causing both cognitive and psychiatric problems, Rutter[16,20,102] and other researchers designed and carried out a careful prospective study of school-age (5 to 14 years of age) children with head injuries. Their study group consisted of 31 children with severe head injuries defined as those resulting in posttraumatic amnesia (PTA) of at least 7 days.

They then matched these with two other groups— 28 children hospitalized for orthopedic injuries and 29 children with less severe head injuries that resulted in PTA of at least 1 hour but less than 1 week. Cognitive deficits were more common in children whose PTA was greater than 2 weeks and nondetectable in those whose PTA was less than 24 hours with somewhat more impairment in performance skills than in verbal ones. Recovery did occur on a descending curve over time. The authors point out that these results do not necessarily predict the same outcomes for younger children, who need to be studied separately. Psychiatric problems were clearly greater in all children with head injuries in a somewhat dose-related fashion: the more severe the injury the more likely the development of disorder. In this case, however, there was a clear influence of premorbid circumstances—behavioral, cognitive, and psychosocial.

In a more recent review of the same subject Duncan and Ment[29] cite four reports[64,69,70,125] that point to traumatic loss of consciousness as a signficant marker for significant sequelae including alterations of intellectual function for "a significant period of time to permanently." Based on these findings they stress the need for early and ongoing counselling of both patient and family. In like manner, Filley et al.,[33] reviewing 53 children and adolescents with closed head injury, also found duration of coma as the single most important factor in determining long-range outcome. They cite coma lasting 1 month as the boundary beyond which all children had persistent cognitive, and likely emotional/behavioral, problems. Using CT scans to determine the location and diffuseness of injury they also concluded that "disordered function of affect and arousal may be caused by injury to frontal systems, either focal cortical injury or damage to the multiple reticular and limbic front connections."

In another attempt to pin down a relationship between location of injury and symptomatology Sollee and Kindlon[112] sorted a group of 32 postinjury children into two groups—17 who were determined to have had injury to the dominant hemisphere (DH) and 15 whose injury had been in the nondominant hemisphere (NDH). Five sources were examined to make the determination of injury location: history, lateralized findings on neurologic exam, EEG, or BEAM, CT or arteriogram, and neuropsychologic assessment. At least three of these had to be available and consistent. For various reasons nine were eliminated, leaving them with 13 in the DH group and 10 in the NDH group; 10 of the 13 and 8 of the 10 scored as having significant problem scores on the Achenbach inventory of behavior. What was of major interest was their finding that "the types of symptoms differ depending on the lateralized site of damage, specifically that DH lesions are associated with externalizing behavior problems" [physical aggression and loss of control, fighting and temper tantrums] "while NDH lesions are associated with internalizing behavior problems" [mood disorders (unhappy, sad, depressed)].

Finally, in the following succinct statement, Craft[23] reported on 300 children with head injury whose preinjury and postinjury behavior patterns were assessed with the Rutter behavior inventory:

The results indicate that children who had a head injury were more likely to have shown abnormal behavior patterns before the accident than the control group. Many children show abnormal behavior both before and after the head injury, but of those who were normal before the accident the incidence of abnormal behavior at 2 years is less than 10 percent. The children exhibiting abnormal postaccident behavior were not only those with the more severe head injuries.

To summarize, in head injuries, as in other kinds of physical trauma in children, children who are already in psychologic difficulty or who come from disorganized homes or environments are more likely than other children to be injured and to suffer serious psychologic sequelae as a result. In this instance, however, in somewhat different fashion from other forms of trauma, the severity of the injury seems also to play some role in determining the likelihood and severity of subsequent psychologic damage, particularly where prolonged coma has been a feature of the posttraumatic period.[75]

Amputation

The loss of part or all of an extremity presents a special set of problems for the child and family to cope with—distortion or corruption of the child's body image. The concept of body image (Hartman,[46] A. Freud,[35] and others) is an important one for physicians to understand. It is, as Kyllonen[63] describes it, "one's subjective perception of self, . . . what we think we look like." This image is built up in infancy and early childhood by the innumerable interactions—tactile, visual, auditory, and so forth—between the infant and his or her environment, both persons and things. In the earliest periods touching, cuddling, rubbing, and other tactile interactions are the most important. Through this process the infant gradually establishes the perimeters of his or her own body. The image developed is not only a psychic one but also a neurophysiologic one on which is based most of the individual's spatial orientation.

Provence and Lipton[91] have shown how the development of body image is distorted by inadequate handling and stimulation in infancy. Kyllonen[63] describes the "disturbances in the integration of body image (which) probably occur in children with physical or neurologic defects (from birth)." In this group of children, for whom amputation is a congenital fact of life, the way in which the child develops a body image depends greatly on the degree of comfort with which the parents can view the defect and handle the child physically as well as psychologically.

For this group of congenital amputees it is important to fit prostheses as early as possible, particularly in the upper extremities. Kyllonen[63] offers the following viewpoint:

Fitting upper extremity amputees at 5, 6, or 7 months is ideal. This is about the time that children are using both hands in palmar prehension, which corresponds to their state of physiological readiness. This is also the time when the pattern of hand use is established, and our experience has been to see the children rapidly acquire a sense of possessiveness toward the prosthesis as if it were literally a part of themselves. If the fitting is delayed they have the opportunity to establish a pattern of use of the stump, which has to be unlearned in order for them to get good use from the prosthesis. . . . The chief criterion used to evaluate progress is the child's maturational state of readiness, not age.

Although early fitting is important in the lower extremities also, "the advantages of bipedal ambulation will quickly outweigh any reluctance to use the device,"[63] and even up to 12 years of age the prosthesis is readily accepted and used.

In instances of traumatic amputation in previously intact children the issues are somewhat different and revolve around the child's need to revise a preexisting body image. How this is managed will depend on many factors including the age and developmental level of the child, the pretraumatic personality of the child, and the parental strengths and reaction to the loss being the most important. In studies of adult amputees Noble et al.[82] and Cone and Hueston[22] both report the almost universal existence of psychologic shock in their patients. Easson[30] and Szasz[119] point out that all patients, whatever the age, will experience grief and mourning after the loss of an extremity. This is, as Kyllonen[63] says,

a normal and necessary adaptive process in which the patient "heals over" his psychic wounds. In this, there will be an inevitable sense of anger and rage at the loss, which is also part of the normal mourning process. Adults who mourn exhibit symptoms of depression, which are clearly understood. Children, however, do not show such signs; we see more often somatic symptoms, regression to more infantile levels, outbursts of temper and the like.

All the authors just cited agree with Kolb,[61] who states that the phenomenon of the phantom limb is universal, even in young children. This fact is masked because many patients, adults and children alike, will not mention their awareness of the sensation unless they are asked about it directly. All recommend that this fact be recognized in the management of amputation and that the patient be assisted in dealing with the phenomenon as soon as possible so that his or her response to it does not become fixed in some unuseful neurotic mode. In dealing with this phenomenon, as well as with the general process of mourning, the role of the parents is critical, and their understanding and support of the child should be actively pursued by the staff.

At the same time the reactions of the staff itself can be most important to the health recovery of the child. Physicians and nurses, especially young ones, can become quite upset themselves by trauma cases, and they need help in understanding their own feelings so that these will not interfere in their care of the child. In a more positive sense, Plank and Horwood[90] describe in detail the process by which a physician or other hospital staff member can work to help the child, family, and staff itself adjust to the preparations for and the reality of amputation. Key aspects of that process include the following:

1. Working with the parents to help them accept the loss and to help them agree to allow themselves and the staff to be open and honest with the child.
2. Helping the child develop a warm and trusting relationship with one particular staff member, particularly one who may not be directly involved in painful treatments.
3. Being honest with the child in explaining, in detail and in ways the child can understand, what has happened and what is going to happen. This may involve using a variety of play tools or other aids to help increase the child's understanding. It also involves respecting the child's sense of time and anticipation and not trying to explain too far in advance to a young child.
4. Accepting the feelings of both parents and child and helping them to work through those feelings to a mature, or maturing, acceptance of the reality. In this respect it is important to note that the authors state, "Our methods and goals were different from a treatment situation in a psychiatric setting. We had to work with this child not in individual interviews, but as part of a group program for many children. . . . Our work was geared to the needs immediately resulting from the illness and its management, but not to uncovering the child's deeper emotional problems." Although more intensive work may occasionally be necessary with some children in some circumstances, these limited goals of psychologic management are more likely to be appropriate most of the time in working with traumatized children in general hospital settings.

In discussing this same approach, Kyllonen notes that such preparation does not, in fact, require the services of a psychiatrist, but merely of a physician who will take the time to be available for the child and make the child as fully aware of procedures as possible. He recommends asking what the child thinks is going to happen as a good way to expose misconceptions that can then be handled. Finally, he issues a strong warning against the casual conversations that occur at children's bedsides during rounds or other times, in which staff members unfeelingly discuss the child's condition and care as though the child were not there or could not understand.

Although some of these authors have suggested that such injuries can be managed without intensive psychiatric intervention, modern practice and knowledge indicate that some form of therapy is useful to both child and parents, especially in the posthospital period. In particular this is true for reducing later feelings of guilt and for shortening the period of disability and dependency that often follows amputation, even when followed quickly by the application of a prosthesis.

Psychosocial Antecedents of Accidental Injury

The discussion to this point has highlighted most of the significant issues that might be considered in any type of injury in children. Consideration of other specific types will add little to these issues. The following three major themes present themselves for consideration in any evaluation of the psychologic impact of a given injury on a given child:

1. Age and developmental level of the child
2. Relative seriousness of the injury
3. Preexisting personality and family and environmental relationships of the injured child

The first two already have been discussed in this chapter; the third requires further discussion. For whatever reasons it seems abundantly clear that some children (and adults) are more likely to become injured than others. However, it has been difficult to determine why that is so, and arguments rage back and forth in the accidental injury literature. For a long time the search for a cause focused on identifying a child's individual characteristics that caused him or her to be more susceptible to accidental injury. This concept was called "accident proneness," a term coined by Farmer and Chambers in 1926[32] and first introduced into the pediatric literature by Bakwin and Bakwin[2] in 1948. In one attempt to summarize this syndrome Cummings and Molnar[24] in 1974 proposed a seven-point list that characterized both the personal and family attributes associated with the child who has recurrent accidents. They developed this list from their own work and that of a number of others.* Much of their list still pertains, but other parts of it now seem too simplistic. McKenna[80] is cited by Bijur[10] as pointing out that

Rather than a single, well-defined theory, accident proneness has been variously conceptualized as a unitary personality characteristic, a general cross-situational behavioral characteristic, and, alternatively, a combination of multiple psychologic factors that lead to increased accident risk. What is shared by all conceptualizations of accident proneness is the importance of the role played by personal factors in accident causation.

Jones[58] prefers the term "accident repeater," defined as "(a child) who has a least three accidents that come to medical attention within a year." Although still describing the child as having a "sus-

ceptible personality, (in whom) a tendency for accident repetition may be due to a breakdown in adjustment due to a stressful environment," he does at least add questions about the environment. Cohen[21] also prefers the term "accident repeater" and lists age, sex, behavior, personality, and also socioeconomic background as risk factors.

The most thorough review of the concept is that of Langley,[67] who in his very title ("The 'Accident-Prone' Child—the Perpetration of a Myth") makes his bias quite clear. He cites a number of reviews that criticize the earlier studies as "undisciplined" and that point out the fallacies in much of the statistical work on this subject including (1) faulty assumptions, (2) misunderstanding the nature of random distribution, and (3) failure to take into account the statistical problems of sample size when dealing with rarely occurring events. He cites Sass and Crook[103] who suggest that the concept of accident proneness "suits those who wish to find fault with the victim and thus decrease the probability of questions concerning hazards." He also quotes Klein[59] as saying that the concept of accident proneness is counterproductive in two ways: "First, it diverts our attention away from the removal or modification of environmental hazards—hazards that are usually implicated directly in injuries attributed to accident proneness. Second, it diverts research resources from relevant and well designed studies to further wild goose chases." Langley concludes by stating, "In view of the mythical nature of the "accident-prone" person, the lack of utility of the concept, and the inhibitory effects it may have on the adoption of effective preventive strategies, the use of the term "accident prone" should be given the last rites."

In place of this concept more recent work has used the process and methods of epidemiology to approach the question of psychosocial causality in childhood accidents. Guyer and Gallagher[41] suggest that "injuries are no more likely to occur by chance than are diseases." They propose the following agent-host-environment model, in which

the agent of injury is the form of energy that damages body tissues . . . kinetic energy . . . thermal energy. . . . The host, or injured individual can be described not only by age and sex, but also by developmental level. . . . Finally, the environment includes not only the physical situation in which injuries occur, but also the psychosocial one. . . . Injuries occur when the elements of host, agent, and environment come together in a critical manner and within a precise time period.

---

*References 1, 36, 62, 66, 76, 123.

However, many studies are still looking at the individual characteristics of the child albeit in a more disciplined way. Nyman[84] undertook a prospective study of "the role of infant temperament in predicting the incidence of hospitalization and accidents of children under the age of five." He obtained temperament measurements on 1855 infants 6 to 8 months of age, of whom 270 were later hospitalized for illness or accident. A disproportionate number of these had been characterized as difficult, with the accident group differing from the illness group by showing more activity and more difficulty with new situations. McCormick and her colleagues[79] also looked at injuries in the first year of life. In a sample of 4989 infants they found that 8.6% had an injury in that first year but relatively few of the injuries were severe. The major risk factor in their sample was the development of walking. There was also a slightly increased risk associated with young and isolated mothers.

Male sex is clearly a risk factor—boys are more commonly and severely injured than girls at all ages. Rivara et al.[95] analyzed data from 197,516 consumer injuries to show that sex differences in injury rates begin as early as the first year of life in most kinds of injuries and the differences get larger with age. Bauchner et al.[3] add to this that injury among teenagers is more common among males and that the risk of injury is heightened by the use of alcohol and drugs.

In a different approach Bijur et al. used data obtained in parent interviews by health visitors from a British 1970 birth cohort of almost 12,000 children for three epidemiologic studies. In the first study[9] they examined the social and behavioral characteristics of the children at 5 years of age to look for risk factors. Aggressive behavior was the single most powerfully associated factor. Overactivity was mostly associated with aggressiveness but seemed independently associated with less severe injuries. In the second study the same group studied whether the occurrence of earlier injury could predict later injury. Using data on the 10,394 children from the original cohort who could still be found at 10 years, they found that children who were reported to have had three or more separate injury events before 5 years of age were approximately six times more likely to have three or more injuries between 5 and 10 years. Injuries requiring hospitalization before 5 years of age similarly predicted likelihood of hospitalization later, only at a lower level, 2.5 times. Although this study sug-

gested earlier injury as the best predictor of late injury, other factors—"male sex, aggressive behavior, young maternal age, many older, and few younger siblings"—were also risk determinants.[10] Finally, the same group using the same data find that the risk of serious injury between 5 and 10 years increased directly with aggression and overactivity scores at age 5. Once again the aggressive behavior seemed the more important component of the risk factor. Although there was some tendency for girls with aggressive behavior also to have more injuries, the same degree of association did not occur. This time the authors[11] also report that

Highly significant linear trends indicated that levels of aggression and overactivity were higher in children of low socioeconomic status and who lived in crowded and deteriorated housing, in children from families that moved frequently, in children whose mothers were employed full time and who were distressed and unhappy, and in children who had high rates of hospitalization for causes not related to injuries.

Davidson[25] has carefully reviewed 13 studies that investigated the relationship between hyperactivity and antisocial behavior and injury. He finds design and methodologic problems with most of the studies and concludes that "the relationship between hyperactivity and injury is still under question" but that "there would appear to be general agreement that antisocial behavior (aggressiveness and control problems) emerges as a definite risk factor for injury." It is possible that hyperactivity is a risk factor only in its association with aggressive behavior.

Other studies have focused more on the families. Larson and Pless[68] studied 918 children who were 82% of a 3-year-old birth cohort. For accidents serious enough to require visits to a physician or treatment, they found that three maternal factors were dominant as risk factors. These involved mothers who were single, who were unemployed, and who smoked. "The presence of all three (of these), as well as the absence of a younger sibling, increases the probability of an injury from 20% to over 60%."

In another study of the same British cohort examined by Bijur, Wadsworth et al.[122] found that children living in step-families were 62% more likely to have had two or more accidents and children living in both step-families and one-parent families were almost twice as likely to have been admitted to a hospital for an accidental injury. Davidson et al.,[26] using a cohort in South Wales, examined the hospital records of 951 children from 5 to 8 years of age. They did not find an expected relationship between overactive behavior and decreased concentration (ADDH syndrome) and injury, but they did find an association between increased injury risk and male sex and children with discipline problems. The latter in particular increased the risk of injury by one third. In this they declare agreement with Bijur and her associates.

Brown and Davidson,[17] in another study of British children, focused mainly on the parents when examining the injury factors of children of a random sample of 458 women in inner-city London. In this case the accident risk was strongly associated with both working-class status and mental illness (most often depression) in the mothers. Klonoff,[60] looking specifically at children with head injuries, found that he could not sustain the old sense of "accident proneness," but rather that his results pointed more at the background characteristics of the parents, specifically congested and poor housing, marital instability, and lower occupational status of the fathers.

Schor[104] goes even further to report that in data from 693 families a small percentage of them accounted for most of the injuries:

Individual members of the families tended to have similar rates of injury, and these rates are stable over time. Individual accident experience is influenced by the family to which one belongs. . . . Patterns of frequent injury should be regarded as possible evidence of poor functioning of a family as a social support system.

Horwitz and her colleagues,[50] in a prospective follow-up study of 532 children in a prepaid health plan, found four factors associated with risk of injury: (1) high activity in the child, (2) high use of pediatric services for noninjury-related problems during the follow-up period, (3) occurrence of a previous injury in the year before the index injury, and (4) a negative attitude toward health care providers by the mother. (Numbers *2* and *3* in addition to the mother working more than 15 hours a week outside the home and also reporting more life stress events during the observation period were related to more severe injuries.) Finally, Marsh and Channing[77] report that, even among children living in the same urban area, deprived children have more psychological illness and more hospital admissions for illness and accidents. Their families were characterized by unemployment, social class IV or V, more children, maternal mental illness, parental smoking and alcohol use, crowded housing, and poor diet.

It seems quite clear that the old concept of the accident-prone individual, as most of us have understood it and used it, is outdated and no longer deserves room in the literature or in our clinical thinking. Nevertheless, the accumulated evidence seems to point out that certain characteristics (specifically male sex, aggressive behavior or conduct disorders, poor impulse control, and, perhaps, overactive physical behavior) are found more often in those individuals who tend to have more accidents. It also seems clear that these factors as well as the existence of preinjury cognitive or psychological problems predispose to worse cognitive and psychologic sequelae of injury. As Hartman[46] pointed out, "Each individual shows a different capacity to adapt to the stress of injury; some regain social integration, well-being and productivity, others fail to adapt and manifest a chronic psychogenic disability or residual maladaptive response." Inasmuch as these findings seem to emerge as early as the first year of life, it seems not unfair to suggest that some biologic neurologic defect, whether genetic or due to intrauterine or birth injury, underlies this. More research is needed to support this suggestion, and it may be forthcoming with the use of the newer, noninvasive tools for studying the central nervous system.

It is essential not to ignore the other compelling evidence that indicates that a number of psychosocial and physical environmental factors are also involved in predisposition to injury. The large epidemiologic studies fail to agree exactly as to which characteristics are the most critical in this relationship. These differences may be due to differences in the cultural attributes of the samples, the differing definitions used by different investigators, the different methodologies, or other factors. When examined carefully, however, all the results seem to agree that families who are more disorganized than most (whether because of single parentage, mental illness, or substance abuse in the parents— stress factors that make it more difficult for them to supervise the daily activities of their children), who live in areas where room for children to play safely is less available and where environmental hazards are more available, and who have more accidents themselves are more likely to have children who have more accidental injuries.

More work needs to be, and will be, done to define these issues more precisely. In the meantime there is enough, and clear enough, evidence for us to begin to plan much more accurately how to prevent accidents and thereby reduce the most important source of disability and death in children of all ages. It is not blaming the children or the families to point out these vulnerabilities; we can only blame ourselves if we fail to act on the increasingly clear evidence presented.

SUMMARY

The accumulation of data in recent years has elucidated and clarified many of the issues relating to the psychologic implications of physical trauma in children. We can no longer claim as Tomlinson[120] and Mattson[78] asserted in the 1970s that the lack of research and discussion of the subject has hampered the care and recovery of patients with physical trauma. Mattson has offered a physiologic analogy for the psychologic implications: "The physiologic outcome of local healing has three alternatives: a) normal or satisfactory repair; b) inadequate or retarded repair; and c) overhealing by scar and contracture. These alternatives are self-explanatory and are directly applicable to psychological healing." This conceptualization has the potential to help physicians and surgeons comprehend more clearly the need to pay more attention to the psychologic implications of their work.

In reporting to a workshop in children's trauma in 1970, Haller,[47] a pediatric surgeon, made almost the *only* reference of the entire meeting to psychologic issues:

Finally, serious injuries in an immature child may have disastrous effects upon his emotional well-being at this impressionable age. The terror of separation from familiar faces is greatly magnified by the usual busy and impassionate environment of a major emergency room. Serious emotional aftereffects are not uncommon from even minor injuries which are treated under threatening circumstances by physicians who are not aware of this important additional insult to a child.

In their work on the PICU, Cataldo et al.[19] conclude the following:

The necessity for an ICU stay and the primary objective of medical procedures . . . are not easily communicated to children; this is especially true for those children whose critical care has had an acute onset and who have not been prepared for the ICU admission (e.g., trauma cases). For children in a PICU, well-programmed contingency procedures can be an effective method for mitigating the unintended results of quality medical care, and consequently help to avoid converting a medical triumph into a psychological trauma.

In furtherance of this point a study at the New England Medical Center by Harris et al.[45] looked at 54 children and their families a year after their discharge for serious multisystem injuries. They found emotional and cognitive problems in the children, emotional problems in the siblings, marital disturbances, and serious financial problems arising from the costs of medical care. They concluded the following:

There is a hidden morbidity in pediatric trauma. It manifests years after injury not only as physical disability, but also as changes in cognition, personality, behavior, and as family stress. Since success in pediatric trauma care is the restoration of the child as nearly as possible to his premorbid state these data suggest that more attention and resources should be directed to the late consequences of multisystem injury in children.

If we can no longer say that the psychologic roots and sequelae of trauma are largely neglected, we still cannot doubt that management of the psychosocial aspects of physical trauma lags well behind management of the medical and surgical aspects. This is not because they are less important or because we do not know how to manage them. The knowledge and skills needed to ameliorate those "serious emotional aftereffects" are available in the hands of many children's pediatric and mental health professionals. The blame must lie in the failure of communication between and among health care professionals, each of whom has his or her eye on only one part of the process. It is unconscionable, and may soon be considered malpractice, for this fractionation of services to stand in the way of better services for children.

The psychologic and physical aspects of the child have been divided too long by disciplinary divisions. For the good of children and their parents those aspects must be brought together. This will not happen easily or casually. Careful planning is required to integrate into the sophisticated physical care of children a humanistic environment and service approach that arises out of the knowledge of developmental issues, the psychologic life of the child, and the needs of their families. Such planning is long overdue. If undertaken it promises to provide the most fruitful approach in the near future to relieving suffering and improving healing.

REFERENCES

1. Ackerman NW and Chidester L: "Accidental" self-injury in children, Arch Pediatr 53:711, 1936.
2. Bakwin RM and Bakwin H: Psychologic aspects of pediatrics, J Pediatr 32:749, 1948.
3. Bauchner H et al: Alcohol, drugs, and nonfatal teenage injuries, Am J Dis Child 142:387, 1988.
4. Beautrais AL, Fergusson DM, and Shannon FT: Childhood accidents in a New Zealand birth cohort, Aust Paediatr J 18:238, 1982.
5. Benians RC: A child psychiatrist looks at burned children and their families, Guy's Hospital Reports 123:149, 1974.
6. Bernstein NR: Disfigurement and social role: the living reproach, Delivered at the Yale Child Study Center, 1976.
7. Bernstein NR, Sanger S, and Fras I: The functions of the child psychiatrist in the management of severely burned children, Am J Child Psychiatry 8:620, 1969.
8. Beverly BI: The effect of illness upon emotional development, J Pediatr 8:533, 1936.
9. Bijur PE, Stewart-Brown S, and Butler N: Child behavior and accidental injury in 11,966 preschool children, Am J Dis Child 140:487, 1986.
10. Bijur PE, Golding J, and Haslum M: Persistence of occurrence of injury: can injuries of preschool children predict injuries of school-aged children? Pediatrics 82:707, 1988.
11. Bijur PE et al: Behavioral predictors of injury in school-age children, Am J Dis Child 142:1307, 1988.
12. Black P et al: The posttraumatic syndrome in children: characteristics and incidence. In Walker AE, Caveness WF, and Critchley M, editors: The late effects of head injury, Springfield, Ill, 1969, Charles C. Thomas.
13. Bochner AK: Psychiatric evaluation of posttraumatic syndrome of head injury. Western Reserve University, Law-Medicine Center: Head: law-medicine problem, Cleveland, 1957, Multi-Stat Company.
14. Brazelton TB: Neonatal behavioral assessment scale, Spastics International Medical Publications, Philadelphia, 1973, JB Lippincott Co.
15. Brodie B and Matern S: Emotional aspects in the care of a severely burned child, Int Nurs Rev 14:19, 1967.
16. Brown G et al: A prospective study of children with head injuries. III. Psychiatric sequelae, Psychol Med. 11:63, 1981.
17. Brown GW and Davidson S: Social class, psychiatric disorder of mother, and accidents to children, Lancet I:378, 1978.
18. Byrne C et al: The social competence of children following burn injury: a study of resilience, J Burn Care Rehabil 7:247, 1986.
19. Cataldo MF et al: Behavioral assessment for pediatric intensive care units, J Appl Behav Anal 12:83, 1979.
20. Chadwick O et al: A prospective study of children with head injuries. II. Cognitive sequelae, Psychol Med 11:49, 1981.
21. Cohen GJ: Factors that may put children at risk for accidents, Pediatric News 17:29, 1983.
22. Cone J and Hueston JT: Psychological aspects of hand injury, Med J Aust 1:104, 1974.
23. Craft AW: Head injury in children, Arch Dis Child 49:827, 1974.
24. Cummings V and Molnar G: Traumatic amputation in children resulting from "train-electric burn" injuries: a socioenvironmental syndrome? Arch Phys Med Rehabil 55:71, 1974.
25. Davidson LL: Hyperactivity, antisocial behavior, and childhood injury: a critical analysis of the literature, J Dev Behav Pediatr 8:335, 1987.
26. Davidson LL, Hughes SJ, and O'Connor PA: Preschool behavior problems and subsequent risk of injury, Pediatrics 82:644, 1988.
27. Deutsch H: Some psychoanalytic observation in surgery, Psychosom Med 4:105, 1942.
28. Dillon H and Leopold RL: Children and the postconcussion syndrome, JAMA 175:110, 1961.
29. Duncan CC and Ment L: Management of pediatric head injury, Conn Med 48:282, 1984.
30. Easson WM: Body-image and self-image in children, Arch Gen Psychiatry 4:619, 1961.
31. Edwinson M, Arnbjornsson E, and Ekman R: Psychologic preparation program for children undergoing acute appendectomy, Pediatrics 82:30, 1988.
32. Farmer E and Chambers EG: A psychological study of individual differences in accident rate, Medical Research Council—Industrial Fatigue Research Board, Report #38, 1926.
33. Filley CM et al: Neurobehavioral outcome after closed head injury in childhood and adolescence, Arch Neurol 44:194, 1987.
34. Freud A: The role of bodily illness in the mental life of children, Psychoanal Study Child 7:69, 1952.
35. Freud A: Normality and pathology in childhood, New York, 1965, International Universities Press.
36. Fuller EM: Injury-prone children, Am J Orthopsychiatry 18:708, 1948.
37. Galdston R: The burning and healing of children, Psychiatry 35:57, 1972.
38. Gofman H, Buckman W, and Schade GH: The child's emotional response to hospitalization, Am J Dis Child 93:157, 1957.
39. Gofman H, Buckman W, and Schade GH: Parents' emotional response to hospitalization, Am J Dis Child 93:629, 1957.
40. Gutierrez FA and Raimondi AJ: Acute subdural hematoma in infancy and childhood, Childs Brain 1:269, 1975.
41. Guyer B and Gallagher SS: An approach to the epidemiology of childhood injuries, Pediatr Clin North Am 32:5, 1985.
42. Haller JA: Trauma workshop report: trauma in children, J Trauma 10:1052, 1970.
43. Hamburg DA, Hamburg B, and deGoza S; Adaptive problems and mechanisms in severely burned patients, Psychiatry 16:1, 1953.
44. Harrington JA and Letemandia FJJ: Persistent psychiatric disorders after head injuries in children, J Mental Sci 104:1205, 1958.
45. Harris BH et al: The hidden morbidity of pediatric trauma, J Pediatr Surg 24:103, 1989.
46. Hartman H: Ego psychology and the problem of adaptation, New York, 1958, International Universities Press.
47. Herndon DN et al: The quality of life after major thermal injury in children: an analysis of 12 survivors with ≥ 80% total body, 70% third-degree burns, J Trauma 26:609, 1986.

48. Hjern B and Nylander I: Acute head injuries in children: traumatology, therapy, and prognoses, Acta Pediatr Scand [Suppl] 152:67, 1963.

49. Hoch S: Problems associated with surgical emergencies and brief elective procedures. In Oremland EK and Oremland JD, editors: The effects of hospitalization on children, Springfield, Ill, 1973, Charles C. Thomas.

50. Horwitz S et al: Determinants of pediatric injuries, Am J Dis Child 142:605, 1988.

51. Huschka M and Ogden O: The conduct of a pediatric prophylaxis clinic, J Pediatr 12:6, 1938.

52. Jackson EB: Treatment of the young child in hospital, Am J Orthopsychiatry 12:56, 1942.

53. Jackson K et al: Problem of emotional trauma in hospital treatment of children, JAMA 149:1536, 1952.

54. Jessner L: Some observations on children hospitalized during latency. In Jessner L and Pavenstedt E, editors: Dynamic psychopathology in childhood, New York, 1959, Grune & Stratton.

55. Jessner L, Blom GE, and Waldfogel S: Emotional implications of tonsillectomy and adenoidectomy in children, Psychoanal Study Child 7:126, 1952.

56. Jessner L and Kaplan S: Reaction of children to tonsillectomy and adenoidectomy—preliminary report. In Senn MJE, editor: Problems of infancy and childhood, New York, 1949, Josiah Macy Jr. Foundation.

57. Johnson R: How parents' attitudes affect children's illnesses, Bull Inst Child Study 17:5, 1955.

58. Jones JG: The child accident repeater: a review, Clin Pediatr 19:284, 1980.

59. Klein D: Societal influences on childhood accidents, Accid Anal Prev 12:275, 1980.

60. Klonoff H: Head injuries in children: predisposing factors, accident conditions, accident proneness, and sequelae, Am J Public Health 61:2405, 1971.

61. Kolb LC: The painful phantom, Springfield, Ill, 1954, Charles C. Thomas.

62. Kroll V: Personality characteristics of accident repeating children, J Abnorm Soc Psychol 48:99, 1953.

63. Kyllonen RR: Body image and reaction to amputation, Conn Med 28:19, 1964.

64. Lanfin TW: Measuring the outcome from head injuries, J Neurosurg 48:673, 1978.

65. Langford WS: Physical illness and convalescence: their meaning to the child, J Pediatr 33:242, 1948.

66. Langford WS et al: Pilot study of childhood accidents, Pediatrics 11:405, 1953.

67. Langley J: The "accident-prone" child—the perpetration of a myth, Aust Paediatr J 18:243, 1982.

68. Larson CP and Pless IB: Risk factors for injury in a 3-year-old birth cohort, Am J Dis Child 142:1052, 1988.

69. Levin HS and Eisenberg HM: Neuropsychological outcome of closed head injury in children and adolescents, Childs Brain 5:281, 1979.

70. Levin HS et al: Long-term neuropsychological outcome of closed head injury, J Neurosurg 50:412, 1979.

71. Levy DM: Psychic trauma of operation in children, Am J Dis Child 69:7, 1945.

72. Long RT and Cope O: Emotional problems of burned children, N Engl J Med 264:1121, 1961.

73. Loomis WG: Management of children's emotional reactions to severe body damage (burns), Clin Pediatr 9:362, 1970.

74. Love B et al: Adult psychosocial adjustment following childhood injury: the effect of disfigurement, J Burn Care Rehabil 8:280, 1987.

75. Lundholm J, Jepsen BN, and Thornval G: The late neurological, psychological, and social aspects of severe traumatic coma, Scand J Rehabil Med 7:97, 1975.

76. Marcus IM et al: Interdisciplinary approach to accident patterns in children, Monogr Soc Res Child Dev 25:2, 1960.

77. Marsh GN and Channing DM: Comparison in use of health services between a deprived and an endowed community, Arch Dis Child 62:392, 1987.

78. Mattson EI: Psychological aspects of severe physical injury and its treatment, J Trauma 15:217, 1975.

79. McCormick MC, Shapiro S, and Starfield BH: Injury and its correlates among 1-year-old children, Am J Dis Child 135:159, 1981.

80. McKenna FP: Accident proneness: a conceptual analysis, Accid Anal Prev 15:65, 1983.

81. Morse TS: On talking to bereaved burned children, J Trauma, 11:894, 1971.

82. Noble D, Price DB, and Gilder R Jr: Psychiatric disturbances following amputation, Am J Psychiatry 110:609, 1954.

83. Nover R: Pain and the burned child, J Am Acad Child Psychiatry 12:499, 1973.

84. Nyman G: Infant temperament, childhood accidents, and hospitalization, Clin Pediatr 26:398, 1987.

85. Parmelee AH Jr: Children's illnesses: their beneficial effects on behavioral development, Child Dev 57:1, 1986.

86. Pearson GHJ: Effect of operative procedures on the emotional life of the child, Am J Dis Child 62:716, 1941.

87. Peet MM and Kahn EA: Subdural hematoma in infants, JAMA 98:1851, 1932.

88. Peterson BH: Psychiatric sequelae of head injuries, Med J Aust 1:689, 1956.

89. Plank EN: Working with children in hospital, Cleveland, 1962, Western Reserve University.

90. Plank EN and Horwood C: Leg amputation in a four-year old: reactions of the child, her family, and the staff. Psychoanal Study Child 16:405, 1961.

91. Provence S and Lipton RC: Infants in institutions, New York, 1962, International Universities Press.

92. Prugh DG et al: A study of the emotional reactions of children and families to hospitalization and illness, Am J Orthopsychiatry 23:70, 1953.

93. Quinby S and Bernstein NR: Identity problems and the adaptation of nurses to severely burned children, Am J Psychiatry 128:90, 1971.

94. Ravenscroft K: Psychiatric consultation to the child with acute physical trauma, Am J Orthopsychiatry 52:298, 1982.

95. Rivara FP et al: Epidemiology of childhood injuries. II. Sex differences in injury rates, Am J Dis Child 136:502, 1982.

96. Robertson J: A mother's observations on the tonsillectomy of her four-year-old daughter, Psychoanal Study Child 11:410, 1956.

97. Robertson J: Young children in hospital, New York, 1958, Basic Books.

98. Roskies E et al: Emergency hospitalization of young children: some neglected psychological considerations, Med Care 13:570, 1975.

99. Rowbotham GF et al: Analysis of 1400 cases of acute injury to head, Brit Med J 1:726, 1954.
100. Rune V: Acute head injuries in children. A retrospective epidemiologic, child psychiatric, and electroencephalographic study of primary school children in Umea. Acta Paediatr Scand [Suppl] 209:3, 1970.
101. Rutter M, Graham PJ, and Yule W: A neuropsychiatric study in childhood. Clinics in developmental medicine, no 35/36, London, 1970, SIMP with Heineman.
102. Rutter M et al: A prospective study of children with head injuries. I. Design and methods, Psychol Med 10:633, 1980.
103. Sass R and Crook G: Accident proneness: science or nonscience, Int J Health Serv 11:175, 1981.
104. Schor EL: Unintentional injuries, Am J Dis Child 141:1280, 1987.
105. Seligman R, Macmillan BG, and Carroll SS: The burned child: a neglected area of psychiatry, Am J Psychiatry 128:84, 1971.
106. Seligman R, Carroll SS, and Macmillan BG; Emotional responses of burned children in a pediatric intensive care unit, Psychiatry Med 3:59, 1972.
107. Senn MJE: Emotional aspects of convalescence, The Child 10:24, 1945.
108. Shaffer D: Psychiatric aspects of brain injury in childhood: a review, Dev Med Child Neurol 15:211, 1973.
109. Sherwood D: Chronic subdural hematoma in infants, Am J Dis Child 39:980, 1930.
110. Shorkey CT and Taylor JE: Management of maladaptive behavior of a severely burned child, Child Welfare 52:543, 1973.
111. Slater EJ and Bassett SS: Adolescents with closed head injuries: a report of initial cognitive deficits, Am J Dis Child 142:1048, 1988.
112. Sollee ND and Kindlon DJ: Lateralized brain injury and behavior problems in children, J Abnorm Child Psychol 15:479, 1987.
113. Solnit AJ: Hospitalization: an aid to physical and psychological health in childhood, Am J Dis Child 99:155, 1960.
114. Solnit AJ and Priel B: Psychological reactions to facial and hand burns in young men, Psychoanal Study Child 30:549, 1975.
115. Spitz RA: Hospitalism: an inquiry into the genesis of psychiatric conditions in early childhood, Psychoanal Study Child 1:53, 1945.
116. Still GF: Some abnormal psychical conditions in children, Lancet I:1008, 1902.
117. Stoddard FJ: Coping with pain: a developmental approach to treatment of burned children, Am J Psychiatry 139:736, 1982.
118. Stone LJ, Smith HT, and Murphy LB, editors: The competent infant, New York, 1973, Basic Books.
119. Szasz TS: Pain and pleasure, New York, 1957, Basic Books.
120. Tomlinson WK: Psychiatric complications following severe trauma, J Occup Med 16:454, 1974.
121. Vaughan GF: Children in hospital, Lancet 272:1117, 1957.
122. Wadsworth J et al: Family type and accidents in preschool children, J Epidemiol Community Health 37:100, 1983.
123. Wheatley GM and Richardson SA: Social approaches to research in childhood accidents, Pediatrics 25:343, 1960.
124. Wright L and Fulwiler R: Long-range emotional sequelae of burns: effects on children and their mothers, Pediatr Res 8:931, 1974.
125. Young B et al: Early prediction of outcome in head-injured patients, J Neurosurg 52:300, 1981.
126. Zuckerman BS and Duby JC: Developmental approach to injury prevention, Pediatr Clin North Am 32:17, 1985.

8

Imaging of Childhood Trauma

Nancy S. Rosenfield, Marc S. Keller, and Richard I. Markowitz

Since the previous edition of this book there has been a technical revolution in the methods of imaging children. Refinements have been made in nuclear medicine imaging, and ultrasound (US) with Doppler, computed tomography (CT), and magnetic resonance imaging (MRI) have been introduced. We will elaborate on the advantages and disadvantages of each of these imaging modalities, as well as conventional radiography, and highlight the role of each in imaging injured children.

HEAD

It is known that the presence or absence of skull fracture correlates poorly with the extent of a child's brain injury.[59] Roberts and Shopfner[59] found that the discovery of a linear skull fracture did not affect the child's treatment. Therefore plain skull radiographs need not be taken routinely on children with head trauma. The only possible exception to this is if there is a clinical suspicion of child abuse and a description of injury is needed as evidence (see chapter 10). CT has enabled us to look directly at the brain to detect abnormalities. In addition, bone windows of the CT scan demonstrate depressed skull fractures but may miss small linear fractures, which as noted above, are not clinically significant. Therefore children who are clinically stable and have neurologic findings should have a CT scan.[12,59] Intravenous contrast is usually not used for CT scanning in acute injury so that blood may be detected.[48] CT may show evidence of skull fractures (Fig. 8-1), but it also can demonstrate epidural bleeding, acute subdural bleeds, subarachnoid bleeding, intracerebral hemorrhages, and cerebral contusions.[85] Hemorrhagic contusions are most frequently found and may lead to focal neurologic deficits[86] (Figs. 8-2 and 8-3), diffuse swell-

ing,[83] diffuse infarction of the white matter,[84] focal decreased densities representing edema or early infarction, and hydrocephalus[86] (Figs. 8-2 and 8-3).

The CT scan may be normal in some children with brain injury, and it was found to be normal in 10% to 26% of children with brain injuries in different series.[12,43] Although some studies have shown that the findings on a CT scan correlate with the clinical outcome of the child,[42,77,87] others have demonstrated no detectable correlation.[58,70] CT has been found very helpful for follow-up of brain-injured children and has elucidated the temporal sequence of evolution of pathologic changes. In patients who remained unconscious, 50% to 75%

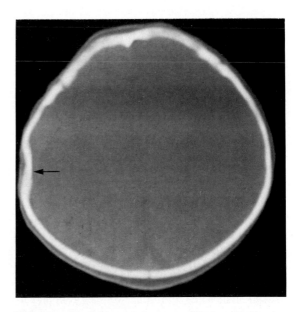

Fig. 8-1   Skull fracture shown on CT scan. Bone windows from a CT examination of the brain demonstrate a depressed fracture *(arrow)* in a 9 month old who fell from a changing table.

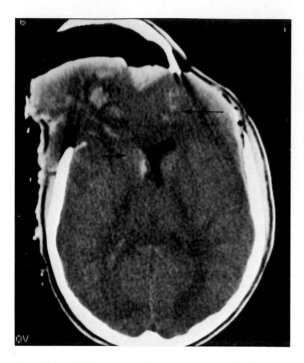

Fig. 8-2   CT demonstration of severe head injury. A 16-year-old boy was hit by an automobile and suffered a severe skull fracture and brain injury. Note the hemorrhage *(arrow)* and mass effect on the frontal horn of the right lateral ventricle *(crossed arrow).*

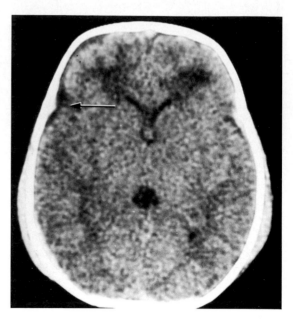

Fig. 8-3   Small chronic subdural hematoma. CT shows an extraaxial low attenuation collection in the right frontal region of the brain *(arrow)* in a 1-month-old baby who had been abused.

of the CT scans showed evidence of an extracerebral cerebrospinal fluid density over one or both frontal lobes 10 to 30 days after the trauma. Subsequently a generalized ventricular enlargement with sulcal dilatation suggested brain atrophy. In one half of these cases the CT scan may show normal findings in 9 to 12 weeks.[12] Follow-up CT scans have also been found helpful to determine which children need intracranial pressure monitors.[40,71,78]

One limitation of CT is that small hematomas close to the bone may be difficult to visualize. However, the overall superiority of CT in detecting the above listed abnormalities has been demonstrated and has superceded more invasive methods of brain imaging. Zimmerman[86] found an 84% decrease in the use of angiography, a 58% decrease in surgical intervention, and a 24% decrease in the use of plain skull films, as well as a significant decreased mortality, since the advent of brain CT.

Recently, comparison has been made between CT imaging of the brain and images made with magnetic resonance (MR). Magnetic resonance has been found by some authors[21,22,27] to be even more sensitive than CT in detecting intracranial lesions of brain injury, but a study by Zimmerman[88] comparing CT scanning with MRI at 1.5 Tesla showed equal sensitivity of CT and MR in detecting acute lesions of intracranial injury. However, these authors found that MRI was better for subacute and chronic injuries.[88] The addition of the paramagnetic contrast material gadolinium may increase the sensitivity of MRI magnetic resonance imaging of the brain even further.

Several studies have shown the necessity for brain CT imaging in children who are suspected of having been abused. Brain abnormalities have been detected in children who had no evidence of skull fracture.[13,17,74] In one series, 38% of patients had skull fracture, and of these 65% had an intracerebral injury demonstrated by CT. However, 78% of those children with no obvious fracture had evidence of intracranial injury. The most frequent abnormality encountered in this series was a parietoccipital acute subdural hematoma. Interhemispheric subdural hematoma with associated parenchymal injury was found in 58% of the patients.[87] Follow-up CT in these patients with acute interhemispheric subarachnoid hemorrhage showed infarction in half and cerebral atrophy in all the patients. CT of the head has been used after strangulation of infants and showed the presence of infarction associated with small subdural hematomas.[7] Other authors have reported finding subarachnoid hemorrhage, cerebral edema, cerebral hemorrhage, subdural hematoma, and late infarctions.[13]

Facial fractures may be demonstrated by plain radiographs. Blowout fractures or fractures of the floor of the orbit are common injuries after blunt trauma to the orbit. On a Water's view, one may see evidence of blood within the maxillary sinus or even the mass of orbital contents herniating downward into the sinus. The actual fracture line may not be visualized on the plain radiograph, but one deduces its presence from the associated findings. Nasal fractures, midfacial fractures and mandibular fractures follow direct blows to these areas.

CT scanning has been shown to be useful in detecting and delineating the extent of facial fractures.[49] The reformatted oblique view was found to be helpful in delineating orbital fractures,[47] but more recently, direct oblique views have been found to complement direct coronal views to show fractures of the orbital wall.[3] High-resolution CT scanning of the temporal bone, using contiguous 1.5 mm CT sections with target reconstructions and dynamic scans, has been helpful for detecting fractures in this area.[35] CT is ideal for detecting maxillary facial fractures[20] and is superior to plain tomography[84] in detecting injury to intraorbital contents[46,75] and orbital foreign bodies.[80]

In conclusion, CT scanning should be used in the child with suspected intracranial injury because of its ease of monitoring and speed. For evaluating children with subacute or chronic injuries, MRI is the method of choice.

SPINE

Significant spinal injuries in infants and young children are very unusual but, just as in the older child or young adult, can result in severe deficits and long-term chronic disability. Prompt recognition and treatment are essential, although at times the presence of a significant spinal injury may be overlooked because of more obvious hemodynamic, respiratory, or neurologic damage.

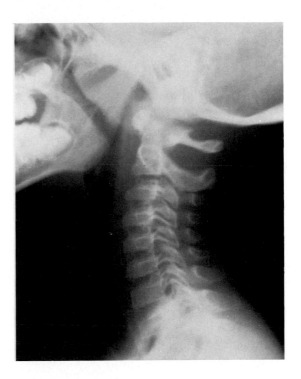

Fig. 8-4   Normal cervical spine, lateral view. Note the alignment of the posterior aspects of the vertebral bodies marking the spinal canal. (Courtesy A. Hubbard, Philadelphia.)

Cervical spine injuries are the most common and most critical. Because of this, it is not unreasonable to try to eliminate the possibility of cervical spine injury in every seriously injured patient before further manipulating the head and neck. A lateral view of the cervical region has therefore become a routine procedure in almost all trauma patients. Usually the patient's neck is splinted or in some way immobilized, and the patient is lying supine. Achieving a true lateral film without distortion and including all seven cervical vertebral bodies is not always easy and may require several exposures.

If the patient's arms are not injured, they should be fully extended and stretched caudally toward the feet allowing the shoulders to drop down, thus exposing the lower cervical region to view. Patients with large shoulders or patients in whom traction of the arms is contraindicated may require a "swimmer's" (Twining) view to fully visualize all seven cervical vertebral bodies (Fig. 8-4).

The vertebral bodies should be assessed for height and configuration and the relationship between adjacent vertebrae carefully checked. Distraction injuries with widening of the apparent disk spaces are most commonly seen with birth trauma and can indicate underlying cord disruptions. Several lines can be drawn that may help evaluate the upper cervical region. The posterior cervical line connects the posterior laminar line of C1 to the posterior laminar line of C3. In the neutral position, the posterior laminar line of C2 should be within 1 mm of this line (Fig. 8-5). Because of increased ligamentous laxity in infants and younger children, the vertebral bodies of C2, C3, and C4 will normally slide forward on one another when the patient's neck is flexed. This normal physiologic motion has been termed "pseudosubluxation" and is nonpathologic.[2,66]

The space between the anterior arch of C1 and the odontoid is also carefully assessed. A distance larger than 4 mm should suggest atlantoaxial subluxation (Fig. 8-6). Swelling of the soft tissues anterior to the vertebral bodies can be a helpful sign, but care should be taken in young infants in whom these tissues are normally very loose and redundant (Fig. 8-7).[32] A Jefferson fracture may be suggested by the normal enlargement of C1 compared with C2 in children under 4 years of age.[67]

The posterior elements, as well as the connections to their respective vertebral bodies, should also be systematically assessed. Remember that the dens or odontoid represents the combination of elements from C1 and C2. The horizontal synchondrosis that connects these two parts should not be mistaken for a fracture line.

Often the normal lordotic curve of the cervical spine will be lost, especially when the patient is lying flat or when there is muscle spasm.

Bohlman et al.[8] discuss the etiology of cervical fractures in children and also correlate different types of fractures with different types of vector forces.[16] Ligamentous disruptions may be as serious as fractures in terms of potential neurologic deficit.

Although the lateral cervical spine examination is extremely useful, it does not in itself constitute

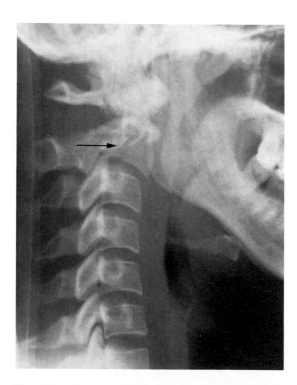

Fig. 8-5   Fracture of C2. There is separation of the posterior and anterior components of C2 caused by fractures of the pedicles. Note that although the posterior spinal canal line remains intact at this level, C1 and the body of C2 are displaced forward *(arrow)*. (Courtesy A. Hubbard, Philadelphia.)

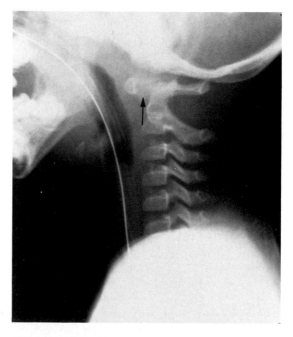

Fig. 8-6   C1-2 dislocation. There is marked anteroposterior widening of the space between the body of C1 anteriorly and the odontoid process of C2 *(arrow)*, indicating ligamentous disruption. (Courtesy A. Hubbard, Philadelphia.)

a complete and comprehensive examination. Frontal views, including an open mouth odontoid projection, are helpful especially for inspecting the lateral relationships of the vertebrae.[60] In some cases, tomography or a CT scan may be required to evaluate this area fully.

CT scans of the cervical region can be extremely helpful in assessing fractures of the vertebrae.[28,32,33,44] Thin sections are usually necessary and require the patient to be still throughout the scanning period. When indicated, the spinal subarachnoid space may be visualized on an MR scan, making the instillation of subarachnoid contrast an obsolete procedure.[1] Newer CT software programs have now made it possible to do three-dimensional reconstructions of the cervical spine and can provide excellent demonstrations of anatomy.[82] They do not, however, demonstrate otherwise undetectable fractures, although they may make complex abnormalities more comprehensible.

Because of the complexity of the anatomy in the cervical region, as well as the pitfalls in diagnosis in children, it is important for those involved in the care of pediatric trauma cases to develop some familiarity with the normal anatomy and common lesions. Harris and Edeiken-Monroe[32] have written an excellent treatise on the radiographic approach to acute cervical spine trauma. Swischuk[65,66] has also provided excellent teaching material on the specific problems in children in several of his articles and books, and reader is directed to those sources for a more comprehensive discussion.

Injuries to the spine below the cervical region are far less common and may occur in a variety of ways. Hyperflexion or compression injuries may result in wedge compression fractures of the vertebral bodies. When these are noted in children after minor or minimal trauma, underlying pathology should be questioned. Children on steroids for chronic arthritis may develop diffuse osteopenia and be prone to such fractures. Likewise, children with leukemia may complain of back pain due to compression fractures. Lap-belt injury to the lumbar spine may be subtle and produce

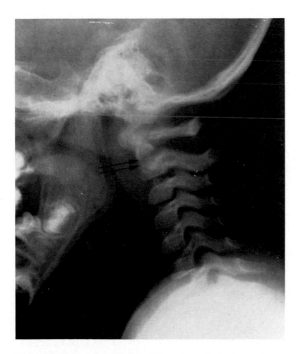

Fig. 8-7   Fracture of C2. There is a slight irregularity to the anterior cortical margin of the odontoid close to the synchondrosis, which is assymetrically widened *(arrows)*. Anterior soft tissue swelling is also present. (Courtesy A. Hubbard, Philadelphia.)

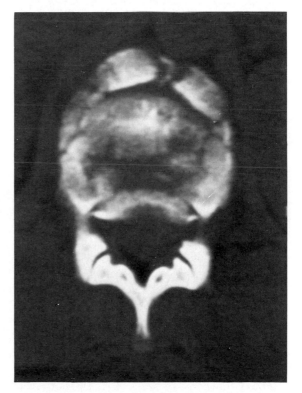

Fig. 8-8   Burst fracture of L1. CT scan of the first lumbar vertebral body shows multiple fracture lines intersecting and slight overall expansion of the fracture fragments. This type of injury is caused by severe compression of the vertebral body. (Courtesy A. Hubbard, Philadelphia.)

symptoms that are at first not readily explainable. Facet subluxation, anterior dislocations, and compression fractures have been described and are believed to be caused by a hyperflexion mechanism (Fig. 8-8).[69]

When a neurologic deficit is present, MRI may be helpful in evaluating the soft tissue components, that is, the cord, the disks, and the surrounding soft tissue spaces.[68] It is not an examination that is suitable for hemodynamically unstable, restless, or uncooperative patients and occasionally will have to be performed under sedation or general anesthesia.

IMAGING ASSESSMENT OF THORACIC TRAUMA IN CHILDREN

Although the circumstances of injury to the chest in infants, children, and young adults may vary considerably, the mechanisms of injury are similar and include direct penetrating wounds, direct nonpenetrating blows, and diffuse crush or rapid deceleration injury. Internal trauma by way of aspiration, inhalation of noxious fumes or gases, as well as asphyxia, may occur independently or as part of an external mechanism of injury. Nevertheless, the initial steps in the diagnosis work-up are similar.

A frontal supine radiograph of the chest is often the first study and should be obtained as a portable examination in the emergency room when the patient's clinical stability is uncertain or when other injuries preclude moving the patient. Immediate attention should be focused on the status of the heart and lungs. A large tension pneumothorax or hemothorax on one side will often cause the mediastinum to shift toward the opposite side because of increased air or fluid pressure. Because of the supine position and vertical beam projection, airfluid levels or the presence of a meniscus sign will not be seen. Blood collecting along the dependent posterior chest wall may be manifest as an overall increase in density rather than as a focal collection. Apical capping and peripheral pleural opacity will be seen as the amount of fluid within the chest increases.

Free intrapleural air will collect anteriorly and inferiorly when the patient is lying flat on his or her back. Distension and displacement of the pleura medially may simulate the presence of pneumomediastinum. Hyperlucency with absence of pulmonary vascular markings has been called the deep

sulcus sign and can suggest a small to moderate pneumothorax. When in doubt, decubitus views of the chest may help confirm a pneumothorax or significant pleural fluid collection. Appropriate therapeutic measures should be performed before the patient is moved and additional diagnostic studies obtained.

If the patient requires respiratory support via endotracheal intubation, postintubation radiographs should be obtained to confirm the position of the tube. Ideally the tip of the tube should lie midway between the larynx and the carina, which usually means at the level of the thoracic inlet or slightly lower. With the tube firmly affixed to the skin about the nose or mouth, a change in the patient's head position will cause the tube to slide up or down relative to the trachea. Hyperextending the patient's neck will cause the tube to ride upwards, whereas flexion will push the tube further down into the trachea.

The position of a thorocostomy drainage tube can also be confirmed on the supine frontal film; however, a lateral view may be extremely helpful in showing whether the tube lies anteriorly or posteriorly. Adequate drainage of a pneumothorax may be difficult when the tip of the tube lies superiorly and posteriorly with the patient in the supine position.

Erect frontal and lateral views of the chest ultimately should be requested as soon as the patient's clinical condition permits. In the face of a probable penetrating injury to the heart (causing cardiac tamponade or massive exsanguination) radiographic examination is superfluous and will waste valuable time. However, once the patient has been hemodynamically stabilized, additional radiographic studies can be helpful. When fully upright projections cannot be obtained, decubitus views are useful in detecting and following residual air and fluid collections.

Pneumomediastinum can be the result of air from a ruptured alveolus dissecting along the interstitial bronchovascular spaces into the hilus and then into the mediastinum. This can occur when the pressure within the airway acutely increases to very high levels. Blunt trauma to the chest or sudden compression of the thorax due to a rapid deceleration injury, especially with the glottis closed, can result in such sudden high pressure and alveolar rupture. Asthmatics can experience the same phenomenon from vigorous coughing and air trapping. Pneumomediastinum can be recognized radiographically by linear streaks of air outlining various mediastinal structures (for example, vessels, thymus, and fascial planes) and will often extend upwards into the soft tissues of the neck and shoulders. Unlike pneumothorax pneumomediastinum itself rarely causes hemodynamic or respiratory compromise, although it certainly can cause pain and discomfort. However, its continued presence, especially in large amounts, may be an indicator of direct trauma to and disruption of the larger airways. Direct blows to the trachea causing fracture, rupture, or both may present as subcutaneous emphysema and may require tracheostomy on an emergency basis.

Occasionally, CT of the chest may be indicated in the evaluation of the child with chest trauma and is a very sensitive method for detecting small amounts of air and fluid.[5,72] Unstable or uncooperative patients, however, are not suitable candidates for CT, and adequate hemodynamic and respiratory control should be achieved before sending the patient off for such studies. Contrast CT can be useful in detecting injuries to the great vessels, especially injuries to the aortic arch.[51] Angiography, however, remains the most sensitive tool for detecting subtle tears in the aortic wall.[24] Very small amounts of air or fluid may be discernible by CT. Whereas these in themselves may not be significant, they might be the only radiologic indicators that reveal that trauma to the chest has occurred. Rapid bolus injections of contrast with dynamic scanning at relatively small thickness contiguous slices will be best able to demonstrate subtle lesions and requires state-of-the-art equipment.

Real-time ultrasound of the heart and pericardial space may be extremely helpful in identifying pericardial effusion and early tamponade. This examination can be performed at the bedside and used to direct the insertion of pericardial catheters and drainage tubes. Likewise, pleural fuid can be localized by ultrasound, but this kind of technical assistance is usually not required in the acute situation. The role of MRI in acute chest trauma is yet to be determined.

Trauma to the rib cage may result in painful fractures; however, these injuries are sometimes difficult to detect on conventional radiographs. It is usually much more important to detect the complications associated with rib fractures than to go to extraordinary lengths to detect their presence. Nevertheless, well-penetrated oblique views are usually the most sensitive in detecting subtle rib fractures. Fractures of the last four ribs may be easier to see on films obtained using abdominal technique rather than on conventional chest radiographs. The presence of periosteal reaction or overt callus about a fracture obviously implies that healing is taking place and a considerable length of time has elapsed since the initial injury. In infants and young children, the presence of healing rib fractures should be viewed as a possible manifestation of child abuse.

Fractures of the first and second ribs are distinctly more uncommon and usually imply larger forces were applied to this part of the chest wall. They may be associated with internal injury to the brachiocephalic vessels or aortic arch (especially fractures of the left first and second ribs) or to the tracheobronchial tree.

Pulmonary contusion may be associated with adjacent rib fractures; however, it may also occur as a result of rapid deceleration injury to the chest without bony fracture.[25] Ill-defined, homogeneous fluid density within the lung parenchyma may mimic pneumonia and similarly show air bronchograms and fluffy air space infiltration. Unlike bacterial pneumonia, pulmonary contusion usually has a regional distribution, rather than lobar or segmental, and therefore may involve portions of lung on both sides of a fissure. Overt hemorrhage into the lung may have a similar radiographic appearance but usually causes longer-lasting infiltrates than simple edema.

Fractures of the tracheobronchial tree are uncommon in children.[54] They can occur on an iatrogenic basis, usually as the result of vigorous intubation or catheter manipulation. Rarely, they can occur as a direct complication of bronchoscopy or endobronchial biopsy. Nevertheless, this type of injury can also occur because of rapid deceleration and high shearing forces generated within the thorax. Persistence of pneumothorax often associated with lung opacification may lead one to suspect this diagnosis several days after the initial trauma has occurred. Erect views of the chest may show the dropped lung sign, whereby the whole lung is situated lower within the left hemithorax and the hilus in the mediastinum does not correlate with the hilus of the lung. Direct bronchoscopic visualization of the tear is the best way to establish the diagnosis, but a CT scan can suggest the diagnosis noninvasively. Repair is often difficult, and persistent atelectasis from occluding granulation tissue is often the result of the untreated injury.

ABDOMINAL TRAUMA

Various imaging techniques have been used in patients with blunt abdominal trauma, including ultrasound,[31,34,41] scintigraphy,[76] excretory urography,[26] and CT.* CT has become the method of choice for examining children with serious blunt upper abdominal injury.[6,39] Kaufman et al.[39] reported on a prospective evaluation of 100 children with severe abdominal trauma in which CT was compared with liver-spleen scintigraphy and sonography. They found CT to provide the most information of any single imaging modality and to be more accurate than nuclear medicine or ultrasound studies. Similarly, Berger and Kuhn[6] performed CT on 23 children following moderate to severe blunt abdominal trauma and found CT superior to excretory urography, sonography, and radionuclide imaging because of better anatomic delineation and the ability to image all organs, the peritoneum, and retroperitoneum simultaneously. The extent of injury is easily seen, and follow-up is accurate. Angiography is still necessary for direct visualization of vascular injury, and there is potential for therapeutic embolization using this technique.[6]

Clinically unstable children are not candidates for CT examinations. Occasionally, sedation of a young child will be required to obtain a satisfactory CT.

In Kaufman's study,[39] liver-spleen scintigraphy

---

*References 10, 11, 18, 36-38, 52-54, 61, 79, 81.

was found to be nearly as accurate as CT, both in the spleen and the liver. Scintigraphy is easier to perform than CT and is less affected by patient motion. Therefore liver-spleen scanning may be used when injury to those organs alone is suspected.

LIVER

Liver injuries are well demonstrated by CT and range from transection to explosive liver rupture to focal intraparenchymal injury (Fig. 8-9). Kaufman[39] found one false negative with CT, four with scintigraphy, and four with sonography in 19 patients with liver injury studied by all three modalities.

SPLEEN

Spleen injuries may similarly range from massive rupture and subcapsular hemorrhage to fragmented rupture to focal intraparenchymal injury (Fig. 8-10). In Kaufman's study,[39] there were no false negatives with CT, three with scintigraphy, and twelve with sonography. Four false positives were found using CT, five with scintigraphy, and one with sonography in 24 patients with splenic injury.

RENAL INJURIES

Posterior scintigraphy during bolus administration can show the presence or absence of renal

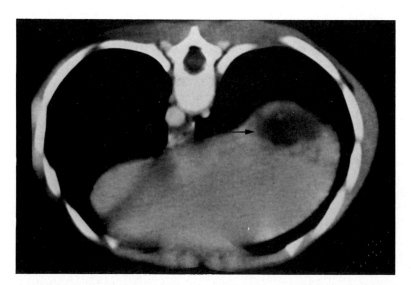

Fig. 8-9 Liver hematoma. CT shows a low attenuation area high in the dome of the right lobe of the liver *(arrow)* in a 6-year-old boy who had fallen off his bicycle.

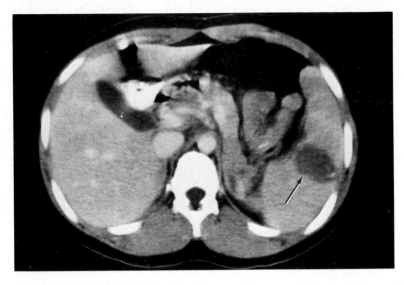

Fig. 8-10   Spleen injury. A fractured spleen *(arrow)* is shown on CT of a 17-year-old girl who was involved in a motor vehicle accident.

refusion. The spectrum of renal injuries demonstrated by CT includes disruption and fragmentation of renal tissue and focal parenchymal damage.[39] Damage to renal vessels is inferred by a nonfunctioning kidney, just as it is when using intravenous urography. In 12 injured kidneys in 11 children, there was one false negative CT scan and two false negative sonograms. There was also one false positive CT scan and two false positive sonograms.

INTRAPERITONEAL FLUID

Free intraperitoneal fluid is shown nicely on CT (Fig. 8-11). In Kaufman's study,[39] 28 of 30 patients with free peritoneal fluid diagnosed by CT had organ injury. Of those patients with injury to one or more organs, 46% had free fluid.

OTHER ORGANS

Duodenal hematoma was better shown by gastrointestinal series in both Kaufman's and Berger's

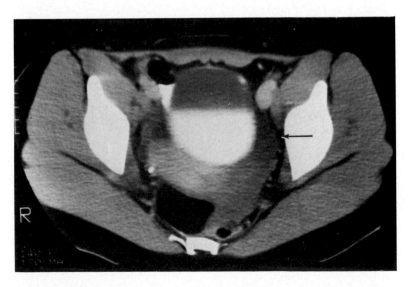

Fig. 8-11   Free fluid in the pelvis. Sections through the pelvis of the same patient show evidence of blood in the peritoneum *(arrow)*.

studies than by CT. Pancreatic injuries may be well demonstrated by CT, as are injuries of the lung bases, retroperitoneum, soft tissues, and bones.[6,39]

It must be pointed out that whereas CT gives superb delineation of intraabdominal injury, it is not used to make the decision as to which children should be taken to surgery, except for two findings: pneumoperitoneum or absent renal perfusion. This continues to be a clinical decision. Recently the trend is toward more conservative treatment, with stable children being followed by sequential imaging studies to follow the course of healing of organ injuries.

PELVIS AND HIPS

The pelvic bones, sacrum, and sacroiliac joints create a relatively rigid ring. The concept of a ring helps in the understanding of pelvic fractures. Fracture of such a ring will seldom occur only at one site.

Generally, one must search for at least a second fracture in the pelvis or diastasis of a sacroiliac joint. The use of CT has been of great value in more accurate diagnosis for orthopedic management.[23]

In major trauma a pelvic radiograph is an important and necessary item in initial patient eval-

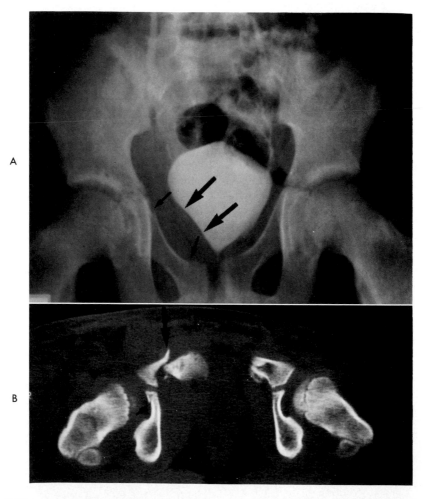

Fig. 8-12   A, Excretory urogram shows right pubic ramus fractures *(small arrows)* causing an extraperitoneal hematoma that displaces the right bladder base *(large arrows)*. **B,** CT scan reveals not only the obvious pubic ramus fracture *(large arrow)* but also a subtle intraarticular acetabular fracture of the ischium *(small arrow)*.

uation, since significant hemorrhage may occur from pelvic fractures and should be anticipated by physicians. Retroperitoneal venous bleeding may be considerable but usually will cease, whereas arterial hemorrhage may require angiography and transcatheter embolization for diagnosis and control.

Pelvic fractures or perineal trauma may cause lacerations of the bladder and urethra. Rectal injuries are less frequent but may occur from partic-

ularly violent trauma. With pubic fractures, retrograde urethrography should be considered before bladder catheterization, since a partial urethral tear might be made complete by a difficult catheterization. Integrity of the bladder is best examined by cystography (Figs. 8-12, 8-13, and 8-14).

At the hip joints, dislocations may occur from violent injury. CT scans are helpful in demonstrating small intraarticular or marginal bone fragments likely to be missed by plain radiographs.[30,45]

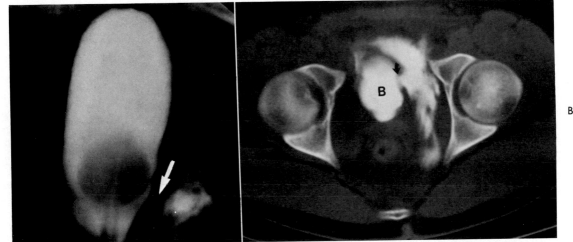

Fig. 8-13   **A,** Cystogram of adolescent unable to urinate following lower abdominal trauma. Site of bladder wall rupture *(arrow)* is identified with contrast flowing into the extraperitoneal space. **B,** CT scan shows leakage of contrast from bladder *(B)* across rent in left bladder wall *(arrow)*.

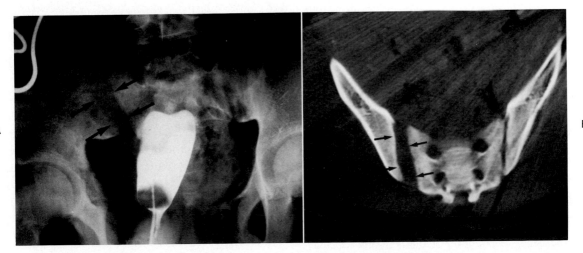

Fig. 8-14   **A,** Massive perineal trauma in an adolescent resulting in diastases of the pubic symphysis and right sacroiliac joint *(arrows)*. Rectal tear has resulted in bubbly retroperitoneal emphysema. Pelvic hemorrhage compresses and elongates contrast-filled bladder. **B,** CT scan more clearly depicts sacroiliac joint diastasis *(arrows)*.

Aside from most severe trauma, proximal femoral fractures are rare in children. However, slippage of the capital femoral epiphysis occurs in preadolescents and adolescents. Children with slipped capital femoral epiphysis tend to be overweight and have suffered a Salter-Harris I displaced fracture of the growth plate. The lateral view of the hip is the single most sensitive radiograph in its detection.

EXTREMITIES

Growing children are subject to differing injuries of their developing musculoskeletal systems. Patterns of pediatric extremity injury have been well described.[62] Although newer imaging modalities are occasionally being used to evaluate extremity trauma in children, the mainstay for examination of suspected skeletal injury remains plain radiography. The smaller size of children often tempts both physicians and radiologic technologies to include unnecessarily large portions of the child on films, but film quality and radiation protection are better achieved by limiting radiographic examination to the injured area. In the great majority of pediatric extremity injuries, experienced observers seldom need comparison views, which add radiation, cost, and time to the evaluation.[50] Although the routine use of comparison radiographs is not recommended, selective and thoughtful use of a comparison view may prove helpful.

SHOULDER

Clavicular fractures are common. Almost all occur in the middle third of the clavicle, with cephalad displacement of the medial fragment owing to the pull of the sternocleidomastoid muscle. This injury occurs in neonates as a result of shoulder dystocia during delivery. From the time children begin to toddle and walk, clavicle fractures may occur throughout childhood as the result of falls on the shoulder. The only other frequently seen fracture at the shoulder in children is that of the proximal humeral metaphysis extending into the growth plate, a Salter-Harris II injury.

Dislocation of the glenohumeral joint, although common in adults, is extremely rare before mid-adolescence. Disruption of the acromioclavicular articulation also is rare and is best demonstrated by simultaneous bilateral shoulder views obtained with and without weights in the hands while the child is standing.

Pitfalls to accurate diagnosis may be caused by normal adolescent apophyses occurring at the tips of the acromion or coracoid processes and at the inferior angle of the scapula. The growth plate of the proximal humerus is irregular and often mistaken for a fracture. An irregular depression along the inferior aspect of the medial end of the clavicle, the normal rhomboid fossa, may be mistaken for bone destruction.

HUMERUS

Fractures of the humeral midshaft generally present no diagnostic difficulty. When these fractures are seen in infants, they should raise suspicions of

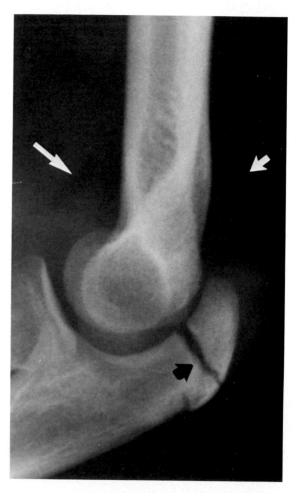

Fig. 8-15 Adolescent hit by car fell on elbow and sustained intraarticular olecranon fracture *(black arrow)*. Elbow joint hemarthrosis distends the joint space and displaces fat pads *(white arrows)*.

child abuse. A history of an infant rolling over on the arm in the crib or of getting an arm caught between crib slats does not adequately explain this injury.

ELBOW

The multiplicity of ossification centers and their changing radiographic appearances make diagnosis of elbow trauma difficult and challenging. From the time toddlers begin walking, elbow trauma may be seen throughout childhood as a result of falling on the forearm or elbow. During the first decade, supracondylar fractures of the distal humerus predominate. Fractures of the proximal radius may also occur, and particularly violent falls may result in olecranon fractures.

Hemarthrosis is present in all intraarticular fractures at the elbow, and radiographic detection of elbow joint effusion is extremely important in the diagnosis of subtle fractures. In fact, the detection of posttraumatic elbow joint effusion, even in the absence of a demonstrable fracture, usually leads to the assumption that a subtle fracture is present, though not radiographically apparent.

Radiographic technique is very important in the diagnosis of elbow trauma. Survey views of the entire upper extremity in internal and external rotation are insufficient. Accurate diagnosis is facilitated by films centered at the elbow, with views in the frontal projection with the elbow extended and in the lateral projection with the elbow flexed to 90 degrees. This lateral view allows demonstration of juxtaarticular fat pads, which become displaced from the humeral margins when the elbow joint capsule is distended with blood or other fluid (Figs. 8-15 and 8-16).

Gross dislocation of the pediatric elbow joint is rare and presents no diagnostic problem. Less obvious subluxations at the ulnatrochlear articulation may be different to appreciate. However, the radiocapitellar joint is easier to evaluate, since the long axis of the radius should point to the capitellum in all views. Small children with radial head subluxation from its anulus as a result of pulled or nursemaid's elbow have no positive radiographic

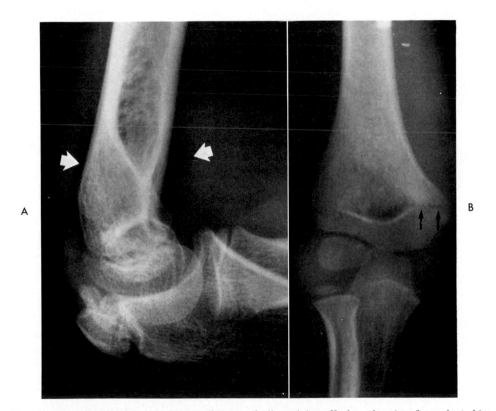

Fig. 8-16   Lateral view **(A)** shows evidence of elbow joint effusion elevating fat pads *(white arrows)*. Frontal view **(B)** images subtle linear supracondylar fracture *(black arrows)*.

findings. In many instances the examining physician or the radiologic technologist will inadvertently reduce this subluxation by supination of the forearm, which results in instantaneous recovery of painless elbow motion.

FOREARM

Falls on outstretched hands commonly result in distal forearm buckle fractures of either the radius alone or of the radius and ulna together (Fig. 8-17). The same mechanism may also result in fracture of the growth plate cartilage alone (Salter-Harris I) or with an attached metaphyseal fragment (Salter-Harris II). Whereas the Salter-Harris II injury is easily diagnosed, the Salter-Harris I injury is subtle. The distal radial epiphysis may be noted to be displaced from its expected position, or if no

displacement has occurred, this diagnosis must be inferred by the combination of mechanism of injury, significant clinical and radiographic soft tissue swelling, and no demonstrable osseous fracture.

Other types of incomplete fractures may occur, including the well-known greenstick fracture and the lesser-known plastic bowing fracture,[9] in which a series of juxtaposed transverse microfractures result in a bowing deformity but not an appreciable fracture line.

Whereas complete fractures of both forearm bones are common and easily appreciated, midshaft fracture of only one bone must generate a search for a dislocation of the other bone at the elbow or the wrist. Monteggia's fracture-dislocation is a midshaft ulna fracture associated with dislocation of the radiocapitellar joint (Fig. 8-18).

WRIST

Before adolescence, carpal bone injuries are not only extremely rare, but almost impossible to diagnose radiographically owing to a lack of carpal bone ossification. Starting in the second decade, a fall on an outstretched hand may result in a fracture of the navicular bone. Since the fracture line may disrupt the recurrent blood supply to the proximal pole, avascular necrosis or nonunion may result (Figs. 8-19 and 8-20). MRI has shown promise in the early diagnosis of this complication.[57] A fall on a flexed hand may cause an avulsion fracture of the dorsal aspect of the triquetral bone, which is best appreciated from the lateral view.

HAND

Crush injuries of the distal fingers are common and often result in subungual tuft fractures, which technically are open fractures. Although survey views of the hand usually include frontal and oblique projections, finger injuries need to be examined in the lateral projection to uncover subtle avulsion fractures, which often occur along the insertion of the volar tendinous expansions.

Punching may result in the boxer's fracture of the distal fifth metacarpal. This fracture always results in volar tilt of the distal fragment and may extend into the growth plate as a Salter-Harris II injury. Another common Salter-Harris II fracture may occur at the base of the proximal phalanx of the thumb as a subtle finding following a fall on the hand.

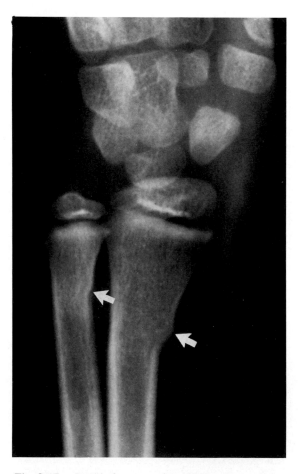

Fig. 8-17 Buckle fractures of the distal radius and ulna *(arrows)* from a fall on an outstretched hand.

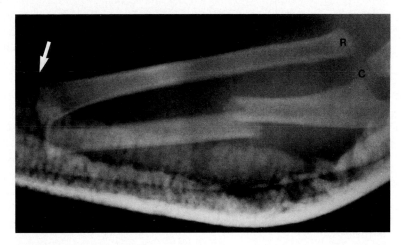

Fig. 8-18   Monteggia fracture-dislocation. In addition to the overriding ulnar midshaft fracture, the radiocapitellar joint is dislocated. A Salter-Harris II distal radius fracture is also seen *(white arrow)*. *R,* Radial head; *C,* capitellum.

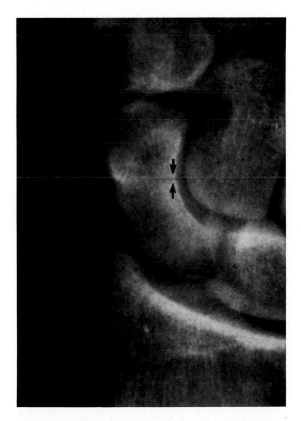

Fig. 8-19   Transverse fracture of the waist of the navicular is often difficult to see *(arrows)*. Disruption of recurrent blood supply to proximal pole may lead to complications of avascular necrosis and nonunion.

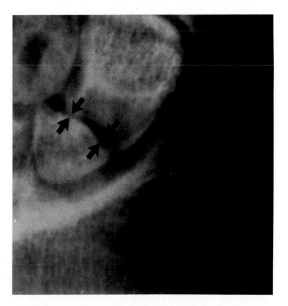

Fig. 8-20   Navicular fracture complicated by nonunion *(arrows)*.

FOREIGN BODIES

Although radiography is an excellent way to localize radioopaque foreign bodies, radiolucent foreign material presents a challenge. The use of CT, xeroradiography, and ultrasound may prove helpful in some cases.[4,29] Removal of small radioopaque foreign bodies may be expedited through the use of intraoperative fluoroscopy.

THIGH

Diagnosis of femoral fractures is not difficult. Most often a history of violent trauma with clinical disability and deformity makes the diagnosis before radiography. In nonwalking infants, the discovery of a femoral fracture should lead to a high suspicion of child abuse.

In teenagers the distal femoral epiphysis may become avulsed and displaced as a Salter-Harris I or II fracture, usually as a result of a sports injury in which the adolescent falls backward or twists on a fixed lower leg. This fracture carries a high risk of injury to the popliteal artery, with the potential for vascular occlusion; therefore immediate assessment of vascular integrity is important, and emergency arteriography may be needed.

KNEE

Joint effusions of the knee are a common feature of many soft tissue injuries, few of which can be diagnosed by radiography. An exception includes the demonstration of pneumarthrosis, which clearly indicates a puncture or tear into the knee joint. Although contrast arthrography had been the imaging standard for the diagnosis of miniscal and cruciate ligament injuries, trends have been changing in recent years, with imaging by MRI[15] and the liberal use of arthroscopy.

In young children, twisting injury to the leg may cause avulsion of the tibial spine by the cruciate ligament. Violent knee traumas may rarely result in Salter-Harris I or II fractures of the proximal tibial growth plate.

A pitfall in knee diagnosis may occur as a result of misinterpretation of the normally irregular medial femoral epiphysis as a fracture in children 2 to 6 years of age. Similarly, in adolescents the normal maturation of the tibial tuberosity and its irregular contours of ossification are frequently miscalled fractures.

Patella fractures and dislocations are rarely seen before adolescence. Some normal variant lucent lines and secondary patella ossification centers may mimic fractures that are often displaced and are invariably associated with large joint effusions. Patellar dislocations are always lateral.

LEG

Fractures of the tibia and the fibula resulting from violent injuries, such as those incurred from a motor vehicle accident or skiing, present no diagnostic difficulty. Toddlers and early-walking children may have leg pain and refuse to stand following a short jump from several stairs or from a car to a curb. The classic toddler's fracture is a subtle linear oblique fracture of the midshaft of the tibia.

Because the periosteum may be intact, no swelling may be evident over the fracture. Another type of fracture that presents a diagnostic challenge in this age group occurs transversely along the posteromedial proximal tibial metaphysis. In both cases, if the initial fracture is overlooked and the child continues to have pain and disability, radiographic reexamination in several weeks will show localized patchy increased density and some periosteal reaction of healing bone that may lead to suspicion of bone neoplasm. Worse yet is that the biopsy of a healing fracture at this stage may be interpreted as sarcoma. Caution and restraint must be exercised in evaluating subtle localized areas of increased tibial bone density in young children so as not to mistake a healing fracture for a bone neoplasm.

ANKLE

In the first decade, ankle fractures are infrequent. At this age, distal tibial and fibular fractures might occur from the child being run over accidentally by an older child's bicycle or inadvertently stepped on by an adult. Inversion and eversion injuries from running usually result in sprains in this younger group.

In the second decade, the child's increased weight and level of activity may lead to fractures, often occurring through the growth plates. Traction and avulsion fractures of the malleoli caused by pulls of the collateral ligaments tend to be transverse, whereas the subsequent pushing motion of the unstable talus against the opposite malleolus creates oblique fractures.

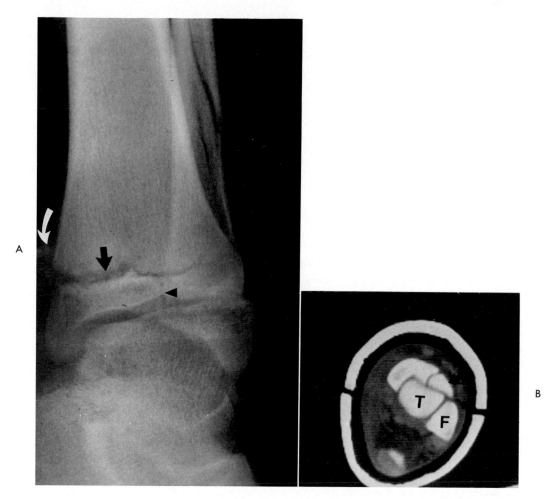

Fig. 8-21   **A,** Triplanar Salter-Harris IV fracture of distal tibia. Fracture extends through metaphysis *(curved arrow)*, physis *(straight arrow)*, and epiphysis *(arrowhead)*. Spiral fracture of fibula is also seen. **B,** CT scan of ankle in plaster shows the nondisplaced anterolateral tibial epiphyseal fragment *(arrow)*. *T,* Talus; *F,* fibula.

The great majority of adolescent ankle fractures are satisfactorily diagnosed and followed by plain radiography. An important exception is the fracture that involves the distal tibial metaphysis, growth plate, and epiphysis—a triplanar Salter-Harris IV injury (Fig 8-21). CT should be used to evaluate these fractures, since the anterolateral part of the epiphysis may be displaced as a free fragment (juvenile Tillaux fracture) requiring internal fixation.[14,19]

FOOT

Foot fractures are rare in young children. Injuries caused by heavy objects falling on young feet may occasionally fracture metatarsals or phalanges. The dense ossification center of the first cuneiform bone in the preschool or early school-age child may appear disturbingly irregular in its normal maturation.

In toddlers, subtle fractures of the calcaneus may be a cause for pain and refusal to bear weight. Early radiographs often do not show this fracture, but radionuclide bone scans may help by showing localized abnormal uptake at this site.[64]

Older children may fracture phalanges by stubbing toes. An association of great toe stubbing followed by distal phalangeal osteomyelitis has occurred in the presence of growth plate injury. Presumably the proximal nail is dislodged, resulting in the deep entrapment of organisms.[56]

In the adolescent, inversion injury may result in the *transverse* avulsion fracture of the fifth metatarsal base. The normal developing apophyseal ossification center at this site is oriented *longitudinally* with smooth edges but remains an occasional source of confusion.

Puncture wounds by foreign material may involve soft tissue and bone. Radiography, fluoroscopy, CT, and ultrasound may play roles in foreign body localization and removal. The question of early osteomyelitis is best addressed by radionuclide bone scan.[73]

REFERENCES

1. Allen RL, Perot PL Jr, and Gudeman SK: Evaluation of acute nonpenetrating cervical spinal cord injuries with CT metrizamide myelography, J Neurosurg 63:510, 1985.
2. Bailey DK: The normal cervical spine in infants and children, Radiology 59:713, 1952.
3. Ball JB Jr: Direct oblique sagittal CT of orbital wall fractures, AJR 148:601, 1987.
4. Bauer AR and Yutami D: Computed tomographic localization of wooden foreign bodies in children's extremities, Arch Surg 118:1084, 1983.
5. Bender TM et al: Pediatric chest trauma, J Thorac Imag 2:60, 1987.
6. Berger PE and Kuhn JP: CT of blunt abdominal trauma in childhood, AJR 136:105, 1981.
7. Bird CR et al: Strangulation in child abuse: CT diagnosis (1), Radiology 163:373, 1987.
8. Bohlman HH, Rekate HL, and Thompson GH: Problem fractures of the cervical spine in children. In Houghton GR and Thompson GH, editors: Problematic musculoskeletal injuries in children, London, 1983, Butterworths.
9. Borden S: Roentgen recognition of acute plastic bowing of the forearm in children, AJR 125:524, 1975.
10. Bretan PN Jr et al: Computerized tomographic staging of renal trauma: 85 consecutive cases, Urol 136:561, 1986.
11. Brick SH et al: Hepatic and splenic injury in children: role of CT in the decision for laparotomy, Radiology 165:643, 1987.
12. Bruce DA and Schut L: The value of CAT scanning following pediatric head injury, Clinical Pediatr (Phila) 19:719, 1980.
13. Cohen RA et al: Cranial computed tomography in the abused child with head injury, AJR 146:97, 1986.
14. Cone RO et al: Triplane fracture of the distal tibial epiphysis: radiographic and CT studies, Radiology 153:763, 1984.
15. Crues JV et al: Meniscal tears of the knee: accuracy of MR imaging, Radiology 164:445, 1987.
16. Daffner RH, Deeb ZL, and Rothfus WE: "Fingerprints" of vertebral trauma—a unifying concept based on mechanisms, Skeletal Radiol 15:518, 1986.
17. Ellison PH, Tsai FY, and Largent JA: Computed tomography in child abuse and cerebral contusion, Pediatrics 62:151, 1978.
18. Federle MP and Jeffrey RB Jr: Hemoperitoneum studied by computed tomography, Radiology 148:187, 1983.
19. Feldman F et al: Distal tibial triplane fractures: diagnosis with CT, Radiology 164:429, 1987.
20. Fujii N and Yamashiro M: Computed tomography for the diagnosis of facial fractures, J Oral Surg 39:735, 1981.
21. Gentry LR, Godersky JC, and Thompson B: MR imaging of head trauma: review of the distribution and radiopathologic features of traumatic lesions, AJR 150:663, 1988.
22. Gentry LR et al: Prospective comparative study of intermediate-field MR and CT in the evaluation of closed head trauma, AJR 150:673, 1988.
23. Gill K and Bucholy RW: The role of computerized tomographic scanning in the evaluation of major pelvic fractures, J Bone Joint Surg [Am] 66A:34, 1984.
24. Godwin JD and Tolentino CS: Thoracic cardiovascular trauma, J Thorac Imag 2:32, 1987.
25. Greene R: Lung alterations in thoracic trauma, J Thorac Imag 2:1, 1987.
26. Halsell RD et al: The reliability of excretory urography as a screening examination for blunt renal trauma, Ann Emerg Med 16:1236, 1987.
27. Han JS et al: Head trauma evaluated by magnetic resonsance and computed tomography: a comparison, Radiology 150:71, 1984.
28. Handel SF and Lee Y: Computed tomography of spinal fractures, Radiol Clin North Am 19:69, 1981.
29. Harcke HI, Grissom LE, and Finklestein MS: Evaluation of the musculoskeletal system with sonography, AJR 150:1253, 1988.
30. Harder JA et al: Computerized axial tomography to demonstrate occult fractures of the acetabulum in children, Can J Surg 24:409, 1981.
31. Harkanyi Z et al: Gray-scale echography of traumatic pancreatic cysts in children, Pediatr Radiol 11:81, 1981.
32. Harris JH Jr and Edeikin-Monroe B: The radiology of acute cervical spine trauma, ed 2, Baltimore, 1987, Williams & Williams.
33. Harwood-Nash CD: Computed tomography of the pediatric spine: a protocol for the 1980s, Radiol Clin North Am 19:479, 1981.
34. Hoelzer DJ et al: Selection and nonoperative management of pediatric blunt trauma patients: the role of quantitative crystalloid resuscitation and abdominal ultrasonography, Trauma 26:57, 1986.
35. Holland BA and Brant Zawadzki M: High-resolution CT of temporal bone trauma, AJR 143:391, 1984.
36. Jeffrey RB, Federle MP, and Crass RA: Computed tomography of pancreatic trauma, Radiology 147:491, 1983.
37. Karp MP et al: The role of computed tomography in the evaluation of blunt abdominal trauma in children, J Pediatr Surg 16:316, 1981.
38. Karp MP et al: The impact of computed tomography scanning on the child with renal trauma, J Pediatr Surg 21:617, 1986.
39. Kaufman RA et al: Upper abdominal trauma in children: imaging evaluation, AJR 142:449, 1984.
40. Kishore PRS et al: Significance of CT in head injury: correlation with intracranial pressure, AJR 137:829, 1981.
41. Lam AH and Shulman L: Ultrasonography in the management of liver trauma in children, J Ultrasound Med 3:199, 1984.
42. Lobato RD et al: Outcome from severe head injury related to the type of intracranial lesion: a computerized tomography study, J Neurosurg 59:762, 1983.
43. Lobato RD et al: Normal computerized tomography scans

in severe head injury: Prognostic and clinical management implications, J Neurosurg 65:784, 1986.

44. Lynch D, McManus F, and Ennis JT: Computed tomography in spinal trauma, Clin Radiol 37:71, 1986.

45. Mack LA, Hardy JD, and Winguist RA: CT of acetabular fractures: analysis of fracture patterns, AJR 138:407, 1982.

46. Mafee MF and Peyman GA: Choroidal detachment and ocular hypotony: CT evaluation, Radiology 153:697, 1984.

47. Marsh JL and Gado M: The longitudinal orbital CT projection: a versatile image for orbital assessment, Plast Reconstr Surg 71:3 308, 1983.

48. McMicken DB: Emergency CT head scans in traumatic and atraumatic conditions, Ann Emerg Med, 15:274, 1986.

49. Mendelsohn DB and Hertzanu Y: Intracerebral pneumatoceles following facial trauma: CT findings, Radiology 154:115, 1985.

50. Merten DF et al: Comparison radiographs of extremities in childhood: recommended usage, Pediatrics 65:646, 1980.

51. Mirvis SE et al: Role of CT in excluding major arterial injury after blunt thoracic trauma, AJR 149:601, 1987.

52. Mohamed G et al: Computed tomography in the assessment of pediatric abdominal trauma, Arch Surg 121:703, 1986.

53. Nelson EW et al: Computerized tomography in the evaluation of blunt abdominal trauma, J Surg 146:751, 1983.

54. Oh KS, Fleishner FG, and Wyman SM: Characteristic pulmonary findings in traumatic complete transection of a mainstem bronchus, Radiology 92:371, 1969.

55. Peitzman AB et al: Prospective study of computed tomography in initial management of blunt abdominal trauma, J Trauma 26:585, 1986.

56. Pinckney LE, Currarino G, and Kennedy LA: The stubbed great toe: a case of occult compound fracture and infection, Radiology 138:375, 1981.

57. Reinus WR et al: Carpal avascular necrosis: MR Imaging, Radiology 160:689, 1986.

58. Rivara F et al: Poor prediction of positive computed tomographic scans by clinical criteria in symptomatic pediatric head trauma, Pediatrics 80:579, 1987.

59. Roberts F and Shopfner CE: Plain skull roentgenograms in children with head trauma, Am J Roentgen 114:230, 1972.

60. Shapiro R, Youngberg AS, and Rothman SLG: The differential diagnosis of traumatic lesions of the occipitoatlantoaxial segment, Radio Clin North Am 11:505, 1973.

61. Sherck JP, McCort JJ, and Oakes DD: Computed tomography in thoracoabdominal trauma, J Trauma 24:1015, 1984.

62. Silverman FN: The limbs. In Silverman FN, editor: Caffey's pediatric x-ray diagnosis, ed 8, Chicago, 1985, Year Book Medical Publishers, Inc.

63. Stalker HP, Kaufman RA, and Towbin R: Patterns of liver injury in childhood: CT analysis, AJR 147:1199, 1986.

64. Starshak RJ, Simons GW, and Sty JR: Occult fracture of the calcaneus: another toddler's fracture, Pediatr Radiol 14:37, 1984.

65. Swischuk LE: Anterior displacement of C^2 in children: physiologic or pathologic?: a helpful differentiating line, Radiology 122:759, 1977.

66. Swischuk LE: Emergency radiology of the acutely ill or injured child, ed 2, Baltimore, 1986, Williams & Wilkins.

67. Suss RA, Zimmerman RD, and Leeds NE: Pseudospread of the atlas: false sign of Jefferson fracture in young children, AJR 140:1079, 1983.

68. Tarr RW et al: MR imaging of recent spinal trauma, JCAT 11:412, 1987.

69. Taylor GA and Eggli KD: Lap-belt injuries of the lumbar spine in children: a pitfall in CT diagnosis, AJR 150:1355, 1988.

70. Taylor SB et al: Central nervous system anoxic ischemic insult in children due to near-drowning, Radiology 156:641, 1985.

71. Timming R, Orrison WW, and Mikulka JA: Computerized tomography and rehabilitation outcome after severe head trauma, Arch Phys Med Rehabil 63:154, 1982.

72. Tocino IM and Miller MH: Computed tomography in blunt chest trauma, J Thorac Imag 2:45, 1987.

73. Treves S et al: Osteomyelitis: early scintigraphic detection in children, Pediatrics 57:173, 1976.

74. Tsai FY et al: Computed tomography in child abuse head trauma, J Comput Tomogr 4:277, 1980.

75. Unger JM: Orbital apex fractures: the contribution of computed tomography, Radiology 150:713, 1984.

76. Uthoff LB et al: A prospective study comparing nuclear scintigraphy and computerized axial tomography in the initial evaluation of the trauma patient, Ann Surg 198:611, 1983.

77. Van Dongen KJ, Braakman R, and Gelpke GJ: The prognostic value of computerized tomography in comatose head-injured patients, J Neurosurg 59:951, 1983.

78. Van Der Sande JJ et al: Hemostasis and computerized tomography in head injury, J Neurosurg 55:718, 1981.

79. Vock P, Kehrer B, and Tschaeppeler H: Blunt liver trauma in children: the role of computed tomography in diagnosis and treatment, J Pediatr Surg 21:413, 1986.

80. Weisman RA et al: Computed tomography in penetrating wounds of the orbit with retained foreign bodies, Arch Otolaryngol 109:265, 1983.

81. Wing VW et al: The clinical impact of CT for blunt abdominal trauma, AJR 145:1191, 1985.

82. Wojcik WG, Edeikin-Monroe BS, and Harris JH Jr: Three-dimensional computed tomography in acute cervical spine trauma, Skeletal Radiol 16:261, 1987.

83. Yoshino E et al: Acute brain edema in fatal head injury: analysis by dynamic CT scanning, J Neurosurg 63:830, 1985.

84. Zilkha A: Computed tomography in facial trauma, Radiology 144:545, 1982.

85. Zimmerman RA, Bilaniuk LT, and Genneralli T: Computed tomography of shearing injuries of the cerebral white matter, Radiology 127:393, 1978.

86. Zimmerman RA et al: Cranial computed tomography in diagnosis and management of acute head trauma, J Roentgenol 131:27, 1978.

87. Zimmerman RA et al: Computed tomography of craniocerebral injury in the abused child, Radiology 130:687, 1979.

88. Zimmerman RA et al: Head injury: early results of comparing CT and high-field MR, AJR 147:1215, 1986.

9

Birth Injury

John M. Driscoll, Jr. and John N. Schullinger

A marked recent decline in neonatal mortality secondary to birth injury is attributable to refinements in obstetric techniques, including the more frequent use of cesarean section in selected instances when vaginal delivery, complicated forceps, or version and extraction would increase the risk of injury to the baby.[20]

A historical review of birth injury reveals a high risk of intracranial hemorrhage. During the first quarter of this century, a 40% incidence of fatal intracranial injury was reported in various autopsy series.[120] An excellent summation of these early studies may be found in Ehrenfest's monograph on birth injury, first published in 1922 and again in 1931.[63]

Potter's review of 2000 autopsies found that injury accounted for only 14% of the deaths and stillborn by 1940,[189] and more recent studies have shown a further reduction in mortality to 2 percent or less.*

However, despite this reduction in mortality, birth injury still occasionally and unavoidably occurs. It is most frequently found in large babies (those over 3800 grams) and in cases of protracted labor and precipitous, breech, or otherwise complicated delivery. Gresham[92] reported that for every death due to birth trauma to least 20 babies incur a major birth injury. At the Columbia-Presbyterian Medical Center in New York City in the years 1963 through 1966, there were 113 significant injuries among 17,649 deliveries, or an average of 6.4 injuries per 1000 live births and stillborns.[157] More recently, Kottmeier,[124] at Downstate Medical Center State University of New York, has reported 437 injuries among 59,963 deliveries, or 7.3 injuries per 1000 live births. The incidence of birth injury has also been shown to be lower among private patients in voluntary hospitals than among ward patients or patients in municipal and proprietary hospitals.[7,263]

Although by strict definition birth injury refers to injury sustained during the processes of labor and delivery, we have also included certain lesions incurred before and in the days immediately following the actual birth of the infant. This chapter, therefore, is divided into three sections—antepartum, intrapartum, and postpartum injury.

ANTEPARTUM INJURY
Intrauterine Transfusions

Although still in use since Liley's[138] first reported successful case in 1963, the need for intrauterine transfusion of the fetus for hemolytic disease has steadily diminished as measures for the prevention of Rh sensitization are more widely applied. There is, however, the occasional case in which the procedure is required, and in experienced hands the risk to the fetus is estimated at about 5%.[145] Many deaths are unexplained, and although various structures may be penetrated without serious result, such as pleura, pericardium, bladder, liver, bowel, and spinal canal,[73,77,260] definite procedure-related fatalities do occur. These have been reported by Queenan,[195] Girling et al.,[80] Price et al.,[192] and Karnicki[115] and include cord laceration with gas infection of fetus and uterus, bowel perforation with gangrene and meconium peritonitis, lacerations of the spleen, hemothorax, and tension pneumothorax with bronchopleural fistula.

Of extreme importance is the unusually hazardous situation observed by Gordon et al.,[84] when delivery occurs soon after transfusion. The abdomen is distended with blood, and unless the paracentesis, which is required to allow respiration, is performed in the *left* lower quadrant, the enlarged

---

*References 33, 114, 143, 163, 190, 201, 208, 241, 256.

130

liver may be inadvertently lacerated with serious and often fatal results.

More recently, infants requiring intrauterine transfusions have been transfused using a new procedure, percutaneous umbilical cord sampling (PUBS). With this technique ultrasonically guided percutaneous umbilical vessel puncture allows both direct blood sampling and catheter insertion for transfusions. The procedure is possible as early as 24 weeks and offers more effective treatment for infants still afflicted with erythroblastosis. The risks of the procedure are still not well defined, but preliminary results have had surprisingly few incidents of fetal trauma.[54,266]

Amniocentesis

Since the introduction of amniocentesis, clinical use and research applications of the technique have multiplied. The now widely accepted value of diagnostic and therapeutic amniocentesis must be weighed against the risks of placental hemorrhage and trauma to the fetus. Numerous reports have stressed the safety of the procedure when in experienced hands and the relatively low complication rates.

A recent collaborative study[161] compared the outcomes of pregnancy in 1040 women undergoing amniocentesis during the second trimester of pregnancy with outcomes in 992 women who did not undergo amniocentesis. The data showed no significant differences in fetal death, prematurity, or birth defects. Newborn physical examination showed no evidence of fetal injury attributable to the procedure. The British collaborative study has reported a higher incidence of fetal loss following amniocentesis and more severe morbidity, including respiratory problems and orthopedic postural abnormalities.[43]

However, as pregnancy progresses, the risks of amniocentesis increase even in experienced hands, and the number of complications multiplies. Although infection is a potential fetal risk, particularly with intrauterine transfusions, it has not been a common complication in reported series.[194] Nevertheless, isolated case reports have been recorded.[137,268]

Peddle[183] reported a 4% incidence of fetal to maternal transfusion following amniocentesis, whereas Cassady et al.[40] noted an 11% incidence. However, authorities generally agree that amniocentesis, when compared with a normal pregnancy, does not increase the likelihood of sensitization in an unsensitized Rh-negative woman.[194] Zipursky et al.[276] and Queenan and Adams[196] have documented significant rises in maternal antibody titer following amniocentesis in sensitized women. However, this maternal-fetal risk is outweighed by the benefits of the procedure.

Fetal blood loss is another risk accompanying this procedure, with fetal exsanguination into the amniotic fluid having been reported. Perforation of the umbilical vein with subsequent blood loss and stillbirth,[39] death secondary to abruptio placenta,[151] and perforations of spleen and liver with subsequent blood loss have all been recorded. As experience with the technique has expanded, the incidence of traumatic blood loss has decreased but still remains a potentially lethal complication.

Puncture of the fetus was originally felt to be a rare event of little significance. MacKay[148] and McLain,[156] in reviewing their individual experiences with amniocentesis, suggested that fetal puncture was a rare event. Mandelbaum,[150] Bener,[22] and Wiltchik et al.[271] reported examples of fetal puncture without significant morbidity. Creasman et al.[50] suggested that fetal injuries were more common than appreciated but suggested that rapid healing left no evidence of injury at birth. Andrews[10] reported only two incidents of fetal morbidity related to puncture following 350 amniocenteses. However, more recent reports have included pneumothorax, pneumopericardium, splenic rupture, skin scars, eye trauma,[51] gangrene of a fetal limb,[128] development of an arteriovenous fistula,[85] and ileal atresia with ileocutaneous fistula.[204]

With the addition of ultrasonography, the placenta can be localized in 98% of the patients. Disappointing results with almost all the prior methods of localization have led in many institutions to their substitution by ultrasonography. With clinical examination for placental site and location of fetal small parts, the obstetrician can select a site for amniocentesis. Ultrasonography can then confirm or negate the selected site prior to the procedure. With these improvements subsequent risks to the fetus should be further minimized.

Scalp Abscess

Although more generally seen as a consequence of scalp vein infusion, scalp abscess occasionally occurs as a complication of fetal electrocardiographic monitoring or scalp sampling during labor. Cordero and Hon[49] recently reported seven such abscesses among 2003 cases in which scalp electrodes were employed. Treatment consists of prompt recognition, surgical drainage, and appropriate antibiotic therapy.

INTRAPARTUM INJURY
Soft Tissue Injury
Caput succedaneum and scalp hemorrhage

Molding of the head or parts of the face caused by unusual fetal positions, uterine fibroids, and pressures sustained during labor is a common finding among newborn infants. Particularly common in the primiparous mother with a large fetus is the development of a caput succedaneum. Because of pelvic rigidity and a long labor, the head is noted to be misshaped (that is, long and narrowed) at the time of delivery. The sutures will usually be overriding, and the anterior fontanel may be closed to palpation. The soft tissues of the skull are edematous, boggy, and occasionally hemorrhagic. The edema and hemorrhage, when present, are located between the aponeurotic layer of the scalp and the periosteum. Because the edema or hemorrhage is external to the periosteum, the caput frequently crosses the midline of the skull, a differentiating feature from the more localized cephalohematoma.

In rare instances, significant scalp hemorrhage can occur in a caput, with subsequent development of anemia requiring transfusion.[175,257] When there is no other evidence suggesting disseminated intravascular coagulation, the infant should be checked for specific coagulation disorders, such as hemophilia. Jaundice may also be a complicating feature when significant hemorrhage occurs.

The edema generally recedes in 7 to 10 days, whereas the ecchymoses clear in several weeks. No treatment is required for caput succedaneum, and aspiration of the swelling is contraindicated because of the risk of infection.

Scalp sampling in the antepartum and intrapartum period has been associated with bleeding and breakage of the blade within the fetal scalp. Bleeding can generally be stopped with pressure but occasionally requires sutures. The broken blade can be removed either by a magnet attached to a small forceps or by excision following localization.

Cyanosis, ecchymosis, and edema

Areas of edema, cyanosis, and hemorrhage may be present over the buttocks when the infant has been a breech presentation. One or both lower extremities may have extensive edema, ecchymosis, and cyanosis in instances of footling presentation. Occasionally an edematous cyanotic arm may be the presenting part, with gangrene having been reported as a rare complication of prolonged circulatory obstruction by the cervix. Generally, no treatment is required for these local findings that are secondary to compression of soft tissue during labor, although jaundice may be a complication of the absorption of extensive ecchymoses.[55] Rarely, small areas of cutaneous necrosis may develop in severely compromised tissues requiring topical skin care.

Subcutaneous fat necrosis

Subcutaneous fat necrosis is becoming an uncommon finding as modern obstetrics minimizes trauma to the fetus. Sharply demarcated, firm, subcutaneous nodules or plaques are noted generally on the extremities, face, trunk, or buttocks during the first 6 weeks of life. Lesions have been noted as early as the second day, but usually the intial ones are noted between the seventh and tenth day of life, with late lesions noted at 6 weeks. The chest and abdomen generally are not involved. The lesions vary in size from a few millimeters to 10 centimeters in diameter. The skin overlying these areas may have a deep red or purple discoloration, but most often it is colorless. There is no local heat.

Most of the affected infants are large and often have a history of difficult delivery requiring manual manipulation or application of forceps. The lesions generally occur in areas of local trauma, such as beneath the forcep marks overlying the mandibular ridge.

There is no treatment required for subcutaneous fat necrosis. The lesions persist for several weeks to months and then gradually regress. Fluctuation and cyst formation are unusual complications. Calcification within lesions is rare, and x-ray studies of the lesions are not indicated. Rarely, residual atrophy is noted.

Petechiae

Following difficult or traumatic deliveries, petechiae are commonly noted in the delivery room, particularly involving the presenting part. In infants with cord occlusion, petechiae are often noted proximal to the occlusion, whether the cord is nuchal or wrapped around an extremity. When petechiae are present on the trunk, they are most readily explained by changes in venous pressure during passage of the trunk through the birth canal.

In an infant with an early appearance of petechiae who is otherwise normal by physical examination and whose perinatal history is negative, no further evaluation may be necessary. With localized distribution of petechiae, neonatal thrombocytopenia is unlikely. However, in the presence of bleeding from other sites and a widespread distribution of petechiae, thrombocytopenic purpura or thrombocytopenia secondary to disseminated intravascular coagulation and sepsis must be excluded. Thrombocytopenia also may be caused by maternal use of quinine or thiazides. With traumatic petechiae no specific therapy is needed, and the lesions disappear within several days.

Muscle trauma

In 1966 Rudolph and Gross[209] noted a frequent rise within 24 hours in the serum creatinine phosphokinase (CPK) activity of newborn infants, especially after breech presentations, secondary uterine inertia with oxytocin stimulation, and emergency cesarean section following a trial of labor. This rise in CPK activity was independent of the maternal enzyme level and only slightly elevated in babies born by simple vertex delivery to multiparous mothers. It was lowest in those born by elective cesarean section. As indirect evidence of muscle damage incurred during the birth process, its significance was emphasized by Ralis,[197] who in 1975, following a 10-year study of babies born by breech and vertex presentation, was impressed by the extensive muscle damage that could occur, especially in the buttocks and lower extremities, following breech delivery. In some of the more severely damaged babies there were findings at necropsy of crush syndrome and disseminated intravascular coagulation. Frequently, there was no sign of injury to the skin or subcutaneous tissues overlying the severely damaged muscle mass. Of interest was the fact that the severity of muscle trauma was greater in the preterm than in the term infant.

One may conclude from these studies that muscle damage can present a serious threat to the breech-born infant, and consideration of its possible consequences must be included among the many other complications that may be seen with breech delivery.

Torticollis and sternocleidomastoid tumor

The incidence of torticollis and sternocleidomastoid tumor is about 0.4% of all births. Its etiology is poorly understood, but one of the many possibilities is that of birth injury, first postulated by Stromeyer[243] in 1938. Jones[110], however, points out that tumors have been found at birth in infants born by cesarean section. He also notes that in other instances fully established tumors have been found on the first day of life with microscopic sections showing considerable maturity of the fibrous tissue. He favors an intrauterine cause, possibly related to mechanical factors associated with cramped or distorted fetal positions.

Pathologically, there is marked fibrosis around muscle fibers, which is usually more extensive than appreciated clinically. The fibrosis may involve the entire muscle even though only a localized tumor is palpable.

Clinically the condition presents as a 1 to 2 cm firm, well-circumscribed, round or ovoid mass in the sternocleidomastoid muscle associated with rotation of the infant's head to the opposite side. Occasionally the tumor is bilateral (2% to 3%), and a history of breech delivery may be found in about 20% of the cases. About a third of patients with torticollis have only fibrosis and shortening of the muscle and no palpable tumor.[110] Plagiocephaly, a cranial deformation commonly associated with torticollis, may be present at birth or may develop later.

Typically the tumor is first noted by the parents or pediatrician in the second or third week of life and, in some cases, enlarges slightly during the next 4 to 6 weeks. With physical therapy it usually diminishes in size and slowly disappears over the ensuing 6 months. Plagiocephaly, if present, gradually stops its progress and, as the years go by, may become less noticeable or even regress. According to Jones,[110] this favorable sequence occurred in 45% of the 66 patients he studied, whereas in 9% the tumor persisted or increased in size during the first year, leading to severe torticollis and facial hemihypoplasia. In 35% of his cases some fibrosis was still palpable at a year of age without torticollis, whereas another 11% showed initial complete resolution followed by the appearance of noticeable fibrosis later in childhood.[110]

The treatment of torticollis is primarily nonoperative and is successful in 80% of cases.[111] With the infant supine and both shoulders held flat against a firm surface, the head is gently rotated six to eight times at least four times a day so that the chin touches alternately each acromion process.

The patient should be placed prone for sleeping, and if possible, the crib should be positioned next to the wall in such a way that sources of external stimulation in the room will encourage the infant to turn its head away from the wall and toward the side of the tumor.

Should passive rotation still be limited after 6 months and there is persistent thickening or tension in the muscle, the development of facial hemihypoplasia is of prime concern, and the patient should be considered a candidate for surgery. Through a transverse incision the muscle is divided in its middle third below the exit of the spinal accessory nerve. According to Jones, the fascia colli also must be divided from the anterior border of the trapezius muscle to the midline anteriorly. Postoperative physical therapy, active or passive, is important and should be instituted on the third or fourth day. The prognosis following surgery is usually excellent, with relief of the torticollis and diminution, if not complete disappearance, of the facial asymmetry.

Abrasions and lacerations

Abrasions and lacerations occasionally occur after difficult forceps delivery or emergency cesarean section. Abrasions are best treated by gentle cleansing and the application of antibiotic ointment. Healing is usually rapid and without scarring.

Lacerations through full thickness skin should be cleansed with a mild antiseptic, such as a povidone-iodine solution, and carefully closed with interrupted sutures of 6-0 to 7-0 nylon. The wound may be either left uncovered, especially in the perineal area, or a simple collodion dressing applied. The sutures are removed in 5 to 7 days. Small, superficial wounds may be closed with adhesive butterfly strips. In either case, healing proceeds rapidly and with minimal scarring.

Skull Injury
Molding

Molding of the head is a common finding in the first-born infant and becomes less common with subsequent pregnancies. Molding actually represents the parietal bones overriding the occipital and frontal bones and is usually associated with caput succedaneum. The molding may not be initially noted because of the caput, but as the caput resolves, the overriding sutures may then be appreciated. No treatment is required, since spontaneous resolution occurs during the first several weeks of life. In an otherwise normal infant, no further diagnostic testing is indicated. X-ray studies of the skull to find associated fractures are unnecessary and unproductive.

Skull fractures

Skull fractures are uncommon in the newborn. Because of the demineralization of the skull, the cranial vault is more pliable and compressible than at any other age. In addition, the membranous sutures allow further changes in the contour of the skull during labor and delivery.

Most fractures that occur are a result of the application of forceps or prolonged or traumatic labor and delivery. In such cases, there is repeated battering of the skull against the maternal symphysis, sacral prominence, or the ischial spines. Most frequently, the observed fracture is linear, but depressed fractures may be seen after the application of forceps. The depressed fracture is not usually a true fracture, since an actual break in the cortex is uncommon. Rather, there is an inward bowing of the thin, resilient bone without disruption of the cortex. Occipital fractures were often described in the past in association with breech delivery and were associated with a high infant mortality and an equally severe neurologic morbidity in survivors. With modern obstetric practice, such fractures seldom occur. In the instance of an occipital fracture, the squamous portion of the occipital bone is fixed beneath the maternal symphysis and, when the infant is lifted upward with hyperextension of the spine, the basilar part of the occipital bone moves with the spine and separates from the fixed squamous portion. The line of fracture represents a suture that is normally present in early fetal life and is, therefore, the weakest portion of the occipital bone.

Clinically, there may be no associated findings with a linear fracture, the fracture often being detected during skull x-ray studies ordered for another purpose. Most commonly, there is soft tissue swelling or a cephalohematoma noted during the newborn examination. The infant is otherwise healthy, except in the instance of an occipital fracture when the infant is usually in shock secondary to disruption of the underlying vascular sinuses by the fractured occiput.

In linear fractures no immediate treatment is required, and the long-term prognosis is excellent. However, the infant should be followed for the development of a leptomeningeal cyst from an associated tear of the dura with protrusion of the meninges or part of the brain into and through the fracture. An incidence figure for this association is impossible to obtain, but it is an uncommon occurrence. If the fracture line widens or a defect in the skull is noted at several months of age, cyst formation should be suspected. Because of this rare association, detected linear fractures should be followed with repeated skull films to detect healing of the fractures at 2 to 3 months of age.

Depressed fractures require immediate elevation of the involved portion of the bone. Surgical intervention is necessary only when manual techniques to elevate the depressed fracture have been unsuccessful. Firm, manual pressure on opposite margins of the fracture with exertion of this pressure toward the middle of the depression rather than in an inferior direction frequently causes elevation of the depressed area. A breast pump[219] or vacuum extractor[108] applied around the margins of the fracture (with a seal created by the application of a lubricant around the same margin) has also been reported as a successful means for elevation of depressed fractures. With early recognition and treatment the prognosis for a depressed fracture is good. When the diagnosis or treatment is delayed, death may result in the most severe cases, and subtle neurologic sequelae may be noted in later infancy.

Occipital fractures, as noted, are associated with a high mortality, and successful treatment of the associated shock and blood loss results in salvage of infants with extremely high rates of neurologic morbidity.

Cephalohematoma

The incidence of cephalohematoma is estimated between 0.5% and 2.5% of live births, with the highest frequency among male infants of primiparous mothers. The hematoma represents an accumulation of blood between the surface of the calvarial bone and its pericranial membrane. Since each skull bone is completely surrounded by its own membrane, any blood that accumulates within this membrane is limited in surface area to the involved bone. Thus blood may be present over either parietal bone or the squamous portion of the occipital or frontal bones. Repeated battering of the skull against the maternal symphysis, sacral prominence, or ischial spines during labor, or mechanical trauma associated most commonly with the application of forceps, results in rupture of blood vessels that cross the periosteum with bleed-

ing into the pericranial membrane. Because the membrane is limited to a single bone, the bleeding is sharply demarcated by the periosteal attachments of the cranial bone involved. The area is generally not discolored, although it may be edematous. Unlike the caput, which is usually noted at the time of delivery, the cephalohematoma may not be detected until a subsequent examination in the nursery. Slow subperiosteal bleeding results in delay in the initial appearance of swelling and also explains the frequently noted increase in size of the cephalohematoma over the first several days of life. The hematomas are initially soft and fluctuant, but they eventually become surrounded by a slightly elevated ridge that gives the false impression of a depressed skull fracture. This ridge represents organizing tissue that is formed as the hematoma clots and absorbs.

In our experience, x-ray examination of the involved bone uncommonly reveals associated fracture. Although prior reports[117] have recorded underlying skull fractures in 25% of cephalohematomas, a more recent report by Zelson et al.[275] noted a 5.4% incidence.

The differential diagnosis between a cephalohematoma and caput succedaneum is determined by the sharp demarcation, normal overlying skin, delayed onset, and longer duration of the cephalohematoma. The cranial meningocele can usually be differentiated by its pulsatile character, its increase in size with crying, and an underlying associated defect in the skull.

Cephalohematomas usually require no treatment. Aspiration of the hematoma is contraindicated because of the risk of introducing infection. Rarely, infection of a cephalohematoma[135] occurs in association with systemic bacterial infection. It is accompanied by sudden changes in size of the hematoma and in the appearance of erythema of the overlying skin. In such cases, diagnostic aspiration may be indicated. Hyperbilirubinemia and blood loss severe enough to require transfusion have been reported as complications of large cephalohematomas. With modern obstetric practice, intracranial hemorrhage associated with large cephalohematomas is a rare occurrence.

Most cephalohematomas are resorbed within the first 6 weeks of life. The rate of absorption is usually related to the original size of the hematoma, complete absorption occurring within 2 weeks for smaller hematomas and as long as 3 months for larger ones.

Facial fractures

Facial fractures (nose and mandible) are rare occurrences with modern obstetric practices but may occur with the application or misapplication of forceps or during obstetric manipulation for breech presentations. Clinically, fracture of the mandible[109] may result in facial asymmetry, whereas nasal fractures[229] may cause mild respiratory distress that increases during and immediately after feedings.

Prompt diagnosis and early treatment of facial fractures are important, since healing with rapid, firm union is reported as early as 7 to 10 days. With proper treatment prompt healing without complications is the usual rule, but misdiagnosis or inadequate treatment may result in nasal asymmetry or ankylosis of the mandible.

Long Bone Fractures

Clavicle

The clavicle is the most frequent site of fracture during labor and delivery. This fracture is most commonly associated with shoulder dystocia, requiring obstetric manipulation for delivery, with complete extension of the arms in breech presentations, and with large infants. In many instances, the obstetrician suspects the diagnosis when he or she feels a snap during delivery. Occasionally, however, clavicular fracture is diagnosed following a completely normal spontaneous vertex delivery.

The clinical presentation ranges from the asymptomatic infant with a greenstick fracture of the clavicle to the irritable child with a complete fracture. It is not uncommon to diagnose fracture of the clavicle retrospectively by palpation of callus formation in the second week of life. With complete fractures, the clinical course is marked by irritability, decreased motion of the ipsilateral arm, crepitus, tenderness over the fracture site, crying with movment, and an asymmetric Moro reflex. Radiologically the fracture is most commonly located at the midportion of the clavicle or at the junction of the middle and outer third. The clinical picture of these infants, particularly those with pseudoparalysis and the asymmetric Moro reflex, requires exclusion of a fractured humerus and/or brachial plexus injury in the differential diagnosis. Radiologic studies will exclude the former diagnosis, but infants with fractured clavicles should be examined carefully to exclude a concomitant brachial plexus palsy from the same birth injury.

Greenstick fractures require no specific treatment other than advising the parents about the development of a lump over the fracture site. With complete fractures, the ipsilateral arm and shoulder are immobilized with the elbow flexed at 90 degrees or greater and the arm adducted. Alternately a figure eight dressing can be applied. Either treatment generally may be discontinued within 7 to 10 days when callus formation is present. The prognosis is uniformly good in these infants, with return of the bone to normal contour after 2 to 3 months.

Humerus and femur

Fractures of the humerus occur much less frequently than clavicular fractures, and femoral fractures are rare. Both humeral and femoral fractures are generally associated with one or all of the following clinical situations: prolonged labor, breech presentation with complete extension of the fractured extremity, and rapid extraction of the infant because of fetal distress. Fractures seldom occur below the knee or elbow even during complicated deliveries. The extremity fracture most commonly occurs through the diaphysis or through the epiphysial plate with separation of the plate from the metaphysis.

In the diaphyseal fractures, either humeral or femoral, the fracture usually occurs in the middle third and is usually a diagonal break. Clinically, there is marked overriding of the fracture with lateral displacement. The infants have pain with motion, pseudoparalysis, tenderness, and crepitus to palpation over the fracture site.

Following confirmatory x-ray studies, the humerus can be immobliized by strapping and wrapping the arm to the side with the elbow flexed at 90 degrees. The maximal period for immobilization is generally 4 weeks, with 2 weeks being sufficient in many infants. The long-term prognosis is excellent.

The fractured femur is immobilized by a posterior splint that extends from the buttock to below the knee. Some orthopedic surgeons prefer traction suspension of both lower extremities with the legs immobilized in a spica cast. With either treatment, the infant is immobilized for 2 to 4 weeks until adequate callus formation is present radiologically. Prognosis with this treatment is excellent without shortening of the involved extremity.

Epiphyseal separations

Epiphyseal injuries happen less commonly than complete fractures and usually occur during breech deliveries requiring manual extraction or version with extraction. The proximal femoral epiphysis is most commonly involved with the proximal humerus next.

Clinically, signs usually develop during the second day and include irritability, low-grade fever, pseudoparalysis, tenderness, erythema, crepitus, and swelling over the involved bone. These signs and symptoms clear within 7 to 10 days. X-ray studies of the involved extremity are normal when clinical findings are present and become abnormal after 7 to 10 days when subperiosteal calcification is noted.

Treatment of these injuries requires early closed reduction with immobilization before callus formation prevents corrective manipulation of the epiphysis. With proper diagnosis and early treatment, union occurs within 2 weeks. The misdiagnosed or poorly treated injury may lead to growth disturbance.

Central Nervous System Injury
Intracranial hemorrhage

Central nervous system hemorrhage is a frequent finding at postmortem examination in the newborn with an overall incidence of between 9% and 30%.[99,238] In the past decade the distribution of these hemorrhages has changed dramatically. Previously, trauma was frequently involved in the pathogenesis of intracranial hemorrhage, but with better obstetric care hypoxia is now assumed to be the leading cause. Thus the incidence of subdural and subarachnoid bleeding has diminished. Similarly the incidence of periventricular hemorrhage has also decreased but not to the same extent. More recently, reports of intracerebellar hemorrhage with a possible traumatic basis have been recorded.

During this same past decade, overall neonatal mortality in many newborn intensive care units has fallen below 10%. With this improvement the number of infants surviving intracranial hemorrhage has also increased. However, the morbidity of those infants surviving periventricular hemorrhage is severe. With the advent of computerized tomography of the cranium, a precise diagnosis and location of intracranial hemorrhage can now be made. This advance in diagnostic technique and the recognized severe morbidity of recently surviving infants with periventricular hemorrhage may allow physicians, in consultation with parents, to discontinue heroic therapy.

There are four types of intracranial hemorrhage:

subdural, primary subarachnoid, periventricular, and intracerebellar. The now recognized causes of hemorrhage are trauma and hypoxia, with hypoxia being the primary insult in periventricular hemorrhage. There are also instances in which both mechanisms are involved in the pathogenesis of the hemorrhage. Before the advent of tomography, the diagnosis of intracranial hemorrhage, regardless of location, involved the interpretation of cerebrospinal fluid ((CSF) changes: protein, red blood cells, xanthochromia, and glucose. There are wide ranges of normal for CSF protein, with accepted differences between the full-term and the preterm infant. A level of between 90 and 110 mg/100 ml is generally accepted as normal for term infants, although ranges between 32 and 240 mg/100 ml have been recorded.[167] In preterm infants, the level is higher, with 110-120 mg/100 ml being the more common values. Here, again, there is a wide range of "normal." With intracranial hemorrhage, the protein generally increases at least twofold.

Similarly, broad ranges of normal have been reported for red blood cells, but more recent reports would restrict normal values to less than 30 red blood cells per cubic millimeter.[213]

The development of xanthochromia after hemorrhage is rapid (6 to 12 hours) in an adult or older child, but the appearance in the newborn is generally believed to be slower. Some reports of normal CSF in full-term and preterm infants record 90% to 97% of all fluid as being xanthochromic at delivery, so its usefulness in detecting intracranial hemorrhage is limited.

The accepted ratios of CSF to blood sugar in full-term and preterm infants are 0.81 and 0.75,[213] respectively. With intracranial bleeding, the CSF glucose drops in as many as 60% of the infants within the first 24 hours following the hemorrhage.[56] In the past, combinations of laboratory abnormalities, rather than an isolated abnormality, were emphasized in the clinical setting in attempting to confirm the clinical impression of intracranial hemorrhage. As the application of tomography in the neonatal intensive care unit increases, it is apparent that this technique will confirm or negate the suspected diagnosis.[259]

Because trauma is felt to be of primary importance in subdural, subarachnoid, and intracerebellar hemorrhage, we will discuss those lesions without commenting specifically on the more common periventricular hemorrhage, which is a hypoxic lesion.

Subdural hemorrhage

There are three major types of subdural hemorrhage: a tentorial laceration with rupture of the straight sinus, vein of Galen, or the lateral sinus; laceration of the falx with rupture of the inferior sagittal vein; or the most common lesion, rupture of the superficial cerebral veins. Approximately 20 years ago the first two types were the most common subdural hemorrhages, but with modern obstetric practice both are unusual.

With a tentorial tear, the hemorrhage is usually infratentorial with rapid extension of the blood into the posterior fossa and subsequent compression of the brain stem.[99] Significant infratentorial hemorrhage can also occur without a tentorial tear by rupture of the vein of Galen. The factors involved in the pathogenesis of this hemorrhage include the size of the fetus, the size and rigidity of the pelvis, the duration of labor, and the method of delivery. With a large baby, a rigid pelvis, a short or prolonged labor, and an abnormal presentation (breech or footling), there is excessive vertical molding, frontal-occipital elongation, or both. These external changes and events lead to stretching of the tentorium, falx, or both, with tearing usually occurring near their junction. Such infants are seriously ill from the moment of birth, have low Apgar scores, and require aggressive resuscitation. Early onset of lethargy progresses rapidly to coma. There is deviation of the eyes with absence of the Doll's eye maneuver. Frequently the pupils are unequal and do not react to light. Apneic episodes progressing to respiratory arrest, bradycardia, and decerebrate posturing may quickly develop. The prognosis for these infants, even when treated aggressively with repeated lumbar punctures and surgery, is poor with the mortality rate usually exceeding 90%. The rare survivor often has hydrocephalus secondary to obstruction either at the tentorial notch or over the cerebral convexities.[259]

Tears of the falx occur most often at the junction with the tentorium and usually rupture the inferior sagittal sinus. This variety of hemorrhage is very uncommon. At delivery the infant is generally not as severely depressed as the infant with a tentorial tear. In the nursery the infant is initially lethargic, depressed, and subsequently develops seizures. With infratentorial extension of the hemorrhage, the infant becomes critically ill similar to the newborn with a tentorial tear. The etiology and prognosis of this type of subdural hemorrhage is the same as with a tentorial lesion.

The most common subdural hemorrhage involves tears of the bridging superficial cerebral veins with hemorrhage over the cerebral hemispheres, usually greater over the lateral aspects of the temporal lobes. Volpe[259] has recently described three clinical groups with this type of subdural hemorrhage. The most common variety, or first group, involves minor bleeding without any associated clinical symptoms in the infant. In the second group are infants with significant hemorrhage that produces symptoms, most commonly seizures, that begin between the second and third day of life The seizures are often focal in nature and may be associated with other focal cerebral signs, such as hemiparesis, deviation of the eyes to the contralateral side, and dysfunction of the third cranial nerve. In the third group are infants who have subdural bleeding during the neonatal period with few signs and who subsequently develop subdural effusions over the first several months of life.

Management of the infant with a subdural hemorrhage requires careful observation. Serial subdural taps should be used on the symptomatic patient to reduce intracranial pressure and to prevent development of cephalocranial disproportion with further bleeding. Surgery is necessary only when subdural taps cannot control the complications. Unlike infants with tears of the falx and tentorium, the prognosis for infants with superior convexity hemorrhage is better. Roberts[205] and Schipke et al.[216] have reported that 50% to 80% of these infants are neurologically normal at follow-up.

Subarachnoid hemorrhage

Subarachnoid hemorrhage is probably the most common type of intracranial hemorrhage and, by definition, indicates primary subarachnoid bleeding as opposed to hemorrhage that extends into the space from a subdural, intraventricular, or intracerebellar hemorrhage. In infants this hemorrhage is generally venous blood unlike the arterial source of most subarachnoid hemorrhages in adults. At postmortem examination subarachnoid hemorrhage is a frequent finding in infants without clinical symptoms. Even with significant subarachnoid hemorrhage symptoms are unusual because of the venous origin of the bleeding and the unlikely development of increased intracranial pressure. The most serious long-term consequence of this bleeding is hydrocephalus from adhesions overlying the cerebral convexities with impairment of cerebrospinal flow and decreased absorption of fluid. Adhesions may also develop around the fourth ventricle, again with secondary obstruction to flow.

Descriptions of infants with subarachnoid hemorrhage are difficult because this hemorrhage is often associated with other forms of intracranial hemorrhage. Volpe[259] described three distinct clinical syndromes. The first, minor bleeds without signs or symptoms, occurs frequently in premature infants, who constitute 75% of all infants with subarachnoid hemorrhage.[99] The full-term infant with neonatal seizures[207] seen after 48 hours accounts for a large percentage of those infants with the second type of subarachnoid hemorrhage. The massive bleeding encountered in the third category commonly results in a rapidly fatal course in a severely hypoxic term infant who has usually sustained a traumatic delivery. This variant is also occasionally seen in premature infants with severe respiratory distress syndrome and marked hypoxia.

The management is purely supportive (blood transfusions and anticonvulsants) in the second and third types of bleedng. The prognosis in the second is generally good. Rose and Lambroso[207] reported that 90% of the infants with neonatal seizures in association with intracranial hemorrhage were neurologically normal at follow-up examination. The infant with the first type of hemorrhage does equally well. The rare survivors of the third type have serious neurologic sequelae.

Intracerebellar hemorrhage

The most recently reported variant of intracranial hemorrhage was diagnosed through retrospective analyses and postmortem examinations. All infants were premature[97,153] and had respiratory distress syndrome that was treated with continuous distending pressure. In Pape et al's.[178] original report, distending pressure had been applied with a face mask that was attached by a band wrapped around the occiput. This band was known to cause occipital molding, and the original authors suggested a traumatic etiology to this hemorrhage. Subsequent reports have noted the same site of bleeding, but without the use of face masks for continuous distending pressure. Of the 18 reported cases in the literature, 13 infants also had periventricular hemorrhage. Clinically, all infants had a sudden, catastrophic change in clinical course between the first and twenty-first day of life, with death occurring in 12 to 36 hours. Although trauma may play a role in some of these infants, hypoxia seems more

likely than trauma in the pathogenesis of intracerebellar hemorrhage.

Eye Injury
Subconjunctival hemorrhage

Subconjunctival hemorrhage is a common physical finding in newborns, more frequently noted after difficult deliveries but often observed after normal deliveries. The hemorrhage is noted in the bulbar area and varies in size from less than 1 mm to involvement of a large aspect of the conjunctiva. In an otherwise healthy infant no treatment is required. The blood is generally resorbed within the first 2 weeks of life. When a large subconjunctival hemorrhage is present, the question of other associated intraocular injuries should be raised, particularly in the instance of a forceps delivery.

Intraocular hemorrhage

Retinal hemorrhage is the most common site for intraocular bleeding, but hyphemas and vitreous hemorrhage are also reported. Sezen[227] has estimated that as many as 50% of vaginally delivered infants will have a retinal hemorrhage, if all infants are examined in the first several days of life. This bleeding is the result of repeated compression of the fetal head during labor with subsequent development of venous congestion and retinal hemorrhage. These hemorrhages are usually multiple small lesions scattered throughout the retina and usually resolve within the first 5 days of life without any residual effect on vision. The flame-shaped or streak hemorrhage, which is less common, is generally found near the disc and does not involve the macula or the periphery of the retina. However, hemorrhages adjacent to or in the macula should be noted and carefully followed because of their later association with decreased visual acuity.

With misapplication of forceps or occasionally with face presentations, blunt injury to the eye produces hyphema (blood in the anterior chamber). This injury is frequently associated with rupture of Descemet's membrane. Without rupture, blood is usually resorbed from the anterior chamber in 5 to 7 days. During that critical period, the infant should be fed more frequently to minimize crying, which may predispose to further hemorrhage into the chamber. If the hyphema persists after 7 days, surgery may be indicated.

Rupture of Descemet's membrane may not be detected until after the hyphema is resolved and a corneal haziness (leukoma) persists. Leukoma is secondary to fluids entering through the rupture with interstitial damage of the substantia propria by the fluid. Leukoma frequently becomes permanent with secondary amblyopia.

Vitreous hemorrhage should be suspected clinically when there is absence of the red reflex. The diagnosis is confirmed by slit-lamp examination, which demonstrates the presence of blood pigment. When resolution occurs, it is within the first 6 months, and surgery, which is occasionally required, is reserved for the second 6 months of life.

Peripheral Nerve Injury

Facial nerve palsy

The most common peripheral nerve palsy involves the facial nerve and is usually associated with the application of forceps or a difficult, traumatic delivery. It is difficult in some instances to distinguish an upper motor neuron lesion from a lower motor neuron lesion. Examination of the facial nerve is accompanied by observing the symmetry of facial movements when the child grimaces or cries. Flattening of one nasolabial fold indicates homolateral lower motor pathology. The coexistence of a simultaneous ipsilateral hemiparesis makes an upper motor lesion very likely. These central lesions cause a paralysis of the lower half or two thirds of the face and are usually associated with additional cranial nerve injuries, most frequently the sixth nerve. Fortunately, upper motor lesions constitute a minority of the facial palsies noted at the time of delivery. Agenesis of the facial nerve nucleus (Möbius syndrome) is a rare cause of upper motor neuron lesion. In such instances a careful history may reveal a family history of facial palsies, but more commonly the occurrence is sporadic.

The lower motor neuron lesion is usually associated with compression of the nerve during delivery or with forceps application. The compression most frequently occurs either at the stylomastoid foramen through which the peripheral portion of the nerve passes or along the ramus of the mandible, the normal anatomic course of the nerve. Differentiation of the more frequently noted lower motor or peripheral facial palsy from a contralateral ptosis can be troublesome. Ptosis may be posttraumatic, congenital, or one of the manifestations of a Horner's syndrome, which includes myosis of the pupil, ipsilateral facial loss of sympathetic function, enophthalmos, and heterochromia iridis. In Horner's syndrome due to cervical injury, an associated lower brachial plexus palsy (Klumpke's palsy) may be encountered. The prognosis of Horner's syndrome depends on whether damage to the nerve is transient (secondary to edema) or permanent.

Peripheral facial paralysis may involve the entire side of the face. With complete paralysis the eye is open during sleep. When the involvement spares the orbicular muscle of the eye, the differential of upper from lower motor lesion is based on history, lack of other neurologic findings, and the statistical likelihood of a peripheral etiology.

Most facial palsies require no treatment and show spontaneous improvement over the first 2 weeks of life.[67] With complete paralysis, the open eye should be patched and the cornea kept moist with regular (every 3 to 4 hours) application of methyl cellulose drops. When there is no improvement in the paralysis and anatomic interruption of the facial nerve is suspected, surgery may be indicated. The prognosis of infants who require surgery is better with earlier intervention.

Traumatic submental palsy, involving the ramus mandibularis of the facial nerve, can also occur at birth. When such an infant cries, the involved corner of the mouth fails to pull down. This rare palsy usually resolves within several days. However, it must also be remembered that the same symptom may be caused by a congenital hypoplasia of the depressor angularis oris muscle or a rare congenital nerve paralysis.[5,177]

Brachial plexus palsy

Brachial plexus palsies also coincide most frequently with difficult deliveries. Erb's upper brachial palsy (C5-C6) is far more common than Klumpke's type (C6-T1), but the two types not uncommonly may coexist.[68] About 10% to 15% of Erb's palsies are bilateral. In the upper plexus injury (Erb's lesion) the infant lies with the affected extremity extended, prone, and internally rotated. The Moro reflex is asymmetric, the scarf maneuver is easier, and the biceps and brachioradialis reflexes are abolished or diminished as compared with the opposite side. There may be x-ray evidence of clavicular fracture and, rarely, with the most severe injuries, homolateral diaphragmatic paresis may also be present. In the lower plexus injury (Klumpke's lesion), the muscles of the hand are involved with loss of grasp on the involved side. With either lesion, if the infant shows evidence of improvement while in the nursery, the prognosis is usually good. Between 70% to 90% of patients do well.

Infants who will fully recover have some degree of improvement by 2 weeks. Most will fully recover by 1 month but no later than 5 months. With partial recovery, the initial improvement may be as late as 4 to 6 weeks, with a reduced rate of recovery between 12 and 24 months. There is seldom improvement after 2 years.[90]

Electrodiagnosis may be helpful in differentiating neuropraxis from root avulsion, with no improvement expected with avulsion. Attempts at surgery have had little success to date, although newer microsurgical techniques may offer new promise.[4]

Phrenic nerve palsy

Naunyn,[168] in 1902, is credited with the first reported case of unilateral diaphragmatic paralysis in a newborn infant. In his case, as in the majority of cases since reported, there was an associated ipsilateral injury of the brachial plexus.[24,75,239] Isolated phrenic nerve injury does, however, occur in about 25% of the cases, the first report having been made by Dyson[60] in 1927.

The etiology of phrenic nerve injury is almost certainly due to overstretching of the anterior third, fourth, and fifth cervical nerve roots, a situation most likely to occur when the neck becomes laterally hyperextended during breech or difficult forceps delivery. The incidence of breech delivery is high, and in one reported series of 12 cases, all were breech deliveries.[239] If injury to the nerve roots is mild, recovery may occur within a few weeks; if severe, it may take as long as 4 to 5 months.[8] Nerve regeneration is probably impossible when avulsion of the roots is complete.

The diagnosis of phrenic nerve injury should be considered in any newborn infant with respiratory distress, but it should be especially suspect in those infants in whom there is a history of breech or other complicated delivery or there is an associated Erb's palsy. It is important to note that a chest x-ray film made in the first few days of life may fail to show an elevated diaphragm, even in the presence of significant respiratory difficulty,[21] and in some cases an erroneous diagnosis of cyanotic congenital heart disease has been made.[2,8]

The symptoms and signs are well described by Behrman and Mangurten[21] and include respiratory distress, tachypnea, and episodes of apnea and cyanosis. Dullness with diminished breath sounds may be found on the affected side, and the normal diaphragmatic thrust, frequently felt just under the costal margin, may be absent. Where the left side is involved there may be feeding difficulties with recurrent regurgitation and aspiration. This occurs when there is elevation of the stomach beneath the affected diaphragm with varying degrees of pyloric or cardioesophageal obstruction. There may also be inversion of the stomach with partial or complete volvulus.[160]

Symptoms commonly begin on the first day of life, and although usually in evidence by the end of the first week, their appearance can be delayed for as long as a month.[240]

As noted earlier, the chest x-ray films may appear normal during the first few days, and diagnosis depends on a high clinical index of suspicion and fluoroscopy. In these instances cine fluoroscopic examination will show paradoxic movement of the involved diaphragm (that is, a rise on inspiration and a fall on expiration). Most cases, however, will show in addition to paradoxic movement an obviously elevated diaphragm with a shift of the mediastinum toward the uninvolved side, especially during inspiration. Stauffer and Rickham[240] have noted that the severity of the eventration does not always correspond to the severity of the symptoms, some patients showing a marked eventration but having little respiratory difficulty. In these cases the diaphragm is only partially paralyzed, and there is no paradoxic motion on fluoroscopy.[240]

Patients with congenital diaphragmatic eventration may be difficult to differentiate from those with isolated phrenic nerve injury (acquired eventration). The clinical and radiologic features can be very similar, although Baffes[17] has stated that in the former condition there is no paradoxic movement of the involved diaphragm. In view of the aforementioned observations of Stauffer and Rickham, this sign may not help to distinguish the two conditions in which partial diaphragmatic paralysis exists. Furthermore, not all authorities would agree with Baffe's observation.

The treatment of acquired eventration is controversial. Some authors recommend a prolonged period of nonoperative management for as long as 4 to 6 months with the expectation of phrenic nerve recovery in a high percentage of cases.[8,215,265] These patients are maintained in reverse Trendelenburg position and fed upright, by gavage, if necessary.

In 1958 Bishop and Koop[24] reported the case of a neonate with left phrenic nerve paralysis who died at 14 days of age of diffuse pneumonia and atelectasis. They made a plea for early operative intervention, an approach that has since been supported by other authors who have reported similar experiences.[29,89,240] By restoring the diaphragm to a more normal position, the mediastinum is stabilized, ventilation improved, and feeding problems diminished.

There is no question that these infants are at risk from not only pneumonia and atelectasis but also from recurrent, and occasionally massive, aspiration from regurgitation. With these considerations in mind, it seems reasonable to recommend surgical intervention in any baby whose symptoms are severe and unimproved after 2 to 3 weeks of medical management or in whom assisted ventilation is required.[129,221]

When symptoms are mild and paradoxic movement of the diaphragm minimal, prolonged and careful observation *in the hospital* is justifiable. If, however, after 4 to 5 months there is no sign of recovery, operation is indicated. The persistence of feeding problems with regurgitation and failure to thrive may preclude this nonoperative approach. It must also be remembered that dangerous and severe symptoms may develop at any time and, occasionally, not until the infant is several weeks of age.

Operation consists of either plication alone or plication combined with partial excision of the diaphragm. Thoracotomy through the seventh or eighth intercostal space affords good exposure and is probably the best approach to the right diaphragm. In left-sided lesions a case can be made for repairing the diaphragm transabdominally through a subcostal incision, adding at the same time a complementary feeding gastrostomy. The diaphragm is plicated to the position of midexpiration, and care is taken not to injure the phrenic nerve.[158,160,224]

Parenthetically, although it may be occasionally difficult to differentiate congenital diaphragmatic eventration from phrenic nerve paralysis, it should be emphasized that treatment is similar. It should be individualized, and the operation should be performed early for severe symptoms.

Sciatic nerve palsy

Sciatic nerve palsy is a rare complication of birth injury, but it may be caused iatrogenically after intramuscular injection into the buttocks. Obturator paralysis involving the adductor muscles of the lower extremity has been reported.

Cord injury

Cord injuries are rare at birth and occur most frequently after breech delivery when version and extraction are used. Other predisposing factors include brow and face presentations, dystocia, and precipitous delivery. There is paresis or flaccid paralysis in all muscles below the cervical level, the usual site of injury. Horner's syndrome may be present, but the facial musculature is otherwise spared. Bladder distention with overflow incontinence, as well as decreased sphincter tone and anal paralysis, differentiate this entity from other causes of severe quadriparesis. There is no treatment available for the severe morbidity associated with this injury.

Intrathoracic Injury
Hemothorax

Hemothorax is rare as a direct result of birth injury, but it may occur occasionally as the result of overly enthusiastic attempts at cardiac resuscitation. As noted previously, it has also been reported as a complication of intrauterine blood transfusion.[84,260] In cases of vitamin K deficiency or other coagulopathic states, it may be a spontaneous occurrence without other definable causes.[232] In 1930 Lundquist[146] reported three cases with intrathoracic hemorrhages, of which two were thymic in origin and apparently unrelated to trauma. More recently, Woolley et al.[272] have reported two additional cases in which thoracotomy and thymectomy were performed for hemorrhage from the thymus gland. In neither case was the birth weight above average nor the delivery difficult.

Hemothorax is best treated initially by tube thoracostomy. If bleeding persists after correction of any existing disturbances in blood coagulation, open thoracotomy with attempt to define and correct the source of hemorrhage is indicated.

Pneumothorax

Pneumothorax, like hemothorax, is rarely a direct result of birth injury but may be seen in the immediate postnatal period as the result of overinflation of the lungs during cardiopulmonary resuscitation or assisted ventilation, deep tracheal suctioning, perforation of the esophagus, or, as previously mentioned, it may occur following intrauterine transfusion with puncture of the fetal lung.[192] Treatment depends largely on etiology but almost always requires tube thoracostomy. (Pneumothorax is discussed in greater detail at the end of this chapter.)

Chylothorax

Chylothorax has been reported in the newborn infant,[28,199,273] but as yet there is no agreement as to its etiology. Trauma to the thoracic duct is a possible cause, but the usual history of normal delivery argues against this as the sole explanation. A true congenital fistula due to improper fusion of the primordial duct structures, as suggested by Randolph and Gross,[199] is also a possibility. Moreover, as these authors point out, it may be a combination of both the normal strain of birth plus a congenital weakness at some point in the thoracic duct that leads to its rupture.

Initial treatment consists of multiple thoracenteses or closed thoracostomy. The use of formulas containing medium-chain triglycerides, as recommended recently by Kosloske et al.,[123] may also be tried during this period. If these methods of management fail, open thoracotomy with closure of the points of leakage by fine nonabsorbable sutures is indicated. The use of Evans blue dye administered subcutaneously in the thighs at operation, as suggested by Merrill[159] and again by Randolph and Gross,[199] may aid in identifying the sites of leakage. Total parenteral nutrition is of value in the depleted infant who is too sick to undergo immediate thoracotomy and may in some instances effect a cure.

Esophageal perforation (spontaneous)

Esophageal perforations in the newborn are uncommon and usually appear as isolated case reports.[100,166,249] They represent emergency situations that can have successful outcomes if recognized early and treated promptly. In 1975 Aaronson et al.[1] reviewed 12 cases in the literature and reported a case of their own. In speculating as to the cause of this lesion, they suggested that spasm or incoordination of the cricopharyngeus muscle might be an important factor in allowing a momentarily high intraluminal pressure to be reached within the esophagus. This could occur during vomiting or as a result of the compression forces of birth on a stomach and esophagus filled with amniotic fluid. They were impressed by the absence of resuscitative attempts and nasogastric intubation (or other instrumentation) in the case histories they reviewed. They did note one 1400-g infant with pathologic findings similar to those of necrotizing enterocolitis at the site of perforation and three others who showed esophagitis.

The condition usually is seen as progressive respiratory distress, cyanosis, and shock on the first or second day of life. A chest x-ray film shows a pneumothorax and, frequently, a hydropneumothorax. The perforation is almost always into the right chest, possibly because of the protective position of the aorta along the left side of the esophagus, as suggested by Harrell et al.[100] Usually the tear is in the distal third.

Diagnosis is established by the instillation of water-soluble contrast material into the esophagus, with fluoroscopy or portable chest x-ray film confirming the suspected intrapleural leak.

Treatment consists of prompt thoracotomy, closure of the perforation with interrupted fine nonabsorbable sutures, and chest tube drainage to underwater seal and low suction. Complementary gastrostomy is recommended, although maintenance of nutrition by parenteral means may be considered. Should signs of tension pneumothorax exist preoperatively, immediate tube thoracostomy may be lifesaving.

Intraabdominal Injury
Hemoperitoneum

Although injury to intraabdominal organs is not common,[203] it does occur and must be considered by any physician involved with the care of sick neonates. The liver is the organ most frequently damaged, followed by the adrenal glands, spleen, and kidneys.[53,102,142,146] Causative factors include breech or otherwise difficult delivery, closed cardiac resuscitation, unusually large babies, and pathologic enlargement of the involved organs. An important contributing factor is asphyxia with its associated visceral congestion and alterations in blood coagulation.[13,96,146] These derangements in platelet function and other clotting factors are most pronounced in the premature and erythroblastotic infant.[104,173]

Early diagnosis of intraperitoneal hemorrhage is important, since deterioration can be rapid, and only through early detection can treatment be effective. Hemoperitoneum should be suspected in any newborn infant with abdominal distention, anemia or falling hematocrit, and evidence of intraperitoneal fluid, clinically or by x-ray film. Shock is a late sign and frequently irreversible. Although normal size and delivery do not preclude the diagnosis, a baby of above average birth weight or with a history of breech or difficult delivery is especially suspect. Diagnosis can frequently be confirmed by early paracentesis (in the left lower quadrant) with the recovery of nonclotting blood.[206,236]

Hepatic injury

As noted previously, the liver is the most commonly injured abdominal organ, the incidence ranging from 1% to 9% in autopsies on newborn infants.[42,53,182,215] Subcapsular hematoma is the most common form of liver injury, and causative factors encompass all those already mentioned in the previous section, including livers pathologically enlarged in infants with erythroblastosis fetalis or born of diabetic mothers. The presence of hemagiomatosis presents a particularly precarious and predisposing situation.[87]

The diagnosis should be suspected in any pale, distended baby with signs of intraperitoneal fluid and a history of breech or otherwise difficult delivery. The significant incidence of prematurity in some reported series may be related to an increased bleeding tendency in these babies.[42,52] Unless the liver is severely lacerated, onset of symptoms depends on the time of rupture of the more frequently found subcapsular hematoma. This may occur at any point up to a week following delivery but most commonly occurs between the second and fifth days.[35,53,142,165] Occasionally, if the hematoma is large, there may be early nonspecific symptoms and signs before rupture, such as poor feeding, lethargy, jaundice, tachypnea, tachycardia, and a slow progressive anemia without external signs of blood loss. A mass may be palpable in the right upper quadrant of the abdomen.

Treatment includes prompt resuscitation followed by laparotomy, evacuation of the hematoma, and repair and drainage of the lacerated or otherwise damaged liver. The application of bovine collagen, fibrin glue, or thrombin spray may be of help in controlling persistent ooze from a broadly denuded area. Cywes,[53] in his excellent treatise on intraabdominal hemorrhage in the newborn, emphasizes the importance of recognizing and treating any associated coagulation defect before operation. Exchange transfusion has been reported to be of value in this regard.[237] In selected cases in which the infant is stable and the laceration or hematoma small, careful observation and follow-up with serial ultrasonography may be practiced. A secure intravenous line should be maintained during this period with provision for immediate transfusion if necessary.

Adrenal injury

Clinically significant or massive hemorrhage into the adrenal glands is caused primarily by trauma and occurs most frequently in large babies and those born by breech or difficult delivery. There are, in addition, many contributing factors, one of which concerns the large size of the adrenal glands at birth and the process of involution, which begins almost immediately after delivery.[65,118] The inner part of the cortical portion of the adrenal gland, also known as the provisional or fetal cortex, undergoes extremely rapid growth toward the termination of pregnancy, constituting up to 85% of the newborn cortex.[244] This portion of the cortex is composed of cells with a high sinusoidal vasculature that may become greatly distended with blood in the presence of asphyxia and other causes of visceral congestion.[190] These large congested glands, destined to become half their size by 2 to 3 months through involution of the fetal cortex,[247] are singularly susceptible to injury. In addition, there is progressive postnatal loss of the sinusoidal supporting structure,[16,118] and the reported increased incidence of postmaturity in cases of adrenal gland hemorrhage may reflect placental dysfunction with inappropriate prenatal involution.[27] The glands also receive a rich blood supply from the renal arteries and aorta, and lying between the diaphragm and upper pole of the kidney they are exposed to compression and traction during the birth process.[181]

About 90% of the reported cases have been unilateral, with 75% of these occurring on the right side.[103,215] The venous drainage of the right adrenal gland directly into the inferior vena cava may make it more susceptible to congestion from increased venous pressure than the left adrenal gland, where the vein is longer and drains into the renal vein. This, plus the position of the right adrenal gland between liver and spine (making it more vulnerable to compression during delivery), may account for the predominantly right-sided involvement.[83]

Symptoms usually arise between 2 and 7 days after birth[66,103,152] and are primarily related to the degree of adrenal hemorrhage. They include poor feeding, fever, lethargy or irritability, abdominal distention, vomiting, and diarrhea. When blood loss is severe there will be signs of shock with tachypnea, bradycardia or tachycardia, pallor, and peripheral vasoconstriction. When both glands are involved, adrenal insufficiency may occur with ac-

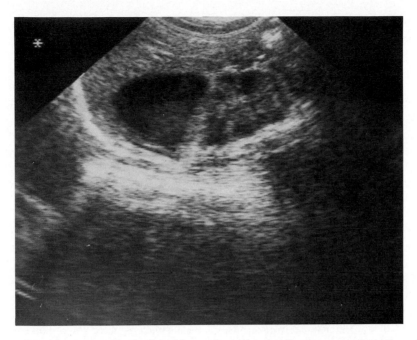

Fig. 9-1   Ultrasound of neonatal adrenal hemorrhage showing large suprarenal sonolucent mass with echogenic debris and flattening of the upper pole of kidney. The ultrasound was normal 1 month later.

companying pyrexia, purpura, coma or convulsions, hypoglycemia, and hyponatremia. A flank mass and unexplained jaundice may be present. An intravenous pyelogram or abdominal ultrasound (Fig. 9-1) will show downward displacement of the kidney on the involved side with flattening and compression of the upper pole.[37] Occasionally, there will be no visualization of the ipsilateral kidney,[106] and differentiation from renal vein thrombosis may be difficult. In the latter condition, however, hematuria is a more prominent feature. Calcification may occur as early as 12 days[261] and is usually rimlike in distribution, as opposed to the more general distribution seen throughout the gland in neuroblastoma. Both types of calcification may be seen early in calcific thrombi of the inferior vena cava, but there is no renal displacement.[116,220,231] Other conditions that may have symptoms similar to those of adrenal hemorrhage include intracranial hemorrhage[215] and intraperitoneal bleeding from other organ injuries.

Treatment depends on the degree of blood loss; when loss is mild and contained within the capsule of the gland, the patient can be managed nonoperatively. When bleeding is massive and continued,

transfusion and operation are mandatory. The first successful attempt was by Corcoran and Strauss[47] in 1924, and since then similar successes have been reported. Operation consists of evacuating the hematoma and carefully ligating all bleeding points. Occasionally, it is difficult to identify and save the adrenal gland when it is involved and surrounded by hemorrhage, and adrenalectomy must be performed.[142] Removal of one gland is well tolerated, however, and decreases adrenal function by only 30%.[95] Where both glands are involved, adrenal insufficiency may be a contributing factor to shock when present, and hydrocortisone should be administered to all patients not responding to volume replacement.[25] Dosages of 25 to 50 mg can be administered intravenously every 8 hours. In one reported case steroid therapy had to be continued postoperatively for 15 days for persistent vomiting, lethargy, hyponatremia, and hypochloremia.[95] However, both glands are rarely affected to the same degree, and although destruction may be extensive, a small island of functioning tissue is likely to survive.[25] Nevertheless, these infants require close follow-up for possible delayed development of adrenal insufficiency.

Splenic injury

Rupture of the spleen is rare in the newborn infant,[215] probably because of its high and well-protected location beneath the diaphragm. It does, however, occur and unless recognized and treated early can lead rapidly to shock and death. It is seen most frequently in large babies, and although a history of difficult or breech delivery is not uncommon, in most reported series the deliveries have been normal and atraumatic.[133,142,222,228,254] The injured spleen itself is also frequently normal, or it may be pathologically enlarged and friable, as in cases of erythroblastosis fetalis and syphilis. Of interest is a report by Philipsborn et al.[186] of three cases of splenic rupture occurring during or just after exchange transfusion. A similar case was reported by Sirola.[233]

The symptoms and signs of splenic rupture are similar to those of hepatic injury. Frequently, there is a latent period of several days if subcapsular hematoma with delayed hemorrhage is present. In addition to pallor and abdominal distention, a mass may be palpable in the left upper quadrant. On x-ray films there may be signs of ascites (blood), and medial displacement of the gastric air bubble may be noted.[78]

In certain infants in whom the situation is stable and bleeding has ceased, careful observation as described earlier under hepatic injury may be justified. In cases of significant and continued blood loss, treatment consists of transfusion, correction of any coagulation defect, and laparotomy. In most instances splenectomy will be required, but because of the recognized risks of fulminating postsplenectomy infection in infants,* an attempt at splenic repair with fine nonabsorbable 6-0 to 7-0 sutures may be justified in certain selected instances. The feasibility of splenic repair has been demonstrated clinically by Mishalany[162] and experimentally in rats by Grosfeld and Ranochak.[94] Matsuyama et al.[154] reported the successful repair of an almost transected spleen in a 2900-g infant, and Simmons et al.[230] were able to control torn capsular bleeding successfully in two infants by cautery and by application of oxidized cellulose to the denuded surface. The use of bovine collagen, fibrin glue, or thrombin spray may also be of help in such instances. Selective ligation of the segmental blood supply to the involved portion of spleen may also be helpful. Considerable caution

*References 30, 36, 71, 72, 105, 119, 131, 225, 234.

and judgment must be exercised in these nonextirpative methods of managing splenic trauma. When splenectomy is performed, long-term prophylaxis with penicillin, as advised by Horan and Colebach[105] in 1962 is urged because of the aforementioned incidence of postsplenectomy sepsis, usually caused by encapsulated pneumococci, meningococci, and Hemophilus influenzae. In selected instances in which the infant is stable and bleeding has ceased, careful observation as described earlier for hepatic injury may be justified.

Renal injury

Renal injury is extremely rare in the newborn infant, but it has been reported as a cause of extensive hemorrhage and death.[53,70] The symptoms of renal injury are those of blood loss, poor feeding, and vomiting. A mass may be palpated in the flank, and an intravenous pyelogram may show distortion or displacement of the involved kidney with or without extravasation of contrast material.

Treatment depends on the degree of injury and blood loss. When blood loss is mild, a nonoperative approach may be feasible; when the loss is great or associated with a significant degree of urinary extravasation, operation with attempt to repair the kidney, plus drainage, is indicated. When damage is extensive, nephrectomy may be necessary. Foreknowledge of a normally functioning opposite kidney is needed in this situation.

Genital injury

Injury to the genitalia, especially in breech presentations, may be seen as postnatal swelling, ecchymosis, or actual hematomas of the scrotum and labia. Although occasionally progressing to gangrene,[170] spontaneous resolution usually occurs over the ensuing 4 to 5 days.

When the scrotal contents are involved, differentiation must be made between an injured testicle (hematoma, hematocele) and testicular torsion. The former condition is usually bilateral and associated with a history of breech delivery and accompanying edema and ecchymosis. Testicular torsion is almost always unilateral, but occasionally bilateral torsion has been reported.[76,132,140,176,200] The involved testicle is seen as a large, firm, scrotal mass with red or purple discoloration, which in the presence of edema of the overlying skin may make distinction from the purely traumatized testicle impossible. When doubt as to the correct diagnosis exists, exploration of the testicle is indicated. If torsion is found and the testicle is viable, simple derotation and fixation are indicated. Where "wet" gangrene is present, orchiectomy should be performed.[235] Contralateral orchiopexy may be delayed but should ultimately be done.[217]

Testicular torsion in the newborn is almost always extravaginal.[107,184] The cause of the twist is unknown but is presumed by at least one author to be caused by the stress of delivery.[107] This possibility receives some support in that many of the reported cases have involved large babies.[76,200,217]

POSTPARTUM INJURY

Pharyngeal Injury

At a meeting of the European Society of Pediatric Radiology in 1968, Eklöf et al.[64] presented the first known report of esophageal pseudodiverticula in newborn infants secondary to submucosal perforation of the esophagus. Since then several other reports of similar injuries have appeared.*

The cause of this lesion, as indicated in a review of the reported cases, is almost certainly due to postpartum suctioning or attempts to pass nasogastric tubes or intubate the trachea. In one case, a breech delivery, the obstetrician felt something "give way" when he inserted his finger in the infant's mouth to help deliver the after-coming head.[79] The site of injury is almost always in the posterior wall of the upper esophagus or pharynx and usually extends inferiorly only a short distance. Occasionally, it may reach the level of the diaphragm (Fig. 9-2). The injury must be differentiated from a high full-thickness perforation of the pharynx or esophagus with penetration into the mediastinum or free pleural cavity.

The symptoms of excessive oropharyngeal secretions and obstruction to the passage of a nasogastric tube are similar to those of esophageal atresia. However, carefully performed x-ray studies using radiopaque contrast material should differentiate the two conditions. As noted by Ducharme et al.,[58] the distance between trachea and opacified tract is much greater in perforation and the tract more elongate and irregular. Also, an upright x-ray film shows a fluid level in atresia that is not seen in cases of perforation. Wells et al.[267] have added the observation that aspiration of contrast material is easily done from an atretic pouch and impossible from a pseudodiverticulum. They also

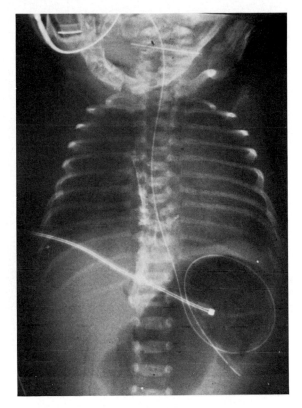

Fig. 9-2   Submucosal perforation of pharynx treated conservatively with nasogastric feeding tube and antibiotics.

note that whereas a dilated, air-containing blind pouch is frequently seen in esophageal atresia on plain lateral x-ray films of the chest, such a structure is absent in cases of perforation.

Treatment is controversial and must be individualized.[26,164] A nonoperative approach with antibiotics and parenteral nutrition or feedings through a carefully placed in-dwelling soft nasogastric tube has been successful in otherwise well-appearing infants in whom injury is diagnosed early.* When there is extensive extravasation of contrast material and a delay in recognition, drainage of the posterior mediastinum and gastrostomy or parenteral nutrition may be the safest treatment (Fig. 9-3). A low right transverse cervical incision with insertion of a small Penrose drain between the carotid sheath and esophagus provides a direct and satisfactory approach to the upper posterior mediastinum. Low and extensive extravasations may require paravertebral, retropleural drainage. Perforations into the

---

*References 14, 58, 61, 79, 134, 147, 267.

*References 61, 64, 125, 147, 164, 252.

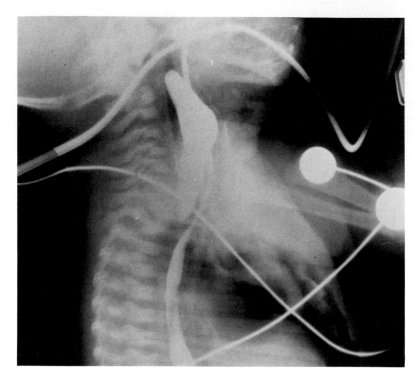

Fig. 9-3   Posterior pharyngeal perforation requiring transcervical drainage and feeding gastrostomy.

free pleural cavity are best managed by closed tube drainage and antibiotics. If the perforation is large with a persistent leak, thoracotomy with attempted repair may be necessary. Rarely will cervical esophagastomy be required.

Pneumoperitoneum

Pneumoperitoneum, as the direct result of birth injury, is a rare occurrence. Traumatic perforation of the gastrointestinal tract is, however, seen in the postnatal period where it is usually the result of therapeutic or other procedures related to infant care. Nasogastric tube perforations of the stomach have been well documented.[258,262] Mask ventilation with overdistention may also lead to gastric rupture. Perforation by feeding tubes have occurred in the duodenum and jejunum.[32,44,141] Perforation of the rectum by thermometers[74,88,180,264,274] and the colon and rectum by therapeutic and diagnostic enemas have also been reported.[74,210] Prevention of these problems is important, and in the case of thermometer perforations it must be remembered that the point of reflection of the parietal peritoneum onto the rectosigmoid colon is only 2 to 3 centimeters from the anus, depending on the size

of the infant. Insertion of a thermometer beyond this point is an invitation to disaster. Some authors have advised against taking rectal temperatures in infants,[74,264] and it has been shown that axillary temperatures properly taken are extremely accurate and usually less than half a degree Fahrenheit lower than simultaneous rectal measurements.[92]

Perforations of the gastrointestinal tract may also be the indirect result of asphyxia incurred by the infant during and immediately following delivery.[139,251] It has been postulated that the asphyxic state evokes a primitive protective reflex seen in certain diving birds and mammals whereby arterial blood is shunted away from the peripheral, renal, and mesenteric circulations to the brain and heart. This reflex, described by Scholander[218] as the "master switch of life," is thought to produce localized areas of ischemia in the gastrointestinal tract, some of which may progress to perforation. By the same mechanism, both asphyxia and cold stress may, through the production of mucosal ischemia and decreased mucous production, set the stage for necrotizing enterocolitis, an important cause of pneumoperitoneum in the newborn period.[18,19,212] These changes in circulation have been shown by Touloukian et al.[253] to occur in asphyxiated neonatal piglets in which diminished segmental and mucosal perfusion was noted in all areas of the gastrointestinal tract except the esophagus.

The symptoms of pneumoperitoneum are those of abdominal distension and vomiting. Respiratory distress, secondary to the upward pressure of massive amounts of free air upon the diaphragms, may be severe enough to require immediate needle decompression. The diagnosis is made by x-ray study, a left decubitus view being less traumatic than an upright in a sick infant.

Treatment consists of expeditious resuscitation followed by prompt laparotomy, the operative procedure itself depending on the pathologic findings. Stomach perforations, usually found high along the greater curvature, should be carefully closed and a gastrostomy performed. Multiple perforations may occur, and the posterior aspect of the stomach must always be inspected by opening the lesser sac.

Perforations of the small intestine are best managed by segmental resection with end-to-end anastomosis. Simple closure is not advisable unless the hole is extremely small and the surrounding bowel viable and free from signs of necrotizing enterocolitis. In selected cases, an end-to-side anastomosis with proximal end-type enterostomy, as described by Santulli and Blanc[211] is both safe and effective.

Colonic perforations may be either closed primarily, with protection by a proximal colostomy, or exteriorized. Treatment by primary closure alone or resection with anastomosis is probably not wise. The possible presence of aganglionic megacolon as a cause of colonic perforation should be borne in mind.

In the presence of advanced peritonitis or necrotizing enterocolitis, resection with establishment of an end-enterostomy and distal mucous fistula may be the quickest and safest procedure.

Pneumoperitoneum in the newborn infant without associated perforation of the gastrointestinal tract has been reported as a complication of severe respiratory disease.* Although this sudden development of free intraperitoneal air may be preceded by the appearance of pneumomediastinum and pneumothorax,[12,57] it has also been noted to occur in the absence of these two conditions.[38,136,188] Most of the reported cases have been in infants requiring

*References 12, 38, 57, 69, 136, 188.

ventilatory support, and almost all have ended fatally. However, occasional survivors have been reported.[69,151] We have had one survivor.

Theory as to pathogenesis and experimental evidence suggests that air from a ruptured pulmonary alveoli dissects its way along vascular sheaths to the mediastinum, from whence it may rupture into the pleural space or progress downward along the aorta and esophagus to enter the retroperitoneum and peritoneal cavity.[57,149] The air may also be carried to the mediastinum by the pulmonary lymphatics, as suggested by Brown and Keenan.[38]

Distinguishing this type of pneumoperitoneum from that caused by perforation of the gastrointestinal tract can be extremely difficult and depends largely on the experience and judgment of the physicians in charge of the case. Leonidas et al.[136] have suggested that x-ray films showing an absence of intraperitoneal air-fluid levels (hydropneumoperitoneum) or signs of necrotizing enterocolitis may be regarded as evidence for a pulmonary origin rather than a perforation. They also recommend the instillation of water-soluble contrast material into the stomach and colon in an attempt to document the presence or absence of perforation. However, even with these diagnostic aids in his or her favor, the surgeon who elects not to operate does so only after careful consideration of all aspects of the case and with the knowledge that pneumoperitoneum in the overwhelming majority of newborn infants is secondary to perforation of the gastrointestinal tract.

Nonoperative treatment consists of controlling any existent pneumothorax by closed-tube drainage and aspirating the intraperitoneal air if it is sufficient enough to cause respiratory embarrassment. Abdominocentesis can be safely accomplished by cautious percutaneous insertion of an angiocatheter in the midline between the xiphisternum and umbilicus.

Endotracheal Tube Complications

The past decade has been marked by an improved understanding of the pathophysiology and treatment of infants with respiratory distress syndrome (RDS). With these advances, neonatal mortality in infants with RDS has decreased in our institution from 50% in the early 1970s to less than 10% today.

Before the introduction of the nasotracheal tube as a way to provide prolonged intubation, tracheostomy was commonly used. With the development of a better understanding of long-term mechanical ventilation, there was renewed interest in alternate methods for providing effective artificial airways. This interest initially led to prolonged orotracheal intubation and subsequently to the use of nasotracheal intubation. The complications associated with tracheostomy in infants and children had been significant[23,171] and included sepsis, erosion of the carotid artery, dislodgement of the tube, tracheal granulomas, and tracheal strictures. There was also mortality related to both insertion of the tube and accidental extubation. Before the use of an orotracheal airway during the insertion of the tracheostomy tube, the intraoperative complications included a 16% incidence of pneumothorax and pneumomediastinum. With an airway in place during tracheostomy, the incidence of these complications was reduced to 5% in Oliver's report.[171] The difficulties of decannulation were related to anatomic damage to the upper airway and larynx with development of obstructive lesions.

With the development of pliable, nontoxic (polyvinyl chloride) materials for tracheal tubes, the therapeutic approach to upper airway maintenance was modified. Following Branfondstater's[34] initial experience, Allen and Steven[6] and McDonald and Stocks[155] also reported successful use of the polyvinyl chloride tube for prolonged intubation. In a review of their initial experience with nasotracheal intubation in 116 infants and children, Striker et al.[242] noted 10 patients with anatomic complications including subglottic stenosis,[256] subglottic granuloma,[120] and papilloma of the vocal cord.[20] The technique was not limited to use in the newborn in this series, and the majority (7 out of 10) of the anatomic complications were in older children with laryngotracheobronchitis. Despite these complications, the authors concluded that nasotracheal intubation was extremely valuable in treating patients with respiratory failure by mechanical ventilation and was, in their opinion, the method of choice for establishment of an artificial airway in infants.

Since these original reports, nasotracheal intubation has been the most commonly used artificial airway. It is preferred by many physicians to orotracheal intubation because there is minimal movement with swallowing, ease in fixation of the tube, and infrequent accidental dislodgement. However, regardless of preference, complications of endotracheal tubes, both oral and nasal, include obstruction by secretions or inadvertent physical kinking of the tube, extubation, malplacement of the tube

into one bronchus with secondary atelectasis on the contralateral side, infection, tracheal ulceration, subglottic edema, granuloma formation, and vocal cord injury. The advantages of orotracheal intubation have been reported by Gregory[91] and include (1) an easier and faster method of intubation, (2) infrequent required tube changes in prolonged intubations, and (3) decreased likelihood of infection from the endotracheal tube. Reported complications of orotracheal tubes include acquired palatal groove and cleft palate. Palatal grooves were noted in two infants who required orotracheal intubation for 70 and 78 days. Saunders et al.[214] suggested rotation of right and left nares and the mouth as sites of intubation to minimize this complication when prolonged intubation is required. Duke et al.[59] reported two cases of acquired cleft of the hard palate in prolonged orotracheal intubation. Similar recommendations regarding rotation of intubation sites were suggested.

In a review of 172 postmortem examinations of infants dying with respiratory distress syndrome within the first 7 days of life, Joshi et al.[112] described acute lesions of the larynx, trachea, and bronchi in the intubated newborn infant. There were histologically demonstrable lesions in 79% of the cases reviewed. The relationship of these lesions to the duration of intubation was examined. In 21%[36] of the infants no lesions were noted: intubation was not conducted in 83% of the group. The most frequent and mildest lesions were detected in 109 infants (63%), with intubation having occurred in 99 of 109 of these patients. The remaining patients (16%) had the most severe lesions and all had been intubated. There was a direct relationship between the severe anatomic lesions and the duration of intubation, the most severe lesions being noted in infants who had longer periods of intubation. The most common site of involvement was the vocal cords, with the subglottic region and trachea next in declining order. The authors reasonably postulated that the mild lesions seen in the 109 infants would have healed completely without any residual damage to the upper respiratory tract. Harrison[101] had reached similar conclusions in a small group of infants who had survived RDS with intubation and died several months later of unrelated causes. He also recognized a relationship between long-term anatomic complications and prolonged intubation. Such reports have been recorded, but the number of large follow-up series of infants surviving intubation with RDS is limited.[86] The factors that would be implicated in the development of the acute lesions and subsequent complications are the method of intubation, experience and technique of the operator, infection, size of the tube, frequency and duration of intubation, and possible toxic substances in the tube itself.

A recent report has cited tracheal perforation as another complication of endotracheal intubation.[226] The perforation was most likely a result of vigorous attempts at intubation. Other etiologic factors that could not be excluded were hyperextension of the head and neck, failure to rotate the tip of the endotracheal tube when an obstruction was noted distal to the cords, and external tracheal compression. The authors suggested that routine chest films, particularly a lateral view after intubation to verify tube position, would have demonstrated the abnormal tube position and allowed a lifesaving tracheostomy to be performed. At least one subsequent report of the same complication cited similar etiologies.

Nasal erosion is still another complication of nasotracheal intubation. Pettet and Merenstein[185] have suggested the following refinements in patient care to prevent this problem: (1) the use of the smallest nasotracheal tube that provides adequate ventilation without excessive air leaks; (2) adequate tube fixation allowing the nasotracheal tube to exit the nose in the same direction that the nares are oriented; and (3) alternation of nares for prolonged or repeated nasotracheal intubation. Most infants requiring mechanical ventilation can be adequately ventilated and suctioned through either a 3.0 or 3.5 mm tube. In a prior report, attachment of the respirator to the nasotracheal tube directly above the infant's nose had been suggested without realization of the excessive pressure and traction placed on the nose by this method.

Stricture of the nasal vestibule has been observed by Jung and Thomas[113] after prolonged nasotracheal intubation. These authors suggest pressure, friction, and chemical irritation of the tube as possible initial insults to the external nares followed by subsequent development of fibrous stricture and stenosis during the healing process. In the reported cases, the strictures involved only the nasal vestibule, but should the scarring involve other nasal structures, chronic serous otitis could become a problem. One of the infants required surgical repair to restore the nasal vestibule to normal size at 2 years: the other child will also eventually require surgical correction. Prevention of this complication includes: (1) the use of a nasotracheal tube that will pass the anterior nares without difficulty or distention of the nasal vestibule but will still allow proper ventilation without excessive air leak; (2) proper fixation of the tube to minimize motion and subsequent friction; (3) changing the tube when there is evidence of irritation, distention, or infection of the external nares; and (4) the use of disposable tubes to prevent tissue irritation secondary to resterilization.

With the introduction of nasal prongs as a method of applying continuous distending pressure, the likelihood of nasal complications is ever present. In our institution, we have noted several infants with nasal erosion secondary to prolonged use of nasal continuous positive airway pressure (CPAP) and others with abnormal unilateral dilatation of the anterior nares. Although the incidence of these complications is low relative to the frequent use of nasal CPAP, precautions must be taken to prevent abnormal degrees of distention, irritation, infection, and friction of the anterior nares. We believe that with compulsive attention to technique and continuous observation of the nasal prongs and the anterior nares these complications can be prevented. Application of CPAP by head box has been associated with severe neck ulceration from failure to support the infant's head while in the hood.[126] Obviously, complications are associated with all artificial airways, but as experience with the techniques increases and proper precautions to prevent complications are followed, these complications can be continually reduced and hopefully eliminated.

Umbilical Catheter Complications (Arterial and Venous)

Catheterization of the umbilical artery in the sick neonate has been an accepted and widely used procedure during the past decade. The atraumatic method of blood sampling, the means for continuous monitoring of blood pressure, and a convenient route for newborn fluid administration have made umbilical artery catheterization a routine practice in many intensive care units. However, as with any other frequently used procedure, complications have been noted.

Optimal position for the umbilical artery catheter has been the subject of controversy in the literature. The two most commonly recommended positions are 1 cm above the diaphragm[98] or just below the inferior mesenteric and renal arteries and above the bifurcation of the aorta.[121] There are few problems in blood sampling and only rare episodes of lower extremity blanching with either position. However, there is some evidence that suggests that the high position of the catheter may be less desirable. Goetzman et al.[81] studied thrombotic complications of high umbilical artery catheterization with aortograms and found a 24% incidence. In comparing the clinical courses of the infants, he noted that only 7% of the patients with normal aortograms had blanching of the leg, whereas 39% of the infants with abnormal studies had blanching. Powers and Swyer,[191] studying possible limb flow changes with the umbilical artery catheter in the lower position, demonstrated no flow deficiencies. Williams et al.[270] and Neal et al.,[169] reviewing 18 positive aortograms out of 21, also suggested placement of the umbilical artery catheter in the distal aorta would be the safest method. This assumption was arrived at after their detection of pericatheter fibrin sleeves and pericatheter and mural clots in the aorta. Wigger et al.[269] also suggested that the location of thromboses corresponded to the level of insertion of the catheter. Boros et al.[31] reexamined 14 children 4 years after demonstration of radiologic evidence of umbilical artery catheter–associated thrombus formation and did not note any long-term sequelae. Femoral length, tibial lengths, leg length measurements, and pulse pressures were not significantly different between the two extremities. The authors presumed that recruitment of fibrinolytic systems and collateral blood supply combined to ensure normal and equal growth of the lower extremities.

Thrombotic complications, clinically suggested and pathologically proven, appear to be the largest contributors to umbilical artery catheter morbidity and mortality. Cochran et al.[45] reported an 8% overall complication rate among 387 infants studied and a 21% incidence of thromboses among 86 infants who came to autopsy. Goetzman et al.[81] also found a 21% incidence of thrombotic complications among 42 necropsies. Symanski and Fox[245] studied 335 umbilical artery catheter insertions over a 4-year period and demonstrated a thrombotic complication rate of 10%. They also noted a higher frequency of aortic thromboses in infants whose birth weight was less than 1000 g. Egan and Eitzman[62] reported a 9.6% total complication rate, but among their 68 autopsies, 17.6% had catheter-related complications. Williams et al.[270] and Neal et al.[169] had a 95% incidence of thrombotic complications found at postmortem examination. Larroche[130] found a 48% incidence of

thrombosis at autopsy, although he could document only one necrotic toe as a clinical sign.

The high incidence of thrombotic complications was explained by Wigger et al.[269] as the result of the catheter tip traumatizing the vessel wall at branching points or as a result of the catheter itself rubbing against the vessel wall. The damaged wall releases ADP, causing platelet aggregation. Catheter-caused spasm reduces blood flow, further exacerbating platelet aggregation and leading to thrombus formation. Many of the above investigators used heparin in the umbilical artery catheter fluid solution in an attempt to prevent thrombosis. Egan and Eitzman[62] used 0.3 U/cc, Williams et al.[270] and Neal et al.[169] used 0.2 U/cc, and Tooley[250] used 1 U/cc. However, the incidence of thrombotic complications did not appear to be reduced significantly among the infants treated with heparin. Williams et al.[270] postulated that heparin therapy is effective in preventing thrombi in the venous circulation because fibrin plays a major role in initiating and maintaining the clot. They commented, as did Wigger, that in arterial thrombosis the initial step is the adherence of platelets to the damaged vessel wall and that "fibrin formation plays a later and less prominent role." They suggested that inhibition of platelet adhesiveness may be more effective than the use of an antifibrin agent, such as heparin, in preventing thrombosis. A recent report[187] of lethal hypertension due to thrombotic complications of umbilical artery catheterization recommends prompt diagnostic evaluation. This report underlines the need for careful monitoring of blood pressure after removal of umbilical artery catheters, a practice not uncommonly overlooked in intensive care units. Response to medical management is generally poor, leading to the recommendation of nephrectomy in patients with occlusion of the renal artery.

Other reported complications include gangrene and infarction of abdominal viscera, paraplegia, false abdominal aortic aneurysm, septic arthritis, hemorrhage, infection, air embolism and potential electrical hazards. Thus the decision to use the umbilical artery demands constant observation of the umbilicus for bleeding, meticulous care of the catheter to prevent propagation of thrombus or air embolism, continuous scrutiny of the lower extremities for evidence of arterial spasm (cyanosis or blanching), and limitation of the duration of catheterization to as short a period as the clinical course requires. The catheter should be removed cautiously to permit proximal arterial spasm and to minimize bleeding. Both the acute and chronic risks of the umbilical artery catheter demand careful evaluation of each patient as to its need and should contraindicate its routine use solely for parenteral therapy. The reports of complications emphasize the dangers involved if there is laxity when using a carefully controlled routine for the placement and subsequent care of catheters.

Realizing the complications of the umbilical artery catheter and assuming that there is virtually no risk in using the umbilical vein, many physicians have adopted this route for routine parenteral therapy. In fact, some authors[48] have failed to note any significant incidence of complications. The accessibility, the technical ease of inserting the catheter, and the longevity of the umbilical vein catheter are obvious advantages to this site. However, the umbilical vein catheter may easily pass into the portal vein, and the administration of sodium bicarbonate[255] or tromethamine (THAM) through the catheter poses the risk of infusing a hypertonic and strongly alkaline solution directly into the liver. The necropsy studies of Goldenberg et al.[82] showed a significant incidence (33%) of hemorrhagic liver necrosis in patients receiving THAM via the umbilical vein. Subsequently, Adamsons[3] documented these findings in laboratory animals. Umbilical vein phlebitis, pyemia, and pulmonary embolus were noted by Scott[223] in infants whose fluid therapy was delivered via umbilical vein catheter. There have also been reports[41,172] of colonic perforation and peritonitis in infants following exchange transfusions via the umbilical vein.

Symanski and Fox[245] noted that umbilical vein catheters had a twofold increase in complications compared with umbilical artery catheters. At autopsy, 44% of their patients with venous catheters were found to have serious thrombi, as opposed to a 6% incidence in those with umbilical artery catheters. Symchych's report[246] of endocarditis, both infected and nonbacterial, confirms the risk of umbilical vein catheterization. In eight of the ten cases reported, documented evidence showed that the vein catheter lay within the heart as a result of misplacement. Symchych et al.[246] postulated that endocardial injury induced by the catheter was followed by the development of endocarditis. Proper placement of catheters should prevent this complication.

Although prophylactic use of antibiotics has been suggested as a means to decrease the risk of infection with umbilical vein catheterization, a recent study[11] clearly demonstrated that such prophylaxis is ineffective. Furthermore, until a large number of infants who have received fluids via the umbilical vein has been followed for several years to exclude the development of portal vein obstruction,[174] it appears wise to follow Lucey's advice[145] that "in the present state of ignorance, it seems best to recommend this route (umbilical vein) of intravascular therapy only when no other is available."

More recently, several studies[127,193,202] have reported successful resolution of aortic thromboses in very low–birth weight infants through the local infusion of streptokinase directly into the clot. The infusion through the arterial catheter in place activates plasminogen, which is converted to plasmin, which, in turn, causes clot dissolution through direct proteolytic enzyme activity. Richardson et al.[202] noted that direct infusion achieved the desired effect at lower and safer doses than previously recommended.

Regardless of the vessel selected for therapy, the following certain recommendations apply universally:

1. Weighing the advantages of the selected route against its risk
2. Using the proper technique when starting the infusion to minimize hazards, to safeguard its continuation, and to promote its longevity
3. Proper nursing observation during the infusion, including maintenance of intravenous flow records and frequent inspection of the infusion site
4. The use of peristaltic pumps to ensure constant flow and to prevent overhydration of a sick infant

The physician who approaches each instance of parenteral therapy with precise knowledge of its practical aspects safeguards the interests of his or her patient and enhances the likelihood of therapeutic success.

Peripheral Nerve Injury (Secondary to Arterial Blood Gas Sampling)

In an attempt either to prevent umbilical artery catheterization or to monitor blood gases after removal of an umbilical catheter, samples of peripheral arterial blood are being obtained by intermittent puncture or by catheterization.

The risks of arterial cannulation include air embolism, sepsis, or injection of incorrect solutions. Todres et al.[248] have described a technique for percutaneous catheterization of the radial artery. In their original report the authors noted occasional occurrences of small necrotic areas at the catheter site but no life-threatening or seriously morbid complications.

Before and since catheterization of peripheral arteries in many intensive care units, repeated arterial punctures have been, and still are, performed to obtain blood samples to monitor oxygen therapy. A recent report[122] documented two cases of carpal tunnel syndrome, one related to multiple radial artery punctures and the other to radial artery catheterization. Both cases were documented by nerve conduction studies, and one was confirmed at autopsy.

Pape et al.[179] prospectively followed 89% (146 out of 167) of the surviving infants in an intensive care unit whose blood gases had been monitored initially with umbilical artery catheterization and then with right brachial artery sampling after removal of the umbilical catheter. All infants were seen until the age of 18 months. Eighteen infants (12%) had evidence of median nerve damage with mild to moderate impairment of the pincer grasp. Thirteen infants (9%) had unilateral impairment; bilateral impairment was noted in five. The incidence of this complication was directly related to the frequency of sampling and indirectly to the birth weight. These two recent reports reemphasize the fact that no procedure in medicine is benign, particularly in the newborn infant. However, the fact remains that at present the risks of peripheral artery catheterization are less than the risks of umbilical artery cannulation.[198]

Pneumothorax

Pneumothorax is a frequent complication of respiratory distress syndrome (RDS). Recent reviews indicate that the incidence rises with the severity of the disease and varies with the mode of mechanical ventilation. In our institution between 1962 and 1975 8% to 10% of all patients with RDS developed a pneumothorax requiring pleural drainage. The most commonly accepted theory of pathogenesis is that when overdistended alveoli rupture, the air dissects along the perivascular sheaths in a retrograde manner to the mediastinum and then breaks into the pleural space. Other causes of pneumothorax include trauma to the lung by sharp instruments during jugular vein puncture,[15] subclavian vein catheterization,[93] and amniocentesis.[46] Recently, bronchial suction catheters[9] have been implicated in perforation of both segmental bronchi and lung parenchyma resulting in pneumothorax.

Regardless of the etiology of the pneumothorax, prompt drainage of the pleural space with a chest tube or catheter is indicated. However, in a postmortem survey of the cases in our institution, we noted a number of iatrogenic lung perforations in infants with RDS and pneumothorax. A review of the clinical courses of 209 infants with RDS over a 40-month period detected 28 infants with pneumothorax requiring pleural drainage, an incidence of 13.4%; 21 of these died, and 20 were examined postmortem. A perforation of the lung directly related to pleural drainage was found in seven of the 20 patients (35%). If we assume that the survivors were free of this complication, the incidence of lung perforation following pleural drainage was 25%. This finding prompted a careful examination of the technique of pleural drainage in the newborn, with particular attention being given to the method of tube insertion, location of the chest tube, and the experience of the operator.

REFERENCES

1. Aaronson IA, Cywes S, and Louw JH: Spontaneous esophageal rupture in the newborn, J Pediatr Surg 10:459, 1975.
2. Adams FH and Gyepes MT: Diaphragmatic paralysis in the newborn infant simulating cyanotic heart disease, J Pediatr 78:119, 1971.
3. Adamsons K: The treatment of acidosis with alkali and glucose during asphyxia in foetal rhesus monkeys, J Physiol 169:679, 1963.
4. Alanen M et al: Early surgical exploration and epineural repair in birth brachial palsy, Z Kinderchir 41:335, 1986.
5. Alexiou D et al: Frequency of other malformations in congenital hypoplasia of depressor anguli oris muscle syndrome, Arch Dis Child 51:891, 1976.
6. Allen TH and Steven IM: Prolonged endotracheal intubation in infants and children, Br J Anaesth 37:566, 1965.
7. Altemus LA and Ferguson AD: The incidence of birth injuries, J Natl Med Assoc 58:333, 1966.
8. Anagnostakis D et al: Diaphragmatic paralysis in the newborn, Arch Dis Child 48:977, 1973.
9. Anderson KD and Chandra R: Pneumothorax secondary to perforation of segmental bronchi by suction catheter, J Pediatr Surg 11:687, 1976.
10. Andrews BJ: The small-for-date infant, Pediatr Clin North Am 17:49, 1970.
11. Aragnostakes D, Kamba A, and Petrochelou V: Risk of infection associated with umbilical vein catheterization, J Pediatr 86:759, 1975.
12. Aranda JV, Stern L, and Dunbar JS: Pneumothorax with pneumoperitoneum in the newborn infant, Am J Dis Child 123:163, 1972.
13. Arden F: Rupture of the liver in the newborn: recovery after blood transfusion and laparotomy, Med J Aust 1:187, 1946.

14. Armstrong RG et al: Traumatic pseudodiverticulum of the esophagus in the newborn infant, Surgery 67:844, 1970.
15. Arnold S, Feathers RS, and Gibbs E: Bilateral pneumothoraces and subcutaneous emphysema: a complication of internal jugular venopuncture, Br J Med 1:211, 1973.
16. Baar HS: Foetal cortex of the adrenal glands, Lancet 1:670, 1954.
17. Baffes TG: Diaphragmatic hernia. In Mustard WT et al., editors: Pediatric surgery, ed 2, Chicago, 1969, Year Book Medical Publishers.
18. Barlow B and Santulli TV: Importance of multiple episodes of hypoxia or cold stress on the development of enterocolitis in an animal model, Surgery 77:687, 1975.
19. Barlow B et al: An experimental study of acute necrotizing enterocolitis—the importance of breast milk, J Pediatr Surg 9:587, 1974.
20. Behrman RE and Mangurten H: Birth injuries. In Behrman RE, editor: Neonatology: diseases of the fetus and infant, St Louis, 1973, The CV Mosby Co.
21. Behrman RE and Mangurten H: Neonatology. In Behrman RE, editor: Neonatology: diseases of the fetus and infant, St Louis, 1973, The CV Mosby Co., p 83-84.
22. Bener HW Jr: Amniography: an accurate way to localize the placenta, Obstet Gynecol 29:200, 1967.
23. Bigles JA: Tracheostomy in infancy, Pediatrics 13:476, 1954.
24. Bishop HC and Koop CE: Acquired eventration of the diaphragm in infancy, Pediatrics 22:1088, 1958.
25. Black J and William DI: Natural history of adrenal hemorrhage in the newborn, Arch Dis Child 48:183, 1973.
26. Blair GK, Filler RM, and Theodorescu D: Neonatal pharyngoesophageal perforation mimicking esophageal atresia: clues to diagnosis, J Pediatr Surg 22:770, 1987.
27. Bolande RP: Adrenal changes in postterm infants and the placental dysfunction syndrome, Am J Pathol 34:137, 1958.
28. Boles TE and Izant RJ Jr: Spontaneous chylothorax in the neonatal period, Am J Surg 99:870, 1960.
29. Bonelli A and Fiocchi A: Unilateral paralysis of the diaphragm following birth injury: surgical treatment, Riv Chir Pediatr 9:234, 1967.
30. Bonyala JM and Aubrespy P: Spontaneous peritoneal hemorrhage of splenic origin in newborn infants, Ann Chir Infant 7:49, 1966.
31. Boros SJ, Nystrom JF, and Thompson TR: Leg growth following umbilical artery catheter-associated thrombosis formation: a 4-year follow-up, J Pediatr 87:973, 1975.
32. Boros SJ and Reynolds JW: Duodenal perforation: a complication of neonatal nasojejunal feeding, J Pediatr 85:107, 1974.
33. Bound JP, Butler NR, and Spector WG: Classification and causes of perinatal mortality, Br Med J 2(suppl):1191, 1956.
34. Branfondstater B: Prolonged intubation. An alternative to tracheostomy in infants, Proc First Europ Congr Anesth (Vienna) 1962.
35. Bret J, Jamain B, and Coupe C: Les hemoperitoines du nouveau-né secondaires a la rupture d'hématome sous capsoulaire du foie, Arch Fr Pediatr 13:1043, 1956.
36. Broberger O, Gyulai F, and Hirschfeldt J: Splenectomy in childhood: a clinical and immunologic study of 42 children splenectomized in the years 1951-1958, Acta Paediatr (Upps)49:679, 1960.
37. Brown B St J, Dunbar JS, and MacEwan DW: The radiologic features of acute massive adrenal hemorrhage of the newborn, J Canad Assoc Radiol 13:100, 1962.
38. Brown DR and Keenan WJ: Pneumoperitoneum without gastrointestinal perforation in a neonate, J Pediatr 85:377, 1974.
39. Burnett RG and Anderson WR: The hazards of amniocentesis, J Iowa Med Soc 58:130, 1968.
40. Cassady G et al: The hazard of fetal maternal transfusion after transabdominal amniocentesis, Am J Obstet Gynecol 99:284, 1967.
41. Castor WR: Spontaneous perforation of bowel in newborn following exchange transfusion, Can Med Assoc J 99:934, 1968.
42. Charif P: Subcapsular hemorrhage of the liver in the newborn: an inquiry into its causes, Clin Pediatr 3:428, 1964.
43. Chayen S: An assessment of the hazards of amniocentesis: report to the medical research council by their working party on amniocentesis, Br J Obstet Gynecol 85:(suppl 2)221, 1978.
44. Chen JW and Wong PWK: Intestinal complications of nasojejunal feeding in low–birth weight infants, J Pediatr 85:109, 1974.
45. Cochran WD, Davis IIT, and Smith CA: Advantages and complications of umbilical artery catheterization in the newborn, Pediatrics 42:769, 1968.
46. Cook LN, Shots RJ, and Andrews BF: Fetal complications of diagnostic amniocentesis: a review and report of a case with pneumothorax, Pediatrics 53:321, 1974.
47. Corcoran WJ and Strauss AA: Suprarenal haemorrhage in the newborn, JAMA 82:626, 1924.
48. Cordero L, Scheig RL, and Orzalesi MM: Umbilical vein infusion. Lancet 2:492, 1969.
49. Cordero L Jr and Hon EH: Scalp abscess: a rare complication of fetal monitoring, J Pediatr 78:533, 1971.
50. Creasman WT, Laurence RA, and Thiecle HA: Fetal complications of amniocentesis, JAMA 204:91, 1968.
51. Cross HE and Maumenee AE: Ocular trauma during amniocentesis, Ophthalmologica 90:303, 1973.
52. Cuadros J, Tovar JA, and Monereo J: Neonatal rupture of the liver: report of 10 cases, Au Exp Pediatr 6:265, 1973.
53. Cywes S: Haemoperitoneum in the newborn, S Afr Med J 41:1063, 1967.
54. Daffos F, Capella-Pavlovsky M, and Forestier F: A new procedure for fetal blood sampling in utero: preliminary results of 53 cases, Am J Obstet Gynecol 146:985, 1983.
55. Davis JA and Schiff D: Bruising as a cause of neonatal jaundice, Lancet 1:636, 1966.
56. Deonna T et al: Neonatal intracranial hemorrhage in premature infants, Pediatrics 56:1056, 1975.
57. Donahoe PK et al: Pneumoperitoneum secondary to pulmonary air-leak, J Pediatr 81;797, 1972.
58. Ducharme JC, Bertrand R, and Debie J: Perforation of the pharynx in the newborn: a condition mimicking esophageal atresia, Canad Med Assoc J 104:785, 1971.
59. Duke PM et al: Cleft palate associated with prolonged orotracheal intubation in infancy, J Pediatr 89:990, 1976.
60. Dyson JE: Paralysis of right diaphragm in newborn due to phrenic nerve injury, JAMA 88:94, 1927.
61. Edison B and Holinger PH: Traumatic pharyngeal pseudodiverticulum in the newborn infant, J Pediatr 82:483, 1973.

62. Egan AE and Eitzman DV: Umbilical vessel catheterization, Am J Dis Child 121:213, 1971.
63. Ehrenfest H: Birth injuries of the child, ed 2, New York, 1931, D Appleton & Co.
64. Eklöf O, Löhr G, and Okmian L: Submucosal perforation of the esophagus in the neonate, Acta Radiol 8:187, 1969.
65. Elliott TR and Armour G: The development of the adrenal cortex and its condition in hemicephaly, J Pathol Bact 15:481, 1911.
66. Emery JR and Zachary RB: Hematoma of the adrenal gland in the newborn, Br Med J 2:857, 1952.
67. Eng GD: The value of electrodiagnosis in facial palsies affecting infants and children, Clin Proc Child Hosp 10:279, 1971.
68. Eng GD: Brachial plexus palsy in newborn infants, Pediatrics 48:18, 1971.
69. Ensing G et al: Pneumoperitoneum in the newborn, J Pediatr Surg 9:547, 1974.
70. Eraklis AJ; Abdominal injury related to the trauma of birth, Pediatrics 39:421, 1967.
71. Eraklis AJ et al: Hazards of overwhelming infection after splenectomy in childhood, N Engl J Med 276:1225, 1967.
72. Erickson WD, Burgert EO Jr, and Lynn HB: The hazard of infection following splenectomy in children, Am J Dis Child 116:1, 1968.
73. Fong SW et al: Intrauterine transfusions: fetal outcome and complications, Pediatrics 45:576, 1970.
74. Fonkalsrud EW and Clatworthy W: Accidental perforation of the colon and rectum in newborn infants, N Engl J Med 272:1097, 1965.
75. France NE: Unilateral diaphragmatic paralysis and Erb's palsy in the newborn, Arch Dis Child 29:357, 1954.
76. Frederick PL, Duschku N, and Eraklis AJ: Simultaneous bilateral torsion of the testes in a newborn infant, Arch Surg 94:299, 1967.
77. Friesen RF: Intrauterine transfusion and erthyroblastosis fetalis. In Lucey JF and Butterfield TJ, (editors): Report of the Fifty-third Ross Conference on Pediatric Research, Columbus, Ohio, 1966, Ross Laboratories.
78. Giedion A: Die Geburtstraumatische Ruptur Parenchymatöser Bauchorgane (Leber, Milz, Nebenniere, and Niere) mit massivem Blutverlust und Ihre Radiologische Darstellung, Helv Paediatr Acta 18:349, 1963.
79. Girdany BR, Sieber WK, and Osman MZ: Taumatic pseudodiverticulums of the pharynx in newborn infants, N Engl J Med 280:237, 1969.
80. Girling DJ, Scopes JW, and Wiggleworth JS: Babies born alive after intrauterine transfusions for severe rhesus haemolytic disease, J Obstet Gynaecol Br Cwlth 79:565, 1972.
81. Goetzman BW et al: Thrombotic complications of umbilical artery catheterization: a clinical and radiographic study, Pediatrics 56:374, 1975.
82. Goldenberg VE, Wiegenstein L, and Hopkins GB: Hepatic injury associated with tromethamine, JAMA 205:71, 1968.
83. Goldzieher MA and Gordon MD: Syndrome of adrenal hemorrhage in a newborn, Endocrinology 16:165, 1932.
84. Gordon H, et al: Experiences with intraperitoneal transfusion, J Obstet Gynaecol Brit Cwlth 73:917, 1966.
85. Gottdiener JS, Ellison RC, and Lorenzo RL: Arteriovenous fistula after fetal penetration at amniocentesis, N Engl J Med 293:1302, 1975.

86. Goumaz CF: Laryngotracheal sequelae of prolonged intubation in newborn infants, Otorhinolaryngologie 35:1, 1973.
87. Graivier L, Votteler TP, and Dorman GW: Hepatic hemangiomas in newborn infants, J Pediatr Surg 2:299, 1967.
88. Greenbaum EI et al: Rectal thermometer–induced pneumoperitoneum in the newborn. Pediatrics 44:539, 1969.
89. Greene W and Hunt CE: Paralysis of the diaphragm, J Pediatr 84:913, 1974.
90. Greenwald AG, Schute PC, and Shiveley JL: Brachial plexus birth palsy: a 10-year report on the incidence and prognosis, J Pediatr Orthop 4:689, 1984.
91. Gregory GA: Respiratory care of newborn infants, Pediatr Clin North Am 19:311, 1971.
92. Gresham EL: Birth trauma, Pediatr Clin North Am 22:317, 1975.
93. Groff DB and Ahmed M: Subclavian vein catheterization in the infant, J Pediatr Surg 92:171, 1974.
94. Grosfeld JL and Ranochak JE: Are hemisplenectomy and/or primary splenic repair feasible? J Pediatr Surg 11:419, 1976.
95. Gross M, Kottmeier PK, and Waterhouse K: Diagnosis and treatment of neonatal adrenal hemorrhage, J Pediatr Surg 2:308, 1967.
96. Gruenwald P: Asphyxia, trauma, and shock at birth, Arch Pediatr 67:103, 1950.
97. Grunet ML and Shields WD: Cerebellar hemorrhage in the premature infant, J Pediatr 88:605, 1976.
98. Gupta JM, Roberton NRC, and Wigglesworth JS: Umbilical artery catheterization in the newborn, Arch Dis Child 43:382, 1968.
99. Haller ES, Nesbitt RE Jr, and Anderson GW: Clinical and pathologic concepts of gross intracranial hemorrhage in perinatal mortality, Obstet Gynecol Surv 11:179, 1956.
100. Harrell GS, Friedland GW, and Daily WJ: Neonatal Boerhaave's syndrome, Radiology 95:665, 1970.
101. Harrison V: Prolonged endotracheal intubation in the newborn infant, Br J Anesth 39:645, 1967.
102. Henderson JL: Hepatic hemorrhage in stillborn and newborn infants: a clinical and pathological study of 47 cases, J Obstet Gynaecol Br Emp 48:377, 1941.
103. Hill EE and Williams JA: Massive adrenal hemorrhage in newborn, Arch Dis Child 34:178, 1959.
104. Honig GR: Disorders of the blood and vascular system. In Behrman RE, editor: Neonatology: diseases of the fetus and infant, St Louis, 1977, The CV Mosby Co.
105. Horan M and Colebatch JH: Relation between splenectomy and subsequent infection, Arch Dis Child 37:398, 1962.
106. Hughes PD and Wiles HB: Adrenal hematoma in a newborn infant simulating renal tumor, Med J Aust 2:370, 1965.
107. Hyams BB: Torsion of the testis in the newborn, J Urol 101:192, 1969.
108. Jan KL: Elevation of congenital depressed fractures of the skull by vacuum extractor, Acta Paediatr Scand 63:562, 1974.
109. Jaworski S and Dudkiewicz A: Mandibular fractures in the course of labor in a newborn infant, Pediatr Pol 48:1501, 1973.
110. Jones PG: Torticollis in infancy and childhood, Springfield, Ill, 1968, Charles C Thomas.

111. Jones PG: Torticollis. In Welch KJ et al, editors: Pediatric surgery, ed 4, Chicago, 1986, Year Book Medical Publishers.

112. Joshi VV et al: Acute lesions induced by endotracheal intubation, Am J Dis Child 124:646, 1972.

113. Jung AL and Thomas GK: Structure of the nasal vestibule: a complication of nasotracheal intubation in newborn infants, J Pediatr 85:412, 1974.

114. Kaern T: Perinatal mortality, Acta Obstet Gynecol Scand 39:392, 1960.

115. Karnicki J: Results and hazards of prenatal transfusions, J Obstet Gynaecol Br Cwlth 75:1209, 1968.

116. Kassner EG et al: Calcified thrombus in the inferior vena cava in infants and children, Pediatr Radiol 4:167, 1976.

117. Kendall N and Woloshin H: Cephalohematoma associated with fracturing of the skull, J Pediatr 41:125, 1952.

118. Kern H: Ueber den Umbau der Nebenniere im Extrauterinen Leben, Dtsch Med Wsch 37:971, 1911.

119. King H and Schumaker HB Jr: Splenic studies: susceptibility to infection after splenectomy performed in infants, Ann Surg 136:239, 1952.

120. Kissane JM: Pathology of infancy and childhood, ed 2, St Louis, 1975, The CV Mosby Co.

121. Kitterman JA, Phibbs RH, and Tooley WH: Catheterization of the umbilical vessels in newborn infants, Pediatr Clin North Am 17:895, 1970.

122. Koenisberger MR and Moessinger AC: Iatrogenic carpal tunnel syndrome in the newborn, J Pediatr 91:443, 1977.

123. Kosloske AM, Martin LW, and Schubert WK: Management of chylothorax in children by thoracentesis and medium-chain triglyceride feedings, J Pediatr Surg 9:365, 1974.

124. Kottmeier PK: Birth trauma. In Randolph JG et al, editors: The injured child: surgical management, Chicago, 1979, Year Book Medical Publishers.

125. Krasna IH, Rosenfeld D, and Bonna, BG: Esophageal perforation in the neonate: an emerging problem in the newborn nursery, J Pediatr Surg 22:784, 1978.

126. Krauss DR and Marshall RE: Severe neck ulceration from CPAP head box, J Pediatr 86:286, 1975.

127. Lacey SR, Zaritsky AL, and Azizkhan RG: Successful treatment of candida-infected caval thrombosis in critically ill infants by low-dose streptokinase infusion, J Pediatr Surg 23:1204, 1988.

128. Lamb MP: Gangrene of a fetal limb due to amniocentesis, J Obstet Gynaecol Br Cwlth 82:829, 1975.

129. Langer JC et al: Plication of the diaphragm for infants and young children with phrenic nerve palsy, J Pediatr Surg 23:749, 1988.

130. Larroche JCL: Umbilical catheterization: its complications, Biol Neonate 16:101, 1970.

131. Laski B and MacMillan A: Incidence of infection in children after splenectomy, Pediatrics 24:523, 1959.

132. Leape LL: Torsion of the testes: invitation to error, JAMA 200:669, 1967.

133. Leape LL and Bordy MD: Neonatal rupture of the spleen: report of a case successfully treated after spontaneous cessation of hemorrhage, Pediatrics 47:101, 1971.

134. Lee SB and Kuhn JP: Esophageal perforation in the neonate: a review of the literature, Am J Dis Child 130:325, 1976.

135. Lee Y and Berg RB: Cephalohematoma infected with bacteroides, Am J Dis Child 121:77, 1971.

136. Leonidas JC et al: Pneumoperitoneum associated with chronic respiratory disease in the newborn, Pediatrics 51:933, 1973.

137. Liley AW: Technique and complications of amniocentesis, New Zeal Med J 59:581, 1960.

138. Liley AW: Intrauterine transfusion of foetus in haemolytic disease, Br Med J 2:1107, 1963.

139. Lloyd JR: The etiology of gastrointestinal perforations in the newborn, J Pediatr Surg 4:77, 1969.

140. Longino LA and Martin LW: Torsion of the spermatic cord in the newborn infant, N Engl J Med 253:695, 1955.

141. Loo SWH, Gross I, and Warshaw JB: Improved method of nasojejunal feeding in low–birth weight infants, J Pediatr 85:104, 1974.

142. Louhimo I, Pasila M, and Sulamaa M: Abdominal birth injuries, Z Kinderchir 4:141, 1967.

143. Low JA, Wesley Boston R, and Gonzalez-Crussi F: Classification of perinatal mortality, Can Med Assoc J 105:1044, 1971.

144. Lucey JF: Colonic perforation after exchange transfusion, N Engl J Med 280:724, 1969.

145. Lucey JF: Diagnosis and treatment: current indications and results of fetal transfusions, Pediatrics 41:139, 1968.

146. Lundquist B: Intraabdominal and intrathoracic hemorrhages in the newborn, Acta Obstet Gynecol Scand 9:331, 1930.

147. Lynch FP et al: Traumatic esophageal pseudodiverticula in the newborn, J Pediatr Surg 9:675, 1974.

148. MacKay EV: The management of isoimmunized pregnant women with particular reference to amniocentesis, Aust N Zeal J Obstet Gynecol 1:78, 1961.

149. Macklin MT and Macklin CC: Malignant interstitial emphysema of the lungs and mediastinum as an important occult complication in many respiratory diseases and other conditions: an interpretation of the clinical literature in the light of laboratory experiment, Medicine 23:281, 1944.

150. Mandelbaum B: Amniocentesis technic: applications and complications, Mich Med 69:209, 1970.

151. Mangurten HH, Ippoliti J, and Besser AS: Pneumoperitoneum in the extremely low–birth weight infant: successful nonoperative treatment, Am J Dis Child 131:422, 1977.

152. Marin HM, Graham JH, and Kickham CJE: Adrenal hematoma simulating tumor in a newborn: report of a case and review of the literature, Arch Surg 71:941, 1955.

153. Martin K, Roessmann W, and Fanaroff A: Massive intracerebellar hemorrhage in low–birth weight infants, J Pediatr 89:290, 1976.

154. Matsuyama S, Suzuki N, and Nagamachi Y: Rupture of the spleen in the newborn: treatment without splenectomy, J Pediatr Surg 11:115, 976.

155. McDonald IH and Stocks JG: Prolonged nasotracheal intubation: a review of its development in a pediatric hospital, Br J Anesth 37:161, 1965.

156. McLain CR: Amniography: a versatile diagnostic procedure in obstetrics, Obstet Gynecol 23:45, 1969.

157. Mellin GW: Unpublished data.

158. Merendino KA et al: The intradiaphragmatic distribution of the phrenic nerve with particular reference to the placement of diaphragmatic incisions and controlled segmental paralysis, Surgery 39:189, 1956.

159. Merrill K; The use of Evan's blue to outline the course of the thoracic duct, J Thorac Surg 29:555, 1955.

160. Michelson E: Eventration of the diaphragm, Surgery 49:410, 1961.

161. Milunsky AL: Risk of amniocentesis for prenatal diagnosis, N Engl J Med 293:932, 1975.

162. Mishalany H: Repair of the ruptured spleen, J Pediatr Surg 9:175, 1974.

163. Mitchell JR et al: An analysis of the causes of perinatal death, Can Med Assoc J 80:796, 1959.

164. Mollitt, DL, Schullinger, JN, and Santulli TV: Selective management of iatrogenic esophageal perforation in the newborn, J Pediatr Surg 16:989, 1981.

165. Monson DO and Raffensperger JG: Intraperitoneal hemorrhage secondary to liver laceration in a newborn, J Pediatr Surg 2:464, 1967.

166. Myers NA: Neonatal rupture of the esophagus, Ann Chir Infant 13:213, 1972.

167. Naidoo T: The cerebrospinal fluid in the healthy newborn infant, So Afr Med J 42:933, 1968.

168. Naunyn B: Ein Falle von Erb'scher Plexuslähmung mit Gleichseitiger Sympathicuslähmung, Dtsch Med Wschr 28:52, 1902.

169. Neal WA et al: Umbilical artery catheterization: demonstration of arterial thrombosis by aortography, Pediatrics 50:6, 1972.

170. Nelson HK, Ferris DO, and Logan DB: Injury of penis, scrotum, and buttocks of the newborn resulting in gangrene, Am J Dis Child 75:85, 1948.

171. Oliver P: Tracheostomy in children, N Engl J Med 267:631, 1962.

172. Orme RLE and Eader SM: Perforation of bowel in newborn as complication of exchange transfusion, Br Med J 4:349, 1968.

173. Oski FA: Hematological problems. In Avery GB editor: Neonatology: pathophysiology and management of the newborn, Philadelphia, 1981, JB Lippincott.

174. Oski FA, Allen DA, and Diamond LK: Portal hypertension: a complication of umbilical vein catheterization, Pediatrics 31:297, 1963.

175. Pachman DJ: Massive hemorrhage into the scalp of the newborn infant: hemorrhagic caput succedaneum, Pediatrics 29:907, 1962.

176. Papadatos C and Moutsouris C: Bilateral testicular torsion in the newborn, J Pediatr 71:249, 1967.

177. Papadatos C et al: Congenital hypoplasia of depressor anguli oris muscle, Arch Dis Child 49:927, 1974.

178. Pape K, Armstrong D, and Fitzhardinge P: Intracerebellar hemorrhage as a possible complication of mask-applied mechanical ventilation in low–birth weight infants, Ped Res 9:383, 1975.

179. Pape KE, Armstrong DL, and Fitzhardinge PM: Peripheral median nerve damage, secondary to brachial arterial blood gas sampling, Ped Res 11:539, 1977.

180. Parker JJ, Mikity VG, and Jacobson G: Traumatic pneumoperitoneum in the newborn, Am J Roent 95:203, 1965.

181. Parmelee AH: Management of the newborn, ed 2, Chicago, 1959, Year Book Medical Publishers.

182. Pasternak P and Hjelt L: Hepatic rupture in the newborn, Ann Paediatr Fenniae 7:131, 1961.

183. Peddle LJ: Increase of antibody titer following amniocentesis, Am J Obstet Gynecol 100:567, 1968.

184. Peterson CG Jr: Testicular torsion and infarction in the newborn, J Urol 85:65, 1961.

185. Pettet G and Merenstein GB: Nasal erosion with nasotracheal intubation, J Pediatr 87:149, 1975.

186. Philipsborn HF Jr, Traisman HS, and Greer D Jr: Rupture of the spleen: a complication of erythroblastosis fetalis, N Engl J Med 252:159, 1955.

187. Plumer LB, Kaplan GW, and Mendoza SA: Hypertension in infants: a complication of umbilical artery catheterization, J Pediatr 89:802, 1976.

188. Porter A: Spontaneous pneumoperitoneum in the newborn, N Engl J Med 254:694, 1956.

189. Potter EL: Fetal and neonatal deaths: a statistical analysis of 2000 autopsies, JAMA 115:996, 1940.

190. Potter EL and Craig JM: Pathology of the fetus and the infant, ed 3, Chicago, 1975, Year Book Medical Publishers.

191. Powers WF and Swyer PR: Limb blood flow following umbilical artery catheterization, Pediatrics 55:248, 1975.

192. Price HV, Andrews J, and Laurence KM: Bronchopleural fistula following intrauterine transfusion, Thorax 27:386, 1972.

193. Pritchard SL, Gordon Culham JA, and Rogers PCJ: Low dose fibrinolytic therapy in infants, Pediatrics 106:594, 1985.

194. Queenan JR: Modern management of the Rh problem: amniocentesis, New York, 1967, Harper & Row.

195. Queenan JR: Intrauterine transfusion: a cooperative study, Am J Obstet Gynecol 104:397, 1969.

196. Queenan JR and Adams DW: Amniocentesis for prenatal diagnosis of erythroblastosis fetalis, Am J Obstet Gynecol 25:302, 1965.

197. Rális ZA: Birth trauma to muscles in babies born by breech delivery and its possible fatal consequences, Arch Dis Child 50:4, 1975.

198. Randel SN et al: Experience with percutaneous indwelling peripheral arterial catheterization in neonates, Am J Dis Child 141:848, 1987.

199. Randolph JG and Gross RE: Congenital chylothorax, Arch Surg 74:405, 1957.

200. Reeves HH et al: Torsion of the spermatic cord in the newborn, Amer J Dis Child 110:676, 1965.

201. Rennard M: Perinatal mortality: review of 450 consecutive perinatal deaths, Am J Obstet Gynecol 104:727, 1969.

202. Richardson R et al: Effective thrombolytic therapy of aortic thrombosis in the small premature infant, J Pediatr Surg 23:1198, 1988.

203. Rickham PP and Johnston JH: Neonatal surgery, New York, 1969, Appleton-Century-Crofts.

204. Rickwood AMK: A case of ileal atresia and ileocutaneous fistula caused by amniocentesis, J Pediatr 91:312, 1977.

205. Roberts MH: Intracranial hemorrhage in the newborn, JAMA 113:280, 1939.

206. Rogers G: Hemoperitoneum resulting from hepatic birth traumatism, Am J Obstet Gynecol 27:841, 1934.

207. Rose AL and Lombroso CT: Neonatal seizure states: a study of clinical, pathological, and electroencephalographic features in 137 full-term babies with a long-term follow-up, Pediatrics 45:404, 1970.

208. Rubin A: Birth injuries: incidence, mechanisms, and end results, Obstet Gynecol 23:218, 1964.

209. Rudolph N and Gross RT: Creatinine phosphokinase ac-

tivity in serum of newborn infants as an indicator of fetal trauma during birth, Pediatrics 38:1039, 1966.

210. Santulli TV: Perforation of the rectum or colon in infancy due to enema, Pediatrics 23:972, 1959.

211. Santulli TV and Blanc WA: Congenital atresia of the intestine: pathogenesis and treatment, Ann Surg 154:939, 1961.

212. Santulli TV et al: Acute necrotizing enterocolitis in infancy: a review of 64 cases, Pediatrics 55:376, 1975.

213. Sarff LD, Platt LH, and McCracken GH: Cerebrospinal fluid evaluation in neonates: comparison of high-risk infants with and without meningitis, J Pediatr 88:473, 1976.

214. Saunders BS, Easa D, and Slaughter RJ: Acquired palatal groove in neonates, J Pediatr 89:988, 1976.

215. Schaffer AJ and Avery ME: Diseases of the newborn, ed 3, Philadelphia, 1971, WB Saunders.

216. Schipke R, Riege D, and Scovelle W:Acute subdural hemorrhage at birth, Pediatrics 14:468, 1954.

217. Schneider RE, Laycob LM, and Griffin WT: Testicular torsion in utero, Am J Obstet Gynecol 117:1126, 1973.

218. Scholander PF: Master switch of life, Sci Am 209.92, 1963.

219. Schraeger GO: Elevation of depressed skull fracture with a breast pump, J Pediatr 77:300, 1970.

220. Schullinger JN et al: Calcific thrombi of the inferior vena cava in infants and children, J Pediatr Surg 13:429, 1978.

221. Schwartz MZ and Filler RM: Plication of the diaphragm for symptomatic phrenic nerve paralysis, J Pediatr Surg 13:259, 1978.

222. Schwartz O and Cohn BD: Rupture of the normal spleen in the newborn with survival, Surgery 59:1124, 1966.

223. Scott JM: Iatrogenic lesions in babies following umbilical vein catheterization, Arch Dis Child 40:426, 1965.

224. Scott R: Surgical aspects of innervation of the diaphragm, Thorax 20:357, 1965.

225. Sera Y et al: The hazard of penumococcal meningitis following splenectomy in the newborn infant, J Jpn Soc Pediatr Surg 7:149, 1971.

226. Serlin SP and Daily WJR: Tracheal perforation in the neonate: a complication of endotracheal intubation, J Pediatr 86:596, 1975.

227. Sezen F; Retinal hemorrhage in newborn infants, Br J Ophth 55:248, 1971.

228. Sieber WK and Girdany BR: Rupture of the spleen in newborn infants: recovery after splenectomy. N Engl J Med 259:1074, 1958.

229. Silverman SH and Liebow SG: Dislocation of the triangular cartilage of the nasal septum, J Pediatr 87:456, 1975.

230. Simmons MA et al: Splenic rupture in neonates with erythroblastosis fetalis, Am J Dis Child 126:679, 1973.

231. Singleton EB and Rosenberg HS: Intraluminal calcification of the inferior vena cava, Am J Roent 86:556, 1961.

232. Sinniah D and Nagalingam I: Hemothorax in the newborn, Clin Pediatr 11:84, 1972.

233. Sirola K: Subcapsular bleeding of the spleen with rupture in a newborn infant with erythroblastosis fetalis, J Pediatr Surg 2:155, 1967.

234. Smith CH et al: Hazards of severe infection in splenectomized infants and children, Am J Med 22:390, 1957.

235. Snyder WH Jr, Brayton D, and Greaney EM Jr: Torsion of the testis. In Mustard WT et al, editors: Pediatric surgery, ed 2, Chicago, 1969, Year Book Medical Publishers.

236. Sokol DM, Tompkins D and Izant RJ Jr: Rupture of the spleen and liver in the newborn: a report of the first survivor and a review of the literature, J Pediatr Surg 9:227, 1974.

237. Srouji MN, Williams ML, and Werner JH: Neonatal rupture of the liver: use of exchange transfusion to correct associated coagulation defects, J Pediatr Surg 6:56, 1971.

238. Srsen S: Intraventricular hemorrhage in the newborn and "low birth weight", Devel Med Child Neur 9:474, 1967.

239. Stauffer UG: Diaphragmatic paralysis due to birth trauma, Helv Pediatr Acta 27:253, 1972.

240. Stauffer UG and Rickham PP: Acquired eventration of the diaphragm in the newborn, J Pediatr Surg 7:635, 1972.

241. Steer CM and Moore JG: The course of perinatal mortality: a review of etiologic factors in the Sloane Hospital 1888-1967, Obstet Gynecol 34:113, 1969.

242. Striker TW, Stool S, and Downes JJ: Prolonged nasotracheal intubation in infants and children, Arch Otolaryngol 85:210, 1967.

243. Stromeyer GF: Beiträge zur Operativen Orthopadik, oder Erfahrungen über die Subcutane Durchschneidung Verkürzter Muskeln und Deren sehnen, Hannover, Helwing, 1838.

244. Swinyard CA: Growth of the human suprarenal glands, Anat Rec 87:141, 1943.

245. Symanski MR and Fox HA: Umbilical vessel catheterization: indications, management, and evaluation of technique, J Pediatr 80:820, 1972.

246. Symchych PS, Krauss AN, and Winchester P: Endocarditis following intracardiac placement of umbilical venous catheters in neonates, J Pediatr 90:287, 1977.

247. Tahka H: On the weight and structure of the adrenal glands and the factors affecting them, in children of 0-2 years, Acta Pediatr (Upps) 40 (suppl 81):371, 1951.

248. Todres ID et al: Percutaneous catheterizations of the radial artery in the critically ill neonate, J Pediatr 87:273, 1975.

249. Tolstedt GE and Tudor RB: Esophagopleural fistula in a newborn infant, Arch Surg 97:780, 1968.

250. Tooley WH: What is the risk of umbilical artery catheterization? Pediatrics 50:1, 1972.

251. Touloukian RJ: Gastric ischemia: the primary factor in neonatal perforation, Clin Pediatr 12:219, 1973.

252. Touloukian RJ, Beardsley GP, and Ablow R: Traumatic perforation of the pharynx in the newborn, Pediatrics 59:1019, 1977.

253. Touloukian RJ, Posch JN, and Spencer RP: Selective gut mucosal ischemia in asphyxiated neonatal piglets: a model for the pathogenesis of "ischemic gastroenterocolitis" of the neonate, J Pediatr Surg 7:194, 1972.

254. Tovar JA, Cuadros J, and Monereo J: Neonatal rupture of the spleen : report of seven cases, An Esp Pediatr 6:273, 1973.

255. Usher R: Reduction of mortality from respiratory distress syndrome of prematurity with early administration of intravenous glucose and sodium bicarbonate, Pediatrics 32:966, 1963.

256. Valdes-Dapena MA and Arey JB: The causes of neonatal mortality: an analysis of 501 autopsies on newborn infants, J Pediatr 77:366, 1970.

257. VanderHorst RL: Exsanguinating cephalohematoma in African newborn infants, Arch Dis Child 38:280, 1963.

258. Vargas LL, Levin SM, and Santulli TV: Rupture of the

stomach in the newborn infant, Surg Gynecol Obstet 101:417, 1955.

259. Volpe JJ: Neonatal intracranial hemorrhage, Clin Perinat 4:77, 1977.

260. Wade ME et al: Intrauterine fetal transfusions: experience with 101 transfusions in 48 mothers, Am J Obstet Gynecol 105:962, 1969.

261. Wagner AC: Bilateral hemorrhagic pseudocysts of the adrenal glands in the newborn, Am J Roent 86:540, 1961.

262. Wagner EA et al: Polyethylene tube feeding in premature infants, J Pediatr 41:79, 1952.

263. Wallace HM, Hoenig L, and Rich H: Newborn infants with cogenital malformations or birth injuries, Am J Dis Child 91:529, 1956.

264. Warwick WJ and Gikas PW: Neonatal transanal perforation of rectum, Am J Dis Child 97:869, 1959.

265. Wayne ER et al: Eventration of the diaphragm, J Pediatr Surg 9:643, 1974.

266. Weiner CP: Cordocentesis, Obstet Gynecol Clin North Am 15:283, 1988.

267. Wells SD et al: Traumatic prevertebral pharyngeoesophageal pseudodiverticulum in the newborn infant, J Pediatr Surg 9:217, 1974.

268. Westbury JA and Margolis AJ: Amniotic fluid evaluation and intrauterine transfusions for erythroblastosis fetalis, Am J Obstet Gynecol 92:583, 1965.

269. Wigger HJ, Bransilver BR, and Blanc WA: Thrombosis due to catheterization in infants and children, J Pediatr 76:1, 1970.

270. Williams HJ et al: Vascular thromboembolism complicating umbilical artery catheterization, Am J Roentgen Radium Ther Nucl Med 116:475, 1972.

271. Wiltchik SG, Schwartz RH, and Emich JD: Amniography for placental localization, Obstet Gynecol 28:641, 1966.

272. Woolley MM et al: Spontaneous thymic hemorrhage in the neonate: report of two cases, J Pediatr Surg 9:231, 1974.

273. Yancy WS and Spock A: Spontaneous neonatal pleural effusion, J Pediatr Surg 2:313, 1967.

274. Young DG: "Spontaneous" rupture of the rectum, Proc Roy Soc Med 58:615, 1965.

275. Zelson C, Lee SJ, and Pearl M: The incidence of skull fracture underlying cephalohematomas in newborn infants, J Pediatr 85:371, 1974.

276. Zipursky A et al: Transplacental fetal hemorrhage after placental injury during delivery or amniocentesis, Lancet 2:493, 1963.

10

Battered Child Syndrome

Barton D. Schmitt and Michael R. Clemmens

Child abuse and neglect can be broadly defined as the maltreatment of children and adolescents by their parents, guardians, or other caretakers. The physician has two main responsibilities in these cases—detection and reporting. He or she must be able to diagnose abuse in his or her own patients, as well as confirm the diagnosis in patients referred by other professionals. Case-finding is especially important in the first 6 months of life because the risk of a fatal outcome is high if an early diagnosis is not made. In addition, laws concerning the reporting of child abuse are clear. In all 50 states the physician must report suspected cases of child abuse and neglect to the local Child Protective Services Agency. The law protects the physician from liability suits if his or her suspicion should prove to be wrong. Reluctance to report can lead to a recurrence of injuries or even death. In this chapter, we shall briefly review the full spectrum of child abuse and neglect and then cover the battered child syndrome (physical abuse) in depth, since it is the main focus of the surgeon.

DEFINITIONS OF CHILD ABUSE AND NEGLECT

Physical Abuse

Physical abuse or nonaccidental trauma can be defined as injuries inflicted by a caretaker. These can be rated as *mild* (a few bruises, welts, scratches, cuts, or scars), *moderate* (numerous bruises, minor burns, or a single fracture), or *severe* (large burn, central nervous system injury, abdominal injury, multiple fractures, or any life-threatening abuse). Severe abuse is the most important type because without treatment it is potentially fatal.[20] Often the injury stems from an angry parent who is punishing a child for misbehavior.

Sometimes it is an uncontrolled lashing out at a child who happens to be in the adult's way during some unrelated crisis. Since physical punishment and spanking are acceptable in our society, physicians must have guidelines as to when it is excessive, and, therefore, represents physical abuse. Corporal punishment that causes bruises or leads to an injury that requires medical treatment is outside the range of normal punishment. Bruising implies hitting without restraint. A few bruises in the name of discipline can easily spill over into a more serious injury the next time. Although discipline is necessary to prevent "spoiling" children, harsh discipline is not. Even when there are no signs of injury, an incident that includes hitting with a closed fist or kicking the child represents physical abuse. Likewise, a history of previously inflicted injuries should be reported if the perpetrator still lives in the household.

Failure to Thrive Due to Nutritional Deprivation

Failure to thrive can be defined as an underweight, malnourished condition.[33] A baby who fails to thrive usually weighs below the third percentile, and his or her height and head circumference are above the third percentile on the growth curves. On physical examination, the infants have gaunt faces, prominent ribs, wasted buttocks, and spindly extremities. Failure to thrive is mainly seen in the first 2 years of life because this is the time of rapid growth and of dependency on adults for feeding. Most babies with this disorder are detected before 8 months of age. The causes of failure to thrive are estimated as 30% organic, 20% underfeeding due to understandable error, and 50% underfeeding from parental neglect. The latter type of failure to thrive is called nutritional deprivation, or caloric deprivation, and should be reported to the Child Protective Services Agency. A common error is the misdiagnosis of short stature as failure to thrive. Of the 3% of children who are under the third percentile in height, the majority are short but well nourished.

A nutritional rehabilitation program is the starting point for reaching a definitive diagnosis in infants with failure to thrive. The child should be hospitalized and placed on unlimited feedings of a regular diet according to age. The formula should be identical to the one used at home. Rapid weight gain on a formula free of cow's milk, protein, or lactose would prove nothing. The daily caloric intake should approach 150 to 200 cal/kg/day. This therapeutic feeding trial should last a maximal of 2 weeks. The underweight infant who gains rapidly and easily in the hospital is a victim of underfeeding at home. A rapid weight gain can be defined as greater than 1.5 oz/day sustained for 2 weeks. A gain of over 2.0 oz/day in a 1-week period is also diagnostic. Sometimes the hospital weight gain is less than this, but if it is two to three times greater than in a similar period at home it is diagnostic.

Without detection and intervention, some infants with nutritional deprivation are brought in dead from starvation.[2] Others sustain superimposed physical abuse.[22] In addition to these physical problems, the child with nutritional deprivation usually suffers from prolonged emotional deprivation and subsequent personality disorders.

Sexual Abuse

Sexual abuse can be defined as any sexual exploitation of a child under 18 years of age by an adult.[24] This may include vaginal intercourse, sodomy (anal intercourse), oral-genital contact, or molestation (fondling, masturbation, or exposure). Many of these incidents occur without force. By contrast, rape is usually defined as sexual intercourse forced on a victim by a stranger using violence or threats of harm. Some studies find sexual abuse to account for 25% of child abuse and neglect.[24] In most cases the victimized child is a girl. Over half the children are under 12 years of age at the time of the first offense. A stepfather or a mother's boyfriend living in the home is more likely than the natural father to be involved in sexual abuse.

In some cases the patient will complain of sexual abuse. More often, neither the girl nor the mother mention it, and the physician must take a careful and sensitive history to uncover it. Sexual abuse should be suspected in cases of unexplained vulvitis, vaginitis, anal fissures, pregnancy, or other genital symptoms. Venereal disease in the prepubertal child is very likely to have resulted from sexual exploitation. The diagnosis becomes more probable if the girl also has a history of running away from home or is accompanied by her father when she comes to the physician's office. Often the diagnosis is made only after the child has been interviewed alone.

Every patient needs a general physical examination so that signs of bodily injury or infection can be detected. The mouth, anus, and external genitals should be especially scrutinized for signs of trauma. The hymenal ring should be inspected for intactness. If the throat is inflamed, a throat culture for gonococcus should be plated on the Thayer-Martin medium, since this has been reported with forced oral-genital contact.[1] Selected sexual abuse cases need to be referred to an emergency room with the expertise and equipment to perform a forensic vaginal examination that can stand up in court. All rape cases (postpubertal and prepubertal) should be referred immediately for this procedure. In cases in which significant genital trauma has occurred, a pelvic examination with the patient under anesthesia is sometimes required. Incest cases also should be referred if intercourse has taken place in the last 48 hours (evidence for sperm rarely persists beyond this time period). In most incest cases, laboratory studies are normal and the diagnosis is based on the history and physical examination.

Intentional Drugging or Poisoning

When a parent gives a youngster a harmful prescription drug that is not intended for children (for example, giving adult sedatives to crying children), this needs to be reported for the child's safety.[34] Intentional poisoning is an uncommon form of child abuse. In an unusual case, a caretaker attempted to poison a child even while he was hospitalized. Some parents have deliberately shared hallucinogenic agents with their children. Some children of drug addicts have become addicted to heroin before 10 years of age.

Medical Care Neglect

When a child with a treatable chronic disease has serious deterioration in his or her condition or frequent emergencies because the parents repeatedly ignore medical recommendations for home treatment (for example, neglecting to give insulin to a diabetic child), the case may require reporting for court-enforced supervision or even foster placement.[32] A court order to hospitalize and to treat is also needed in emergency situations that are not acknowledged as such by the parents (for example, refusing a blood transfusion on religious grounds or refusing to hospitalize a child with meningitis). The child's right to live must override the parents' constitutional right to religious freedom. All these problems require attempts to educate and persuade before a legal approach is used. It should be obvious that if the disease is incurable (for example, a cancer), the parents' wishes regarding nonintervention, be they on religious or philosophic grounds, should be respected.

Safety Neglect

Safety neglect should not be reported unless there is gross lack of supervision and the child is under 2 years of age. It is common knowledge that parents have to supervise their child carefully at this age. Beyond 2 years of age, most children exercise a certain amount of freedom, thereby creating the potential for accidents to happen. Gross lack of supervision includes being left in the house without sitters or being left unsupervised to roam the neighborhood. The criteria given apply to far less than 1% of accidents.

Although most accidents are caused by a breach in safety and theoretically could be prevented, the normal parent is already filled with guilt, and reporting these accidents does nothing but accentuate this guilt. The physician would do best to use an educational rather than a punitive approach when confronting parents about an accident. Has anyone's child grown up without at least one "preventable" accident?

Emotional Abuse

Emotional abuse can be defined as the continual scapegoating and rejection of a specific child by his or her caretakers. Severe verbal abuse and berating are always components. This condition is difficult to prove. Psychologic terrorism is present in some cases (for example, locking a child in a dark cellar or threatening to mutilate). The diagnostic criteria of emotional abuse are severe psychopathology in the child, documented by a psychiatrist, plus the continued refusal by the parents to provide treatment for the child. Situations in

which an only parent is either floridly psychotic and hence inadequate to care for the children or severely depressed and therefore a danger to the children should also be included and reported. In addition, lack of supervision, abandonment, physical neglect (grossly inadequate hygiene, clothing, and shelter), and school avoidance are also reportable but usually do not involve physicians.

INCIDENCE AND DISTRIBUTION

The incidence of child abuse and neglect is generally 1%. The prevalence is approximately 1200 cases per million population per year. The types of child abuse seen by physicians are physical abuse (70%), sexual abuse (25%), and failure to thrive due to nutritional deprivation (5%). Approximately 10% of the injuries seen in a hospital emergency room in children under 5 years of age are inflicted.[17] The mortality is about 3%, or 4000 deaths per year, in this country. Physical abuse may be the greatest killer of children between 6 and 12 months of age when compared with any specific cancer, malformation, or infectious disease; from 1 to 6 months of age, it is probably second only to sudden infant death syndrome.

Victim

The abused child is usually an infant. Younger children are at greater risk because they are demanding, defenseless, and nonverbal. Estimates of the usual age for physical abuse are that one third of all cases involve children under 1 year of age, one third involve children from 1 to 6 years of age, and one third of all victims are 6 years of age and older. Lauer et al.[25] found that 63% of the infants were under 2 years of age. Boys are twice as likely as girls to be a victim. Premature infants are at a greater risk of three to one,[21] and stepchildren are also at an increased risk.

Abuser

The abuser is a related caretaker in 90% of the cases, a boyfriend in 5%, an unrelated babysitter in 4%, and a sibling in 1%. Parents who abuse their children come from all ethnic, geographic, religious, educational, occupational, and socioeconomic groups. Those in poverty may abuse their children more frequently because of increased crises (for example, unemployment and overcrowding) and decreased resources. Alcoholics and other substance abusers are more likely to abuse their children. An increased incidence of physical abuse has also been noted on military bases. Women are more likely to be involved in abuse than are men because mothers spend more time with their children; however, there is no difference if the fathers are unemployed.

ETIOLOGY OF PHYSICAL ABUSE

The parent is psychotic in less than 5% of physical abuse cases. These parents are more likely to be involved in cases of deliberate murder. The parent is a sociopath in less than 5% of the cases. Such a parent punishes with little concern for injury and demonstrates little restraint. Often he or she can be recognized by a history of spouse-beating or difficulty with the law.

Over 90% of abusive parents are neither insane nor criminals. They tend to be lonely, unhappy, angry adults under tremendous stress. Often they are married to someone who is neither supportive nor helpful. They are also usually isolated and incapable of using agencies or an extended family in times of crisis. They injure their child in anger after being provoked by some misbehavior. Often they have experienced physical abuse themselves when they were children; their poor self-control is thus a reenactment of what happened to them. They also believe that aggression is necessary in teaching children to respect authority.

Physical abuse requires not only the right parents but also the right child and the right day. The right child has characteristics that make him or her demanding and difficult. He or she may be a handicapped or preterm child requiring extra parenting, a hyperactive child, a strong-willed child, or a precocious child who is brighter than the parents. In some way the injured child is different and stands out from siblings. Misbehavior may range from crying to making a mess to talking back.

The right day usually is a day of crisis. The most common crises involve parents in poverty and include losing a job, being evicted, having the heating turned off and telephone disconnected, having the car break down, or losing food stamps. The second most common crisis concerns marital conflicts. The third most common crisis involves an acute illness in the child that leads to intractable crying. Other crises include a recent move, death in the family, birth of a sibling, diagnosis of an unwanted pregnancy, or responsibility for several young children.

INJURY HISTORIES SUSPICIOUS FOR PHYSICAL ABUSE
Diagnostic History

When a child readily indicates that a particular adult hurt him or her, it is almost always true. A confession by either parent or the report of an eyewitness is also diagnostic but rarely available.

Unexplained Injury

Some parents are reluctant to elaborate on how an injury might have happened. They may state that they "just found him that way" and that there are no witnesses. When pressed, they may become evasive. Some will give a vague explanation, such as "she might have fallen down" or "his brother may have hit him." These explanations are self-incriminating. Parents normally know to the minute where and when their child was hurt. They also show complete willingness to discuss it in detail.

Discrepant History

Sometimes there is a discrepancy between the histories offered by the two parents, or the history changes in regard to dates, times, and causes. Another common contradiction occurs between the history offered and the physical findings, such as a history of a minor accident and the findings of a major injury (for example, a child who allegedly fell against a coffee table and yet is covered with bruises, or a child who allegedly fell on thick carpet but who looks as if he or she had been hit by a car). Children who fall from a crib almost never suffer serious head injuries.[16] Sometimes the parents' dating of the injuries may differ from the clinical dating, or bruises may be of several different ages. Sometimes a discrepancy exists between the history and the child's developmental age (for example, a 1-year-old child allegedly turning on scalding water in the bathtub, or a 6-month-old infant climbing out of the crib). Another contradiction occurs in children who allegedly bruise easily. This history is usually misleading, and no new bruises appear during hospitalization.

Alleged Self-Inflicted Injury

The child who is under 6 months of age is unlikely to be able to induce any accident. Fractures in children younger than this are almost uniformly inflicted. Absurd stories such as "the baby rolled over on his arm" and broke it or "got his head caught in the crib" and fractured it are pure nonsense. Histories implying that the child is masochistic are also uniformly false, such as the child who hurts himself badly during a temper tantrum, suffers subdural hematomas by hitting himself with a bottle, climbs up onto a hot radiator, or burns himself up to the elbow by immersing his arm in hot water. Children rarely deliberately injure themselves.

Alleged Third Party–Inflicted Injury

When the parents blame their child's injuries on a babysitter, neighbor, or sibling, the physician must remain skeptical. Although such a story could be true, the accused abuser must be interviewed in private as early as possible for confirmation. Often the parent will be unable to remember the name of the accused. Sometimes the blame has been projected onto a nonexistent person.

Delay in Seeking Medical Care

Parents generally go to the hospital immediately when their child is injured. Some abused children are not brought in for a considerable amount of time despite a major injury. In its extreme, children are brought in nearly dead. The parents are usually merely hoping that the event never occurred or that the injury will not require medical care. In addition, the time of occurrence may be significant. Accidents occurring between midnight and 6:00 AM are open to question.

History of Repeated Suspicious Injuries

A suspicious injury is one that is unexplained or seems excessive for the described accident. If a child has suspicious bruises on more than one occasion or has a sibling with similar findings, this probably represents inflicted trauma. Many of these children are simply dismissed as "accident prone"—a serious mistake. Certainly no magic number of accidents per year is diagnostic of child abuse. Recurrent accidents (even three in 1 week) can occasionally occur in families. However, the authentic nature of the accident is documented by complete and plausible accounts that are spontaneously offered. Even in these cases, one should be certain that the sudden upsurge in accidents does not stem from a major family crisis.

PHYSICAL FINDINGS PATHOGNOMONIC FOR PHYSICAL ABUSE

Many of the following physical findings are pathognomonic for nonaccidental trauma and speak for the child who is too young to speak for himself. Other nondescript bruises become diagnostic of physical abuse when combined with the vague histories already reviewed.

Diagnostic Bruises, Welts, Lacerations, and Scars

Inflicted bruises are so common at certain sites that finding them there is pathognomonic. Bruises that predominate on the buttocks and lower back are almost always related to punishment (for example, paddling) (Fig. 10-1). Likewise, genital area or inner thigh bruises are usually inflicted for toileting mishaps.[13] Bruises on the cheek or numerous petechiae on the earlobe are usually caused by being slapped or cuffed. If one looks closely, often there are associated fading yellow bruises, which mean this area has been hit on other occasions. Accidental falls rarely cause bruises in the soft tissues but instead involve bony prominences such as the forehead or zygoma. Bruises of the upper lip and labial frenulum are usually caused by impatient forced feedings or by jamming a pa-

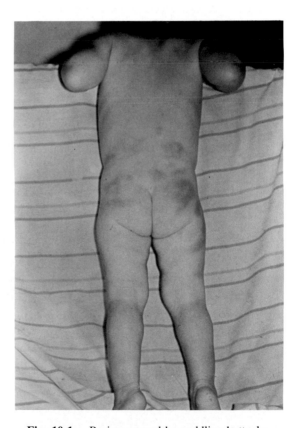

Fig. 10-1   Bruises caused by paddling buttocks.

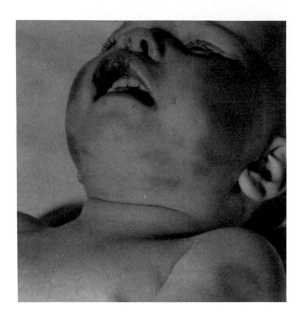

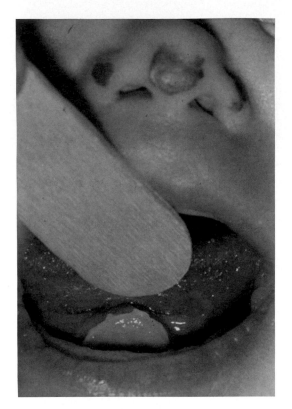

Fig. 10-2   Bruised upper lip and frenulum resulting from forced feeding of a baby.

Fig. 10-3   Laceration of the floor of the mouth from forcible jamming of a bottle against the tongue. Also note the abrasion of the nose.

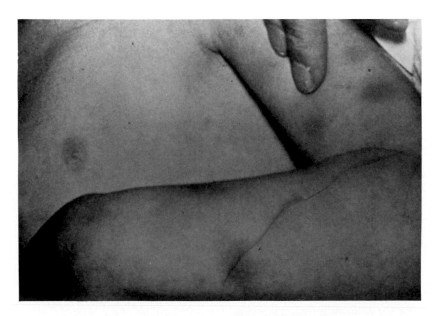

Fig. 10-4   Fingerprint bruises (grab marks) on upper arm.

cifier into the mouth of a screaming baby as a desperate attempt to silence him or her (Fig. 10-2). This bruising may remain hidden unless the inside of the lips is carefully examined. The floor of the mouth may also be torn by similar actions (Fig. 10-3). Bruises in this area cannot be self-inflicted until the baby is old enough to sit up without assistance and inadvertently fall over.

Human hand marks are pressure bruises resembling fingertips, fingers, or the entire hand. Grab marks are oval, fingertip-sized bruises. Several grab marks are often found on the arms or legs where the child was vigorously held during a beating (Fig. 10-4). Encirclement bruises occur when the child is grabbed about the chest or abdomen. This results in eight finger bruises on one side and two thumb bruises on the other side. The examiner's fingers can easily be placed into this pattern. Linear grab marks are caused by pressure from the entire finger. An outline of the entire handprint is sometimes seen on the back or other sites. Such bruises are outlined because only the capillaries at the edges of the injury are stretched enough to rupture. In slap marks to the cheek, two or three finger-width lines are often seen to run through the bruise (Fig. 10-5). Pinch marks are two small crescent-shaped bruises facing each other (Fig. 10-6). Human bite marks are distinctive, paired, crescent-shaped bruises that usually contain individual teeth marks (Fig. 10-7). Sometimes the two crescents meet to form a complete ring of bruising. The size of the arch can distinguish adult from children's bites.[27]

Strap marks are 1- to 2-inch wide rectangular bruises of various lengths, sometimes covering a curved body surface (Fig. 10-8). These are almost always caused by a belt. Sometimes the eyelets or belt buckle can be discerned. Lash marks are narrow straight-edged bruises and scratches, most often caused by beating with a tree branch or switch. Loop marks on the skin are caused by being struck with a doubled-over lamp cord or rope (Fig. 10-9).

Bizarre-shaped bruises are always inflicted. When a blunt instrument (for example, a toy or shoe) is used in punishment, a bruise or welt will often resemble it in shape (Fig. 10-10). Children have displayed tattoos inflicted with a sharp instrument such as a pin or razor (Fig. 10-11). Numerous puncture wounds may be caused by a fork. Choke marks may be seen on the neck (Fig. 10-12) and circumferential tie marks on the ankles or

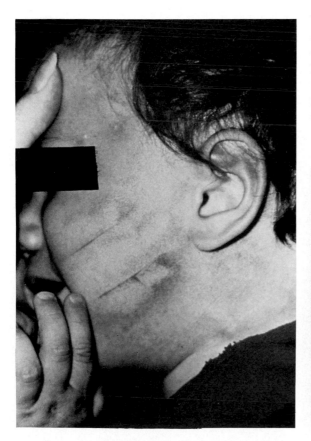

Fig. 10-5   Slap marks bruise of cheek with finger-width lines running through it.

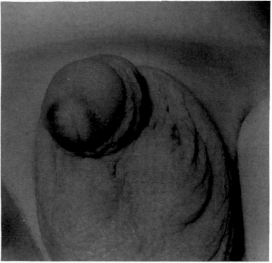

Fig. 10-6   Pinch mark bruise of glans penis for "touching self."

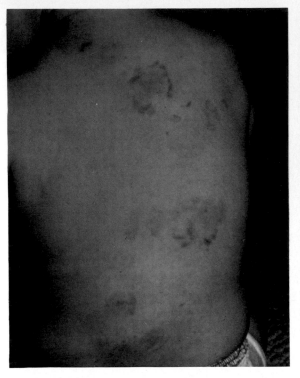

Fig. 10-7 Multiple human bite bruises. Individual tooth marks are visible.

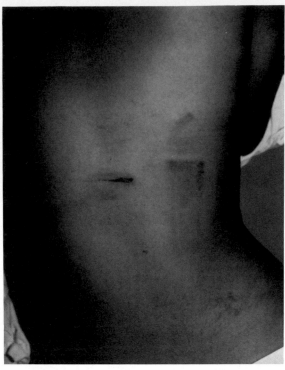

Fig. 10-8 Strap mark bruises of the back.

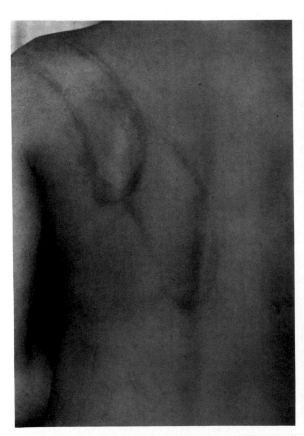

Fig. 10-9 Loop mark from beating with doubled-over cord.

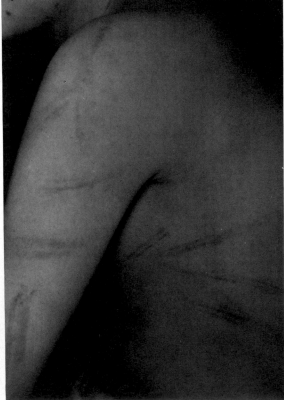

Fig. 10-10 Marks from beating with plastic railroad track.

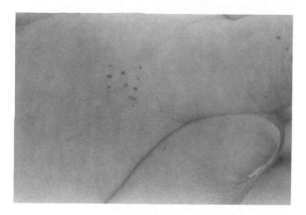

Fig. 10-11   The letter "N" tattooed on child's foot with a pin.

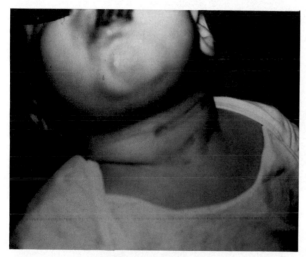

Fig. 10-12   Choke marks on the neck, probably from a cord.

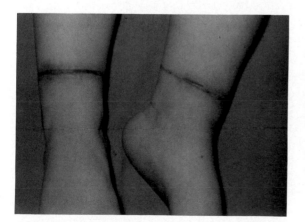

Fig. 10-13   Circumferential marks on the ankles from being tied to a bed with cords while the mother went out.

wrist caused by a rope, cord, or dog leash (Fig. 10-13). Gag marks may be seen at the angles of the mouth.

Bruises and scars found at multiple stages of healing are extremely diagnostic and imply repeated beatings. Most falls cause bruises on just one body surface. Bruises on multiple body planes are usually inflicted unless there is a history of a tumbling accident.[18] True tumbling accidents often cause minimal bruises and abrasions, but if there are many bruises, they will predominate on the elbows, knees, and shoulders. Falling down a stairway is commonly offered as a last-minute explanation for unexplained bruises on the child. However, the lack of bruises in the noted locations makes this explanation doubtful.

Diagnostic Burns

Approximately 10% of the cases of physical abuse involve burns.[13] The most common inflicted burn seen in an outpatient setting is from a cigarette (Fig. 10-14). These are circular, punched-out burns of similar size. These lesions are often found on the palms, soles, or abdomen. A hot cigarette is sometimes applied to the hand to stop the child from sucking his or her thumb or to the genital area to discourage masturbation. Bumping into a cigarette causes only a single burn, unless the ash catches in the clothing. Smaller but similar burns have been inflicted with incense or match tips. Burns have also been inflicted with lighters in an aberrant attempt to teach children not to play with fire. The only differential diagnosis is bullous impetigo. In such a case, the lesions are of various

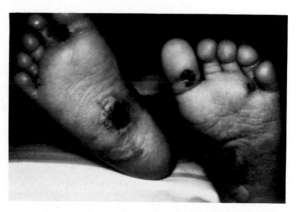

Fig. 10-14   Cigarette burns of the feet.

sizes, occur in groups, have purulent crusts, and increase in number and size while in the hospital.

Dry contact burns can occur as a result of forcibly holding the child against a heating device (for example, a radiator) (Fig. 10-15). This usually causes second-degree burns without any blister formation and usually involves only one surface of the body (for example, the back or both palms).

The shape of the burn is pathognomonic if the child is held against a heating grate, touched with a hot iron, or forced to sit on an electric hot plate (Figs. 10-16 and 10-17). Unexplained linear burns are usually caused by running a heated piece of metal (for example, the heated cover of a cigarette lighter or a hot comb) across the child's skin for punishment (Fig. 10-18).

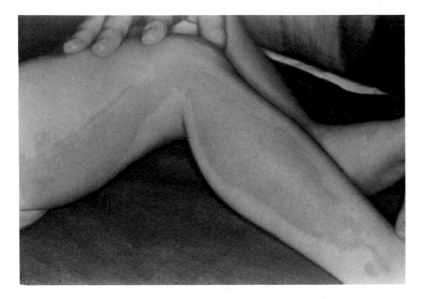

Fig. 10-15 Dry burns of the leg from forcible holding against radiator.

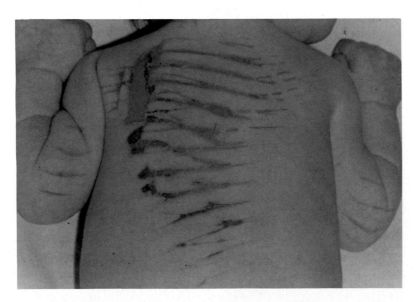

Fig. 10-16 Heating grate burn of the back and upper arms in a 6-week-old baby.

Hot water burns (scalds) are of several types. The most common is a dunking burn in which the offender holds the thighs against the abdomen in a jack-knife position and dunks the buttocks and perineum into a bucket of scalding water. Often this results in a circular burn restricted to the buttocks (Fig. 10-19). With deeper forced immersion, the scald extends to a clear-cut water level on the

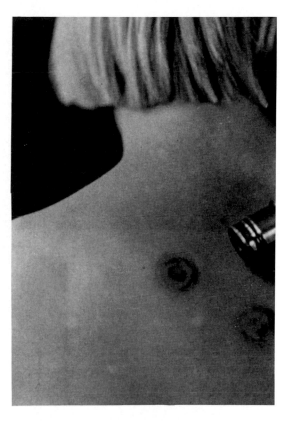

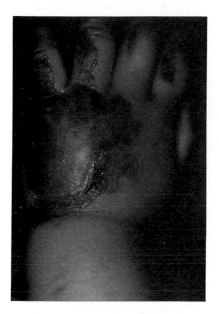

Fig. 10-17   Iron burn on dorsum of hand.

Fig. 10-18   Car cigarette lighter burn of the upper back.

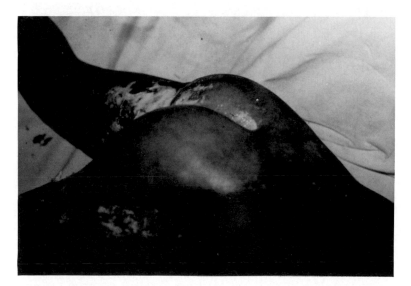

Fig. 10-19   Circular burn of the buttocks from forcible immersion in scalding water as punishment for resisting toilet training.

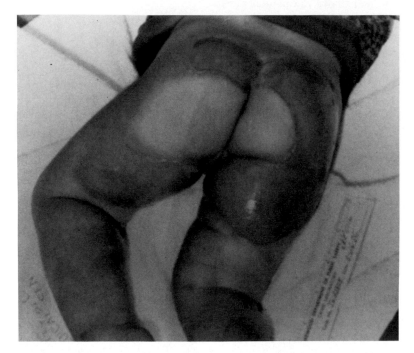

Fig. 10-20   Severe dunking burn of buttocks and posterior thighs from being forced to sit in a bathtub of scalding water. The spared areas on the buttocks were probably pressed against the bottom of the tub at the time of injury.

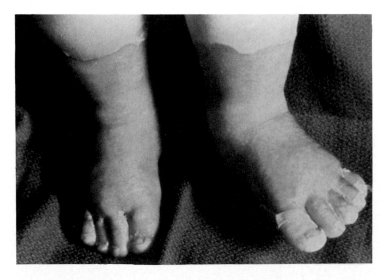

Fig. 10-21   Forced immersion burn of the lower leg.

thighs and waist. The hands and feet are spared, which is incompatible with falling into a tub of hot water or turning the hot water on while in the bathtub. Sometimes the child is forced to sit in scalding water. This causes the dunking-type burn plus scalds of the back of the thighs and legs (Fig. 10-20). Depending on exposure time, the soles may be relatively spared because of their thicker skin. The bottom of the toes, however, are not spared. Of interest, 45% of inflicted burns involve the perineum or buttocks.[19] These sites are almost always chosen as punishment for enuresis or toilet-training resistance. Occasionally the perianal skin will be spared because it was protected by contact against the bottom of the bathtub.

Forcible immersion of a hand or foot as punishment can be diagnosed by the finding of a burn that extends well above the wrist or ankle without splash marks (Fig. 10-21). Children are not foolish enough to place an extremity into hot water to this depth. Whenever a scald of the hand or foot is full thickness and requires grafting, it points to prolonged hot water exposure, and hence forced immersion. Burns due to throwing scalding water at a child are more difficult to diagnose, since so many children acquire splash burns when they pull a pan of hot liquid off the stove. A scald limited to the back may mean that the child was trying to run away from an angry parent.

The only remote differential diagnosis in hot water burns is the scalded skin syndrome (toxic epidermal necrolysis) caused by Staphylococcus aureus. Unexplained blebs are seen, but they occur at such scattered sites that inflicting them with hot water would be nearly impossible; also, they may increase in number during hospitalization.

Eye Injuries

Ocular damage in the battered child syndrome includes acute hyphema, dislocated lens, and detached retinas.[12] Over half of these result in permanent impairment of vision affecting one or both eyes. Retinal hemorrhages are also a clue to subdural hematoma in children with unexplained central nervous system findings. Dilation of the pupil with a mydriatic agent or indirect retinoscopy performed by an ophthalmologist is sometimes required to discover these hemorrhages. Retinal hemorrhage can also occur without clinically important intracranial hemorrhage in children with sudden compression of their chest.[37] This finding is called Purtscher's retinopathy.

Brain Injuries

Subdural hematoma is the most dangerous inflicted injury, often causing death or serious sequelae (Fig. 10-22). Infants often are seen in coma or have convulsions and increased intracranial pressure.[28] In the classic case the subdural hematomas are associated with skull fractures (Fig. 10-23).

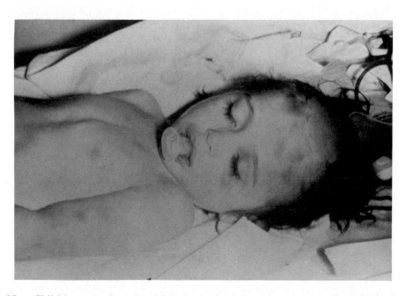

Fig. 10-22   Child in coma from head injuries and subdural hematomas. Note the bruises of the head and grab marks on the upper arm.

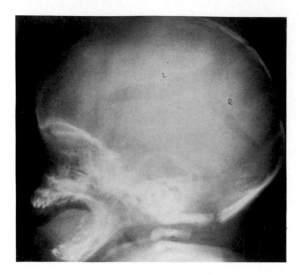

Fig. 10-23   Film of a 2-month-old infant with bilateral parietal fractures and massively spread sutures.

These fractures are caused by a direct blow from the parent's hand or from being hit against a wall or door. Numerous other bruises are usually present (Fig. 10-24).

Inflicted subdural hematomas can also occur without skull fractures, scalp bruises, or scalp swelling. In fact, over one half of the cases do not involve a fracture. These used to be called "spontaneous subdural hematomas," but recent evidence points to violent, whiplash-type, shaking injuries as the mechanism.[8,14] The head is relatively large and the neck muscles weak in children less than 2 years of age. When the child is held by the arms or torso and shaken, the head bobs back and forth. The rapid acceleration and deceleration of the head as it bobs about leads to tearing of the bridging cerebral veins with bleeding into the subdural space, usually bilaterally. The only findings on examination may be retinal hemorrhages and signs of increased intracranial pressure, such as irritability, altered level of consciousness, vomiting, a full fontanelle, or split sutures. Occasionally, bruising of the pinna may be noted.[4,10] In over one half of the cases, a trauma survey reveals bony injury where the child was grasped during shaking. It is important that the physician discard the concept of the "spontaneous subdural hematoma" in young infants lest he send a child home to be reinjured or killed. Likewise, the physician should remain skeptical of the diagnosis of "chronic subdural hematoma" caused by birth trauma. Subdural hematomas due to birth injury will almost always produce acute signs and symptoms within 24 to 48 hours after delivery.

Cephalohematomas are sometimes seen. Occasionally a subgaleal hematoma will be seen as a result of vigorous hair-pulling. This diagnosis is most likely if the child has braids at the site.[15]

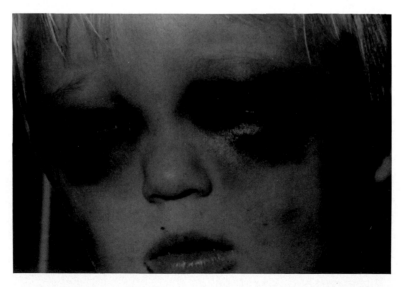

Fig. 10-24   Bilateral severe swelling and bruising of eyes and scalp from repeated cuffing about the head.

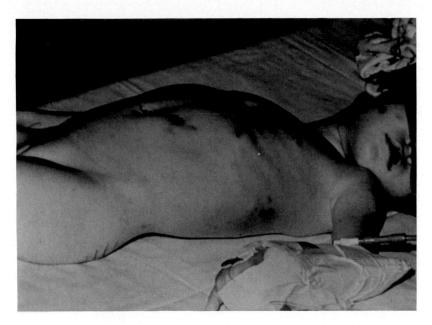

Fig. 10-25   Child with torn mesenteric vein from repeated blows to the abdomen. She had an acute abdomen and hemoglobin of 5 g/dL. Note multiplanar bruises, including switch marks on buttocks.

Abdominal Visceral Injuries

Intraabdominal injuries are the second most common cause of death in battered children.[39] These children have recurrent vomiting, abdominal distention, absent bowel sounds, or localized tenderness (Fig. 10-25). Abdominal wall bruising may be absent. The most common findings are tears or other injuries of the small intestine at sites of ligamental support, such as the duodenum and proximal jejunum. Intramural hematomas, most commonly of the duodenum, are common and lead to temporary obstruction. Rupture of the liver is also seen. These injuries are produced by the whipping force of a punch or blow and are different from the ruptured spleen, kidney, or viscera, which are more common with the crushing or compressing forces present in traffic accidents or falls. Inflicted chylous ascites and pseudocyst of the pancreas also have been reported.[5,30] Trauma to the abdomen is routinely denied in these cases. Therefore the physician must consider child abuse in any abdominal crisis of undetermined etiology.

Bone Injuries

More than 20% of physically abused children have a positive radiologic bone survey. Although some have overt fractures (Fig. 10-26), the most classic early finding is a chip fracture or corner fracture (Fig. 10-27).[7,26,35] The corner of the metaphysis is usually torn off with the periosteum during wrenching injuries to the long bones (for example, during an angry diaper change). From 10 to 14 days later, calcification of the subperiosteal bleeding will become visible, giving the classic double contour lines (Fig. 10-28). By 4 to 6 weeks after injury, the subperiosteal calcification will be solid and start to smooth out and remodel (Fig. 10-29). After several months, the only finding will be cortical thickening and metaphyseal squaring. X-ray findings usually last for 6 months after an injury, and rarely 12.

The most diagnostic x-ray film is one that includes evidence of multiple bone injuries at different stages of healing (Fig. 10-30). Such a film implies repeated assault. Unusual fractures of the ribs, lateral clavicle, scapula, and sternum should arouse suspicion of nonaccidental trauma (Figs. 10-31 and 10-32).[31]

Rare bone disorders, such as osteogenesis imperfecta, infantile cortical hyperostosis, scurvy, syphilis, and neoplasms, may resemble nonacci-

Fig. 10-26   Spiral fracture of the lower humerus.

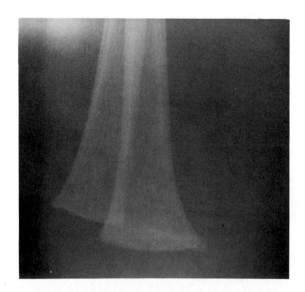

Fig. 10-27   Corner fracture of distal radius caused by a recent wrenching injury.

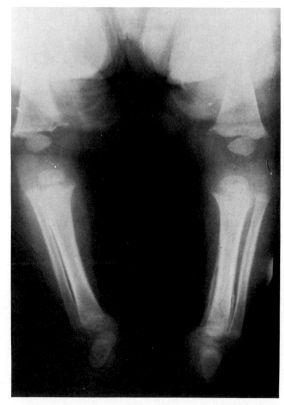

Fig. 10-28   Calcification of subperiosteal hematomas of the left tibia as seen 2 weeks after injury. Also note bilateral medial femoral chip fractures plus metaphyseal fragmentation.

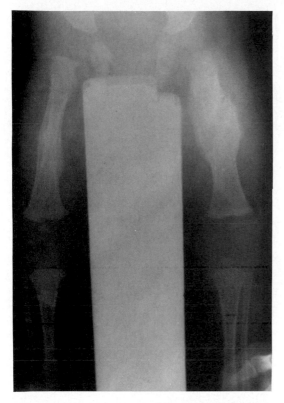

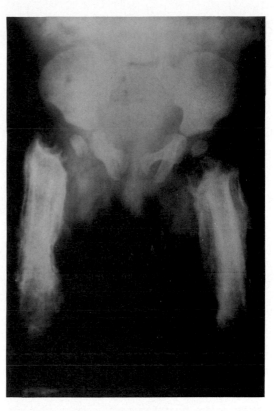

Fig. 10-29   Smooth subperiosteal calcification of the right femur as seen 6 weeks after injury. Reinjury has occurred on left side as evidenced by the irregular surface.

Fig. 10-30   Severe subperiosteal calcification of both femurs caused by repeated trauma and subsequent repeated rents in the periosteum.

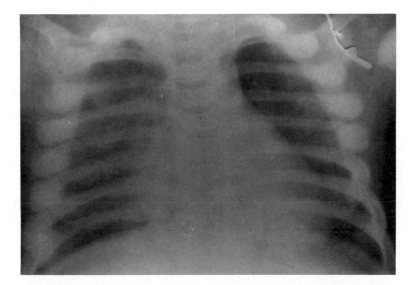

Fig. 10-31   Rib fractures with callus; six on the right and four on the left.

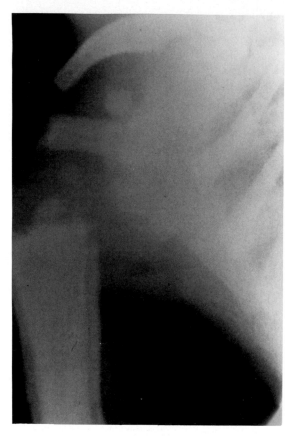

Fig. 10-32   Bizarre inflicted fracture of acromial process of the scapula. Also note fracture of the proximal humerus and subperiosteal calcification of the same.

dental bone trauma.[23] However, a skilled radiologist can easily differentiate these entities.

HOSPITAL BEHAVIOR IN THE PARENT SUGGESTIVE OF PHYSICAL ABUSE

The average parents of an injured child are concerned about their child's injury, are interested in the proposed treatment, and call and visit the hospital frequently. The abusive parents often show a lack of concern regarding the degree of injury, ask very few questions about prognosis, risks, or the treatment to be used, and may disappear from the hospital during admission without giving even an initial history. In extreme cases parents may refuse hospitalization of the child despite a serious injury. Previous use of medical resources may include various doctors and hospitals. Visits and phone calls are unusual. Visits that do occur are brief and include minimal contact with the child. The phone

---

MEDICAL EVALUATION CHECKLIST

1. History of injury
2. Physical examination of patient
3. Trauma x-ray survey on selected patients
4. Bleeding disorder screen on selected patients
5. Color photographs of selected patients
6. Physical examination of siblings
7. Official medical report in writing
8. Behavioral assessment
9. Developmental assessment

---

number that is left at the hospital may turn out to be disconnected.

PSYCHOSOCIAL RISK FACTORS SUGGESTIVE OF PHYSICAL ABUSE

The presence of the factors mentioned in the section on etiology are confirmatory but not diagnostic of child abuse. They are most helpful in cases arousing suspicion of child abuse but not diagnostic by the history or physical findings alone. The combination of a suspicious injury plus a strongly positive psychosocial predisposition in one of the parents permits the physician to reach 99% medical certainty in the correctness of a child abuse diagnosis. These data are usually collected by the hospital social worker, although the physician may collect some of it. A checklist of 10 physical abuse risk factors may help in performing a complete assessment (see box on p. 179).

COMPREHENSIVE MEDICAL EVALUATION OF PHYSICAL ABUSE

The nine tasks listed in the box above represent the medical data base that must be collected in a comprehensive child abuse evaluation.

History of Injury

A complete history should be obtained as to how the injury allegedly happened, including the informant, date, time, place, sequence of events, people present, time lag before medical attention sought, and so forth. If possible, the parents should be interviewed separately. The parents can be pressed for exact details when necessary. No other professional should have to repeat this detailed, probing interview. The physician must talk with the parents

CHECKLIST FOR PHYSICAL ABUSE HIGH-RISK FACTORS

This checklist should be completed only *after* a careful psychosocial history has been elicited. It is not intended as the content for a rapid interrogation. Its main purpose is to help the interviewer with completeness.

Grade the boxes for the mother and father as follows: normal (0), mild (middle number), or severe (highest number) and circle the appropriate number. Notice that some categories have more weight than others. The maximal high-risk raw score a parent can receive is 40. Only one high-risk parent is required to put a family at high risk.

Mother	Father	
0-1-2	0-1-2	1. Parent was repetitively beaten or deprived as a child (e.g., repeated foster homes, no helpful parent model during childhood)
0-2-4	0-2-4	2. Parent has criminal or mental illness record (e.g., record of assault and battery, prison, drug abuse, alcoholism, mental hospitalization, or any current indication of psychosis)
0-2-4	0-2-4	3. Parent suspected of physical abuse in the past (e.g., official reports, mysterious death of a sibling, child abuse reported or suspected in previous marriage)
0-1-2	0-1-2	4. Parent with low-self-esteem, social isolation, or depression (e.g., feelings of worthlessness, no lifelines, no close friends, unable to ask for help, no enjoyment even at home, unlisted telephone, lack of transportation, poor coping skills, suicide threats/attempts(s)
0-2-4	0-2-4	5. Multiple crises or stresses (e.g., generally chaotic life, marital discord, multiple separations, threats of divorce, recent significant loss(es), poor work stability, debts, recent or frequent moves, overcrowded living conditions)
0-3-6	0-3-6	6. Violent temper outbursts in either parent toward child or others (e.g., impulsive acting out, doesn't care if someone gets hurt, physical abuse of spouse, puts fist through walls, throws furniture, breaks up the house, one parent spontaneously states she/he suspects the other because of his/her temper)
0-2-4	0-2-4	7. Rigid and unrealistic expectations of child's behavior (e.g., expects child to perform beyond his capacity in obedience, respect for his parents and developmental milestones; afraid of spoiling the child or sees child as spoiled; intolerance of normal annoying behavior, and expects child to gratify and love them; sees child as extension of self rather than separate individual)
0-3-6	0-3-6	8. Harsh punishment of child (e.g., physical punishment in the early months of life; child seen to be deserving of punishment; current frequent spanking, in its extreme—sadistic punishment)
0-3-6	0-3-6	9. Child is difficult and/or provocative or is perceived to be by parents (e.g., any frequent misbehavior that causes anger in the parent such as excessive crying, temper tantrums, hyperactivity, aggressiveness, destructiveness, negativism, defiance, etc.)
0-1-2	0-1-2	10. Child is unwanted or at risk for poor bonding (e.g., premature baby, caesarian-section baby, out-of-wedlock baby, baby almost therapeutically aborted or relinquished for adoption, any baby with hospitalization in first 6 months of life causing prolonged separation, stepchild or adopted child)
___/40	___/40	Total
%*	%	

Developed by Schmitt BD, Carroll C, and Gray J—Child Protection Team at the University of Colorado Medical Center, 4200 East Ninth Avenue, Denver, Colorado, 80220. May be utilized in direct service settings without authors' permission. Comments will be appreciated and may be sent to the Child Protection Team. Sixth revision, June 1976.

*Percentage can be calculated by multiplying the raw score by 2.5.

directly so that the history will not be considered as hearsay evidence in court. In obvious cases, obtaining the history from the parents on the phone may suffice if they cannot come in. The physician commonly forgets to interview the child, which is often helpful if the child is older than 3 or 4 years of age. This should be conducted in a private setting without the parents present. In failure-to-thrive cases, the history is of little value except to rule out errors in formula preparation or feeding. In sexual abuse cases, the history is usually the most critical datum of all.

Physical Examination of Patient

All bruises should be recorded as to size, shape, position, color, and age. The following information can be used for dating bruises[40]:

Age	Color
0-2 days	Swollen, tender
0-5 days	Red, blue, purple
5-7 days	Green
7-10 days	Yellow
10-14 days (or longer)	Brown
2-4 weeks	Cleared

It should be recorded if they resemble strap marks, grab marks, or marks from a blunt instrument. The oral cavity, eardrums, and genitals should be closely examined for signs of occult trauma. If the anterior fontanelle is open, it should be palpated for fullness. Any splitting of the sutures of the skull should be noted. All bones should be palpated for tenderness and the joints tested for full range of motion. In addition, special attention should be paid to the retina, since hemorrhages there may point to subdural hematomas from a shaking injury.

The height and weight percentiles should be plotted, and if the child appears malnourished, he or she should be given a return appointment for a weight check after 2 weeks, either in the foster home with ad lib meals or in the natural home with specific feeding advice. In sexual abuse cases, the mouth, anus, and external genitals should be carefully inspected for signs of trauma. In selected cases of sexual abuse, laboratory studies should be performed in an effort to diagnose sexually transmitted infections such as gonorrhea, syphilis, chlamydia, or herpes simplex.[24]

Trauma X-ray Survey

Every suspected victim less than 2 years of age should receive a radiologic bone survey consisting of films of the skull (anteroposterior and lateral), thorax (anteroposterior), pelvis (anteroposterior, including lumbar spine), spine (lateral, centered at T8 and including ribs), and long bones (anteroposterior, including hands and feet).[11] These films are of great diagnostic value, since the clinical findings of fracture often disappear in 6 or 7 days even without orthopedic care. A child with multiple fractures may still move about and play normally. For most children 2 to 5 years old, a bone survey is indicated unless the child has a single episode of minor injuries. For children older than 5 years of age, x-ray films need to be obtained only if any bone tenderness or limited range of motion is noted on physical examination or there is a history of frequent trauma. If films of a tender site are initially normal, a radionuclide bone scan should be considered. A bone scan may detect fractures not evident on routine x-ray films. When there is a significant suspicion of abuse but routine radiographs are normal, a bone scan may be performed in an effort to increase the probability of fracture detection.[29] Alternately, x-ray films can be repeated in 2 weeks to detect calcification of subperiosteal bleeding or nondisplaced epiphyseal separations that may have been present. A CT or MRI scan of the head should be considered whenever suspicion exists about intracranial injury.[3,9] Retinal hemorrhages in an apparently battered child should always prompt further radiographic study of the head using one of these modalities. Babies with severe nutritional deprivation need a trauma x-ray survey; approximately 10% of them have associated skeletal injuries. Sexually abused children and siblings of abused children rarely require an x-ray survey.

Bleeding Disorder Screen

A bleeding screen includes a platelet count, bleeding time, partial thromboplastin time, prothrombin time, and thrombin time. On a clinical level, bleeding tests are rarely indicated. However, a normal bleeding panel strengthens the physician's court testimony that bruising could not have occurred spontaneously or as the result of minor injury. Children with subtle bleeding tendencies demonstrate ongoing bruising in the school, office, hospital, and foster home. Screening is not needed for bruises confined to the buttocks, bruises resembling weapons, or hand bruises and is also unnecessary when one parent or the child accuses a specific adult of hitting the child. Screening is primarily indicted for nonspecific bruises that the parent denies inflicting and attributes to "easy bruisability."

Color Photographs

Color photographs are required by law in some states. In most juvenile court cases, they are not essential to the primary physican's testimony. When an expert witness, who has not actually examined the child, is to testify, color photographs are mandatory. When criminal court action is anticipated, they will usually be required and will be taken by the police photographer. In cases of nutritional deprivation, "before" and "after" photographs may occasionally be helpful. In sexual abuse cases that involve physical harm, the police usually arrange for photographs. Whether or not medical photography is available, the physician should carefully diagram the body surface findings in the official medical chart and carefully date and sign the entry.

Physical Examination of Siblings

There is approximately a 20% risk that a sibling of a physically abused child has also been abused at the same point in time.[25] Therefore all siblings should be brought in for total body surface examinations within 12 hours of uncovering an index case. If the parents say they cannot bring them in because of transportation problems, the Child Protective Services Agency will provide transport. If the parents refuse to have their other children examined, a court order can be obtained and police dispatched. In failure-to-thrive cases, examination of siblings is usually unnecessary. In sexual abuse cases, all the patient's sisters should be interviewed within 24 hours because it is not uncommon for more than one child to be victimized.

Official Written Medical Report

An official medical report is required by law and should be written by the examining physician. Since it is an official document, it obviously should be typed, and since it will be used in court, the accuracy and completeness of this report are extremely important. This report should not simply be a copy of the admission workup or discharge summary because the evidence of the diagnosis of child abuse is often lost in those highly technical documents. The report should include the following:

1. History—The alleged cause of the injury (with date, time, place, and so forth)
2. Physical examination—Description of the injury using nontechnical terms whenever possible (for example, "cheek" instead of "zygoma," "bruise" instead of "ecchymosis")

PHYSICAL ABUSE—MEDICAL REPORT

D.F.
BD: 2-26-87
CGH 444555

History

At 8 PM on April 29, 1988 the father decided to bathe his 14-month-old baby because she had "messy" pants. It is known that the parents are currently trying to toilet train this child. Despite her crying, he held her in the bathwater for 15 to 20 minutes straight. When he took her out, he noted the burn. Allegedly, she usually cries during the bath. Also, allegedly the father cannot tell hot from cold water. He states that bruise on cheek is from a fall yesterday.

Physical examination

1. 70% to 80% body burn up to midchest and involving both forearms with huge blisters
2. Rapid fading bruise of left cheek and scattered bruises of left earlobe

Trauma x-ray films

Normal

Conclusion

Inflicted dunking burns were probably a punishment for toilet-training resistance. Forearm burns resulted from struggling to get out. The child is old enough to climb out unless forcibly held. The bruise on the left cheek and ear is from being slapped several days ago. This sadistic burn points to serious psychopathology and the need for long-term foster care.

Betsy Ross, M.D.

---

3. Results of laboratory tests and x-ray films
4. Conclusion—Statements on why this incident represents nonaccidental trauma, on the severity of the incident in terms of long-term handicaps, and on the risk of subsequent fatal abuse

A sample report is shown in the box above.

Behavioral Assessment

The abused child is likely to have associated behavior problems. Some may be primary behaviors (for example, negativism and hyperactivity) that make the child difficult to live with and hence prone to abuse. Other behaviors, such as fearfulness and depression, may result from abusive treatment. Often the abused child's individual need for therapy will be overlooked unless these symptoms are uncovered. The child's behavior should be reviewed.

Developmental Assessment

Abuse and neglect of the infant and preschool child can lead to developmental delays. These problems can be recognized by routine use of the Denver Developmental Screening Test (DDST) or other developmental tests for this age group. A school report may be helpful in the comprehensive assessment of the abused school-age child.

TREATMENT OF PHYSICAL ABUSE

Hospitalization

The highest priority of treatment is to protect the child. Any child suspected of having been abused requires hospitalization until evaluations regarding the safety of the home are complete. All too often a crying baby with a minor inflicted injury is sent home, only to return the next day with subdural hematomas or multiple fractures. The physician justifies hospitalization by convincing the parents that their child's injuries need to be watched. Incriminating questions should be kept to a minimal in the outpatient setting. A more detailed history can be pursued once the child is safely admitted to the ward. If the parents refuse hospitalization, a court hold can be obtained. The above comments do not apply if the Child Protective Services Agency has an on-call worker and a place for the child in an emergency foster home can be arranged.

Reporting

The physician is required by law to report physical abuse cases to the Child Protective Services Agency in the child's county of residence. The report should be made by phone within 24 hours and in writing within 48 hours. This agency is made up of specially trained social workers. Unless these cases are reported, treatment will not occur and abuse will probably continue. Reporting guarantees adequate evaluation, treatment, and follow-up. The physician must tell the family that he or she is obligated by state law to report any unusual injuries. The physician can reassure the parents that everyone involved will try to help them find better ways of dealing with their child. Maintaining a helping approach with these parents is often the most difficult part of therapy. Feeling angry with these parents is natural, but expressing this anger is very damaging to parent cooperation. The physician should keep in mind that the injury occurred in a moment of anger, it was not deliberate, and that these parents already feel inadequate and unloved. Confrontation, accusation, and repeated interrogation must be avoided. The physician should encourage hospital visits by the parents and be certain that the ward personnel treat them kindly.

Consultation

Some surgeons will want to report their cases of physical abuse personally and to carry out the other medical responsibilities described under the comprehensive evaluation. Other surgeons will want to treat the injuries but not be involved in the child abuse aspects. In such circumstances it is imperative that surgeons refer their child abuse cases to the medical consultant on their community child protection team. This should be looked on as a legitimate consultation for a life-threatening disease. Most communities or medical centers have one or two pediatricians with expertise in this area who can help with diagnostic dilemmas, submit the official child abuse report, and testify in court if necessary. This person is comfortable working with angry parents and the multiple agencies involved in this complex psychosocial problem.

Child Protection Teams

Multidisciplinary teams, called child protection teams, are needed to evaluate the cases and coordinate the numerous community agencies involved.[6] Such a team is made up of a physician, hospital social worker, protective service agency social worker, psychiatrist, psychologist, developmental specialist, lawyer, public health nurse, police representative, and others. Within 1 week of admission and after all evaluations are completed, this multidisciplinary, interagency team holds a dispositional conference to decide the best immediate and long-range treatment plans for a family.

Therapy

Treatment modalities must be individually designed for the specific family and should be more expansive than traditional case-work. Some modern types of treatment that have been shown to be successful are lay therapists, or parenting aides, homemakers, parents anonymous groups, telephone hotlines, crisis nurseries, psychotherapy, marital counseling, vocational rehabilitation, and child rearing counseling. The treatment needs of the child should also be considered and may require play therapy, a therapeutic preschool, or day care. The Child Protective Services Agency also makes home visits and is responsible for ensuring that therapy is in progress and the family does not become "lost to follow-up." In about 20% of cases, the child must temporarily be placed in a foster home while the natural home is made safe. This requires a legal action in the juvenile court.

Court Testimony

In some cases the physician will need to appear in court. Good court testimony depends on solid knowledge of the case. The physician must have talked with the parents and examined the child personally. He or she must keep precise medical records of the dates and content of these examinations and interviews. The initial medical report submitted must be composed carefully so that it does not become inconsistent with later court testimony. Before the hearing the physician should review the medical records, including the results of pertinent laboratory tests and x-ray films. It is also helpful to review pertinent medical literature regarding this type of injury. The physician should also confer with the county attorney about the points he or she wishes to stress and about anticipated questions during the cross-examination. On the witness stand, he or she should offer objective data in an impartial and fair manner. An organized presentation of the medical facts, including relevant x-ray films and photographs, makes for a more convincing, yet fair, testimony.[38] In a severe case of child abuse, it is extremely important for the child's well-being that the physician present findings and expert opinion as soundly and convincingly as possible.

PHYSICIAN'S RELUCTANCE TO REPORT PHYSICAL ABUSE

In all 50 states it is mandatory for the physician to report suspected cases of child abuse and neglect to the local Child Protective Services Agency. In many states the physician can be sued for not reporting a clear-cut case. The other risks of not reporting include the probable recurrence of beatings, the further decline of familial harmony, and the likelihood of abused children growing up to become violent members of our society. Despite the legal and humanistic need to report child abuse and neglect, numerous physicians are reluctant to report and often do not. There are several reasons for this resistance.

Failure to Diagnose Child Abuse

Some physicians by training do not have the capacity to detect child abuse. Minor injuries not requiring hospitalization are especially likely to be overlooked by the physician because of their frequent occurrence. The physician may forget to ask even how the injury happened, since all attention and energy are directed toward its treatment. Others do not believe that certain parents, such as those who are educated and respected, would abuse their children. Others suspect abuse but fear making a mistaken diagnosis. They must be reminded that the current problem in our country is gross under-diagnosis by private physicians. These errors are correctable by education or consultation since they are the result of ignorance. Some physicians find child abuse so abhorrent that they deny the possibility that parents would harm their own child. They sometimes can overcome their denial if it is pointed out that these injuries occur in a moment of anger and are rarely deliberate.

Ignorance About the Seriousness of Abuse

Many physicians have not seen a child die from abuse. They do not realize that this disorder kills over 4000 children a year and that many of these deaths were preventable. Child abuse kills more children than any specific cancer or any of the other well-studied fatal diseases. Some look on it as an isolated episode that will pass, yet without intervention abuse has a 50% recurrence rate.

Failure to Identify the Abuser

Sometimes the physician cannot make even an educated guess as to who injured the child. Even with extensive evaluations, it is impossible to determine who did it with certainty on that particular day in perhaps half the cases. By and large, this is unimportant. The question is not who did it but rather if something serious happened. It is the family who injured the child, and it is the family who is responsible.

Extenuating Circumstances

Sometimes a babysitter is not reported, although a report should be made to protect other people's children from her. Sometimes a sibling who injures a child is not reported. Nevertheless, this indicates a family is in trouble. Either the sibling is harshly disciplined or is being grossly undersupervised. Sometimes the parents are not reported because they so readily admit to having inflicted the injury as a result of discipline. This leads to the conflict over parents' and children's rights. Discipline should not lead to bodily injury. The parents have a right to discipline their children, but the child is guaranteed reasonable and safe punishment. In addition, the next time the injury may be worse. An obviously feeble excuse is that the parents were under the influence of alcohol and did not intend to beat up the child, or did not know their own strength, or the child interferred in their quarrel.

Fear of Liability

Fear of liability is unfounded. The laws protect the physician from liability suits if his or her suspicion should prove to be wrong. The law also provides a waiver of patient-physician and husband-wife confidentiality in such cases.

Fear of Damage to Practice

Physicians who practice in a small town or ghetto area where everyone knows each other express concern that their reputation or practice can be hurt if they report child abuse. On the contrary, most parents consider it important that someone does something about child abuse. If a clear-cut case is reported, the physician's reputation should be enhanced.

Dread of Dealing with Angry Parents

Reporting child abuse often brings the parents' wrath down on the physician. The physician must accept the fact that there is little gratitude in most of these cases. Occasionally a distressed parent will say, "Thank God, somebody finally did something." It is obvious that the child's safety is more important than the physician's emotional well-being.

Reliance on Voluntary Therapy

Some physicians believe that a little fatherly talk with both parents is sufficient. Others may decide to see the parents several times for therapy. Some may fear that reporting the case would interfere with this voluntary therapy. In reality, few, if any, physicians can provide the amount of outreach therapy, close follow-up, and constant availability that

these cases require. The physician who "makes a deal" with these parents may never learn that the child suffered additional injury but was taken to a different hospital.

Avoidance of Incompetent Community Resources

In some counties the police are involved in all cases and have a reputation for being excessively harsh. In a few counties the whole approach is punitive, and the parents are prosecuted in the criminal courts. Both of these tactics interfere with the success of any therapeutic intervention. In other counties the juvenile courts intervene in only the blatantly dangerous cases or prematurely return children to homes that are unchanged. They bias their decision toward parental rights. When the system is defective in these ways, it is important that the physician continue to do his or her job well, to report cases, to document inadequacies in the system, and eventually to change the system through pressure based on facts.

Avoidance of Bureaucratic Entanglements

These cases can be rather time-consuming. It is understandable that a physician may not wish to write a report to a public agency or attend numerous meetings and court hearings. Lack of experience in court may lead to a fear of testifying. If a physician feels overwhelmed by such a case, it is critical that he or she refer the case to a pediatrician in the community who is willing to act as a consultant.

PROGNOSIS OF PHYSICAL ABUSE

With comprehensive intensive treatment of the entire family, 80% to 90% of these families can be rehabilitated and can, thereafter, provide adequate care for their child. Approximately 10% to 15% of these families can only be stabilized and require indefinite support services. Termination of parental rights and release of the child for adoption are required in 1% to 2% of the cases.

If abused children are returned to their parents without any intervention, 5% are killed and 35% are seriously reinjured. The child with repeated central nervous system injuries may develop mental retardation, organic brain syndrome, seizures, hydrocephalus, or ataxia. Also, the untreated families tend to produce children who grow up to be juvenile delinquents and violent members of our society,

HIGH-RISK CHECKLIST FOR NEWBORNS AND BABIES

Introduction

Most of the high-risk factors described below can be detected before a newborn baby is discharged from the nursery. Some factors will be evident even before the baby is born. Most of the factors can be detected by the routine observations of nurses and physicians, a special interview not being required. When one of the serious risk factors (*) or a cluster (2 to 4) of the other risk factors are present, the mother should be referred to the hospital social worker for an in-depth interview regarding the safety of the home and the family's specific needs.

Prenatal history and observations

1. The mother conceals the pregnancy (for example, no prenatal care)
2. Abortion is unsuccessfully sought or attempted
3. Relinquishment for adoption is sought, then reversed
4. No "nesting" behavior (for example, preparation of layette)
5. Unwed mother without emotional support
6. History of severe marital discord
7. History of serious mental illness, institutionalization, current depression or repeated foster homes in either parent
8. History of drug addiction or alcoholism in either parent (very high risk if the mother is currently addicted)
9. History of violent behavior or prison sentence in either parent
10. *History of previous abuse or neglect of another child

Delivery room observations

How does the mother look?
1. *Negative appearance (sad, depressed, angry, agitated)
2. Passive, disinterested, apathetic appearance
What does she say?
1. *Negative comments about the baby (expresses disappointment, anger, disparaging remarks)
2. Negative comments about self
3. Negative comments about others (specify relationship)
What does she do?
1. *Does not want to see or look at baby
2. *Does not want to touch or hold baby

Maternity ward observations

1. *Lack of claiming behavior or maternal attachment by 48 hours of age (for example, does not want to hold, feed, or name her baby; no signs of cuddling, rocking, eye contact, or talking to the baby)
2. *Disparaging remarks about the baby (for example, that he or she is ugly, defective, a disappointment, mean, bad, and so forth)
3. Repulsion at the baby's drooling, regurgitation, urine, stools, and so forth
4. The mother feeds her baby in a mechanical or other inappropriate way
5. *A postpartum depression (that is, perhaps the mother is overwhelmed or cannot attach)
6. The mother attempts to sign her sick newborn out of the hospital against medical advice
7. Prolonged separation of the baby from the mother because of neonatal complication, maternal complication, or any severe illness requiring hospitalization in the first 6 months of life (for example, prematurity)
8. *Inadequate visiting or telephoning patterns if the mother is discharged before the baby
9. *Reluctance to come in for the baby when discharge is approved
10. *Spanking of the newborn baby or overt anger directed toward the baby (for example, for crying)

Pediatric office observations

1. *Lack of holding the baby
2. *Holding but no signs of attachment (for example, no eye contact, talking, cuddling, and so forth)
3. *Rough handling
4. *Hygiene neglect
5. *Spanking of a young infant

Prepared by Schmitt BD, Souza B, Gray JD, and Kempe CH, Denver and Honolulu. May be utilized in direct service settings without authors' permission. Revised July 1976.

not to mention child abusers. Child abuse has been correlated with playground, street, marital, and criminal violence.

PREVENTION

Inadequate parenting is the inability of parents to love and to care for their offspring adequately. The delayed recognition of this family problem in the emergency room after the child appears with evidence of physical abuse or starvation is unacceptable. The high-risk group should be identified early and an attempt made to help such people. The logical person to detect this problem is the primary physician or public health nurse. The high-risk checklist for newborns and babies reviews the factors that help to identify such families (see box on p. 185).

These families are not reportable to child protective services. The main focus of intervention is to provide an intensive form of well-baby care. This includes prenatal classes, delivery room contact with the baby, a rooming-in maternity ward, increased parental contact with premature babies, extra help with colic, more frequent office visits, public health nurse visits, crisis nurseries, close follow-up of acute illnesses, numerous telephone lifelines, day care arrangements, and family planning assistance. Educating parents about acceptable means of discipline is critical. Especially needed is an admonition to *never shake a child,* since this may cause severe, though unintentional, injury to the brain. This type of helping, reaching-out approach has been shown to help prevent serious physical abuse.

SUMMARY

The battered child syndrome kills over 4000 children a year in the United States. This condition is not only treatable but often preventable. The surgeon is in a strategic position for diagnosing physical abuse. After detection, it is his or her moral and legal duty to report the family to the Child Protection Services Agency in the community or to immediately seek consultation from a pediatrician who will report it.

ACKNOWLEDGMENT

The authors wish to thank Dr. George W. Starbuck for Figs. 10-7, 10-12, 10-19, and 10-21; Dr. John S. Wheeler for Figs. 10-11, 10-15, and 10-17; Dr. Harry J. Umlauf for Fig. 10-13; the Lakewood Department of Public Safety for Fig. 10-18; and Dr. Jerry J. Tomasovic for Fig. 10-25.

REFERENCES

1. Abbot SL: Gonococcal tonsillitis-pharyngitis in a 5-year-old girl, Pediatrics 52:287, 1973.
2. Adelson L: Homicide by starvation, JAMA 186:458, 1963.
3. Alexander RC, Schor DP, and Smith WL Jr: Magnetic resonance imaging of intracranial injuries from child abuse, J Pediatr 109:975, 1986.
4. Billmire ME and Myers PA: Serious head injury in infants: accident or abuse? Pediatrics 75:340, 1985.
5. Boysen BE: Chylous ascites, Am J Dis Child 129:1338, 1975.
6. Bross DC et al: The new child protection team handbook, New York, 1988, Garland Publishing, Inc.
7. Caffey J: Some traumatic lesions in growing bones other than fractures and dislocation: clinical and radiologic features, Br J Radiol 30:225, 1957.
8. Caffey J: The whiplash-shaken infant syndrome, Pediatrics 54:396, 1974.
9. Cohen RA et al: Cranial computed tomography in the abused child with head injury, Am J Roent 146:97, 1986.
10. Dykes LJ: The whiplash-shaken infant syndrome: what has been learned? Child Abuse Negl 10:211, 1986.
11. Ellerstein NS and Norris KJ: Value of radiologic skeletal survey in assessment of abused children, Pediatrics 74:1075, 1984.
12. Gammon JA: Ophthalmic manifestations of child abuse. In Ellerstein NS, editor: Child abuse and neglect: a medical reference, New York, 1981, John Wiley & Sons.
13. Gillespie RW: The battered child syndrome: thermal and caustic manifestations, J Trauma 5:523, 1965.
14. Guthkelch AN: Infantile subdural hematoma and its relationship to whiplash injuries, Br Med J 2:430, 1971.
15. Hamlin H: Subgaleal hematoma caused by hair-pull, JAMA 204:339, 1968.
16. Helfer RE, Slovis TL, and Black M: Injuries resulting when small children fall out of bed, Pediatrics 60:533, 1977.
17. Holter JC and Friedman SB: Child abuse: early case-finding in the emergency department, Pediatrics 42:128, 1968.
18. Johnson CF and Showers J: Injury variables in child abuse: child abuse and neglect, Child Abuse Neglect: Int J 9:207, 1985.
19. Keen JH, Lendrum J, and Wolman B: Inflicted burns and scalds in children, Br Med J 1:268, 1975.
20. Kempe CH et al: The battered child syndrome, JAMA 181:17, 1962.
21. Klein M and Stern L: Low birth weight and the battered child syndrome, Am J Dis Child 122:15, 1971.
22. Koel BS: Failure to thrive and fatal injury as a continuum, Am J Dis Child 118:565, 1969.
23. Kogutt MS, Swischuk LE, and Fagan CJ: Patterns of injury and significance of uncommon fractures in the battered child syndrome, Am J Roent 121:143, 1974.
24. Krugman RD: Recognition of sexual abuse in children, Pediatr Rev 8:25, 1986.
25. Lauer B, Ten Broeck E, and Grossman M: Battered child syndrome: review of 130 patients with controls, Pediatrics 54:67, 1974.

26. Leonidas JC: Skeletal trauma in the child abuse syndrome, Pediatr Ann 12:875, 1983.

27. Levine LJ: The solution of a battered-child homicide by dental evidence: report of case, JAMA 87:1234, 1973.

28. Ludwig S and Warman M: Shaken baby syndrome: a review of 20 cases, Ann Emerg Med 13:104, 1984.

29. Merten DF, Radkowski MA, and Leonidas JC: The abused child: a radiological reappraisal, Radiology 146:377, 1983.

30. Penna SDJ and Medovy H: Child abuse and traumatic pseudocyst of the pancreas, J Pediatr 83:1026, 1973.

31. Radkowski MA: The battered child syndroeme: pitfalls in radiological diagnosis, Pediatr Ann 12:894, 1983.

32. Schmitt BD: Child neglect. In Ellerstein NS, editor: Medical aspects of child abuse and neglect, New York, 1981, John Wiley & Sons.

33. Schmitt BD: Failure to thrive: the medical evaluation. The new child protection team handbook, New York, 1988, Garland Publishing, Inc.

34. Shnaps Y et al: The chemically abused child, Pediatrics 68:119, 1981.

35. Silverman FN: Unrecognized trauma in infants, the battered child syndrome, and the syndrome of Ambroise Tardieu, Radiology 104:337, 1972.

36. Slosberg EJ et al: Penile trauma as a sign of child abuse, Am J Dis Child 132:719, 1978.

37. Tomasi LG: Purtscher retinopathy in the battered child syndrome, Am J Dis Child 129:1335, 1975.

38. Torrey SB and Ludwig S: The emergency physician in the courtroom: serving as an expert witness in cases of child abuse, Pediatr Emerg Care 3:50, 1987.

39. Touloukian RJ: Abdominal visceral injuries in battered children, Pediatrics 42:642, 1968.

40. Wilson EF: Estimation of the age of cutaneous contusions in child abuse, Pediatrics 60:751, 1977.

PART II

SPECIFIC INJURIES

11

Soft Tissue Injuries

Richard S. Stahl and John H. Seashore

APPROACH TO THE INJURED CHILD

Anyone who cares for children with lacerations or other minor injuries knows what a major ordeal this can be—terrifying for the child, upsetting for the parents, and frustrating for the physician. Although some children react to injury and the necessary repairs with equanimity and even pride in their "battle scars," most children are thoroughly frightened. Fear—of pain, of separation, of punishment and, most of all, of the unknown—is the dominant reaction of the injured child. Children have a remarkable tolerance for pain, and with proper techniques there should be relatively little pain associated with treatment of soft tissue injuries. The anxiety produced in children and their parents by the injury itself and the often unfamiliar, busy, and impersonal environment of the emergency room tend to distort and exaggerate their perception of reality. Overcoming these fears and anxieties is an important and challenging task for the physician.

A calm and unhurried manner is essential. Children respond poorly to the impersonal, all-business, "let's-get-this-over-with-quickly" approach. A few minutes invested at the beginning of the encounter to gain the child's confidence and reassure both the child and the parents will help the child relax and cooperate and may actually save time in the long run. Since children look to their parents for protection and security, it is helpful to talk with the parents first. This time can be used to obtain essential facts about the child, the circumstances of the injury, the immunization status, and so forth. Parents often visibly relax during this discussion, especially if the physician projects a warm, confident, and professional image. Attention should then be directed to the child as a person, not as a laceration, fracture, or foreign body. Children love to talk about themselves and their interests—family, friends, school, pets, and so forth—and can be distracted from their fears and shyness. Younger children enjoy playing with stethoscopes and tongue depressors. Once the child's confidence has been obtained it is possible to examine the injured part slowly and gently.

Assessment of neuromuscular integrity distal to the injured part can be challenging. A wisp of cotton or a paper clip is less threatening than a pin to test sensation. Older children may be willing to play a game of imitating finger (or hand, arm, foot) motions to assess nerve and tendon function. With younger children, it is better to offer an interesting object, such as a pen, and observe how the child reaches and grasps it. Simply demanding that the child move a part is pointless.

Whether the child has a laceration to be sutured, a burn to be debrided and dressed, or a fracture to be set and casted, it is essential to explain everything that will be done, emphasizing that most of it will not hurt. Absolute honesty is imperative to retain the child's trust and cooperation, however. The physician should never lie about things that will hurt, nor should he allow the parents to do so. To the child, everything is threatening; soap and water seem to be some powerful poison, drapes are seen as mouth gags, and any movement of the physician's arm is assumed to bring a needle or some other instrument of torture. A few moments explaining the details of what is to be done will defuse much of this anxiety. Even a 2-year-old child can understand simple explanations.

Explanations should continue throughout the procedure. The physician or an assistant can continue to distract the child with light conversation appealing to the child's self-interest. It is important to warn the child when any painful maneuver is coming. He or she should be allowed to vent fear and anger by crying or screaming, as long as the involved part is not moved.

Whether a parent should be present for the procedure is controversial. If the parent does not wish to stay, is as frightened as the child, or threatens punishment for poor cooperation, the parent should leave. However, we believe that in general the support and security offered by the parents outweigh other considerations. The parent can sit next to the child and provide the distraction that is so helpful in allaying anxiety. The probability of parents fainting is overemphasized. If the office is familiar and the physician has an established rapport with the child, the parents' presence may be less important.

Some sort of physical restraint is necessary for children under the age of 2 years, since it is unreasonable to expect them to understand and to cooperate. A satisfactory method of immobilizing children using a folded sheet is illustrated in Fig. 11-1. The commercially available papoose board shown in Fig. 11-2 is more convenient. Neither system provides adequate immobilization of the head; if the wound is in this area, an assistant must hold the child's head. If the injury involves an extremity, the part should be gently but securely taped to an arm board. Physical restraint of 2- to 5-year-old children should be individualized. The stress of trying to cooperate and please their parents is greater for some children than is the stress of the procedure. These children may be more comfortable if they are immobilized and relieved of the responsibility of holding still. Other preschoolers are quite capable of adequate cooperation and feel threatened or insulted by physical restraints. Immobilization occasionally may be necessary for uncooperative older children, especially those who are mentally retarded and cannot understand explanations or communicate their feelings.

If these precepts are followed, sedation should rarely be necessary for treatment of soft tissue injuries. Sedation should never be given to a child if there is any question of intracranial or thoracic injury, and narcotic analgesics should be avoided if there is a possibility of associated intraabdominal injury. Unusually frightened or uncooperating children, especially infants and toddlers, may benefit from the judicious use of sedation if adequate doses are employed. A little sedation may be worse than none, since it may inhibit whatever cortical control of behavior the child has without altering fear and rage responses. In small children, barbiturates

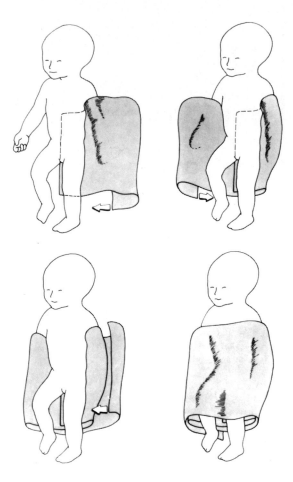

Fig. 11-1   Technique for using a folded sheet to immobilize a child. The method is easily modified to leave an injured extremity free.

alone often have the paradoxic effect of overstimulation. The best sedation is a "lytic cocktail," which is composed of a narcotic analgesic, a tranquilizer, and a sedative. Several effective combinations include the following:

Drugs	Doses
Meperidine (Demerol)	1.0 mg/kg
Chlorpromazine (Thorazine)	0.5 mg/kg
Promethazine (Phenergan)	0.5 mg/kg
Morphine sulfate	0.2 mg/kg
Hydroxyzine (Vistaril)	1.0 mg/kg
Meperidine (Demerol)	1.5 mg/kg
Secobarbital (Seconal)	3.0 mg/kg

Maximal doses are given, and the physician must be prepared to observe the child for 4 to 6 hours in the emergency room or even to admit the child until the effects of sedation subside. Since the ma-

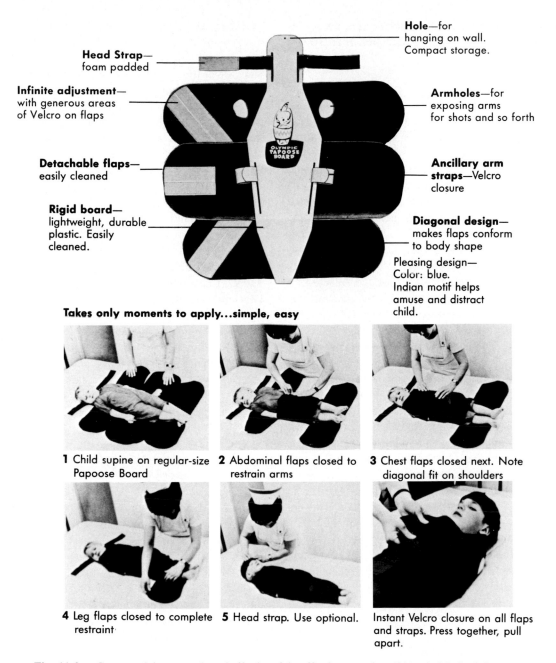

Head Strap—foam padded

Infinite adjustment—with generous areas of Velcro on flaps

Detachable flaps—easily cleaned

Rigid board—lightweight, durable plastic. Easily cleaned.

Hole—for hanging on wall. Compact storage.

Armholes—for exposing arms for shots and so forth

Ancillary arm straps—Velcro closure

Diagonal design—makes flaps conform to body shape

Pleasing design—Color: blue. Indian motif helps amuse and distract child.

Takes only moments to apply...simple, easy

1 Child supine on regular-size Papoose Board

2 Abdominal flaps closed to restrain arms

3 Chest flaps closed next. Note diagonal fit on shoulders

4 Leg flaps closed to complete restraint

5 Head strap. Use optional.

Instant Velcro closure on all flaps and straps. Press together, pull apart.

Fig. 11-2   Commercial papoose board affords quick, effective restraint. (Olympic Medical Corp., 4400 Seventh South, Seattle, Washington 98108.)

jority of injuries to children occur in late afternoon and evening when the child is already becoming sleepy, overnight observation may be necessary. Sedation alone should be reserved for highly selected cases.

Complex and extensive injuries, especially those involving the face, oral cavity, or hand may require general anesthesia for repair. The need for general anesthesia is greater in children than in adults because of greater apprehension and limited ability to cooperate. Vomiting and aspiration of gastric contents are definite risks of emergency operation and general anesthesia. Delaying the procedure for several hours may allow time for the stomach to empty but does not ensure it, since injury and the apprehension may inhibit gastric peristalsis. If there is any question of a full stomach, awake intubation or controlled rapid induction of anesthesia should be used.

INFECTION AND SOFT TISSUE INJURIES

All open wounds are contaminated with bacteria. Pulaski et al.[9] and Altemeier and Gibbs[1] cultured tissue debrided from acute traumatic wounds and obtained bacterial growth in 100% of the wounds, including those seen within 30 minutes of injury. Bacteria may come from the patient's skin or be introduced by the wounding agent. Air-borne contamination, especially from the nose and mouth of personnel caring for the patient, may also occur.

The presence of bacteria is not synonymous with infection. The probability of wound infection is determined by the balance between bacterial growth and host defenses, both local and systemic. In uncompromised hosts, defense mechanisms are generally adequate to control bacterial contamination, and most acute civilian wounds heal uneventfully after appropriate repair. A number of factors may tip the balance in favor of bacterial growth. Devitalized tissue, foreign material, and hematomas in closed wounds impede normal defense mechanisms and encourage bacterial growth.[14] Abundant experience with military injuries has shown that wounds closed in the presence of these factors invariably become infected. The principles of open treatment of wounds with delayed primary closure or healing by secondary intention evolved from these observations. Application of these techniques resulted in a remarkably low incidence of wound infection in recent wars. The same principles obviously apply to comparable civilian injuries.

Quantitative Bacteriology

Recognition that the *quantity* of bacteria present in tissue is of crucial importance has been a major advance in our understanding of the biology of wound infections. Biopsies of wound tissue can be weighed, homogenized, and cultured, and the concentration of bacteria per gram of tissue can be determined by standard colony counting techniques.[14] Wounds that contain 10^5 or more organisms per gram of tissue almost invariably become infected, whereas wounds with fewer than 10^5 organisms per gram usually heal whether treated by primary closure, delayed primary closure, or skin grafting.

Robson et al.[13] used quantitative bacteriology in a study of acute soft tissue wounds in the emergency room. Eighty wounds were cultured before standard closure. Of these wounds, 80% contained 10^5 or fewer organisms per gram of tissue, and all healed without infection. The other 20% contained more than 10^5 organisms per gram, and half of these wounds became infected. The interval from time of wounding to time of culture and repair correlated directly with bacterial concentration. Mean time was 2.2 hours for wounds containing fewer than 10^2 bacteria per gram, 3.0 hours for wounds containing 10^2 to 10^5 organisms, and 5.17 hours for wounds containing greater than 10^5 bacteria. This study confirmed the findings of Altemeier and others that all wounds are contaminated. It also demonstrated clearly that the tissue concentration of bacteria is generally low initially but rises precipitously in the first few hours after injury to levels that are incompatible with primary wound closure.

The clinical implications of these observations are clear. Acute soft tissue wounds must be adequately debrided and mechanically cleaned to remove all devitalized tissue and foreign material. Repeated bulb syringe irrigation with normal saline will free most wounds of clots and debris but will not lower the wound's bacterial count. General anesthesia may be necessary to achieve thorough debridement of deeply imbedded or tattooed material, such as road burns. Pulsating jet lavage is the most effective method of lowering the bacterial count with wound irrigation. Hemostasis must be adequate and the wound should be closed in layers. Soft tissue wounds (bites or other contaminated wounds excepted) that are less than 3 hours old and properly prepared and closed should heal primarily. Wounds seen more than 3 hours after injury must be judged individually. Deep, irregular, and grossly contaminated wounds can be assumed to have a higher initial inoculum of bacteria; *delayed* primary closure may be the best treatment. Wounds that are relatively small and clean and that are located in a well-vascularized area, such as the face or scalp, can be closed primarily during a longer period after injury. Wounds more than 12 hours old are invariably heavily contaminated and should be left open.

Since the tissue concentration of bacteria is the most important factor in the development of wound infections, a rapid technique of bacterial quantification would be clinically useful in dealing with questionable wounds. Heggers et al.[6] developed a rapid slide technique for estimation of bacterial concentration in wound biopsies that can be used in the emergency room. The tissue is weighed, flamed to remove surface bacteria, diluted 1:10 in thioglycolate broth, and homogenized. Exactly 0.02 ml of the suspension is placed on a glass slide in an area of 15 mm. The slide is oven dried for 15 minutes and stained with Gram's stain. The presence of a single organism anywhere on the slide correlates with greater than 10^5 organisms per gram with 98% accuracy. The technique is rapid and simple and should be adopted more widely.

In theory, the administration of appropriate antimicrobial agents might be thought to inhibit bacterial growth in wounds and tip the balance toward the host. Burke[4] demonstrated that antibiotics administered more than 3 hours after inoculation of a wound with bacteria failed to inhibit bacterial growth. It appears that once the critical tissue concentration of greater than 10^5 bacteria per gram is reached, antibiotics are incapable of preventing suppuration in the closed wound. Antibiotics given within 3 hours of wounding may inhibit bacterial growth, but since most of these wounds contain fewer than 10^5 organisms and heal without antibiotic therapy, there is no indication for their use. Antimicrobial agents may have a role in certain wounds that receive a large inoculum of bacteria and that are seen and treated within 3 hours, but adequate debridement and mechanical cleansing to reduce the bacterial load are certainly more important. Circumstances in which "prophylactic" antibiotics are thought to be helpful are discussed in the sections on specific injuries.

Treatment of Established Infections

Infection in wounded soft tissue usually becomes apparent one to several days after the injury and is manifested by cellulitis, abscess, lymphangitis, lymphadenopathy, and occasionally by systemic signs, such as fever or chills. Initial therapy is directed at the local wound. Sutured wounds should be opened through their full extent to provide adequate drainage. Abscesses and infected puncture wounds should be incised and drained. Pus or tissue biopsy material is obtained for culture and sensitivity testing. The wound must be carefully explored to detect any retained foreign material, such as a wooden splinter, rose thorn, or glass fragments. Soft tissue x-ray films are helpful for identifying a radiopaque substance, such as glass or

metal. Warm soaks on *open* wounds aid in the dissolution and removal of wound exudate and prevent formation of an eschar under which bacteria can multiply. Elevation helps to prevent venous and lymphatic stasis. Immobilization by bulky dressings, splints, or bed rest may aid in localization of the infection. The bacterial concentration in burns and other open wounds can be decreased significantly by the use of topical antibacterial agents, such as silver sulfadiazine (Silvadene).

If the wound can be opened and drained and the surrounding cellulitis is minimal, local therapy as outlined previously may be all that is necessary. More extensive cellulitis should be treated with systemic antibiotics. Spreading cellulitis, lymphangitis, and systemic symptoms are indications for hospitalization and intravenous antibiotic therapy. In children, facial cellulitis, especially in the periorbital area, is also an indication for treatment with intravenous antibiotics because of the risk of cavernous sinus thrombophlebitis and meningitis. Since penicillin-resistant Staphylococcus is the most common cause of soft tissue wound infection, the antibiotic of choice is a synthetic penicillin such as dicloxacillin (oral) or oxacillin (intravenous). Antibiotic therapy can be altered as necessary when the results of the culture and sensitivity testing are known.

Tetanus

Clostridium tetani is a ubiquitous organism that is particularly abundant in soil, dust, and human and animal feces. Almost any wound, even a clean minor laceration, can be contaminated with this bacterium. It is not an invasive organism but grows well in anaerobic areas of wounds and liberates a neurotoxin that is absorbed into the bloodstream to cause the clinical syndrome. Tetanus is a devastating disease characterized by generalized, violent, and uncontrolled muscle spasms. Death may result from respiratory failure, exhaustion, or aspiration. Mortality is approximately 30% even with modern management.

Although any wound may be contaminated with *Clostridium tetani,* certain injuries have a greater risk of tetanus than others. Deep wounds by agents contaminated with soil or feces receive a larger inoculum of bacteria than do minor superficial injuries. Puncture wounds and wounds that contain devitalized tissue, foreign material, and/or hematomas have areas of low oxygen tension that favor growth of the organisms. Neglected deep wounds

---

PRIMARY TETANUS IMMUNIZATION

Children 2 months to 7 years of age

Three doses DPT* at 2-month intervals
Fourth dose DPT 1 year after third dose
Booster DPT about age 5
Booster Td† every 10 years

Children older than 7 years of age

Two doses Td 2 months apart
Booster Td 1 year after second dose
Booster Td every 10 years

---

*Diphtheria-pertussis-tetanus vaccine.
†Tetanus-diphtheria toxoid, adult type.

Table 11-1   Tetanus prophylaxis at time of injury

	Tetanus prophylaxis needed for	
Immunization status	Clean/minor wound	High-risk wound
Unimmunized, unknown, or less than three doses	Td, DPT, or DT*	Td, DPT, or DT* 250-500 U TIG†
Immunized		
Last dose within 5 years	None	None
Last dose within 5 to 10 years	None	Td
Last dose more than 10 years	Td	Td

*Td, Adult tetanus-diphtheria toxoid (children 7 years); DPT, diphtheria-pertussis-tetanus toxoid (children 7 years); DT, diphtheria-tetanus toxoid (children 7 years). First dose of primary immunization.
†Human tetanus immune globulin. Equine tetanus antitoxin (TAT) causes more reactions but should be used if TIG is not available.

that are untreated for more than 24 hours are especially likely to have high concentrations of clostridia. Clean wounds less than 6 hours old entail a very low risk of tetanus.

The best prophylaxis against tetanus is adequate preinjury immunization. Recommended schedules of immunization with tetanus toxoid for infants and for school-age children not previously immunized are shown in the box above. After a complete course, protective levels of circulating antibody are present for at least 1 year. Furthermore, there is adequate recall (the ability to raise circulating antibody to protective levels after a booster dose of tetanus toxoid) for a minimum of 10 years and probably for 25 years of more. Although tetanus immunization is considered to be an integral and essential part of routine well-child care, studies have shown that up to 40% of inner-city first-grade children have not received a complete course of primary immunization. The record is even worse among children of migrant workers.

Tetanus prophylaxis at the time of injury is equally important and consists of local wound therapy and measures to ensure adequate levels of circulating antibody. The wound should be debrided and cleaned thoroughly before meticulous layered closure. Wounds more than 6 hours old should usually be left open.

Immunologic therapy at time of injury must be determined individually on the basis of prior immunization, the nature of the wound and wounding agent, and the time since injury. An accurate history of immunization status must be obtained, preferably from written records, which everyone should carry at all times. A telephone call to the patient's primary physician or clinic may be necessary. The

recommendations shown in Table 11-1 have been adapted from reports by the American College of Surgeons Committee on Trauma and the American Academy of Pediatrics Committee on Infectious Diseases. These are guidelines; the final decision regarding treatment is the responsibility of the attending physician. Since *Clostridium tetani* is sensitive to penicillin and oxytetracycline, the use of one of these agents should be considered in patients with high-risk wounds.

Rabies

Rabies is an almost uniformly lethal neurotoxic disease caused by a virus that is transmitted through the saliva of infected animals. Any open wound contaminated by animal saliva is a potential cause of rabies. Bites provide a large inoculum of virus, but even superficial nonbite wounds or mucosal contact may lead to infection. Wild animals, especially skunks, bats, and foxes, are the major reservoir of the disease. Domestic animals are rarely infected because of routine immunization, but unimmunized, stray, or feral dogs and cats can acquire the disease. Although rodents and other small animals can develop rabies, there has never been a reported case of human infection following

Table 11-2 Guide to rabies prophylaxis

Animal species	Condition of animal at time of attack	Treatment of exposed person*
Domestic		
Dog and cat	Healthy and available for 10 days of observation	None unless animal develops rabies†
	Rabid or suspected rabid	RIgH‡ *and* rabies vaccine§
	Unknown	Consultation with public health officials. If treatment is indicated, give RIgH† *and* rabies vaccine§
Wild		
Skunk, bat, fox, coyote, raccoon, bobcat, and other carnivores	Regard as rabid unless proven negative by laboratory test‖	RIgH‡ *and* rabies vaccine§
Other		
Livestock and rodents	Consider individually. Provoked bites of squirrels, hamsters, guinea pigs, gerbils, chipmunks, rats, mice, and other rodents or rabbits and hares almost never call for antirabies prophylaxis. Local or state public health officials should be consulted about questions that arise about the need for rabies prophylaxis.	

Information from references 3, 10, and 11.

*All bites and wounds should immediately be thoroughly cleansed with soap and water. If antirabies treatment is indicated, both rabies immune globulin, human (RIgH) and rabies vaccine should be given as soon as possible, *regardless* of the interval after exposure. If RIgH inadvertently was not given when the vaccination was begun, it can be given up to the eighth day after the first dose of vaccine was given. Persons who have been previously immunized with rabies vaccine and were known to have protective rabies antibody titer should receive only vaccine.

†Begin treatment with RIgH and rabies vaccine at first sign of rabies in biting domestic animals during the usual holding period of 10 days. The symptomatic animal should be killed immediately and tested.

‡If RIgH is not available, use antirabies serum of equine origin. Do not use more than the recommended dosage.

§Discontinue vaccine if fluorescent antibody tests of animal are negative.

‖The animal should be killed and tested as soon as possible. Holding for observation is not recommended.

bites by these animals. Domestic animals that bite without provocation or animals that exhibit unusual behavior are more likely to be rabid, but the virus can be transmitted before the animal is symptomatic.

Children are frequently bitten by dogs, usually their own or that of a neighbor. The attack is often provoked, either by overzealous play or harassment. Cats are more likely to scratch but occasionally inflict bites. Wild animal bites are uncommon unless the animal has been captured as a pet.

Thorough debridement and mechanical cleansing of animal bites effectively reduce the volume of contaminated saliva and are essential parts of rabies prophylaxis. The decision to close the wound is based on the principles outlined in the section on bites. Neither good wound preparation nor leaving the wound open are adequate protection against rabies.

A decision to administer rabies vaccine, hyperimmune antirabies serum, or both must be based on the patient, animal species involved, nature and circumstances of the injury, and local epidemiologic data, which can be obtained from the State Health Department[3,5,10,11] Human diploid cell vaccine and human rabies immune globulin have enabled patients to achieve both passive and active immunity without the many adverse reactions formerly resulting from duck embryo– and horse serum–derived agents. General guidelines for the use of rabies vaccines are shown in Table 11-2 and in the box on p. 198. Wild animals are assumed to be rabid, and treatment with serum and vaccine is begun at once. If the animal is captured, it is sacrificed and the brain examined (usually by the State Health Department) by the fluorescent antibody technique for evidence of rabies. If none is found, the vaccine can be discontinued.

Nonvaccinated or stray dogs and cats should be sacrificed and the brain examined. If the animal has escaped, it is safe to delay therapy for up to 48 hours while attempts are made to catch the animal. If the animal cannot be identified and cap-

---

GENERAL GUIDELINES FOR USE OF RABIES VACCINES

Dosage

Rabies immune globulin human (RIgH): 20 IU/kg body weight

$$\frac{\text{Body weight in lbs}}{2.2} = \text{Body weight in kg}$$

$$\frac{\text{Body weight in kg} \times 20\ \text{IU}}{150\ \text{IU/ml}} =$$
Amount of ml needed for treatment

If possible, up to half the dose should be used to infiltrate the wound.

Rabies vaccine human diploid cell: five (1 ml) doses given on days 0, 3, 7, 14, and 28

Studies conducted at the Centers for Disease Control have shown that a regimen of five doses of rabies vaccine human diploid cell plus RIgH was safe and induced an excellent antibody response in all recipients.*

Administration

RIgH is administered only once at the beginning of antirabies prophylaxis to provide antibodies until the patient responds to vaccination. RIgH, after preparation of the injection site, is injected intramuscularly (for example, in the gluteal region).

Rabies vaccine is administered on days 0, 3, 7, 14, and 28. After preparation of the injection site, immediately inject the vaccine intramuscularly, (for example, in the deltoid region).

Note: Never administer rabies vaccine in the same injection site as RIgH

Information from references 10 and 11.
*Recommendations of the Immunization Practices Advisory Committee (ACIP). MMWR 33:393, July 1984, Centers for Disease Control, US Public Health Service.

---

tured, treatment should be instituted with serum and vaccine for bite wounds and with vaccine alone for nonbite wounds. These recommendations are modified according to local epidemiologic data, however. For example, in Connecticut, rabies has not been reported in dogs or cats for many years, and the wild animal reservoir is small. Therefore treatment is not usually recommended for dog or cat bite even if the animal escapes. Accurate and current data from the State Health Department concerning the prevalence of rabies in the local area is obviously of great importance in making therapeutic decisions. Bites by currently immunized (within 1 year) domestic animals do not require treatment, but the animal should be observed for 10 days. If unusual behavior or signs of rabies appear, the animal is sacrificed. Treatment of the child is started immediately if fluorescent antibody examination of the animal's brain shows evidence of rabies.

SPECIFIC SOFT TISSUE INJURIES

Abrasions

Superficial abrasions require little more than adequate local cleansing. The child may be more comfortable if abrasions in areas exposed to further trauma are covered by a light, nonadherent dressing. Topical antibacterial ointments may not only reduce the bacterial count, but also may serve to minimize coagulum formation and prevent adherence of dressings. Maintenance of a clean wound is the most important factor in proper healing of abrasions; the area should be cleaned by gentle cleansing once or twice daily.

Deep abrasions with embedded foreign material are of far greater consequence. Children typically sustain this type of injury during falls from bicycles or when hit by or thrown from motor vehicles. Dirt, tar, and bits of gravel become deeply embedded in the dermis; if not removed, a permanent and disfiguring tattoo results. The most effective method of removing this material is to debride the wound thoroughly with a stiff brush or pulsating jet lavage with the patient under local anesthesia for small wounds. Larger areas, however, will require general anesthesia (Fig. 11-3). The debrided wound is then comparable to a skin graft donor site and is treated accordingly by application of fine-mesh gauze, biologic dressings, or topical antibacterial agents. Since there is no question of primarily closing the wound, it is appropriate to fast the child for 6 to 8 hours before semi-elective induction of anesthesia.

Contusions and Hematomas

Minor bumps and bruises are sustained almost daily by active children. More severe contusions and hematomas may occur as a result of falls and vehicular accidents. Careful examination for underlying injury (fracture, dislocation, or major vascular disruption) is essential.

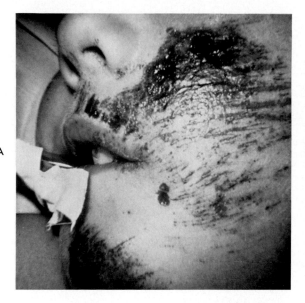
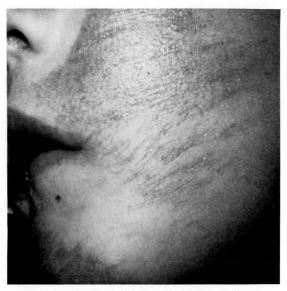

A

B

Fig. 11-3   **A,** Deep facial abrasions in a small child. Dirt and other foreign material are embedded in the wound. **B,** Same patient after vigorous debridement and mechanical cleansing with the child under general anesthesia. The wound, although deep, may now heal with an acceptable cosmetic result.

Hematomas of the abdominal wall are a particular problem since the muscle spasm associated with this injury may be indistinguishable from the signs of local peritonitis caused by rupture of the spleen or a hollow viscus. The most valuable means of differentiating these conditions is careful, serial physical examination. The physical findings of abdominal wall hematoma remain localized and unassociated with other signs, whereas the examination of the patient with significant intraabdominal injury reveals progressive abdominal distension, ileus, and increasing tenderness and spasm. Flank contusions and hematomas may be caused by local trauma or to extension of a retroperitoneal hematoma, but in the latter case flank ecchymosis characteristically does not appear until several hours or days after injury.

The swelling and pain of symptomatic contusions may be reduced by application of ice in the first 24 hours. Thereafter, heat in the form of warm soaks or baths or a heating pad may hasten resolution of the inflammatory process. Immobilization and elevation (sling, bulky dressing, elastic bandage, bed rest) of the injured part may also minimize swelling and provide symptomatic relief.

Subungual hematoma is an acutely painful condition that can be drained readily by drilling a small hole in the nail. Adults welcome the relief afforded by this simple procedure, but children are often terrified by the sight of a drill or hot paper clip. Since children tolerate continuing discomfort better than adults, it may be advisable to leave the hematoma alone unless the child is in severe distress. X-ray films of the underlying phalanges should be obtained in select cases to prevent conversion of a simple phalangeal fracture to a compound fracture equivalent by drainage of an overlying subungual hematoma.

Crush Injuries

More extensive trauma may cause actual destruction and necrosis of tissue. The degree of inflammation and swelling associated with a crush injury is much greater than with simple contusion. Fascial layers investing muscle usually remain intact, and the tension produced within the fascial envelope may exceed arterial pressure leading to ischemic necrosis and contracture. Major vessels supplying parts distal to the injured area also may be occluded. Fasciotomy may be necessary early in the course of this reaction to prevent the late consequences of ischemia. The fascial compartments of the forearm and the anterior tibial component of the leg are especially prone to ischemic complications. If fasciotomy is necessary it should be performed without delay. The fascia should be incised along the entire length of any involved muscle compartment.

A classic example of crush injury in childhood involves injury caused by electric clothes wringers.[15] These injuries occur much less frequently now than in the past, but wringer washers may still be used by some families in poorer socioeconomic groups. The moving rollers of the wringer trap the exploring fingers of a toddler and pull the arm through, exerting tremendous crushing pressure on the tissues. This process usually stops at the elbow but may continue to the axilla. The injury is compounded by the shearing effect of the rollers after the arm stops advancing in the wringer. Deep abrasions may lead to full thickness–skin loss, and the skin may be sheared off the subcutaneous tissue, creating a large dead space and hematoma. Trauma may be intensified by attempts to pull the arm out of the wringer instead of turning the machine off or tripping the release mechanism.

Children who sustain wringer injuries should be hospitalized for local wound care and observation of the arm. X-ray films are obtained, although frac-tures are uncommon. Skin abrasions are cleaned and dressed in the usual manner. The arm is then elevated in a slinglike support most easily made from a piece of stockinette. Bulky dressings should be avoided because they interfere with adequate observation. Elastic bandages do not prevent swelling and may actually compound the tissue tension. Fasciotomy may not be necessary but should be performed promptly if there is evidence of paresthesias, hypesthesias, or progressive local ischemia. Obliteration of the radial pulse is a late finding in this syndrome.

Most children with wringer injuries can be discharged in 24 to 48 hours. Local wound care is continued on an outpatient basis. Split-thickness skin grafting may be necessary at a later date for areas of full-thickness loss.

Lacerations

Few children escape childhood without a scar or two. The face and hands, with which the child meets and explores the world, are the most frequently injured areas. The supraorbital ridge is

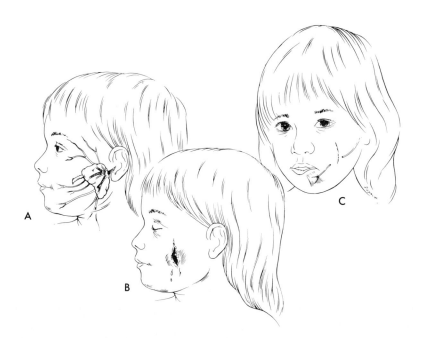

Fig. 11-4   A, The parotid gland or its duct or branches of the facial nerve may be injured by facial trauma. **B,** With salivary gland or ductal injury, saliva may be noted in the wound. A transected salivary duct may be evident on examining the wound. Otherwise, transoral or direct duct cannulation and/or injection of the duct may help localize such an injury. **C,** Facial nerve injury may involve the main trunk of the facial nerve or zygomaticofrontal, buccal, or marginal mandibular branches. Division of the marginal mandibular branch, as depicted, results in the loss of ipsilateral lip depressor muscle function and an asymmetric smile.

probably the single most common site of laceration, followed closely by chin, fingers, scalp, and
knees. Most lacerations result from falls in and
around the home, abetted by the instability of toddlers and the frenetic, nonstop activities of older
children. Falls against coffee tables are the single
most common cause of lacerations. Bumping into
door, falling down stairs, and tumbling from
wheeled toys follow closely behind.

Children with lacerations should be examined
carefully for evidence of injury to deeper structures
(Figs. 11-4 and 11-5). Transection of tendons and
nerves in the extremities may be difficult to detect
in the young patient, but the approach to the injured
child outlined previously should facilitate adequate
examination. If there is serious question of nerve
or tendon injury, exploration of the wound under
general anesthesia is indicated. The possibility of
fracture should be considered, but radiologic examination, especially of the skull, is greatly over-
used. Careful prospective studies have shown that
skull fracture is present in less than 10% of all
children for whom skull films are part of the evaluation of a head injury.[12] Findings from history and
physical examination correlate poorly with the likelihood of fracture. The physician's overall assessment of the degree of injury is the best indicator
of fracture, but even among the most severely injured children (for example, those who are unconscious or who have labored breathing or extensive

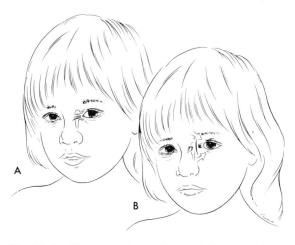

Fig. 11-5 Trauma to the medial canthal and nasal regions may cause disruption of the medial canthus or the
lacrimal collecting system (for example, canaliculi or
lacrimal sac). Severe deformity (traumatic telecanthus)
or dysfunction (epiphora) may result from such injuries.

scalp wound) skull fracture is present in less than
half.[7] The yield in children who sustain minor head
trauma is virtually nil. The practice of obtaining
routine skull series in every child with a scalp laceration or hematoma cannot be justified, notwith-
standing medicolegal implications. When a scalp
laceration is accompanied by any neurologic sequelae, a head CT scan is indicated.

The general principles of repair of lacerations in
children are the same as in adults, but certain details
should be mentioned. Suture of facial lacerations
is particularly upsetting to children. Fear is often
intensified by the bright surgical light glaring in
the face. Directing the light at an angle or centering
it slightly to one side should provide adequate illumination with less distress to the child. Covering
the face with large sterile drapes is also threatening.
Loss of eye contact with the parent or surrogate
exacerbates the child's insecurity and fear that
something awful is about to happen. Fear of suf-
focation is aroused if the nose and mouth are covered. It is often advisable simply to place a sterile
towel on one side of the laceration, leaving at least
one eye and either the nose or mouth uncovered.
Although this may entail some compromise of sterile technique, a clean if not absolutely sterile field
can be achieved. The face fortunately has a rich
blood supply, and wound infections are rare.

Adequate anesthesia is essential to maintain the
child's cooperation and to permit careful repair of
the laceration. Infiltration of the local anesthetic
should be the only painful part of the procedure,
and the pain can be minimized if the agent is injected slowly through a small needle (25, 27, or
30 gauge) directly into the open wound. It is tempt-
ing to hurry at this point to get through the un-
pleasant period, but a slow, patient approach will
cause less pain and ensure adequate anesthesia for
subsequent debridement and repair. Small children
(under 2 years of age) require larger amounts of
local anesthetic in proportion to their size than older
patients. A 0.25% or 0.5% lidocaine solution is
safer in this age group than the 1% solution commonly used in older children, but is is important
to remember that the total dose of local anesthetic
must not exceed 5 mgm/kg (5 mgm/cc in 0.5%
lidocaine). Epinephrine should generally be
avoided in infants because of its systemic effects,
but it may be helpful in controlling bleeding from
scalp and face lacerations in older children.

The wound and surrounding skin should be
washed gently, for example, with an iodine-con-

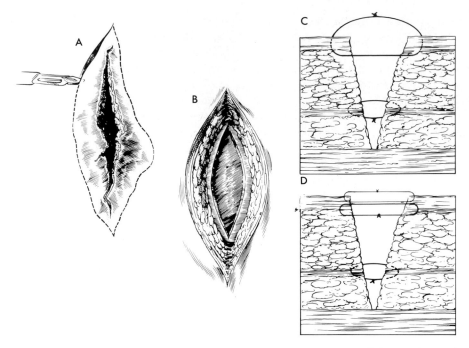

Fig. 11-6   **A,** Untidy, irregular, and contaminated wounds are best repaired if they are first excised. **B,** Thus fresh, sharp, untraumatized tissue margins may undergo layered repair. When several anatomic planes are violated, layered repair is necessitated. Fascia may be repaired with absorbable sutures. More than one technique may be chosen to complete the cutaneous closure: **C,** full-thickness nonabsorbable cutaneous sutures are used; **D,** absorbable, inverted (knots lying on the deeper surface) dermal sutures give the closure its greatest strength, while a final adjustment is made with a fine, nonabsorbable, epithelial suture.

taining solution, before infiltration with local anesthetic. Major cleaning and debridement of extensive lacerations should be deferred until the wound is adequately anesthetized. All foreign material and devitalized tissue must be removed. The wound should be explored and irrigated to its full depth to facilitate debridement and to search for injury to deeper structures. Contused and ragged skin edges should be trimmed (Fig. 11-6). Deep wounds are closed in layers; careful apposition of the subcutaneous tissue is particularly important if the skin will be closed with subcuticular or subepidermal sutures. Meticulous approximation of the skin edges without tension will minimize the ultimate scar. Suture size should be sufficient to give the wound adequate early strength, but not so large as to result in objectionable suture marks. At prominent sites such as the face, 5-0 or 6-0 nylon or prolene is adequate. Fine absorbable sutures such as 6-0 plain catgut or even 7-0 may be used in select cases. This material will usually fragment and fall from the wound in a week or so if they

are regularly cleansed or gently abraded with a cotton-tipped applicator and hydrogen peroxide from the outset. Recommended suture for simple lacerations of the face, scalp, trunk or extremity, and joint surface in a young child are outlined in Table 11-3. Common types of suture placement are depicted in Fig. 11-7.

Dressings are useful to protect, to immobilize the repair, and to absorb any wound drainage. Scalp lacerations are difficult to dress but can be covered with collodion or one of the aerosol plastic films. A piece of gauze cut to the right size and shape and held in place with tincture of benzoin and tape works well for lacerations of the face. Most hand and finger injuries should be wrapped with a bulky, protective, immobilizing dressing made of fluffed gauze and soft flexible gauze rolled around the hand and between the fingers (leaving the tips exposed to monitor circulation). Adequate immobilization is especially important for lacerations near joints. Most children are unable to sit still for any length of time no matter how much they wish to cooperate.

Table 11-3 Type of skin suture and method of placement in a young child with a simple laceration

Site of laceration	Gauge of suture (nylon or prolene)	Placement*
Facial	6-0	Interrupted or running
Scalp	4-0	Running
Trunk (extremity)	4-0 or 5-0	Running
Joint	4-0 or 5-0	Interrupted
Hand (finger)	4-0 or 5-0	Interrupted

*See Fig. 11-7 for type of suture.

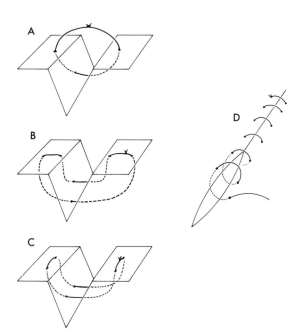

Fig. 11-7 Suture techniques depicted include simple suture **(A)**, vertical mattress suture **(B)**, horizontal mattress suture **(C)**, and running (or continuous) simple suture **(D)**. Mattress sutures are especially useful in achieving a favorable eversion of wound edges. This advantage is especially helpful in hand and foot injuries. Running or continuous sutures are helpful in closing wounds that are long, providing that any necessary set sutures have been placed and that the underlying layers have been securely closed.

Any wound around a joint, especially on the extensor surface, should be dressed to immobilize the joint. Lacerations on or just below the knee in young boys are especially prone to breakdown and secondary infection as a result of repeated flexion. Use of a posterior splint for 7 to 10 days should be routine. Similar splints can be made for wounds around the elbow, wrist, and ankle. Splints provide essential protection and do not seem to interfere greatly with the child's normal activities.

Lacerations in and around the oral cavity in children deserve special comment.[8] Intraoral lacerations result from falls with a stick or other pointed object in the mouth or from dental crush injury. In general, smaller mucosal injuries should not be repaired. The turnover time of oral mucosa is about 3 days, and wounds heal rapidly with little or no scar if left open. The wound is contaminated from the outset because of the high concentration of bacteria in the mouth, and suturing may lead to invasive, closed-space infection. Extensive or gaping lacerations should be repaired if necessary, with the patient under general endotracheal anesthesia to search for injury to a deeper structure (for example, Stensen's duct or the carotid artery) and to allow adequate debridement, irrigation, and accurate reconstitution of muscle layers. Antimicrobial therapy, usually with penicillin, should be given for 5 days for such extensive injuries. Lacerations of the pharynx are of particular concern; perforation of the pharynx or hypopharynx may lead to retropharyngeal abscess or mediastinitis and may be missed on routine oral examination. Pharyngeal perforation should be considered in any child who has a history of falling with a stick in

his or her mouth even if an obvious pharyngeal wound is not seen. A history of persistent severe pain, respiratory distress, dysphagia, or dysphonia is presumptive evidence of perforation, as is palpable crepitus in the neck. Lateral x-ray films of the neck should be obtained to look for extrapharyngeal air (Fig. 11-8). Barium swallow may demonstrate a perforation. Inhospital observation, fasting, and intravenous antibiotic therapy (penicillin) are essential steps in the management of known or suspected pharyngeal perforation. If the wound cannot adequately be seen by direct oral examination, pharyngoscopy should be performed with the patient under general anesthesia. Most simple perforations will heal promptly in a few days. Extensive lacerations may require surgical repair and a longer period of fasting. Feeding gastrostomy may be a useful adjunct in some cases.

Lacerations of the lip caused by the child's teeth occur commonly during falls. Wounds that cross

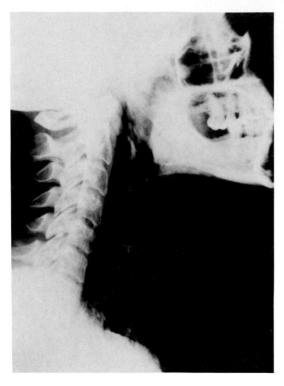

Fig. 11-8   Lateral x-ray films of the neck in a patient who fell with a stick in her mouth. Large amounts of air are present in the retropharyngeal soft tissues. This facial plane is continuous with the mediastinum.

Table 11-4   Schedule for skin suture removal in a young child with a simple laceration

Site of laceration	Optimal time for suture removal (day)	Supplementary care
Facial	5	Steri-strip
Scalp	7-10	?Collodion
Trunk	10-14	
Joint	10-14	?Splint
Hand (finger)	10-14	?Splint

the surface of the lip should be sutured with meticulous alignment of the vermilion border. Through and through lacerations of the lower lip should be repaired by approximation of the muscle and routine debridement and suture of the skin. The mucosal side of the wound is left open if relatively small, or it can be closed with fine absorbable sutures (Fig. 11-9). Similarly, deliberate and precise repair of the grey line of the eyelid, the eyebrow margin, and the nasal alar margin must be accomplished to set the stage for completion of cutaneous closure.

Tongue lacerations, also usually caused by the teeth, may be especially difficult problems because of the highly vascular and mobile nature of the tongue. Most of these wounds stop bleeding spontaneously and do not need to be sutured. If bleeding persists or recurs (a possibility parents should be alerted to) or if the laceration is gaping, repair should be performed with the patient under general anesthesia if necessary and with an endotracheal tube in place. In the very rare event of massive

hemorrhage and acute airway obstruction, temporary emergency control of the tongue can be achieved by placing a heavy stay suture or towel clip through the tip. The tongue is drawn out of the mouth and immobilized. The wound then can be controlled by direct compression or suture. Children with extensive tongue (or floor of mouth) injuries should be hospitalized even if direct operative repair is not performed, since the tongue is predisposed to massive edema and hematoma formation that may obstruct the small child's airway. Equipment for emergency intubation and tracheostomy should be at hand.

Timing of suture removal is critical in achieving primary wound healing with the best possible cosmetic result. If the wound is properly closed, there will not be too much tension or dependence on the removable sutures for strength. The deeper absorbable dermal sutures will retain significant strength to maintain wound approximation. In an apparently healing wound showing no signs of inflammation or infection, sutures may be removed as early as the fifth day in the face and as late as 10 to 14 days in the trunk or extremities (Table 11-4).

Puncture Wounds

Puncture wounds should be left open or debrided to minimize the risk of closed-space infection. Antibiotic therapy should be instituted if cellulitis subsequently appears. Incision and drainage of an abscess may occasionally be necessary. The most important principle of management of puncture wounds is adequate tetanus prophylaxis. These injuries favor growth of anaerobic organisms and are most often caused by stepping on a nail or other sharp object on the ground, which may harbor *Clostridium tetani*.

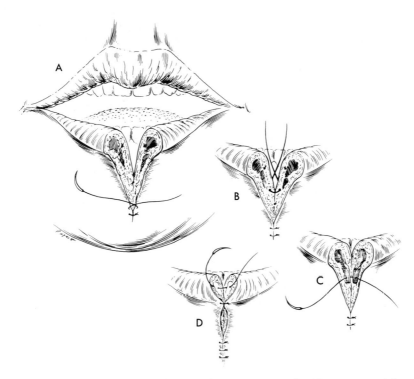

Fig. 11-9   **A,** Repair of lip and eyelid lacerations must proceed with great regard for anatomic landmarks and layers. The sequence of tissue repair should furthermore proceed in such a way as to allow for adequate exposure and access to the tissues as the repair progresses. **B,** The labial mucosal repair is initiated with absorbable sutures (plain catgut) placed with the tied knots lying within the oral cavity. **C,** After several mucosal sutures are placed, the orbicularis muscular repair is begun with 4-0 or 5-0 absorbable sutures (for example, Vicryl, Dexon, or catgut). **D,** Once several cutaneous sutures have been placed and the wound margins are more closely apposed, a crucial set stitch is placed to align the vermilion border. Once the vermilion is repaired, the remaining adjacent mucosa and skin are repaired.

The possibility of joint space penetration should be considered with puncture wounds near joints. Careful physical and radiologic examination for signs of joint trauma (limitation of motion and effusion) should be performed initially and as indicated during close outpatient follow-up.

Foreign Bodies

The possibility of retained foreign bodies should be considered in puncture wounds or lacerations caused by sticks, glass, needles, or other breakable objects. The importance of thorough wound exploration before repair has already been emphasized. Puncture wounds are not routinely explored or closed, and foreign bodies can be missed unless the physician has a high degree of suspicion. The history and appearance of the wound may be suggestive. Most foreign bodies are radiopaque, but cone-down roentgenograms and careful tech-

niques may be necessary to demonstrate subtle differences in radiodensity compared with adjacent soft tissue. Despite these precautions, many foreign bodies are not recognized initially. Some, especially small metallic ones, may become encapsulated in scar tissue and remain asymptomatic. Others, notably wood and glass fragments, tend to become infected and produce a draining sinus tract along the original wound. It is often easier to locate and to remove these foreign bodies after a draining sinus is established. Vigorous attempts to identify and extract foreign bodies at the time of injury are therefore not absolutely indicated and may be much more difficult than initially apparent. Large and easily visible objects should be recovered, but prolonged wound exploration is painful, frustrating, often unnecessary, and may paralyze nearby vital structures. Deep wounds are difficult to anesthetize adequately. Thus injudicious probing and steady enlargement of the wound may result in more extensive tissue destruction than would a policy of watchful waiting.

Foreign bodies in certain locations should be removed promptly, however. Material embedded in the plantar surface of the foot is exposed to repeated trauma as the child walks. This is painful and may cause the object to erode into tendons, bones, or joints. Metatarsal osteomyelitis may ensue. Foreign bodies in the hands, especially the fingers and web spaces, may also be acutely symptomatic and are potentially harmful to the intricate structures of the hand. Foreign bodies near joints should be removed because of the possibility of joint space penetration.

A typical example of retained foreign body in a child is a broken sewing needle in the foot. The barefoot child steps on a needle, which may penetrate and break off so quickly that the child is hardly aware of the injury. After a few days of persistent pain and limping the child is brought to the physician but may not recall the injury until x-ray films demonstrate a needle in the foot. The fragment should be removed, but finding needles and other small, sharp, thin foreign bodies is challenging and frustrating. The entrance wound is too fine to trace, local anesthesia is inadequate, and the field is full of blood. In general, the safest and simplest approach is to obtain true anteroposterior and lateral films (Fig. 11-10) to localize the foreign body in relation to bony landmarks. Then, with the child under general anesthesia and with an operating tourniquet in place to ensure a bloodless field, the object can be found and removed rapidly through a small incision. Placement of the incision is critical and requires careful study of the x-ray films; ideally, it should be perpendicular to the long axis of the foreign body, but it should also follow natural skin lines as closely as possible and avoid weight-bearing areas. An incision in one of the web spaces is often a good choice. In our experience foreign bodies invariably can be found in this manner. The patient is usually discharged the same day.

Attempts to localize foreign bodies with the aid of image-intensified fluoroscopy have become popular in recent years. Fluoroscopy requires work in a darkened room under a large machine. If it is attempted, it should be abandoned if not successful in 10 or 15 minutes. Ariyan has described a stereotactic method of foreign body removal.[2] Using local anesthesia and fluoroscopy, the operator inserts two needles into the skin at right angles to

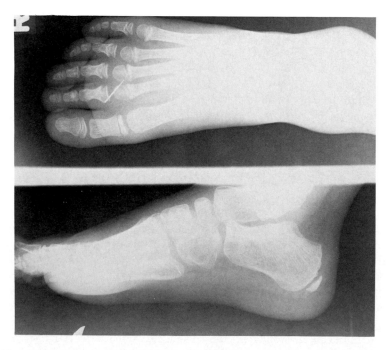

Fig. 11-10   Anteroposterior and lateral films demonstrate a broken needle on the plantar aspect of the foot superficial to the second metatarsal-phalangeal joint. An incision was made in the first web space perpendicular to the needle, which was located and removed.

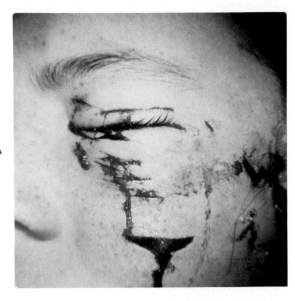
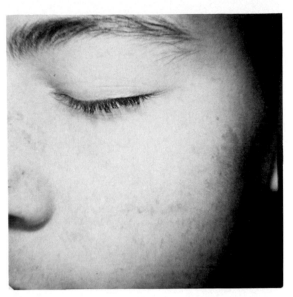

A   B

Fig. 11-11   A, Extensive dog bites of a young girl's face. She was seen immediately after injury. The wounds were carefully debrided, irrigated, and closed with the girl under general anesthesia. **B,** Same patient several weeks after suture removal. The wounds healed primarily without incident. (Courtesy Gary Mombello, M.D.)

each other. These are advanced until their tips are touching the foreign object, which can be removed by cutting down on the locator needles. This technique seems superior to blind wound exploration, even under fluoroscopy, and may prove to be an acceptable alternative to operative removal in older patients.

Bites

Wounds resulting from animal bites must be considered contaminated, in general. Animal bite puncture wounds are common; they need not and should not be closed. The contused edges of the wounds should be debrided. A 2- or 3-day effort at debriding the coagulum and encrustments forming at such sites will minimize the addition of an obstructed collection of serum to the bacterial inoculum. When there is suspicion of violation of joints or tendon sheaths, appropriate specialty consultation should be obtained.

When leaving animal bites open to heal secondarily would result in a significant defect (by virtue of size or location, for example, the face) or exposure of vital structures, primary closure may be performed (Fig. 11-11). In these cases, the wounds are ideally sharply excised and irrigated with pulsatile lavage (syringe and 21-gauge needle) to re-

duce contamination and provide fresh edges of normal tissue for repair. Antibiotic coverage (penicillin) is also instituted for 2 to 5 days.

Human bites are invariably heavily contaminated with virulent organisms and are rarely closed. Vigorous debridement and irrigation, continuing local wound care, and antimicrobial prophylaxis are indicated as the wound heals by secondary intent. Cosmetically unacceptable scars can be revised at a later date.

SUMMARY

Soft tissue injuries are very common in children. A calm, gentle, and unhurried approach to their management is essential. An appreciation of children and their special needs and fears is of inestimable value in achieving optimal results and preventing further emotional trauma.

Adherence to the basic principles of wound management minimizes the risk of infection and leads to acceptable functional and cosmetic results in most cases. Thorough debridement, adequate mechanical cleansing, and layered wound closure are essential. Delayed primary closure or healing by secondary intention are indicated in certain contaminated wounds. An accurate history of tetanus immunization status must be obtained and appropriate tetanus prophylaxis administered.

Management of specific injuries in children is similar, for the most part, to treatment in adults. Certain types of wounds are unique to childhood, however, and the biologic and psychologic response of children to injury may be different.

REFERENCES

1. Altemeier WA and Gibbs EW: Bacterial flora of fresh accidental wounds, Surg Gynecol Obstet 78:164, 1944.
2. Ariyan S: A simple stereotactic method to isolate and remove foreign bodies, Arch Surg 112:857, 1977.
3. Bahmanyar M et al: Successful protection of humans exposed to rabies infection, JAMA 236:2751, 1976.
4. Burke JF: The effective period of antibiotic action in experimental incisions and dermal lesions, Surgery 50:161, 1961.
5. Chait LA and Spitz L: Dogbite injuries in children, S Afr Med J 49:718, 1975.
6. Heggers JP, Robson MC, and Ristroph JD: A rapid method of performing quantitative wound cultures, Milit Med 134:666, 1969.
7. Loop JW and Bell RS: The utility and futility of radiographic skull examination for trauma, N Engl J Med 284:236, 1971.
8. Pickett LK and Stark DB: Trauma in and about the mouth of children, Pediatr Clin North Am 3:905, 1956.
9. Pulaski EJ, Meleny FL, and Spaeth WLC: Bacterial flora of acute traumatic wounds, Surg Gynecol Obstet 72:982, 1941.
10. "Rabies — what to do in an emergency," Miami, 1984, Merieux Institute, Inc.
11. Recommendations of the immunization practices advisory committee, Morbid Mortal 33:393, Rockville, Md, 1984, Centers for Disease Control.
12. Roberts F and Shopfner CE: Plain skull roentgenograms in children with head trauma, Am J Roentgenol Rad Ther Nucl Med 114:230, 1972.
13. Robson MC, Duke WF, and Krizek TJ: Rapid bacterial screening in the treatment of civilian wounds, J Surg Res 14:426, 1973.
14. Robson MC, Krizek TJ, and Heggers JP: Biology of surgical infection, Curr Prob Surg Mar 1973, p. 13.
15. Stone HH, Cantwell DV, and Fulenwider JT: Wringer arm injuries, J Pediatr Surg 11:375, 1976.

12

Maxillofacial Trauma

Margaret A. Kenna

Significant maxillofacial trauma in children, with resultant facial fractures, is uncommon compared with that seen in the adolescent and adult populations. The management of these injuries can be difficult and controversial and may require a team approach involving maxillofacial surgeons, otolaryngologists, neurosurgeons, pediatric radiologists, pediatric general surgeons, and pediatricians to diagnose and treat the child correctly. The effect of trauma on facial development cannot always be predicted, and facial deformity may result from the trauma itself, from bony displacement and impaired growth of developing facial structures, or from both.

INCIDENCE

James[9] reviewed 11 studies evaluating fractures of the facial bones in children up to age 14. The incidence varied from 1.5% to 8.0% of the total population sustaining maxillofacial trauma. Many of these same studies revealed an even lower incidence in children under age 5: 0.87% to 1.2%. Kaban et al.[10] evaluated 109 children with facial fractures secondary to facial trauma and found nasal fractures to be most common (45%), followed by mandibular fractures (32%), orbital (including blowout) fractures (17%), and zygomaticomaxillary complex fractures (5.5%). Hall[8] and McCoy et al.[15] also noted that fractures of the nasal bones and mandible were much more common than other types of facial fractures. All of these studies note a very low incidence of midface fractures (that is, maxilla and maxillary sinus); 0%,[10] 0.5%,[18] 6.5%,[8] 8% (maxilla), and 18% (maxillary sinus).[7] Mid-third fractures are more common in older children and adolescents. In the series of Kaban et al.,[10] Gussack et al.,[7] and Morgan et al.[16] there was a slight male predominance. The incidence of

facial fractures in several series is noted in Table 12-1.

The abused child is a special case. In a 1986 study by Worlock et al.[23] children with fractures (anywhere in the body) caused by child abuse had a much higher incidence of associated head and neck bruising than a control group of children sustaining fractures from accidental injuries. Although the abused children did not have a high incidence of facial fractures, marked head and neck bruising, especially if associated with other injuries, should raise the suspicion of abuse and suggest further investigation.

ASSOCIATED INJURIES

Children who sustain facial trauma frequently have other, sometimes life-threatening, injuries. In the study by Gussack et al.[7] 73% of the children sustaining facial fractures had associated injuries, as opposed to 58% of the adults. The most common associated injuries in both groups were soft tissue, cranial, and orthopedic. In this same series, of the patients with associated injuries, multiple injuries

Table 12-1 Incidence of facial fractures in children

Authors	Age group (years)	Total in series (adults and children)	Percentage of children with facial fractures
McCoy et al. (1966)	0-14	1500	6.0
Morgan et al. (1972)*	0-12	300	4.0
Bochlogyros (1985)†	0-14	853	6.0
Gussack et al. (1987)	3-16	206	14.5

*Midface fractures only.
†Mandibular fractures only.

209

were also found more frequently in children than in adults: 68% versus 39%, respectively. Cranial injuries were found in 55% of the pediatric population compared with 39% of the adult population. In a 1975 study by Morgan,[17] of 63 children with mandibular fractures, 34.9% had associated nondental problems, with problems in the cranial region and central nervous system being the most common (cerebral contusion, coma, skull fracture, intracerebral hematoma). Maniglia and Kline[13] noted a 1% incidence of cervical spine injury, such as subluxation or fractures, in pediatric patients with mandibular symphyseal and subcondylar fractures.

ETIOLOGY

Children are spontaneous, curious, and generally fearless. When learning to walk they fall frequently, and once able to walk they will run, climb, and continue to fall. Fortunately, young children are usually supervised and prevented from falling from great heights. As they get older, children have less supervision and participate in sports and other activities that may cause serious injury.

James[9] found falls, play, and motor vehicle accidents to be the most common causes of facial trauma. Kaban et al.[10] also noted falls to be the most common, followed by being struck by a blunt object (for example, a baseball bat). In the series by Gussack et al.,[7] motor vehicle accidents were the most frequent cause of facial fractures in both children and adults. Gussack et al.,[7] James,[9] and Kaban et al.[10] all found that children injured in motor vehicle accidents were not wearing safety restraints. As previously noted,[23] child abuse appears to be an unfortunate but increasingly recognized cause of facial trauma in children, especially in children under age 5. Facial fractures caused by birth trauma, especially forceps use, are very rare. James[9] reported a left zygomatic arch fracture due to forceps delivery. At birth the facial nerve is very superficial in the posterior auricular area and the mastoid is poorly developed, so forceps can damage the nerve and cause temporal bone fractures. These patients manifest at birth, or shortly thereafter, facial nerve paresis or paralysis; fortunately, these injuries are often of a crushing nature, and some degree of recovery is expected.

There are several anatomic reasons for the low incidence of facial fractures, especially in younger children. At birth, and for the first 2 years of life,

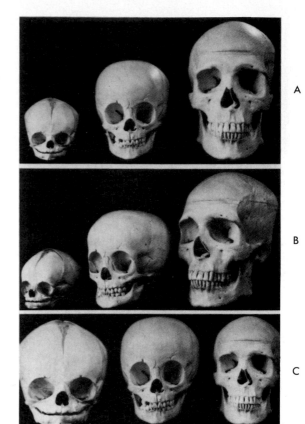

Fig. 12-1 Skulls of a newborn, child, and adult illustrate skeletal changes during growth and development. **A,** Frontal view. **B,** Three quarter view. **C,** The newborn and child skulls have been enlarged to the same size as the adult skull to demonstrate the changes in proportion with growth. (From Bluestone CD and Stool SE, editors: Pediatric otolaryngology, Philadelphia, 1983, WB Saunders Co.)

the cranium is large relative to the face. The forehead is prominent, and as the frontal sinuses have not developed, the cranium is poorly protected (Fig. 12-1). The facial skeleton at this age is elastic and covered by a thick layer of adipose tissue, both factors providing protection. The nose in infancy and early childhood is mainly cartilaginous, and the nasal bones have not fused. Therefore at this stage, if the infant falls from a great distance or is struck by a heavy object, injury will more commonly be sustained by the skull, since it is larger, less protected, and less elastic than the facial skeleton.[7,9,10,18] McCoy et al.[15] pointed out that great force is required to produce facial fractures in small children, as evidenced by the fact that in children there is a higher incidence of serious associated injuries than in adults.

As the facial bones grow, the paranasal sinuses develop. This weakens much of the anterior facial skeleton but may protect the cranium by absorbing some of the energy of anterior blows. This also explains why midface fractures are so uncommon in younger children but increase as the paranasal sinuses enlarge and aerate.

In all patients the three areas of the facial skeleton that project are the nose, the mandible, and the maxilla. It is no surprise, then, that these are the areas most commonly fractured.

SPECIAL CONSIDERATIONS

In the child the facial skeleton is still growing and developing. This fact is the reason not only for rapid healing and extensive remodeling, but also for unpredictable long-term outcome as the result of damage to growth centers. In children, the rapid metabolic rate and high osteogenic potential of the periosteum means that fractures should undergo definitive diagnosis and treatment in the first 7 to 10 days. After that the fragments may be difficult, or impossible, to manipulate. Nonunion, or fibrous union, not uncommon in adults, is rare in children, also making late reduction of fractures inadvisable and unsatisfactory. If early reduction in adults is prevented by other injuries or severe underlying medical problems, revision surgery with osteotomies may be considered, especially for the nose and mandible. However, in children, because of the presence of growth centers and of developing dentition in the mandible, osteotomies are not usually considered an option until adolescence, when the child's facial skeleton has completed growth and reached its adult size.

Disturbance in growth patterns is very difficult to predict. The facial bones themselves grow individually but also in relation to each other. All periosteal surfaces are active in deposition, resorption, or both during growth and reparative processes. For this reason, maintenance of the periosteum is important when considering facial fracture treatment.

The studies of Enlow[4] showed that two processes account for postnatal facial growth: displacement and remodeling. In displacement the entire bone moves, whereas remodeling involves altering the bone itself through resorption and deposition. Re-

cently the concept of a "functional matrix" has developed. This theory suggests that bony displacement occurs as a result of growth of the soft tissues and that displacement triggers remodeling. According to this theory, sutural membranes and cartilage provide growth as bones are displaced, and separation occurs at articular surfaces.[12]

Previous to the functional matrix theory, displacement was thought to occur as a result of growth at certain "centers," especially in the mandibular condyle, nasal septum, and circumaxillary, pterygopalatine, and zygomaticotemporal sutures. However, it is now generally accepted that the condylar cartilage is not an independent growth site. Evidence now indicates that the condylar cartilage is the site of adaptive remodeling processes, and it is possible that this is true for septal cartilage as well.

Injury to the mandibular condyle is common in all age groups and has been extensively evaluated. Fractures of the condyle in the growing mandible may result in severe facial deformity and micrognathia and in functional problems in association with ankylosis of the temporomandibular joint. Studies of surgically created condylar fracture-dislocations in young rhesus monkeys revealed healing with a morphologically and functionally intact structure that was not affected by early mobilization.[3] Several clinical studies, including Kaban et al.,[10] Leake et al.,[11] and Gussack et al.[7] have shown that conservative management of condylar fractures results in normal function and mandibular growth. The condylar area is highly vascular in children and undergoes resorption and remodeling within 6 to 12 months. The physiologic pull and stress of the muscles of mastication are primarily responsible for this healing and realignment, with good results obtained both functionally and radiographically even with bilateral condylar fracture-dislocations.

Development of ankylosis appears to be one of the major factors in impaired mandibular growth and function. Crushing injuries to the condyle, with disruption of the blood supply, fragmentation of the articular surface, and extravasation of blood into the joint may cause considerable injury and eventual ankylosis. This type of injury seems especially damaging before the age of 2 to 2½ years, when the condyle is very vascular. The remodeling process is disrupted, and calcification or ossification of a hematoma in the joint could lead to ankylosis.

Obviously the effect of facial trauma on the growing facial skeleton is still controversial and difficult to predict. In any case, there appears to be marked dependence of each structure on the others, and conservative treatment involving minimal bone, cartilage, and soft tissue removal or mechanical "reshaping" (using osteotomies, for example) should be the rule.

DIAGNOSIS

Since maxillofacial trauma in children, especially with resultant fracture, is relatively uncommon, initial diagnosis must begin with a high index of suspicion. Photographs of the injury are important in treatment planning, in explaining the devastating nature of the injury and possible resultant facial deformity to the parents, and for documenting for medicolegal reasons. Because children have much facial fibro-adipose tissue, skeletal deformity may not initially be as obvious as in an adolescent or adult. As in all trauma patients, the immediate concern should be establishment of an adequate airway and the maintenance and replacement of intravascular volume.

Once the airway is established and the child is otherwise stable, careful physical examination of the head and neck area should be performed. Factors that should be evaluated include bony symmetry, subcutaneous emphysema, obvious bony mobility, ecchymosis, and areas of tenderness. Examination of the nose should include palpating the nasal bones and looking for mobility, crepitus, or telescoping of the bones into the ethmoid region or beneath the frontal bone. The nasal cavity should be inspected for septal deformity, septal hematoma, (indicated by marked widening of the septum), foreign objects, epistaxis and cerebrospinal fluid (CSF) leak. Fracture of the nasal bones is often associated with a "black eye" caused by venous stasis in the lower eyelid area.

The orbital area should be examined for symmetric extraocular mobility, diplopia, irregularity, tenderness, or crepitus to palpation along the bony orbital margins, and the presence of enophthalmos. The globe should be examined for gross vision, subconjunctival hemorrhage, (often found in trimalar ["tripod"] fractures), blood in the anterior chamber, presence of foreign bodies, and global disruption. Periorbital ecchymosis, especially bilateral (raccoon's eyes), is a sign of skull base fracture. An ophthalmologist should examine all patients with severe maxillofacial trauma and *any* other patient if there is suspicion of orbital injury, no matter how minor the facial trauma appears.

Examination of the maxilla includes palpation and visualization of the zygomatic arches for possible flattening and of the zygoma for depression or displacement. Hypesthesia in the area of the infraorbital nerve may indicate fracture of the zygoma or orbital rim or floor. Zygomatic arch fractures may also impinge on the coronoid process of the mandible, causing pain and limiting opening distance. Flattening of the malar eminence may be the result of soft tissue edema or maxillary fracture.

Examination of the oral cavity, maxilla, and mandible should include evaluation of opening and closing ability, determination of whether the mandible shifts consistently to one side, and inspection of how the patient's teeth fit together (occlusion), if teeth are present. Hypesthesia of the mental nerve may indicate a symphyseal fracture.[22] The mucosa of the oral cavity and the gums should be examined for lacerations and open fracture sites. The maxilla should be firmly grasped anteriorly and rocked in an anteroposterior and side-to-side fashion. Any movement may indicate a LeFort (midface) fracture. The alveolar ridges should be examined for fractures and the dentition carefully palpated. Particular attention should be paid to avulsed or fractured teeth, and avulsed teeth should be saved.

Although the temporal bone is not part of the facial skeleton, it should be examined along with the rest of the head and neck. The ear canal may sustain lacerations, fractures, or both as a result of posterior displacement of the mandible. A blow or fall strong enough to fracture the midface may also fracture the skull base. Skull base fractures may be manifested by CSF otorrhea, a perforated eardrum, hemotympanum or Battle's sign (posterior auricular ecchymosis over the mastoid caused by bleeding at a skull base fracture site). Skull base fractures may also be indicated by CSF leaking from the nose or eustachian tube (the patient may complain of a persistent or recurrent salty taste).

Physical examination of the child, especially in the setting of trauma when the child is frightened, in pain, in an altered mental state, in unfamiliar surroundings, and without family support, is difficult at best. Reexamination at frequent intervals, especially after resolution of edema, may be very helpful. Sedation, or even general anesthesia, may be required for complete evaluation or radiographic investigation. Teamwork at this point may be critical. If the child undergoes general anesthesia for any reason and is relatively stable, the otolaryngologist, dentist, oral surgeon, ophthalmologist, or plastic surgeon may be able to complete their physical examinations at that time. Photographs should be taken, both for documentation and later surgical planning. Splints for mandibular and maxillary stabilization can be made, and urgent repairs or reimplantation of dentition can be accomplished.

RADIOGRAPHIC EXAMINATION

In all cases radiographic evaluation of facial fractures should be obtained. Soft tissue swelling, lacrations, abrasions, pain, and altered mental states can interfere with clinical examination, making radiographic examination essential. These films are needed for definitive surgical management and provide documentation of injury for any later medicolegal disputes. They can also be used to discuss treatment strategy with the patient and family.

Plain facial radiographs can be very helpful. The standard views for facial trauma include (1) Water's view, (2) posteroanterior view, (3) lateral view, and (4) submentovertex view.[21] Water's view gives excellent delineation of the orbital rims, zygoma, and maxillary sinuses (Fig. 12-2); it also provides a good view of the nasal bones and septum and may help clarify orbital floor injury. An air-fluid level in the maxillary sinus, in the absence of a history of acute sinusitis, usually indicates a fracture of the maxilla with blood in the sinus and is frequently seen in trimalar fractures. The posteroanterior view is best for evaluation of the ethmoid and frontal sinuses, the frontonasoethmoid complex area, and the orbits.

The lateral view allows evaluation of the frontal sinuses, both for bony architecture and air-fluid levels. Fractures of the sphenoid sinus, hard palate, and pterygoid plates may also be seen with this view.[21]

The submentovertex view can be very helpful, but it is difficult to obtain in most children, and in patients with cervical spine injuries it is contraindicated. It is the best film for viewing zygomatic arch fractures, and skull base fractures are also often clearly seen. If there is subcutaneous emphysema of the head and neck, crepitus over the larynx, hoarseness, or stridor, a soft tissue lateral film of the neck should be obtained at the same time as the facial films. This provides for evaluation of the larynx, trachea, retropharyngeal space, and anterior cervical soft tissue.

Nasal fractures are best evaluated clinically, with

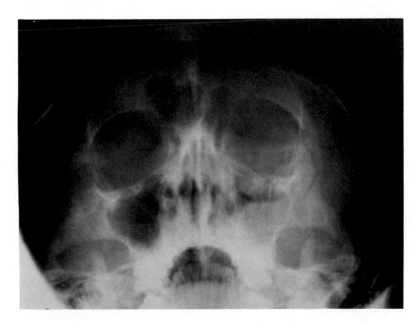

Fig. 12-2 Water's view. This film demonstrates a left zygomaticomaxillary complex fracture (trimalar fracture) in a 16-year-old oriental male. There is an air-fluid level in the left maxillary sinus, frequently seen with fractures involving the maxillary sinus walls.

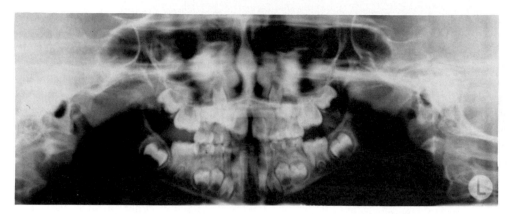

Fig. 12-3 Panorex (orthopantograph). The entire mandible is visualized, including the angles and condyles. The symphyseal area, however, is poorly defined, and intraoral and extraoral dental films and other mandibular views are often necessary to evaluate this area.

films used for confirmation. Since the nasal bones are not fused in young children and the nasal skeleton is primarily cartilaginous films are frequently not helpful. Views often obtained include the lateral nasal film, which can demonstrate the nasal bones and anterior nasal spine, and the superoinferior nasal bone film, which is helpful in evaluating lateral nasal bone displacement.

Fractures of the mandible can be especially difficult to see radiographically in children. The teeth, both deciduous and permanent, occupy most of the mandible in children. Furthermore, since the mandible is more elastic in children, it is predisposed to greenstick fracture, especially in the area of the condyle. In the young child the demarcation between medullary and cortical bone is not as clear, and fractures of the mandible in these children tend to be irregular, passing between or through the crypts of developing teeth.

The posteroanterior view shows the whole mandible, including the entire ramus and symphysis, the nasal spine, and the nasal septum. The modified Towne's view demonstrates the condyles well and is very useful for evaluating displacement of condylar fractures and incomplete or bending fractures of the condyle.[1] The anterior lateral oblique view shows the mandibular body from the canine to second molar. The posterior lateral oblique view shows the condylar head, neck, ascending ramus, and posterior molar region of the body.

For evaluating both the mandible and the teeth, a panoramic film (orthopantograph) is extremely helpful (Fig. 12-3). The entire mandible is seen on one film, with excellent views of the body,

angles, and condyles. The symphyseal area is not well seen, however, because of superimposition of the cervical vertebrae, and is best evaluated on an occlusal film of the mandible. Occlusal views of the maxilla are also useful to look for midline separation of the maxilla, alveolar fractures, and fractures involving the teeth of the upper jaw. For further dental evaluation, intraoral and extraoral dental films can reveal detail of fractured and avulsed teeth and greenstick fractures of the mandible (Fig. 12-4). Deciduous teeth that have sustained a blow along their long axis may be pushed up against a permanent tooth with deflection upward and outward through the thin labial plate, giving the impression of avulsion. These injuries may be diagnosed only on spot dental films.

Computed tomography (CT) is excellent for obtaining information about the sinus, orbit, maxilla,

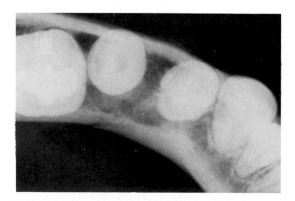

Fig. 12-4 Intraoral dental film showing a crack fracture of the inner table of the mandible.

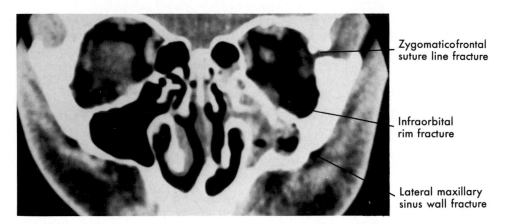

Fig. 12-5   This CT scan of a 16-year-old male reveals a trimalar fracture. The arrows point out the fractures of the infraorbital rim, lateral maxillary sinus wall, and zygomaticofrontal suture line.

skull base, and frontonasoethmoid complex. The relationship between soft tissue, bone, and possible foreign bodies can be assessed (Fig. 12-5).[5]

Because so many children with maxillofacial trauma have associated head trauma, a CT scan is often performed soon after the child arrives at the emergency room, especially if the mental status is altered. It may be possible to include CT of the facial skeleton at this time; if the patient is too unstable, then facial CT can be obtained at a later date. CT can provide information that is not evident on physical examination or plain films. Coronal images and the newer three-dimensional reconstructions can be extremely helpful in both the diagnosis and treatment of complex facial fractures, from both a functional and cosmetic point of view. The most recent CT equipment, using very thin (1.5 to 3 mm) slices, has been found to be superior to plain films for some types of fractures, especially at the skullbase and midface. The type of radiography ordered will obviously depend on the degree of injury and the overall clinical condition of the patient.

SPECIAL CONSIDERATIONS

Facial fractures obviously do not always occur in the same anatomic location but depend on the direction and force of the injury and the age of the patient. Fractures of the zygoma, mandible, and orbit require special care in their assessment.

In evaluating the zygoma it is necessary to realize that the zygoma essentially has four "feet": the lateral orbital wall, the orbital floor, the lateral wall of the maxillary antrum, and the zygomatic arch. Because of this four-footed arrangement, it is very difficult to fracture one foot without fracturing at least one of the others. The zygomatic arch is the most frequently fractured in isolation. A tripod, or trimalar, fracture consists of fractures of the zygomatic arch, infraorbital rim, and zygomaticofrontal suture line. These three fractures are connected by fractures across the anterior, lateral, and posterior walls of the maxillary antrum, the lateral floor of the orbit, and zygomaticosphenoid suture. The zygoma is mobile and displaced posteriorly and medially. When one of these fractures is detected or suspected, the others should be carefully sought, since fractures of the maxilla occur most commonly in this tripod arrangement.

Fractures of the mandible are also often multiple. The mandible itself is rigid and closely connected to the skull at each temporomandibular joint. When injured, therefore, it may behave as a complete ring and fracture in multiple places, especially in older children and adults. For example, symphyseal fractures are often associated with condylar fractures, and fractures of the angle with the opposite mandibular neck. Isolated condyle fractures are quite common in very young children but not in older children. The most common mandible fractures in most series in children are condylar fractures, followed by fractures of the body, angle, and symphysis.[9,17] In adults, fractures of the body are more common.[2] Careful physical examination and multiple radiographic views may be needed to diagnose all mandible fractures accurately.

Fractures of the midface, fortunately very uncommon in children, often require a high index of suspicion and very careful radiographic evaluation, especially CT. These fractures are defined as separation of some or all of the facial skeleton from the cranium and were classified by LeFort as I, II, or III. These can be unilateral or bilateral and mixed (LeFort I on the left and LeFort III on the right, for example). A LeFort I fracture (transverse) involves separation of the hard palate, lower portions of the pterygoid plate, and nasal septum from the rest of the facial and cranial skeleton. A LeFort II fracture (pyramidal) involves separation of the maxilla, including the palate, from the rest of the cranial and facial skeleton. A LeFort III fracture (craniofacial dysfunction) involves separation of the entire facial skeleton—maxilla, zygoma, and nasoethmoid complex—from the cranium.[14] Fractures frequently occur that cannot be fit into the LeFort classification.

Orbital fractures can be roughly classified into blowout and other fractures. The globe becomes compressed and then reexpands, blowing out medially into the ethmoid or inferiorly toward the maxillary antrum. The orbital rim is usually intact in blowout fractures. Entrapment of orbital fat or extraocular muscles may occur with enophthalmos and limitation of extraocular mobility. Fractures of the other orbital walls are less common than blowout fractures and are usually associated with other severe injury.

TREATMENT

Initially, stabilization of the child's airway and repletion of intravascular volume are essential. The airway above the larynx is maintained by the mandible, which supports the tongue and the maxilla (including the nose). Collapse or severe injury to any of these structures can lead to airway compromise. Fortunately, severe midface trauma with craniofacial dysfunction (LeFort III fracture) is rare in children, but nasal and mandibular fractures can cause marked and sudden airway compromise. Infants under the age of 6 weeks to 3 months are obligate nose breathers and may be unable to maintain an oral airway on their own if nasal obstruction occurs. In these children, especially if the mandible is intact, an artificial oral airway can be lifesaving. If the mandible is fractured in a child of any age, opening the mouth and pulling the tongue forward can markedly improve the airway. Placing the child in the prone position and suctioning blood and se-

cretions from the oral cavity can also be useful. If the facial bones are very comminuted, if there is a lot of bleeding, or if the larynx is edematous or fractured, endotracheal intubation may be inadvisable or impossible, and tracheotomy should be considered. In a recent series of 30 children with facial fractures reported by Gussack et al.,[7] intubation was required in five children (17%) and tracheotomy in two (7%). The two children requiring tracheotomy were 14 and 16 years of age and both had midface fractures.

Neurosurgical evaluation for head and cervical spine injury should also be performed as soon after injury as possible. Neurosurgical intervention, including stabilization of the cervical spine, should be accomplished before any extensive radiographic evaluation or repair of facial fractures. This is not only the safest course for the patient, but high quality radiographs can be obtained only in a relatively cooperative and nonmoving patient.

Nasal fractures are common in children, but if they are not adequately treated they can cause permanent deformity. Epistaxis or a CSF leak can usually be stopped by adequate reduction of the nasal fracture. A septal hematoma or abscess requires urgent incision and drainage to prevent cartilage destruction and a saddle-nose deformity. After incision and drainage, a drain can be left in the pocket between the cartilage and mucoperichondrium, or the nasal cavity can be tightly packed for several days. Each method is designed to prevent reaccumulation of blood and resultant infection and cartilage loss.

Reduction of nasal fractures, especially if being performed primarily for cosmetic reasons, should be performed when enough edema has resolved to allow objective evaluation. In young children, general anesthesia is required, but in adolescents sedation and local anesthesia are often adequate. If the fracture involves only the nasal bones, septum, or both, repositioning using gentle but firm external and internal pressure and manipulation is adequate. Resection of septal cartilage or bone should be very limited and only undertaken if an adequate airway cannot be achieved by manipulation alone. Nasal fractures heal rapidly in children. Even if the nasal or septal fracture or dislocation is properly treated at the time of injury, deformity may result. Grymer et al.[6] studied 57 children, ranging from newborns to those 16 years of age, with known nasal fractures. All patients had closed reduction under general anesthesia and were treated for associated complications. All were reevaluated after 16 years of age, when nasal development had been completed. They found several deformities, including deviations of the bony pyramid, a long nose, and hump and saddle deformities, in patients who had had a previous successful closed reduction, as compared with a control group without known nasal fractures. Therefore parents should be cautioned that the child with a nasal fracture may desire or need further revision when he or she reaches adolescence.

Nasoethmoid complex fractures, rare in children, involve telescoping of the nasal bones beneath or over the frontal bone and frequent telecanthus caused by avulsion of one or both medial canthal ligaments. This injury should be repaired with the child under general anesthesia because moderate force may be required for reduction. As this fracture is often associated with other midface fractures, a disimpaction forceps may be needed. If the medial canthal ligaments are avulsed, they should be reapproximated and wired to the nasal bones and the nasal bones stabilized with compression plates.

Injuries to the teeth, especially avulsion injuries, require urgent attention. An avulsed adult tooth, especially an anterior tooth that is not significantly carious, should be reimplanted. The outside limit for this is 48 hours, although the success rate drops dramatically after 2 hours.[20] Avulsed deciduous teeth should not usually be replaced. Consultation from a pediatric dentist should be obtained if injury to the teeth is suspected or documented.

Fractures of the mandible and maxilla usually involve malocclusion, and repair should always include restoring the child to preinjury occlusion if possible. Careful evaluation of the dentition is essential because the method of immobilization depends on the findings. Rowe[19] divided patients into the following four groups based on the state of the development of their dentition at the time of injury:

Age (Years)	Dental Development
Newborn-2	Before completion of eruption of deciduous dentition
2-4	Before the roots of the deciduous incisors show any significant degree of resorption
5-8	Before the roots of the deciduous molars are significantly resorbed or the roots of the permanent incisors are sufficiently developed
9-11	Before eruption of premolars but after eruption of the first permanent molar and final development of the roots of the permanent incisors

Factors that make fixation of the mandible or maxilla difficult include physiologic resorption of deciduous roots, carious teeth, developing teeth within the bone, and incomplete development of the roots of the permanent teeth.

With the above limitations in mind, treatment of mandible and maxillary fractures involves the same techniques as those used in adults. However, drill holes or pins should be used with extreme caution and avoided if possible to prevent injury to developing teeth.

Intermaxillary fixation (IMF) should also be used with caution because children tolerate it poorly, may not have adequate oral intake, and have an increased chance of aspiration if they vomit.

FRACTURES OF THE MANDIBLE

In newborns and children 2 years of age and under, it is usually not possible to use arch bars because of unerupted or partially erupted teeth. Ivy loops with interdental wiring can be considered (Fig. 12-6), but their use is difficult because of the poor retentive shape of deciduous teeth and varying resorption of the existing teeth. Therefore in this age group the use of a Gunning splint, as in the adult edentulous mandible, is advised. After manual reduction of the fracture, the prefabricated acrylic splint, lined with gutta percha, is pressed down over the mandibular dentition and alveolus and held in place with circummandibular wires. If the fracture is within the tooth-bearing area of the mandible, fixation to the maxilla is not needed. If the fracture is proximal to the tooth-bearing area at the mandibular angle, then fixation to the maxilla

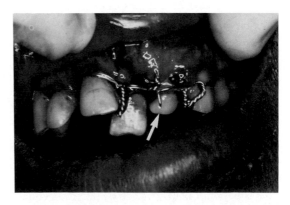

Fig. 12-6 Ivy loops are used here to secure an avulsed tooth *(arrow)* to surrounding intact teeth.

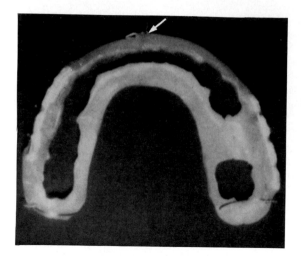

Fig. 12-7 This labiolingual splint fits around existing dentition. It can be opened anteriorly (*arrow*) for application and then fastened closed.

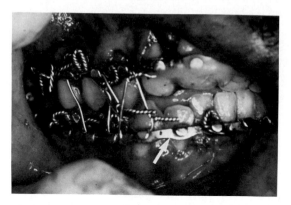

Fig. 12-8 ERICH arch bars (*arrow*) are wired to the remaining maxillary and mandibular teeth. They provide lugs for intermaxillary fixation with wire or rubber bands.

is necessary. The Gunning splint is then modified to allow occlusion with the maxillary molars or alveolus. The mandibular splint can be wired directly to the maxilla via piriform aperture wires or can be affixed to a similar maxillary splint. Generally, 3 to 4 weeks is enough time to allow union. Open reduction and internal fixation should usually be considered if the facilities to make splints are not available. In this case, intermaxillary fixation is obtained via circumandibular and piriform aperture wires.

In the 2- to 4-year age group, interdental wiring with ivy loops may be possible. Labiolingual acrylic splints, made from molds of the child's dentition, can be used, again with circumandibular wiring. (Fig. 12-7). Arch bars (either ERICH or Jelenco) may also be used, especially to bridge a gap left by a deciduous tooth or a tooth lost through trauma.

In children 5 to 8 years of age, the anterior incisors are of little use, either because the deciduous roots are resorbed or the permanent teeth have incompletely formed roots. The deciduous molars can be used, but they may be carious or prematurely extruded. Also the pattern of tooth loss may be such that there are no maxillary teeth for the mandibular teeth to occlude with, or the other way around. Splint construction and usage are crucial in this situation. Fixation can be by circumferential mandibular wires, piriform aperture wires, pernasal wires, or circumzygomatic wires. Circumzy-

gomatic wires should be used with caution, however, as the zygomatic arch at this point is soft and immature, and sawing of the wires may cut through the bone.

In the 9- to 11-year age group, arch bars (Fig. 12-8) can be safely used because the roots of the incisors and first molars have matured. By this age, open reduction and internal fixation using wires or plates can also be considered.[9]

Some mandibular fractures do not require fixation. Undisplaced crack fractures of the angle or body may be treated without immobilization. Condyle fractures, very common in children, are a special case, as ankylosis with limited opening ability and mandibular deformity may result. With unilateral or bilateral condyle fractures or fracture-dislocations, if there is no occlusal abnormality, treatment with soft diet and muscle-training exercises is usually effective. However, if the occlusion is deranged, or there is posterior displacement with an anterior open bite, fixation in centric relationship (the child's normal occlusion) for 2 to 3 weeks may be needed, followed by active encouragement of movement to prevent ankylosis.

FRACTURES OF THE MAXILLA

If the fracture(s) are nondisplaced and the occlusion is stable and reproducible, no active treatment is needed. However, severe functional or cosmetic impairment requires intervention. In treat-

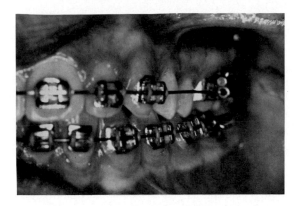

Fig. 12-9   Orthodontic bands can be used to stabilize loose or avulsed teeth.

ment of fractures of both the mandible and the maxilla, it is frequently desirable to fix the fractured and mobile segment to an immobile site. Intermaxillary fixation (IMF) via splints, arch bars, orthodontic bands (Fig. 12-9), or ivy loops will accomplish this. With the maxilla it is usually necessary to fix the fragment to an immobile point above the level of the fracture site after the mandible and maxilla are in IMF. A low-level LeFort I type fracture may be secured by piriform aperture or zygomatic arch wiring; a LeFort II by wiring around the zygomatic arch or zygomatic process

of the frontal bone; and a LeFort III by wiring to the zygomatic process of the frontal bone.

Several external devices have been used for fixation of maxillary fractures. These include a craniomandibular box frame, halo frames (Fig. 12-10), and headcaps with attachment to the maxilla. The disadvantages of most of these is that they are external devices that require fixation to the cranium, which is not possible until the cranium is fairly thick and can support the screws without loosening, about age 10. Headcaps may slip down over the brow, because of the lack of development of the frontal sinuses and supraorbital ridge. External devices are also prone to interference by the small and inquisitive child. The newer methods of open reduction and fixation with metal plates are applicable in older children and adults.

Alveolar ridge fractures can occur in either the mandible or maxilla. The fractured alveolus, along with several teeth, can become impacted or displaced. Fixation can be accomplished by either arch bars or acrylic cap splints (Fig. 12-11). If dentition is missing as a result of trauma or normal shedding, the space between teeth can be maintained by Jelenco bars (Fig. 12-12).

ORBITAL FRACTURES

Blowout fractures, if accompanied by enophthalmos, diplopia, or both, should be treated. In children older than 11 years of age, antral packing, with replacement of orbital contents, is effective.

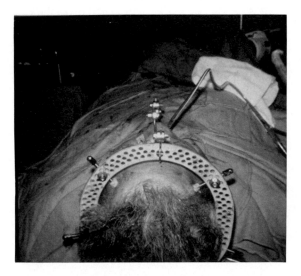

Fig. 12-10   This halo device is fixed to the skull with screws and can provide support for repair of a severe midface fracture. External fixation devices are used when there are no intact points on the body facial skeleton on which the fractured segments can be stabilized.

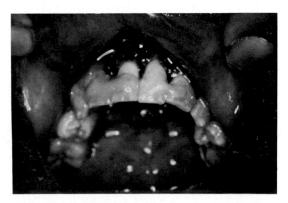

Fig. 12-11   Cap splints (the one shown here is acrylic) are used to stabilize an alveolar rim fragment with teeth. The teeth in the fractured segment are glued to the surrounding intact teeth, holding the fractured alveolus in correct position.

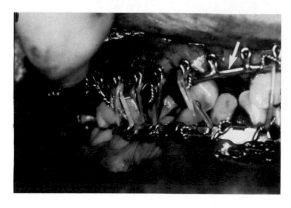

Fig. 12-12 Jelenco arch bars *(arrow)* are used to bridge a gap left by a missing tooth. In this photo, Jelenco bars are used on the maxillary teeth and ERICH arch bars on the mandibular teeth.

In the younger child with a small maxillary antrum and developing tooth roots, direct exploration of the orbital floor is indicated. Comminuted fragments should be preserved if possible, and reconstruction of the floor with Silastic, bone, cartilage, or Gelfilm undertaken.

Fractures of the zygoma can be approached as in the adult. This usually requires open reduction of the orbital rim, zygomatic arch, and zygomaticofrontal suture line fractures. Isolated zygomatic arch fractures can be reduced via an intraoral approach and elevated with a periosteal or other elevator. Reduction via a Gilles incision is also effective. Rarely, open reduction with wire fixation is needed.

COMPLICATIONS OF SURGICAL TREATMENT

Because of the excellent blood supply to the facial region and the excellent remodeling and adaptive ability of the growing bony skeleton, nonunion or malunion is very rare in children. Nonunion may occur because of infection at the fracture site, although infection in the child is also uncommon. In the study by Gussack et al,[7] no infections or malunion were noted in 30 pediatric patients. There were two patients with residual deformity and one with malocclusion and residual deformity combined. Malunion and deformity may result from late or inadequate reduction of the fractures, either because of late identification of injury or

other severe medical problems precluding early intervention.

As previously noted, ankylosis and altered growth may result from mandibular condyle fractures. Nasal fractures may result in bony nasal bridge deformities, septal deviations, and saddle-nose deformity.[6]

SUMMARY

Trauma to the face in children is very common, usually resulting in soft tissue injury. Maxillofacial trauma with resultant facial fractures is fortunately much less common. Diagnosis can be difficult because of the child's age, ability to cooperate, and high incidence of associated injuries. The osteogenic potential in children is high, and fractures heal rapidly and completely over 2 to 3 weeks. For optimal functional and cosmetic results, repair should be undertaken within 3 to 4 days if possible. After 7 to 10 days, healing may have occurred and osteotomies may be needed, causing possible injury to the growing facial skeleton. Conservative management in children should be the rule, with radical reconstruction reserved for residual functional or cosmetic deformity.

REFERENCES

1. Ahrendt D et al: Incomplete (bending?) fractures of the mandibular condyle in children, Pediatr Radiol 14:140, 1984.
2. Bochlogyros PN: A restrospective study of 1521 mandibular fractures, J Oral Maxillofac Surg 43:597, 1985.
3. Boyle PJ: Osseous repair and mandibular growth after subcondylar fractures, J Oral Surg 25:300, 1967.
4. Enlow DH: Handbook of facial growth, Philadelphia, 1975, WB Saunders.
5. Finkle DR et al: Comparison of the diagnostic methods used in maxillofacial trauma, Plast Reconstr Surg 75:32, 1985.
6. Grymer LF, Gutuierrez C, and Stoksted P: Nasal fractures in children: influence on the development of the nose, J Laryngol Otol 99:735, 1985.
7. Gussack GS et al: Pediatric maxillofacial trauma: unique features in diagnosis and treatment, Laryngoscope 97:925, 1987.
8. Hall RK: Injuries of the face and jaws in children, Int J Oral Surg 1:65, 1972.
9. James D: Maxillofacial injuries in children. In Rowe NL and Williams JL, editors: Maxillofacial injuries, New York, 1985, Churchill Livingston.
10. Kaban LB, Mulliken JB, and Murray JE: Facial fractures in children, Plast Reconstr Surg 59:15, 1977.
11. Leake et al: Long-term follow-up of fractures of the mandibular condyle in children, Plast Reconstr Surg 47:127, 1971.

12. Maisel H: Postnatal growth and anatomy of the face. In Mathog RH, editor: Maxillofacial trauma, Baltimore, 1984, Williams & Wilkins.

13. Maniglia AJ and Kline SN: Maxillofacial trauma in the pediatric age group, Otol Clin North Am 16:717, 1983.

14. Marlowe FI: Injuries of the nose, facial bones, and paranasal sinuses. In Bluestone CD and Stool SE, editors: Pediatric otolaryngology, Philadelphia, 1983, WB Saunders.

15. McCoy FJ, Chandler RA, and Crow ML: Facial fractures in children, Plast Reconstr Surg 37:209, 1966.

16. Morgan BDG, Madan DK, and Bergerot JPC: Fractures of the middle third of the face—a review of 300 cases, Br J Plast Surg 25:147, 1972.

17. Morgan WC: Pediatric mandibular fractures, Oral Surg 40:320, 1975.

18. Rowe NL: Fractures of the facial skeleton in children, J Oral Surg 26:505, 1968.

19. Rowe NL: Fractures of the jaws in children, J Oral Surg 27:497, 1969.

20. Sowray JH: Localized injuries of the teeth and alveolar process. In Rowe NL and Williams JL, editors: Maxillofacial injuries, New York 1985, Churchill Livingston.

21. Trapnell DH and Wake MJC: Diagnostic radiography. In Rowe NL and Williams JL, editors: Maxillofacial injury, New York, 1985, Churchill Livingston.

22. Wolford DG and Mathog RH: Development of teeth and fracture of the jaws in children. In Mathog RH, editor: Maxillofacial trauma, Baltimore, 1984, Williams & Wilkins.

23. Worlock P, Stower M, and Barbor P: Patterns of fractures in accidental and nonaccidental injury in children: a comparative study, Br Med J 293:100, 1988.

13

Central Nervous System

HEAD INJURY

Charles C. Duncan and Laura R. Ment

Traumatic brain injury in the young, an important issue from both professional and personal perspectives, has been the topic of many reports. Head injury represents the leading cause of death in children older than 1 year of age and is also the primary cause of mortality and long-term neurodevelopmental morbidity in this patient population.[23,36] In infants less than 1 year of age head injury is the third leading cause of death. Although there have been extensive scientific investigations of head injury in adults and in mature animal models,[17,24,74] little is know about the effects of head trauma on the developing brain.[1,25,70] Notable exceptions include increasingly sophisticated management and outcome studies with detailed neurodevelopmental testing and diagnostic imaging, the hypothesis of Bruce et al.[8-10] of cerebral hyperemia, recognition of the particular occurrence of transient cortical blindness,[27] mechanisms of injury studies,[55,65] and epidemiologic investigations.[5,11,36,52,64] Many of these and other investigations suggest that traumatic injury to the developing brain has basic mechanisms that differ from those of the mature brain.[6,8-10,12,27]

Similarly the ability of the developing brain to recover from injury may also significantly differ from that of the mature brain. Compensatory mechanisms in the developing brain appear quite different than those in the mature brain (for example, in cerebral dominance, with the well-known shift of hemisphere that occurs following damage or destruction of speech areas and the accompanying reduction in intellectual performance).[41] Other less well-recognized processes of recovery are poorly understood with long periods of improved function.[67]

EPIDEMIOLOGY

Although a precise epidemiology of head injury has not been possible, successive approximations have been made over the past 15 years beginning with the most recent studies, which estimate a range of 0.2% to 0.3% per year. The most recent age incidence is thought to be 150 per 100,000 for newborns to children 4 years of age, increasing to 550 per 100,000 for children 15 to 24 years of age, gradually decreasing for those 50 years of age and older, and then increasing with age.[23,37,64,65]

In all age groups, males have twice the incidence of head injury and also appear to have four times the risk of suffering fatal head injuries. Across the age groups approximately two thirds of deaths occur before hospitalization. A number of studies have shown a steadily increasing incidence of head injury in males 5 to 25 years of age, whereas the incidence in females decreases across the first 15 years of life, which has suggested to Frankowski et al.[23] that not only does the risk of injury differ between genders but also the types of injuries differ.

Although agreement on definitions of injury in adult populations has largely followed the suggestions of Teadsdale and Jennett[76] with the Glasgow Coma Scale (GCS) (see left box on p. 223) and Glasgow Outcome Score, there are well-recognized limitations of the former and problems in useful analysis with the latter. Similar problems hold concerning the application of these instruments to children, and they become exceedingly difficult to apply to the very young. As a consequence, surrogates for the scale have been used, which include best guesses of a response in the intubated patient and other scales, such as the Neonatal Arousal

```
        GLASGOW COMA SCALE

Eye opening
  Spontaneous                    E4
  To speech                       3
  To pain                         2
  Nil                             1

Best motor response
  Obeys                          M6
  Localizes                       5
  Withdraws                       4
  Abnormal flexion                3
  Exterior posture                2
  Nil                             1

Verbal response
  Orientated                     V5
  Confused conversation           4
  Inappropriate words             3
  Incomprehensible sounds         2
  Nil                             1

  Coma score (E + M + V) = 3 to 15
```

From Teasdale G and Jennett B: Lancet 2:81, 1974.

```
         NEONATAL AROUSAL SCALE

Best response to bell
  Facial and extremity movements        5
  Grimaces/blinks                        4
  Increases in respiratory and heart     3
    rates
  Seizure/extensor posturing             2
  No response                            1

Best response to light
  Blink and facial and extremity         4
    movements
  Blink                                  3
  Seizure/extensor posturing             2
  No response                            1

Best motor response
  Spontaneous
    Periods of activity alternating      6
      with sleep
    Occasional spontaneous move-         5
      ments
  Sternal rub
    Extremity                            4
    Grimaces/facial movements            3
    Seizures/extensor posturing          2
    No response                          1

Total                                  3-15
```

From Duncan CC et al: Child's Brain 8:299, 1981.

Scale (see box above, right) which attempt to categorize patients similarly.[19] Outcome has been increasingly measured by the scores of sophisticated neuropsychologic evaluations. The approaches of Walker and co-workers[78,79] have addressed the multiple-injury patient with models such as the Modified Injury Severity Scale (MISS) and the Abbreviated Injury Scale (AIS).

The lack of linearity of one score to the next is well recognized as well as is the skew toward lower scores with dominant hemisphere processes. Furthermore, the absence of classical pupillary and respiratory signs is notable, but the GCS has provided a consistently reliable means for broadly categorizing minor, moderate, and severe head injuries, on which the most current management and investigation are based.[52]

CAUSES OF INJURY

The causes of head injury in the young vary widely across age groups, environments, and time periods. Three major groups of vectors for head injury have been formulated based on general mechanisms and the means for data collection and

reporting: abuse, nonmotor vehicle related, and motor vehicle related.[44]

In 1984 1,727,000 cases of child abuse were reported in the United States and in 1985 2.2 million; the substantiation rate in both instances was just below 50%. In 1984 there were 260,871 cases with known types of maltreatment. Of these 0.52% were head injuries. Connecticut recorded 12,186 reports of child abuse in 1980 and 16,804 in 1985, for an incidence of 22.23 per 1000.[4] Fatalities are reported in these data only if the cases are known to local departments of Child and Youth Services; consequently, national and statewide fatality information misses most early inhospital and essentially all out of hospital deaths, since these are reported to law enforcement agencies or are classified as accidental. In 1984 500 deaths from abuse were reported from 23 states. In 1985 223 deaths were reported from five states, although this num-

Table 13-1   1986 Nonvehicular-related accidents*

Age group	Head injury	Overall accidents	Male/female
Newborn-4	335,374	1,516,667	1.46
5-14	252,856	2,362,670	1.79
15-25	114,789	2,317,247	2.12

*Reported to National Electronic Injury Surveillance System.

ber increased to 279 following a telephone survey of the individual states.[4,28,49,85]

The US Consumer Product Safety Commission maintains the National Electronic Injury Surveillance System (NEISS) to track product-related injuries; this serves as a surrogate for nonvehicular-related injuries and also excludes child abuse. The data are based on total population events from a sample of 130 hospital emergency rooms in the US and its territories. The first report of this data was set from 1978, and serial reports have been produced since that time. The most recent data set is from 1986 and contains 9,827,453 injuries with almost two thirds of these occurring in individuals younger than 25 years of age. The data are divided by age as follows: newborn to 4 years, 4 to 14 years, and 15 to 24 years. Table 13-1 describes the

---

CT INDICATIONS IN PEDIATRIC HEAD INJURY

1. Depressed level of consciousness at the time of arrival in the emergency room
2. Focal neurologic signs
3. Penetrating injury or otherwise detectable depression of skull
4. History of progressive headache
5. Unreliable history of injury
6. Special consideration for children less than 2 years of age
7. Signs of basilar skull fracture including hemotympanum, nasal CSF, raccoon eyes, and Battle's sign
8. Serious multiple trauma with evidence of head injury

Note: One continued definite indication for skull films is suspected child abuse.

---

occurrence of injuries and head injuries in particular in these age groups. The gender distribution reflects the total age group.[55,65]

The 1964 report by Hendrick et al.[29] of 4465 consecutive cases of head injuries in children 15 years of age or younger who were admitted to the Hospital for Sick Children revealed that almost two

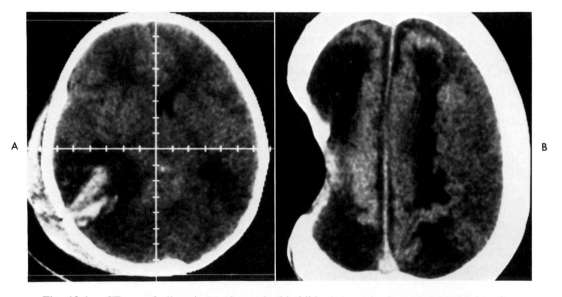

Fig. 13-1   CT scan findings in an 18-month-old child who sustained a severe head injury from a three-story fall out of an open window. **A,** Scan obtained on admission to hospital shows large cerebral contusion. Craniectomy was carried out to remove contusion of parietal lobe and lacerated, herniated temporal lobe. **B,** Scan 3 months later. The child had persistent coma. This scan demonstrates widespread loss of cerebral parenchyma.

thirds of the injuries were caused by nonmotor vehicle accidents, and 53% were the result of falls.[16] This series predated the GCS and CT scanner. As much as 65% of the children had a loss of consciousness and 37% had a period of coma. Fig. 13-1 illustrates the CT scan findings in an 18-month-old child who sustained a severe head injury after a three-story fall out of an open window. The Olmsted County study related 55% of head injuries in children to falls, whereas 78% of head injuries in the newborn to 4 year age group were caused by falls. Others have reported that 80% of head injuries in children less than 2 years of age were caused by falls. Violence has varied between studies, with Olmsted County having 1% violent head injury, compared with 10% in Bronx, New York.[5,36,37,69,70]

Motor vehicle–related accidents constituted 25% of the series by Hendrick[29] but accounted for 92% of severe head injury in children in the 1987 study by Alberico and co-workers.[1] Representative population-based studies have reported that motor vehicle–related accidents accounted for 18% of head injuries in Bronx, 24% in Olmsted County, and 24% in San Diego County.[5,36,37,69,70] Studies by Rimel et al.[62,63] of moderate and minor head injury do not separate the young by cause but show that

motor vehicle–related accidents caused 66% of moderate head injuries and 46% of minor head injuries. The San Diego County study of children less than 15 years of age found 88% minor head injury, 7% moderate head injury, and 5% severe head injury from all causes. In distinction from nonvehicular-related injuries with a 10% hospital admission rate from NEISS data,[55,65] the San Diego County study definitions required hospital admission or death for inclusion. The overall crude death rate in the United States for 1986 was 870.8 per 100,000; the rate of deaths resulting from accidents was 39.7 per 100,000, with 20.1% resulting from a motor vehicle–related accident and 19.6% from another cause. Deaths from motor vehicle accidents increased 5% from 1985 to 1986.[82] The Fatal Accident Reporting System considers one third of the deaths due to injuries to be related to motor vehicles. There was no mortality from motor vehicle accidents involving small children in Tennessee during the first year in which a law required restraints for all passengers less than 5 years of age. This provides a clear indication that the incidence of such injuries could be reduced. Fig. 13-2 shows the CT finding of a posterior fossa epidural hematoma in a 5-year-old child who was an unrestrained passenger in a motor vehicle accident.

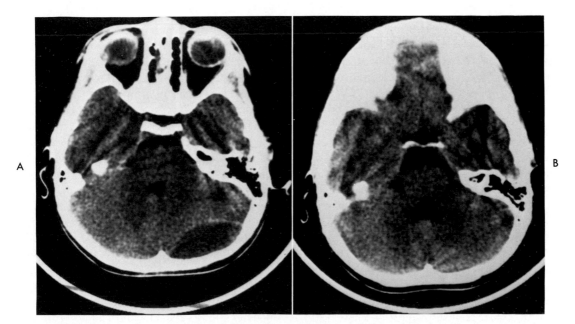

Fig. 13-2 **A,** CT finding of a posterior fossa epidural hematoma in a 5-year-old girl, who was an unrestrained passenger in a motor vehicle accident. She had a transient loss of consciousness then steady improvement. **B,** Scan 8 weeks later without any intervention. She has fully recovered.

Thus head injury represents an important cause of morbidity and mortality in the general population, with clear data that the young are vulnerable to particular types of injury. This includes maltreatment and falls in younger children to high rates of motor vehicle accidents in teenagers. Furthermore, as increasing numbers of head-injured children are followed in detail, increasing evidence shows that preexisting behavioral and cognitive factors play a role in the cause of some head injuries in children.[7,13,67] An obvious example of this is the relationship between alcohol and motor vehicle accidents, although other examples are difficult to ascertain, as noted by Rutter[67] and the pilot study of the National Traumatic Coma Data Bank.[3,7,13,20,52] Data from populations engaged in wars and other conflicts are difficult to obtain and not well reported, but such strife must account for vast numbers of childhood injuries and deaths in those regions.

MANIFESTATIONS OF INJURY

In addition to the differences in epidemiology and causes of head injury in the young there appear to be several differences in manifestations, including acute focal edema of the brain[73] cerebral hyperemia[8-10] impact seizures, cortical blindness, vascular headaches, brain stem preservation, the pressure volume index, and growing fractures.

Perhaps described as early as the end of the last century, acute, flash, or malignant edema following head injury in the young has been well recognized as a clinical entity.[8,81] Bruce has hypothesized that these result because of an acute increase in cerebral blood volume and has therefore renamed the process "cerebral hyperemia" in keeping with these observations.[8-10,73] Such processes have been estimated to occur in between 50% and 5% of head-injured children who are admitted to the hospital and to account for much of the variability in survival between various studies. Bruce's[9] 1979 report was supported by CT scans showing white matter attenuation increasing greater than expected and (in 1981) by limited cerebral blood flow data. The third support for this hypothesis was the dramatic improvement with hyperventilation in this group of patients. Snoek et al.[73] confirmed these observations with similar clinical pictures of head-injured children but considered scanner resolution and characteristics for reliable Houndsfield measurements to have limited reliability. Furthermore cerebral blood volume measurements have not confirmed these proposals. Hence whether such brain swelling is the case of clinical deterioration or a concomitant finding is not resolved. Severe sudden clinical deterioration at an interval following head injury does appear to exist and to occur much too frequently. Diffuse swelling has been noted in 29% of head-injured children, with 41% in severe head injuries and 15% in minor and moderate injuries.

In 1984 Obrist et al.[56] conducted cerebral blood flow studies using intravenous [133]xenon in 74 adults and considered 55% hyperemic, which correlated with raised intracranial pressure, and placed these findings into the general concepts of "vasomotor paralysis." Approximately 37% of that group had relative ischemia. The relationship of hyperemia in the adult to a clinical condition could not be made and remains unknown. Cerebral blood volume was not measured or inferred in this series of 74 patients, as in the original observations by Bruce, and a similar clinical picture has not been observed in adults. Perhaps the general concept of vasomotor paralysis that exposes the cerebrovasculature more directly to the systemic circulation with dramatic posttraumatic hypertension is more consistent with these observations and the changes in autoregulation.[34,54,56]

Transient blindness following head injury in the young has been noted for over 40 years, with Sutter and Essen-Moller giving the earliest reports.[27] This syndrome of transient cortical blindness ordinarily resolves in minutes to hours without sequelae. Its incidence is not known, with small series having been reported in the literature. Most current studies of head injury make no mention of this occurrence. Various mechanisms have been postulated including acute focal edema, vasospasm, or an electrical event, such as the spreading depression of Leao.[50]

The recent review of Haas and Lourie[27] relates a number of complex temporary alterations of brain function following minor head injury to migraine; they called these episodes trauma-triggered migraine. These authors argue that cortical blindness, altered level of consciousness, focal cortical deficits, and transient incoordination all represent various manifestations of trauma-triggered migraine. Impact seizures are considered to be part of the same process and similar if not identical to spreading depression. Patients with trauma-triggered migraine fall into a different spectrum of injury than the comatose child; the former have sustained minor head injury. Propanolol has been beneficial when tried, and calcium channel blockers might be of theorectic benefit if a vascular hypothesis holds.*

In severe traumatic and nontraumatic brain injury in the infant, brain stem preservation has frequently been found. In general, such patients may have patterned motor activity and adequate respirations and cranial nerve functions with concomitant electrical silence on the EEG and CT scans, which show dissolution of the cerebral hemispheres but preservation of diencephalon. Less severe manifestations have shown subtotal hemispheric loss. Preservation of brain stem or diencephalic blood flow appears to have occurred in these instances.†

Shapiro[69-71] has noted that children with head trauma have a less favorable pressure volume index (PVI) than adults. Furthermore, he has correlated this finding with steeper slopes with progressively

younger ages, explaining this on the basis of a shorter spine and a concomitant lower thecal space. This appears to run counter to the expected extra buffering capacity of a fontanel and cranial vault that easily separates at the sutures. One hypothesis is that the rapidity of events in head injury prevent these mechanisms, which are classically thought to provide accommodation for the infant, from benefiting in this setting. Alternatively, the limited range of CSF absorptive capacities of the young along with greater changes in CBF and possibly CBV account for these changes. Marmarou[45] attributed approximately one third of intracranial pressure (ICP) changes in a series of severely head-injured patients to CSF outflow resistance and two thirds to vascular factors.

The other difference in mechanical manifestation of head injury in the very young is the growing fracture or leptomeningeal cyst. Presumably, a wider separation of the fractured bone edges occurs in small children than in older individuals, with a

---

*References 15, 20, 25, 27, 31, 40, 53, 62.
†References 1, 8, 12, 24, 31, 43.

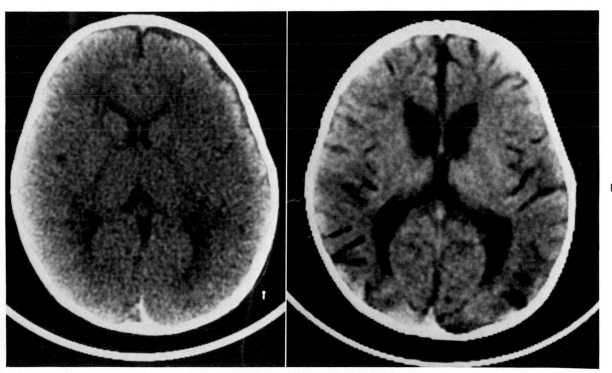

B

Fig. 13-3   CT findings in an infant who suffered a subdural hematoma from abuse and developed hydrocephalus requiring shunt. **A,** Scan obtained on admission. The child had a bulging fontanelle and an altered level of consciousness. The subdural hematoma resolved with serial subdural taps, but then the child developed dilated ventricles (**B**). Lumbar puncture pressure was persistently elevated. The infant was shunted and made an excellent recovery with normal neurodevelopmental testing in follow-up.

resulting dural tear and arachnoidal/CSF herniation. In Ito and co-worker's[34] series, the oldest patient was 2 years old, and Matson's[46] observations were primarily in children less than 3 years old, although he had observed this entity in children 6 years of age.[84]

Finally, hydrocephalus appears to occur more often following head injury in the young than in older populations because of limited absorptive capabilities. Cardoso[10a] considered trauma to be the etiology of hydrocephalus in 5% of their shunted population. Beyerl[6a] noted the incidence of ventriculomegaly to vary between 29% to 72%, depending on the severity of injury, with high pressures being observed in about half. Fig. 13-3 demonstrates the CT findings in an infant with subdural hematoma who developed hydrocephalus requiring shunt. The converse of head injury in the individual with hydrocephalus is well known for severe manifestations with minimal force.[32,42,69]

MECHANISMS OF INJURY

Head injury quite clearly has a broad range of mechanisms ranging from essential differences in cause and severity to the response of the tissue from the primary insult, which has been broadly termed secondary injury.[15,70] Penetrating head injury with direct tissue disruption, mass lesions, and differing magnitudes of generalized force to the brain appear to result in quite different processes in the brain and in differing outcomes.* As a consequence of insult, brain structure and function alter, leading to further events that may increase damage.[15] Alterations in cerebral blood flow (CBF), metabolism, electrical activity, and CSF flow have been critically followed in patients and animal model systems.[45,51] Anatomic alterations have been discerned from diagnostic imaging with computerized tomography and magnetic resonance imaging and pathologically from the light to electron microscopic level. Most recently, detailed analysis of transmitter activity following injury to the brain has become possible, particularly with the availability of magnetic resonance spectroscopy as well as anatomic and physiologic methods for inferences of the blood-brain barrier and axonal and synaptic function.†

The target in brain injury would seem to be identical, whether the injury is from kinetic force, altered circulation, hypoxia, or intracranial mass.[15,72] Particular mechanisms of injury may have unique features, such as tissue disruption in a specific area (for example, a mass lesion), and have variable surrounding tissue response (for example, abscess versus hematoma), but the basic underlying actions of the brain would appear to be limited.[1,9,58]

Despite the early return of CBF, metabolism, and electrical activity with injury to the brain, normal function is not concomitant. Additional parameters must still be disrupted or altered. Anatomically, axons appear to be more vulnerable to kinetic injury than the cortex, but detailed synaptic morphology has been difficult to ascertain.* Changes in the microvasculature from both morphologic and chemical perspectives are poorly understood. Furthermore, the role of neurotransmitters has only recently been approached. Hypotheses regarding their role have extended for many years in conjunction with the autolysis proposal in spinal cord injury.[33,83] Advances in magnetic resonance spectroscopy permit detailed measurement of neurotransmitters as well as high-energy cerebral compounds in samples of brain.[38,59]

The interaction of these events is not clear. Ischemia-induced alterations in calcium homeostasis are believed to be responsible for the initiation of a cascade of events leading to irreversible neuronal damage. These and other insults are known to result in cerebral metabolic disturbances characterized by a decreased concentration of high-energy phosphate compounds.[18,72] Cerebral blood flow falls, adenosine, a putative cerebral smooth muscle relaxant, is released, and secondary failure of the ionic pump results in neuronal depolarization and calcium entry.[61,83] This imbalance in calcium provokes the accumulation of free fatty acids, which in turn uncouple oxidative metabolism and produce additional permeability changes as well as stimulating the release of excitotoxic neurotransmitters.[21,22,33,66]

Since it has now been established that the regional selective nerve cell loss after an ischemic insult is not caused by a lack of local reflow,[39,60,75] the search for biochemical factors common to the most vulnerable areas has intensified. In experimental animals and in man certain neuronal groups

---

*References 1, 9, 14, 16, 26, 40, 41.
†References 6, 47, 48, 56-61, 66, 68, 83.

*References 15, 58, 66, 74, 75, 77, 83.

in the hippocampus, basal ganglia, and cerebral cortex have been known to be especially sensitive to insult. In adult animals this pattern coincides with the occurrence of regions with a high density of aspartate and glutamate binding sites.[47,48] In addition, glutamate and the glutamate analogs kainic acid and ibotenic acid are potent convulsants and neurotoxic agents that destroy neurons. Rothman[66] has demonstrated that fetal neurons placed in culture are much less sensitive to exposure to an anoxic atmosphere but become highly vulnerable after 2 weeks in culture. At 2 weeks the cultures had developed extensive synaptic contact and had shown spontaneous spike activity. Blockage of glutamate receptors with agents such as gamma-D-glutamyl glycine blocked the neuronal degeneration induced by anoxia. Addition to the culture medium of glutamate or aspartate for 1 hour led to neuronal degeneration similar to that induced by anoxia; this toxicity was also blocked by gamma-D-glutamyl glycine. These data appear to indicate that the effect of glutamate and aspartate is probably via receptor sites. Similarly, antagonists of the N-methyl-D-aspartate receptor are known to be potent anticonvulsants, and recently Stahl[68] has examined the effectiveness of peripherally administered MK-801 to protect against neuronal degeneration produced by complete forebrain ischemia in gerbils. Not only did pretreatment with this agent completely prevent neuronal change, but also MK-801 possessed posttreatment protective effects. Finally, both Benveniste et al.[6] and Johnson and Silverstein[33] have utilized intracerebral microdialysis to demonstate elevations of glutamate and aspartate in adult and neonatal animals, respectively, exposed to models for transient cerebral ischemia.

Such hypotheses stress the importance of transmitters and complex interactive roles between local calcium and cellular function for the understanding of brain injury. The immature brain has a particular vulnerability to hemorrhage in the first few days after birth when premature. Rapid and apparently vascular-based changes take place in the child following injury. A variety of seizure and migraine-like phenomena take place in the young. Recovery can include shifts of speech and prolonged improvement. The basis of these obvious differences may provide insight into the mechanisms of brain injury and subsequent function along with strategies to improve them.

MANAGEMENT OF HEAD INJURY

The most important aspect of the care of the head-injured child is appropriate observation. Without question computerized axial tomography (CT scan) has significantly improved management as have advanced monitoring and ventilatory support. The appropriate use of these tools depends on the observations of the patient. Such observations begin at the time of injury from witnesses, family, and emergency medical personnel and extend to hospital arrival and intensive care observations. Such observations, while of the utmost importance in the acute phases of injury, extend at some level until all manifestations have resolved or become permanent.[19,76]

The level of consciousness is far and away the most important parameter to observe, and it must be assessed repeatedly. The Glasgow Coma Scale (GCS) (see the box on p. 223) and the Neonatal Arousal Scale (see the box on p. 223), although imperfect tools, permit the level of consciousness to be determined objectively with good interobserver reliability.[17] Minor head injuries normally score between 15 and 13, moderate head injuries between 12 and 9, and severe head injuries between 8 and 3. Assessment of level of consciousness, although foremost in the evaluation, does not at all replace or lessen the need for neurologic and general physical examination on a continuous basis.[1,2,15]

Skull films have been demonstrated to correlate poorly with the presence or absence of intracranial pathology. In several large studies less than 10% of patients undergoing skull films had fractures. In addition, most patients with fractures did not have posttraumatic intracranial lesions, and many with serious intracranial pathology did not have evidence for fracture. This has led to a general thesis that head-injury management should not ordinarily be based on the presence or absence of fracture. Therefore in an effort to maximize the information available and avoid unnecessary studies the guidelines for CT scan with bone windows (see box on p. 224) have been adopted at several institutions.[1,14,25,29] Fig. 13-4 shows the CT findings in a 14 year old who had a transient loss of consciousness and then a persistent GCS of 13. This scheme has clear imperfections. A fracture crossing the middle meningeal groove may not be seen; widely separated fractures may not be appreciated; and minor depressed fractures may be missed. However, the concepts of management based on neu-

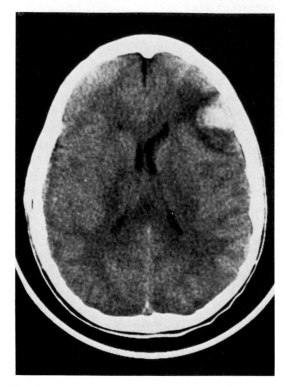

Fig. 13-4   CT findings of a frontal contusion in a 14 year old who was struck by a car while riding a bicycle and subsequently sustained a transient loss of consciousness then a persistent GCS of 13.

rologic assessment appear to be the most reliable approach.*

Any patient whose head is struck with sufficient force should be considered to have an injury that may potentially result in a cervical fracture. Thus the neck should be immobilized until assessment can be carried out. In the alert patient this may require no more than an inquiry into symptoms and a physical examination. With an altered level of consciousness or actual signs and symptoms of fracture, plane films are ordinarily required for screening and a CT scan necessary for resolving questions.[19]

Initial management follows the basic guideline of elementary first aid. The use of MAST suits and endotracheal intubation by emergency medical services should be encouraged. The airway must be maintained with additional care given to the potential for cervical instability and the high likelihood of aspiration in the patient with an altered

*References 10, 14, 25, 43, 78, 79.

level of consciousness. Hypovolemic shock is widely believed not to be the result of head injury, and therefore other sources of bleeding must be sought. The very young are the dramatic exception to this rule, since an infant may have an intracranial or even subgaleal hemorrhage.[15,69,70]

The usual signs of injury to the spine, chest, abdomen, or extremities in terms of guarding or splinting are not present in the unconscious patient and are not necessarily reliable in the child with an altered level of consciousness. As a consequence, suspicion of injury must be entertained in these patients. Abdominal CT scans and survey films should be considered in these settings.[64,70,79]

Basilar skull fractures and maxillofacial injuries require special considerations. With disruption of the skull base nasogastric tubes may enter the brain if they are not placed with direct visualization orally. Positive-pressure mask ventilation where there is a CSF leak or basilar fracture may lead to contamination of the basilar cisterns and meningitis.[8,14,25]

Initial care may blend very rapidly into definitive operative or nonoperative management, depending on the nature of the injury. The timeliness of such intervention will in many instances provide the difference between recovery and death. Fig. 13-5 demonstrates an epidural hematoma in a 9 year old who had an apparent minor head injury and subsequently a declining level of consciousness. Such urgency may occur on arrival to the hospital or later as the patient is undergoing observation.

Medical and surgical management of head injury are certainly not separate or sequential entities in the care of head-injured patients. They must be conjoined or the patient is likely to lose the benefits of both. Appropriately organized observation of the level of consciousness, neurologic examinations, vital signs, CT scans, and laboratory values are the information on which decisions must be based. Such aspects as the use of anticonvulsants, steroids, sedation, muscle relaxants, mechanical ventilation, diuretics, fluid limits, antibiotics, and agents for cerebral protection depend on the critical and experienced evaluation of patient data.

Patients in coma for greater than 6 hours have an incidence of seizure approaching 50%. The routine use of anticonvulsants in this and in less severe head injuries remains controversial. If anticonvulsants are used, they are not expected to be effective unless formal loading is carried out with the continuation of an appropriate maintenance dosage.

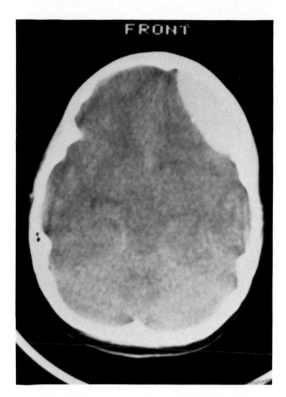

Fig. 13-5   CT appearance of an epidural hematoma in a 9 year old who had an apparent minor head injury from a bicycle fall and experienced a declining level of consciousness.

Phenobarbital is likely to confound assessment of the level of consciousness; as a consequence phenytoin (Dilantin) is the usual drug of choice.[64,70,73,78]

With basilar skull fractures, a CSF leak, or both, prophylactic administration of antibiotics is similarly controversial. Studies do not show a decrease in the incidence of meningitis following antibiotic administration; rather, more frequent resistant organisms are encountered if meningitis does occur and such prophylactic antibiotics have been given. Regardless of the decision made about antibiotics initially, nose and throat cultures are probably worthwhile if there is evidence of a CSF leak.

Steroids have not been shown to be of clear benefit in head injury. Multiple trials have either suggested a benefit or a lack of it without citing clear answers. Stress, including stress-induced gastrointestinal bleeding, is a significant problem regardless of the debate about steroids; antacids, H1 blockers, or both, should be considered in moderate to severe head injuries.[70]

Essentially all patients with an altered level of consciousness have an excessive output of antidiuretic hormone (ADH) and need fluid restriction for a period of time. Measurement of electrolytes and osmolalities is essential for critical management of these parameters.

Intracranial pressure (ICP) after a severe head injury follows an abnormal pattern in most instances with an elevated baseline, brief rises to levels interfering with cerebral perfusion, and more prolonged elevations of ICP, which may also interfere with cerebral perfusion and which are termed "plateau waves." Clinically, patients usually deteriorate toward the end of such plateau waves. As a consequence of such events, patients with posttraumatic coma, that is, a GCS of 8 or less, undergo in many centers ICP monitoring.[1,2,5] Several methods are possible for such pressure measurement including ventriculostomy, tissue pressure measuring devices, and a variety of devices for measuring pressure at the surface of the hemisphere. As with all other invasive monitoring approaches, there are significant risks, and care must be taken to ensure reliable measurement. Whether techniques that do not directly measure ventricular pressure are reliable at elevated pressures has remained a question. The two major risks of such monitoring are intracranial hemorrhage and infection. The elevated ICP tends to tamponade most vessels, which may bleed during such a procedure. There may be an increased risk of such hemorrhage if mannitol has been recently given. Risk of infection appears to increase after 5 to 7 days of monitoring. Prophylactic antibiotics are routinely given during such monitoring and daily ventricular fluid sampling is conducted for cells, protein, sugar, and culture in the case of ventriculostomy.

Once a decision is made to monitor ICP, the ICP at which treatment is required must be decided. For this there are two basic approaches: to set arbitrarily a pressure above which treatment modalities will be instituted (in many centers this is 20 torr and somewhat lower in the very young) and to calculate the cerebral perfusion pressure (CPP), which is the difference between the mean arterial blood pressure (MABP) and the mean ICP, that is, $CPP = MABP - MICP$. 60 to 70 torr are thought to be adequate. Infants with MABP in the range of 40 to 50 torr normally will obviously have a much lower CPP. Hence an understanding of normal ranges according to age is critical. Despite the maintenance of adequate CPP an ICP above 25 torr appears to be deleterious. Thus a combined assessment of CPP and absolute ICP are most often used, and no clear numbers are available to guide care. Trends of ICP are critically important, since increases may indicate, for example, intracranial bleeding. The extent to which rises in ICP should be treated is a matter of both pressure and time. Brief elevation may quickly resolve spontaneously, but more prolonged elevations or an elevated baseline may require considerable intervention and a search for its cause.

Treatment of elevated ICP necessitates additional monitoring and patient control, including an arterial line for constant blood pressure measurement and periodic arterial blood gases, intubation and controlled ventilation, bladder drainage with the frequent need for diuretics, and central venous pressure measurement or in some circumstances pulmonary artery wedge pressures. Increases in ICP may in most circumstances be controlled by the following therapies:

1. Sedation and muscle relaxants
2. Controlled mechanical ventilation to lower the P_{CO_2}. Values in the low twenties appear to be well tolerated, but numbers in the teens likely produce ischemia.
3. Osmotic diuretics such as mannitol and renal diuretics such as furosemide (Lasix) either alone or in combination often reduce ICP for as long as 2 to 6 hours by producing fluid shifts out of the brain and dumping free water. Caution needs to be exercised with fluid restriction when such diuretics are given. Whereas fluid intake is generally restricted to two thirds maintenance, patients receiving diuretics may need considerably more as indicated by outputs, venous pressure, electrolytes, and osmolalities.
4. The effectiveness of barbiturates continues to be controversial. If used, pentobarbital sodium at a loading dose of 5 mgm/kgm and a continuous infusion of 1 to 4 mgm/kgm/h will maintain a blood level of 30 to 50 ug/dL. This agent is more rapidly cleared than phenobarbital sodium, and the level may be more easily controlled. If more than one type of barbiturate is given, measurement of levels becomes confused.
5. Decompressive craniotomy is widely used in some centers as an early measure. When ICP is aggressively treated from a medical stand-point the advantages of craniotomy appear to be limited in the absence of mass.

Withdrawal of such support once elevated ICP resolves should be stepwise with gradual reduction. When diuretics have not been required for 24 hours or more, allowing the p_{CO_2} to rise gradually appears to be effective, allowing spontaneous respiratory control. If ICP again rises as the support stops, then it is reinstituted for at least another 24 hours.

Patients with significant mass lesions ordinarily require operation. Aggressive control of ICP is not likely to be beneficial, since the shift and extra volume consist of hemorrhage. In addition, the structural shift and distortions of brain by such mass are likely to cause irreversible damage. The timeliness of such an operation cannot be overemphasized. Intracerebral hematomas are the most frequent, followed by subdural hematomas and epidural hematomas. The presence of any mass lesion is not itself the indication for operation; rather the patient's level of consciousness and neurologic examination are the determining factors. Unfortunately the operation does not offer absolute protection from further problems, and repetitive evaluation must continue.

Subdural hematomas in the very young present a special opportunity for rapid early treatment with subdural taps. Even acute subdural hematomas in children of this age are likely to be liquid and lower attenuation by CT than blood because of mixing with CSF. Short, beveled subdural tap needles with trochars following appropriate preparation may be used for immediate removal of the mass and reduction in ICP. Both sides should be tapped to prevent brain shifts since most subdural hematomas are bilateral. Certain caution must be exercised because the too rapid removal of the subdural fluid may result in excessive brain shift. Taps ordinarily need to be carried out repetitively over a number of days. Subdural tap peritoneal shunts may be required temporarily if an initial series of taps do not resolve the process.

OUTCOME FOLLOWING HEAD INJURY

The consequences of head injury are wide, ranging from immediately lethal injury to headache and temporary decline in performance. However, dismissing even transient traumatic loss of consciousness as inconsequential is incorrect. Essentially everyone with minor head injury has sequelae. Seizure threshold is likely to have been lowered, headaches may persist for weeks to months, smell is frequently disturbed, and intellectual function is likely to be altered for a significant period of time. Similarly, moderate head injury will produce similar but frequently more prominent signs and symptoms. The pilot study of the Traumatic Coma Data Bank found half of those sustaining severe head injury to survive and only half of these survivors to recover to a neurodevelopmental testable range. These findings indicate the need for counseling of the patient and his or her family early in the course of an injury and the need for organized follow-up care. [7,30,62,63]

Return to contact sports following head injury requires judicious decisions. As an increasing number of individuals have been developmentally tested following sports-related head injuries there appears to be a large proportion whose scores significantly decline following injury. This seems to argue that return to such activities should at least await demonstration of return to usual school function with the consideration for formal testing if problems occur. [62,63]

REFERENCES

1. Alberico AM et al: Outcome after severe head injury: relationship to mass lesions, diffuse injury, and ICP course in pediatric and adult patients, J Neurosurg 67:648, 1987.
2. Alves WM and Jane JA: Mild brain injury: damage and outcome, Cent Nerv Syst Trauma 1:255, 1985.
3. Amacher AL: Pediatric head injury: a national tragedy, Concepts Pediatr Neurosurg 6:76, 1985.
4. American Humane Association: Annual report, Denver, 1985, The Association.
5. Annegers JF et al: The incidence, causes, and secular trends of head trauma in Olmsted County, Minnesota, 1935-1974, Neurology 30:912, 1980.
6. Benviste H et al: Elevation of the extracellular concentrations of glutamate and aspartate in rat hippocampus during transient cerebral ischemia monitored by intracerebral microdialysis, J Neurochem 43:1369, 1984.
6a. Beyerl B and Black PM: Posttraumatic hydrocephalus, Neurosurgery 15:257, 1984.
7. Brown G et al: A prospective study of children with head injuries. III. Psychiatric sequelae, Psych Med 11:63, 1981.
8. Bruce DA et al: Outcome following severe head injuries in children, J Neurosurg 48:679, 1978.
9. Bruce DA et al: Pathophysiology: treatment and outcome following severe head injury in children, Childs Brain 5:174, 1979.
10. Bruce DA et al: Diffuse cerebral swelling following head injuries in children: the syndrome of "malignant brain edema," J Neurosurg 54:170, 1981.
10a. Cardoso ER and Galbraith S: Posttraumatic hydrocephalus: a retrospective review, Surg Neurol 23:261, 1985.
11. Cartlidge NEF and Shaw DA: Head injury, Philadelphia, 1981, WB Saunders Co.
12. Cavazzuti M and Duffy TE: Regulation of local cerebral blood flow in normal and hypoxic newborn dogs, Ann Neurol 11:247, 1982.
13. Chadwick O et al: A prospective study of children with head injury. II. Cognitive sequelae, Psychol Med 11:49, 1981.
14. Chapman PH and Grove AS: Early management of penetrating orbital injuries in children, Concepts Pediatr Neurosurg 5:1, 1985.
15. Cooper PR: Delayed brain injury: secondary insults, Cent Nerv Syst Trauma 1:217, 1985.
16. Coulon RA: Depressed skull fractures in children, Concepts Pediatr Neurosurg 4:253, 1984.
17. Dixon CE et al: A fluid percussion model of experimental brain injury in the rat, J Neurosurg 67:110, 1987.
18. Duffy TE et al: Local cerebral glucose metabolism in newborn dogs: effects of hypoxia and halothane anesthesia, Ann Neurol 11:233, 1982.
19. Duncan CC and Ment LR: Management of pediatric head injury, CT 48:282, 1984.
20. Eisenberg HM and Levin HS: Outcome after head injury: general considerations and neurobehavioral recovery, Cent Nerv Syst Trauma 1:271, 1985.
21. Farber JL: The role of calcium in cell death, Life Sci 29:1289, 1981.
22. Farber JL, Chien KT, and Mittnacht S Jr: The pathogenesis of irreversible cell injury in ischemia, Am J Pathol 102:271, 1981.
23. Frankowski RF, Annegers JF, and Whitman S: The descriptive epidemiology of head trauma in the United States, Cent Nerv Syst Trauma 1:33, 1985.
24. Genarelli TA and Thibault LE: Biological models of head injury, Cent Nerv Syst Trauma 1:391, 1985.
25. Gjerris F: Head injuries in children—special features, Acta Neurochir [Suppl] 36:155, 1986.
26. Gutierrez FA, McLone DG, and Raimondi AJ: Epidural hematomas in infancy and childhood, Concepts Pediatr Neurosurg 1:188, 1981.
27. Haas DC and Lourie H: Trauma-triggered migraine: an explanation for common neurologic attacks after mild head injury, review of the literature, J Neurosurg 68:181, 1988.
28. Hahn YS et al: Traumatic mechanisms of head injury in child abuse, Childs Brain 10:229, 1983.
29. Hendrick EB, Harwood-Nash MB, and Hudson AR: Head injuries in children: a survery of 4465 consecutive cases at the Hospital for Sick Children, Toronto, Canada, Clin Neurosurg 11:46, 1964.
30. Humphreys RP: Outcome of severe head injury in children, Concepts Pediatr Neurosurg 3:191, 1983.
31. Humphreys RP et al: Severe head injuries in children, Concepts Pediatr Neurosurg 4:230, 1984.
32. James HE, Buchta R, and Stein M: A multipurpose infant helmet, Concepts Pediatr Neurosurg 5:41, 1985.
33. Johnson MV and Silverstein FS: New insights into mechanisms of neuronal damage in the developing brain, Pediat Neurosci 12:87, 1985.
34. Ito H, Miwa T, and Onodra Y: Growing skull fracture of childhood, Childs Brain 3:116, 1977.
35. Kanter RH, Carroll JB, and Post EM: Association of arterial hypertension with poor outcome in children with acute brain injury, Clin Pediatr 24:320, 1985.

36. Klauber MR et al: The epidemiology of head injury, Am J Epidemiol 113:500, 1981.

37. Krauss JF: Epidemiology of head injury. In Cooper PR, editor: Head injury, ed 2, Baltimore, 1987, Williams & Wilkins.

38. Langfitt TW, Zimmerman RA: Imaging and in vivo biochemistry of the brain in head injury, Cent Nerv Syst Trauma 1:53, 1985.

39. Laptook A, Stonestreet BS, and Oh W: The effects of different rates of plasmanate infusions upon blood flow after asphyxia and hypotension in newborn piglets, J Pediatr 100:791, 1982.

40. Levin HS and Eisenberg HM: Neuropsychological outcome of closed head injury in children and adolescents, Childs Brain 5:281, 1979.

41. Levin HS et al: Memory and intellectual ability after head injury in children adolescents, Neurosurgery 11:668, 1982.

42. Luerssen TG et al: Posttraumatic hydrocephalus in the neonate and infant. In Raimondi AJ et al, editors: Head injuries in the newborn and infant, New York, 1986, Springer-Verlag.

43. Luerssen TG et al: Magnetic resonance imaging of craniocerebral injury: clinical and research considerations, Concepts Pediatr Neurosurg 7:190, 1987.

44. Lundar T and Nestvold K: Pediatric head injuries caused by traffic accidents, Childs Nerv Syst 1:24, 1985.

45. Marmarou A et al: Contribution of CSF and vascular forces to elevation of ICP in severely head-injured patients, J Neurosurg 66:883, 1987.

46. Matson DD: Neurosurgery of infancy and childhood, ed 2, Springfield, Ill, 1969, Charles C. Thomas.

47. Meldrum B: Excitatory amino acids and anoxic/ischemic brain damage, Trends Neurosci 8:47, 1985.

48. Meldrum B: Possible therapeutic applications of antagonists of excitatory amino acid neurotransmitters, Clin Sci 68:113, 1985.

49. Ment LR, Duncan CC, and Rowe DS: Central nervous system manifestations of child abuse, CT 46:315, 1982.

50. Ment LR et al: Evaluation of complicated migraine in childhood, Childs Brain 7:261, 1980.

51. Ment LR et al: Beagle puppy model of perinatal cerebral infarction: acute changes in cerebral blood flow and metabolism during hemorrhagic hypotension, J Neurosurg 63:441, 1985.

52. Miller JD and Teasdale GM: Clinical trials for assessing treatment for severe head injury, Cent Nerv Syst Trauma 1:17, 1985.

53. Mizjahi EM and Kellaway P: Cerebral concussion in children: assessment of injury by electroencephalography, Pediatrics 73:419, 1984.

54. Muizelaar JP and Obrist WD: Cerebral blood flow and metabolism with brain injury, Cent Nerv Syst Trauma 1:123, 1985.

55. National Electronic Injury Surveillance System: Annual report, Washington, DC, 1987.

56. Obrist WD et al: Cerebral blood flow and metabolism in comatose patients with acute head injury, J Neurosurg 61:241, 1984.

57. Petroff OAC et al: In vivo phosphorous nuclear magnetic resonance spectroscopy in status epilepticus, Ann Neurol 16:169, 1984.

58. Povlishock JT: The morphological responses to head injury, Cent Nerv Syst Trauma 1:443, 1985.

59. Prichard JW et al: Cerebral metabolic studies in vivo by ^{31}P NMR, Proc Natl Acad Sci USA 80:2748, 1983.

60. Pulsinelli WA, Levy DE, and Duffy TE: Regional cerebral blood flow and glucose metabolism following forebrain ischemia, Ann Neurol 11:499, 1982.

61. Raichle M: The pathophysiology of brain ischemia, Ann Neurol 13:2 1983.

62. Rimel RW et al: Disability caused by minor head injury, J Neurosurg 9:221, 1981.

63. Rimel RW et al: Moderate head injury: completing the clinical spectrum of brain trauma, Neurosurgery 11:344, 1982.

64. Ring IT et al: Epidemiology and clinical outcomes of neurotrauma in New South Wales, Aust N Z J Surg 56:557, 1986.

65. Rivera FP: Childhood injuries. III. Epidemiology of nonmotor vehicle head trauma, Dev Med Child Neurol 26:81, 1984.

66. Rothman S: Synaptic release of excitatory amino acid neurotransmitter mediates anoxic neuronal death, J Neurosci 4:1884, 1985.

67. Rutter M et al: A prospective study of children with head injuries. I. Design and methods, Psychol Med 10:633, 1980.

68. Stahl S: MK-801: Novel glutamate antagonist and neuroprotective agent—preclinical data. In Cotman CW, editor: Neuronal plasticity versus disease, New York, 1987, The Institute for Child Development Research.

69. Shapiro K: Head injury in children, Cent Nerv Syst Trauma 1:243, 1985.

70. Shapiro K: Special considerations for the pediatric age group. In Cooper PR, editor: Head injury, ed 2, Baltimore, 1987, Williams & Wilkins.

71. Shapiro K and Marmarou A: Clinical applications of the pressure-volume index in treatment of pediatric head injuries, J Neurosurg 56:819, 1982.

72. Siesjo BAK: Cell damage in the brain: a speculative synthesis, J Cereb Blood Flow Metab 1:155, 1981.

73. Snoek JW, Minderhoud JM, and Wilmink JT: Delayed deterioration following mild head injury in children, Brain 107:15, 1984.

74. Sullivan HG et al: Fluid-percussion model of mechanical brain injury in the cat, J Neurosurg 45:520, 1976.

75. Suzuki R et al: The effects of 5-minute ischemia in Mongonolian gerbils. I. Blood-brain barrier, cerebral blood flow, and local cerebral glucose utilization changes, Acta Neuropathol (Berl) 60:207, 1983.

76. Teasdale G and Jennett B: Assessment of coma and impaired consciousness, Lancet 2:81, 1974.

77. Vannucci RC and Duffy TE: Cerebral metabolism in newborn dogs during reversible asphyxia, Ann Neurol 1:528, 1977.

78. Walker ML, Storrs BB, and Mayer T: Factors affecting outcome in the pediatric patient with multiple trauma: further experience with the modified injury severity scale, Concepts Pediatr Neurosurg 4:243, 1984.

79. Walker ML et al: Pediatric head injury—factors which influence outcome, Concepts Pediatr Neurosurg 6:84, 1985.

80. Walton GL: Subarachnoid serous exudation productive of pressure symptoms after head injuries, Am J Med Sci 116:267, 1898.

81. Walton GL and Brooks WA Jr: Observations on brain surgery suggested by a case of multiple cerebral hemorrhage, Boston Med Surg J 136:301, 1897

82. Wegman ME: Annual summary of vital statistics, Pediatrics 80:817, 1987.

83. Winn HR, Rubio DG, and Berne RM: The role of adenosine in the regulation of cerebral blood flow, J Cereb Blood Flow Metab 1:239, 1981.

84. Winston K, Beatty RM, and Fischer EG: Consequences of dural defects acquired in infancy, J Neurosurg 59:839, 1983.

85. Zimmerman RA et al: Computed tomography of craniocerebral injury in the abused child, Neuroradiology 130:687, 1979.

SPINAL CORD INJURY

Joan L. Venes and Michael A. DiPietro

The epidemiologic studies of pediatric spinal trauma generally agree on the following points[3,14,19,28,36]:

1. The incidence of pediatric spinal trauma varies depending on the location and referral base of the reporting institution and the defined age group, but certainly, pediatric trauma represents less than 10% of all spinal cord injuries. If one limits the study to children less than 8 years of age the incidence is closer to 2%.

2. Lower cervical spine injury is uncommon in children less than 8 years old and almost unheard of in children less than 3 years old.

3. In children less than 8 years old, falls and pedestrian/motor vehicle accidents are the most common cause of injury.

4. Beyond the age of 13 the causes of injury do not differ significantly from those experienced by adults.

CERVICAL SPINE INJURY

Two major pitfalls of radiologic diagnosis wait to trap the unwary: hypermobility of the upper cervical spine produces a false appearance of dislocation known as pseudosubluxation, and the synchondroses of unfused ossification centers may be mistaken for fractures.[7,43] Synchondroses are smooth and regular, and the following information concerning the location of the more commonly encountered ossification centers is helpful to prevent this particular diagnostic pitfall[4]:

1. Closure of the posterior arch of C1 proceeds from extension of ossification centers for the lateral masses and is not complete until about 3 years of age.

2. The anterior arch of C1 does not fuse with the lateral masses until 6 to 9 years of age, and multiple ossification centers are a fairly common normal variant.

3. Fusion of the dens with the centrum of the axis does not occur until sometime between the fourth and seventh year. Persistence of the subdental synchondrosis is not uncommon. Indeed it can be seen even in young adults as a normal variant. The apical ossification center of the dens appear about age 2 and does not fuse with the dens until age 12.

4. The neurocentral synchondrosis persists until fusion between the paired centers for the arches and vertebral body, sometime between 3 and 6 years of age.

5. Other ossification centers that may be confused with traumatic avulsion are those at the tips of the transverse processes and spinal processes.

6. Congenital clefts are uncommon and can be distinguished from fractures by their smooth margins. Sclerosis of bony margins and the location of congenital clefts differentiate them from more common synchondroses (Fig. 13-6). Between 8 and 13 years of age the spine rapidly takes on the conformation and characteristics of the adult spine.

The infant head is disproportionately large, and the paravertebral and trunk musculature is not sufficiently developed to support it. One has only to witness the intuitive care taken in cradling the infant by even the youngest and most inexperienced parent to appreciate the potential for upper cervical spine injury to this age group. Additionally, the facets that even in adults become more horizontal

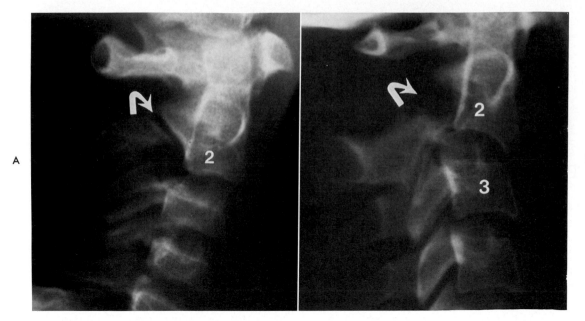

A   B

Fig. 13-6   A, Congenital cleft through the pars interarticularis of C2 *(arrow)* without malalignment, noted as an incidental finding in an 8-year-old child. Note the smooth sclerotic bony margins of the cleft. **B,** 8-year-old child with bilateral pedicle fracture *(arrow)* of C2 with anterior subluxation and flexion.

as one proceeds cephalad provide almost no resistance to forward glide in the infant and toddler. The wedge-shaped, incompletely ossified vertebral bodies contribute further to this propensity for subluxation, and it has been postulated that laxity of the transverse ligament allows the atlas to slide forward on the axis. The remarkable mobility of the upper cervical spine produces a roentgenologic "pseudosubluxation."[7,43] An atlas-dens distance of 3 to 4 mm has been recorded in healthy subjects.[25] Since subluxation of the upper cervical vertebrae with or without fracture is responsible for the majority of cervical spine injuries in young children the differentiation of physiologic "pseudosubluxation" from true subluxation is important. Physiologic subluxation can be seen into late adolescence (Fig. 13-7).

Swischuk[45] has noted that regardless of the extent of anterior displacement of C2 on C3 during flexion, a line drawn along the anterior cortex of the spinous process of C1 to the anterior cortex of the spinous process of C3 will be straight in cases of pseudosubluxation. Posterior deviation of the anterior cortex of C2 spinous process from this line by more than 1.5 mm is pathologic and highly suspect for a hangman's fracture. Prevertebral swelling, pain, and limitation of motion must also be heavily weighted in the diagnosis. Unfortu-

nately, in very young infants the prevertebral space, particularly during crying, is quite wide and should not be mistaken for edema. It can normally be as wide as the anteroposterior diameter of the vertebral bodies under 1 year. The ratios of width, that is, soft tissue to vertebral bodies, decrease to 0.7 (1 to 2 years), 0.5 (4 to 5 years), and 0.4 (8 to 10 years).[34]

Rotary suboccipital dislocation characterized by unilateral disengagement of one of the condyles of the occiput and its corresponding atlantal facet is probably underdiagnosed as a cause of torticollis in young children. Reduction usually occurs without treatment, and the child is presumed to have had viral myositis. Torticollis is an important presenting sign in children with unilateral dislocation and without fracture at other levels of the upper cervical spine. In 1935 Stimson and Swenson[41] reported that 37 out of 66 patients had a dislocation between the C2 and C3 vertebrae, and Donaldsen[11] reported that fully 75% of subluxations occurred at this level.

When one considers only children under 8 years of age, atraumatic, unilateral, subluxation of the atlas on the axis (Fig. 13-8) is the commonest form of dislocation and results in a fairly stereotyped from of torticollis known colloquially as the "cock-robin" tilt, which is virtually diagnostic. Some

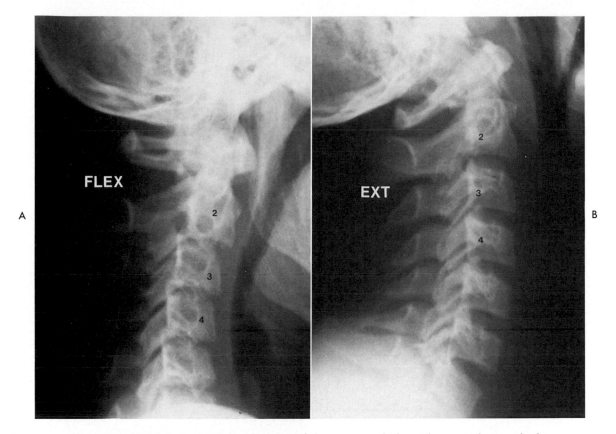

Fig. 13-7   Physiologic anterior subluxation of the upper cervical vertebrae may be seen in the older child, although it occurs far more commonly in the first years of life. **A,** Note anterior subluxation of C2 and C3 in flexion *(flex)*. A line drawn from C1 to C3 along the posterior boundary of the spinal canal will pass along the anterior cortex of the spinous process of C2. **B,** The apparent subluxation is corrected in extension *(ext)*.

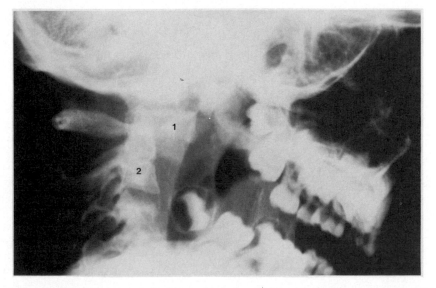

Fig. 13-8   Lateral view showing rotary subluxation of C1 and C2 in a 6-year-old child with torticollis.

authors[18,42] believe that although such spontaneous subluxations are related to infection the incidence of upper respiratory infection in this age group is so high that validating such a relationship would be quite difficult. Computerized axial tomography (CT) may be helpful in establishing the diagnosis.

There is a special case of atlantoaxial dislocation that in recent years has received increasing attention. In 1961 Spitzer et al.[40] first reported the increased incidence of atlantoaxial dislocation in children with Down syndrome. Martel and Tishler[27] reported their observations in 70 children with Down syndrome and noted that such dislocations were fairly common and usually asymptomatic. Children with Down syndrome have extremely loose, hypermobile joints and it was theorized that laxity of the transverse ligament was responsible for the high frequency of atraumatic dislocation. Although this is probably the primary contributing cause in many of the asymptomatic cases, it is likely that the increased incidence of deformity of the dens, for example, ossiculum terminale,[21] is a factor in those children who become symptomatic and require fusion (Fig. 13-9). The active participation of children with Down syndrome in the competitions of the Special Olympics has prompted a position statement by a group of physicians, including experts in sports medicine, legal advisors, and the Surgeon General of the United States.[39] Subsequently these recommendations were supported and more specific recommendations made by the American Academy of Pediatrics.[2] Although the degree of risk posed by the apparent atlantoaxial instability in these children remains to be documented,[10] it is generally agreed[33] that it is judicious to examine children with Down syndrome radiologically and neurologically at regular intervals and take special precautions when atlantoaxial instability is identified.

Fractures through the subdental synchondrosis extending into the vertebral body[13,37,38] are the most common of the cervical spine fractures of childhood and can be well demonstrated with CT.[12] The examiner should suspect a fracture whenever an

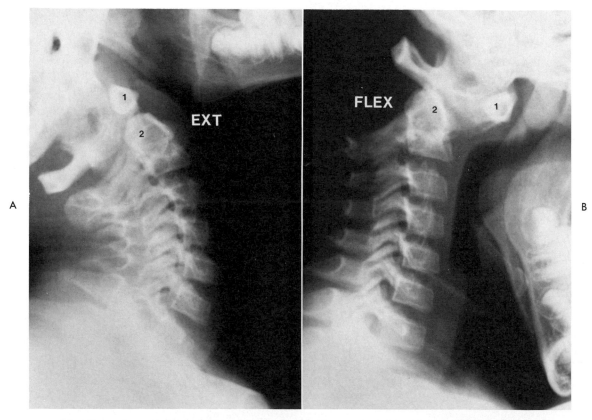

Fig. 13-9   Lateral views of the cervical spine in a 10-year-old child with a hypoplastic odontoid.
A, Extension *(ext)*. **B,** Note the marked anterior subluxation of C1 with flexion *(flex)*.

anterior angulation of the dens appears on lateral spine x-ray films (Fig. 13-10). Fractures through the apex of the dens are exceedingly rare in the preteenager, and the normal apical ossification center should not be mistaken for a fracture.

Pseudospread of the atlas[44] is easily confused with a Jefferson burst fracture and is common in children between 3 months and 4 years of age, with 90% to 100% of 2 year olds exhibiting lateral offsets in excess of 2 mm with some offsets measuring as much as 8 mm bilaterally. This normalizes between 3 and 6 years of age. Zaborowski[53] documented that the rate of growth of the atlas was greater than that of the axis during the first year of life. Suss et al.[44] noted that delayed ossification and limited visualization of the lateral portions of the body of the axis is hollowed out and thinned by the vertebral artery contribute to the apparent disparity. If in doubt the CT scan can be used to image the ring of C1. According to Suss the earliest reported case (1822) of a Jefferson fracture was found at autopsy in a 3-year-old boy. From 1822 to the publication by Suss et al. on pseudospread of the atlas in 1982, not a single documented case

of Jefferson fracture in a preteen appeared in the literature.

In the very young child, cervical fractures below the third cervical vertebra are very uncommon and occur almost exclusively in children older than 8 years of age. As in the adult, hyperextension forces are the major contributing factor.[26]

THORACOLUMBAR SPINE INJURY

Angular bending forces, commonly flexion, are usually accompanied by an axial compression force and result in vertebral body collapse of varying degrees (Fig. 13-11). This appears to be the most common injury mechanism in children.[1] With progressive collapse, the posterior vertebral body and cortex become involved and may protrude into the spinal canal. The long-term outlook of anterior angulation injury with intact posterior elements is almost invariably good, although an occasional

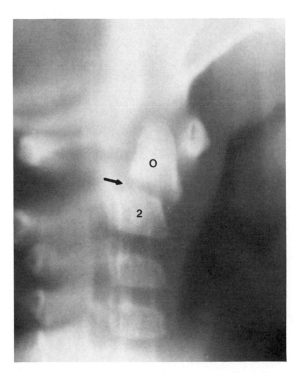

Fig. 13-10   Fracture through the subdental synchondrosis *(arrow)* in a 3 year old. There is anterior subluxation and flexion of the odontoid *(O)* on the body of C2.

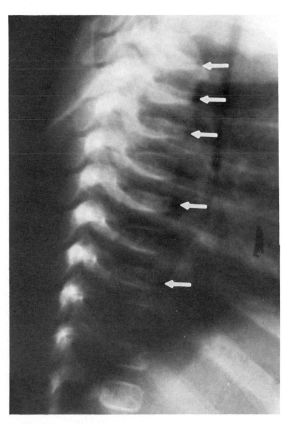

Fig. 13-11   Multiple thoracic vertebral body compression fractures *(arrows)* in an abused 2-month-old infant. Other more common causes of multiple compression fractures in childhood are leukemia and histiocytosis.

older child will complain of chronic lower back pain. Axial loading results in vertebral body burst of varying degrees. Neurologic injury may occur if fragments are driven into the canal. If the posterior elements are intact the injury is stable. Rotational-shear injuries with or without angulation occur most often at the thoracolumbar junction and frequently involve both the conus and cauda equina. These fractures are quite unstable, and spontaneous fusion is infrequent. This injury is rare in children under 8 years of age.

Palpation of the back may reveal a stepoff or sudden angulation in the alignment of the spinal processes. If thoracic spine injury is suspected associated injuries such as rib fracture and hemopneumothorax should be looked for. On occasion avulsion or injury to the great vessels may occur. Lumbar spine fractures are more commonly associated with trauma to the intraabdominal viscera. Multiple transverse process fractures of the lumbar vertebrae are usually unassociated with the neurologic deficit but may cause a large retroperitoneal hematoma with significant fall in hematocrit in the younger child. Urinary retention is common following thoracolumbar spine injuries and may be present in the absence of any demonstrable neurologic deficit. Most often the problem is one of a pain-related spasm of the pelvic floor, although local trauma, particularly in pelvic fractures, may be responsible.

Plain x-ray films will usually demonstrate the injury in the lower thoracic and lumbar region, but the upper thoracic and cervicodorsal areas are difficult to visualize on standard radiographs particularly in the older child. A swimmer's view can be helpful, but CT is the single best study for the demonstration of bony compromise of the spinal canal by either bone fragments or disk material and has supplanted myelography for this purpose in the majority of cases.

A special category of fracture usually occurring in young teenagers deserves mention. This is a fracture through the apophyseal ring with retropulsion into the spinal canal simulating a disk protrusion. These can generally be identified on CT examination.[15,32]

SPINAL CORD INJURY WITHOUT RADIOLOGIC ABNORMALITY (SCIWORA)

Melzak[28] was probably the first to call attention to the high incidence of traumatic spinal cord injury

without radiologic abnormality (SCIWORA) of spine fracture or dislocation (16 out of 29 patients). This high incidence has been confirmed with more advanced neurodiagnostic studies. Plain films, CT scans or myelograms fail to demonstrate fracture or dislocation in roughly half of all children with spinal cord injury,[30] according to a 1982 report from the Children's Hospital of Pittsburgh (CHP). However, it is important that a thorough radiologic evaluation be completed before diagnosis of SCIWORA is made.

In the relatively large series of 24 children with SCIWORA reported from the CHP the authors noted that children younger than 8 years of age tended to sustain more serious neurologic damage and suffer a larger number of upper cervical cord lesions. They postulated that the spine in infants and young children is inherently more deformable and therefore provides less effective protection for the subadjacent spinal cord regardless of whether flexion or extension forces are applied to the spine. 52% of their cases of SCIWORA presented with delayed onset occurring several hours to as long as 4 days following injury. Many children recalled that they had transient numbness, tingling, or subjective paralysis. Once the brief symptom-free period had passed, "sensorimotor paralysis progressed inexorably" evolving into complete transverse myelopathy in 7 out of 24 children and severe central cord syndrome in 4 children. Only one of these eleven severe injuries occurred in children older than 8 years of age, although they comprised one third of patients. Conversely, six out of the seven mild to moderate cases of central cord syndrome occurred in children older than 8 years of age. In a smaller series from the University of Kentucky, Walsh et al.[49] reported their experience with eight children diagnosed with SCIWORA. All injuries occurred in the thoracic region, none had the asymptomatic interval described by Pang and Wilberger,[30] and seven out of eight remained without neurologic function below the level of injury. No child in their series was older than 5 years of age, although children up to 16 years of age had been included in the study protocol. This supports the statement made by Pang and Wilberger that the inherent instability of the pediatric spine is maximal in infancy and decreases as the child reaches the second decade. Both of these studies conclude that the prognosis for children under 8 years of age is poor.

The pathophysiology of SCIWORA remains to be elaborated, and a full discussion of the proposed mechanisms is beyond the scope of this chapter. The following events have been hypothesized as the etiology of this uncommon condition:

1. Transient retropulsion of the disk into the spinal canal[51]
2. Transient subluxation[51]
3. Inward bulging of the ligamentum flavum during hyperextension[46]
4. The infant's vertebral column being more elastic than the spinal cord, allowing it to be distracted and lead to tearing of the cord without demonstrable vertebral injury[24]
5. Ischemic infarction[8]

MANAGEMENT OF PEDIATRIC SPINE INJURIES

As with any injury general principles of airway management and fluid resuscitation apply to the child with spinal cord injury. Hypotension may result from injury to the autonomic relays in the low cervical and thoracic spine. Vasodilatation with rapid expansion of the vascular tree rather than blood loss may be the problem. Injury to the phrenic nerve nucleus in patients with injury to the upper cervical spinal cord will cause them to be ventilator dependent, and hypoxia and anoxia at the time of injury contribute to poor outcome. Even children with lower cervical and upper thoracic cord injury may require short-term ventilatory assistance. Great care must be taken during intubation to prevent further injury and, if feasible, a fiberoptic nasotracheal intubation is the method of choice in these children. Once resuscitative efforts have stabilized the child, rapid priority is generally given to the evaluation and management of life-threatening head, thoracic, and intraabdominal injuries. During this time the assessment of sensorimotor deficit is relatively easy to pursue, and any suggestion of neurologic dysfunction mandates adequate stabilization of the spine during other diagnostic and therapeutic procedures. Diagnosis of sensorimotor loss in the infant and young child can be more difficult than in the adult. Often, asymmetry of movement under observation is the best way to demonstrate motor loss. The use of tickle rather than pin, painstaking repetition, and the effort to ensure cooperation may allow one to estimate a less than total sensory loss. Such a detailed examination is often not possible in the exigencies of an emergency room situation. Unsustained clonus and extensor plantar responses may be normal in the infant before completion of myelination

and, once again, symmetry is the guiding principle. The flaccid, areflexic patient with a sensory level to pin and touch is said to be in spinal shock until return of the superficial reflexes. Spinal shock, first brought to attention in 1917 by Head and Riddoch,[16] remains a poorly understood phenomenon. If the cord injury has not been too severe, reflexes recover, voluntary micturition is reestablished, and motor recovery begins within hours or days of injury. Careful evaluation of those patients' recovery after injury will usually demonstrate some patchy sensation or fragments of motor activity. If after return of such superficial reflexes as the bulbocavernous reflex the patient remains without sensorimotor function the lesion is invariably permanent. In the infant the reflex activity of the isolated cord may be almost indistinguishable from normal motor function. Electrodiagnostic studies may be necessary to confirm the suspicion of total cord transection.

The child with significant head injury should be assumed to have an associated cervical spine injury. In children, negative cervical spine films do not rule out SCIWORA. Fortunately the milder lesions, which occur more commonly in the preteen and teenager than in the younger child, appear to be relatively stable, and maintaining the unconscious patient in a soft collar until evaluation or dynamic studies can be performed to rule out instability is all that is necessary. For the more severely injured child with SCIWORA therapy appears to have no significant effect on outcome. In the CHP series no child with a complete lesion had any neurologic recovery. There was only one child with a severe partial injury, and that child recovered with moderate deficits. Half of the children had mild deficits initially, and all made an excellent recovery. One out of eight children reported by Walsh et al.[49] made a partial recovery. All eight children in that study were rendered either immediately paraplegic or became paraplegic within 48 hours of injury.

The immediate goals of treatment of spine injury are to provide stability, restore alignment, and ensure the adequacy of the spinal canal. As noted, the anterior angulated fracture through the subdental synchondrosis is the commonest cervical spine fracture in children. Generally these are easily aligned, and in the child of 16 to 18 months of age or older a Halo jacket provides adequate stabilization.[22] Immobilization of the cervical spine in the infant can present a real challenge to the orthotist because of the relatively large size of the baby's head, which tends to flex the spine anteriorly even with the child in the neutral position. However, adaptive casts can be molded.[1]

Traction is almost impossible to maintain in the infant and toddler unless the baby is paralyzed. Although traction is a reasonable alternative in the older cooperative child, the Halo jacket is generally preferred for the management of cervical and cervicodorsal spine injuries. If traction is used care must be taken to prevent overdistraction, and unless there is some ligamentous integrity across the fracture site traction is unsafe and should not be used. The mobility of the cervical spine is such that injuries tend to be reduced readily, and the need for open surgical reduction in the young child must be very rare indeed. On occasion, rotary atlantoaxial subluxation is missed, and the torticollis becomes relatively fixed. In these children traction and liberal use of analgesics and antispasmodics may be required to effect realignment.

Atlantoaxial dislocation and simple subluxation without cord injury usually respond well to conservative management. In those cases in which fusion is necessary, posterior fusion by simple wiring is generally all that is required. In the special case of Down syndrome a developmental anomaly of the dens may require a transpalatal approach for removal of the odontoid in addition to the posterior fixation. This procedure is somewhat more difficult in these children because they have a small mouth, a high palate, and a large tongue. Tracheotomy is almost always required during the postoperative period. Traction in these children or in others with limited mental ability can be hazardous. Immobilization in a Halo jacket can provoke much anxiety for the child with Down syndrome. Patience and skill in dealing with mentally handicapped children are necessary to achieve acceptance of the orthosis by the youngster.

Management of the older child with a lower cervical spine and thoracolumbar injury is similar to the adult save that children heal faster and can reconstitute some of the loss of height that is seen with wedged compression fractures. Stable vertebral fractures in children rarely result in progressive or delayed angular deformity. Lateral wedge fractures may result in minimal scoliosis, but progressive spine deformity is quite uncommon. Unfortunately the very growth potential that can be so useful in reducing the kyphosis of wedged compression fractures contributes to a propensity for spinal deformity in the child with severe cord injury.[20,23] Kilfoyle et al.[20] first called attention to the fact that the great majority of patients who sustain a significant spinal cord injury before the adolescent growth spurt will develop a spinal deformity. Laminectomy is rarely indicated and may convert the stable to an unstable fracture. Children who undergo laminectomy without fixation are much more likely to develop kyphosis than those who do not undergo laminectomy.[6,29]

Winter[50] categorically declares that "spinal deformity following spine fractures with or without neurologic deficit is a preventable problem." He suggests early (though not emergent) stabilization, avoidance of ill-conceived laminectomies, and bracing of all children who sustain traumatic paraplegia before the adolescent growth spurt. Surgery is indicated for children with progressive spinal deformity uncontrolled by bracing and for those presenting with spinal angulation of greater than 40 degrees. Discussion of the increasingly varied methods of stabilization is not within the scope of this text, although instrumentation with Harrington rods probably remains the most widely used form of posttraumatic fixation.

The problems associated with early management pale beside a consideration of the long-term problems facing the child with either traumatic paraplegia or quadriplegia. Early involvement in a program of spinal cord rehabilitation is of great importance, and in those centers in which it is available such involvement usually begins on the day of injury. Attention to bladder and bowel function, avoidance of decubiti and contractures, and relief of spasticity are three of the major areas addressed by the rehabilitation team that can be considerably ameliorated by proper early management.

OBSTETRIC TRAUMA

Spinal cord injury as the result of obstetric trauma merits consideration as a separate entity. Injury to the spinal cord during a difficult breech delivery was first described by Parott[31] in 1870. Subsequently, improved obstetric techniques have made this form of spinal cord injury an infrequent event. In a review of 15,000 infants delivered at the University of Pennsylvania Hospital, only one instance of spinal cord injury was recorded.[35] Yates[52] and Towbin,[47] however, suggest that the injury often escapes diagnosis. Both comment on the high incidence of vertebral artery damage and significant epidural hemorrhage in neonates in whom the spinal cord is examined postmortem. Most reported cases of spinal injury have occurred with breech delivery in applying traction to the trunk and manipulating the aftercoming head or in vertex delivery when traction is applied. Cesarean section delivery has been suggested for those infants shown radiographically to be in a hyperextended "star-gazing" breech position.[5,17] Birth injuries occur most commonly at the cervicothoracic junction (Fig. 13-12). As noted by Crothers and Putnam[9] the spinal column of the infant consists of a series of elastic rings joined by relatively brittle disks and ligaments. The dura mater is attached to the vertebral canal by many strong fibrous bands in the cervical and lumbar region, but only very loosely attached in the thoracic region. The cord itself is anchored firmly by the brachial plexus above the cauda equina below and is relatively inelastic and friable. Lateral traction on the head puts an increased tension on the cord at its junction with the brachial plexus and may result in avulsion of the cervical roots. Hyperextension with traction applied to the legs and the head held firmly by a uterine contraction may result in actual rupture of the cord and its meninges, accompanied at times by an audible snap. The elastic cartilaginous spine of the infant may be grossly distorted but does not disrupt because of its relative elasticity. Injuries occurring above the level of the phrenic nuclei are generally rapidly fatal. Survival, however, may be anticipated in the neonate with a lower cervical or cervicothoracic injury. In general the damage extends over several segments, and the infant is noted at birth to be hypotonic with depressed respirations. Prompt resuscitative measures generally are followed by the appearance of reflex movement to stimulation, which sometimes lead to the diagnosis of primary muscle disease. It should be noted that the spinal shock seen in adult patients following severe cord trauma is generally not present in the infant, and recovery of reflex function follows a time course similar to that seen in the recovery of movement following any resuscitative procedure in the newborn. Continued flaccidity is probably caused by cord destruction over many segments, either as a result of intramedullary hemorrhage or infarction. The demonstration of a sensory level is the key diagnostic criterion. The presence of an abnormal skin wheal and flare response or the lack of a cortical-evoked response to lower extremity stimulation may be helpful.

Treatment in these cases is generally supportive. Upper respiratory infections are common, and pneumonia is a frequent cause of death in infancy. Lack of vasomotor and sudomotor control below the level of the lesion may seriously impair temperature regulation in the infant.

Minor degrees of cord damage may account for some of the spastic diplegias now grouped with cerebral palsies. Secondary injuries to the cerebral cortex may occur with hypoxia caused by transient respiratory depression associated with reversible, undiagnosed neonatal cord injury. The true contribution of neonatal traumatic myelopathy to the broad group of neurologic diseases associated with birth injuries remains to be defined.

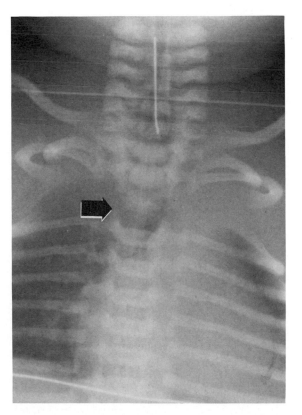

Fig. 13-12   Fractured, distracted, and dislocated upper thoracic spinal column *(arrow)* caused by birth trauma in a 1-day-old infant. Preservation of spinal cord mass reflexes may make clinical diagnosis difficult.

REFERENCES

1. Allen BL and Ferguson RL: Cervical spine trauma. In Bradford DS and Hensinger RM, editors: The pediatric spine, New York, 1985, Thieme Medical Publishers, Inc.
2. American Academy of Pediatrics, Committee on Sports Medicine: Atlantoaxial instability in Down syndrome, Pediatrics 74:152, 1984.

3. Anderson JM and Schutt AH: Spinal injury in children: a review of 56 cases seen from 1950 through 1978, Mayo Clin Proc 55:499, 1980.

4. Bailey DK: The normal cervical spine in infants and children, Radiology 59:712, 1952.

5. Bresnan MJ: Neurologic birth injuries: Part II, Postgrad Med 49:202, 1971.

6. Cattell HS and Clark GH: Cervical kyphosis and instability following multiple laminectomies in children, J Bone Joint Surg 49A:713, 1967.

7. Cattell HS and Filzer DL: Pseudosubluxation and other normal variations in the cervical spine in children, J Bone Joint Surg 47A:1295, 1965.

8. Choi JU et al: Traumatic infarction of the spinal cord in children, J Neurosurg 65:608, 1986.

9. Crothers B and Putnam MC: Obstetric injuries of the spinal cord, Medicine 6:41, 1927.

10. Davidson RG: Atlantoaxial instability in individuals with Down symdrome: a fresh look at the evidence, Pediatrics 81:857, 1988.

11. Donaldson JS: Acquired torticollis in children and young adults, JAMA 160:458, 1956.

12. Geehr RB, Rothman SLG, and Kier EL: The role of computer tomography in the evaluation of upper cervical spine pathology, Comput Radiol 2:79, 1978.

13. Griffiths SC: Fractures of odontoid process in children, J Pediatr Surg 7:680, 1972.

14. Hadley MN et al: Pediatric spinal trauma: reveiw of 122 cases of spinal cord and vertebral column injuries, J Neurosurg 68:18, 1988.

15. Handel S et al: Posterior lumbar apophyseal fractures, Radiology 130:629, 1979.

16. Head H and Riddoch G: The automatic bladder, excessive sweating, and some other reflex conditions in gross injuries of the spinal cord, Brain 40:188, 1917.

17. Hellstrom B and Sallmander V: Prevention of spinal cord injury in hypertension of the fetal head, JAMA 204:1041, 1968.

18. Hess JH, Bronstein IP, and Abelson SM: Atlantoaxial dislocation unassociated with trauma and secondary to inflammatory foci in the neck, Am J Dis Child 49:1137, 1935.

19. Hill SA et al: Pediatric neck injuries, J Neurosurg 60:700, 1984.

20. Kilfoyle RM, Foley JJ, and Norton PL. Spine and pelvic deformity in childhood and adolescent paraplegia, J Bone Joint Surg 47A:659, 1965.

21. Kobori M, Takahashi H, and Mikawa Y: Atlantoaxial dislocation in Down's syndrome: report of two cases requiring surgical correction, Spine 11:195, 1986.

22. Kopits SE and Steingass MH: Experience with the "Halo-Cast" in small children, Surg Clin North Am 50:935, 1970.

23. Lancourt J, Dickson J, and Carter R: Paralytic spinal deformity following traumatic spinal cord injury in children and adolescents, J Bone Joint Surg 63A:47, 1981.

24. Leventhal HR: Birth injuries of the spinal cord, J Pediatr 56:447, 1960.

25. Locke GR, Gardner JI, and VanEpps EF: Atlas-dens interval (ADI) in children: a survey based on 200 normal cervical spines, Am J Roentgenol Radium Ther Nucl Med 98:135, 1966.

26. Marar BC: Hyperextension injuries of the cervical spine: the pathogenesis of damage to the spinal cord, J Bone Joint Surg 56A:1655, 1974.

27. Martel W and Tishler JM: Observations of the spine in mongolism, Am J Roentgenol 97:630, 1966.

28. Melzak J: Paraplegia among children, Lancet 2:45, 1969.

29. Morgan R, Brown JC, and Bonnett C: The effect of laminectomy on the pediatric spinal cord–injured patient, J Bone Joint Surg 56A:1767, 1974.

30. Pang D and Wilberger J: Spinal cord injury without radiographic abnormalities in children, J Neurosurg 57:114, 1982.

31. Parott T: Note sur un cas de repture de la moelle, chez un nouveau ne par suite de manouevres pendant l'accouchement, L'Union Med 11:137, 1870.

32. Petterson H et al: The CT appearance of an avulsion of the posterior vertebral apophysis, case report, Neuroradiology 21:145, 1981.

33. Pueschel SM: Atlantoaxial instability and Down syndrome, Pediatrics 81:879, 1988.

34. Rivero HJ, Young LW, and Flom L: Reliability of retropharyngeal soft tissue measurements in infants and children: new standards based on 586 normals, Presented at the Twenty-Ninth Annual Meeting of the Society of Pediatric Radiology, Washington, DC, April 10-13, 1986.

35. Rubin A: Birth injuries: incidence, mechanisms, and end results, Obstet Gynecol 23:218, 1984.

36. Ruge JR et al: Pediatric spinal injury: the very young, J Neurosurg 68:25, 1988.

37. Seimon LP: Fracture of the odontoid process in young children, J Bone Joint Surg 59A:943, 1977.

38. Sherk HH, Nichoson JT, and Chung SMK. Fractures of the odontoid process in young children, J Bone Joint Surg 60A:921, 1978.

39. Special Olympics Bulletin: Participation by individuals with Down syndrome who suffer from atlantoaxial dislocation condition, Washington, D.C., March 31, 1983, Special Olympics, Inc.

40. Spitzer R, Rabinowitz JY, and Wybar KC: A study of the abnormalities of the skull teeth and lenses in mongolism, Can Med Assoc J 84:567, 1961.

41. Stimson BB and Swenson PC: Unilateral subluxations of the cervical vertebrae without associated fracture, JAMA 104:1578, 1935.

42. Sullivan AW: Subluxation of the atlantoaxial joint: sequel to inflammatory process in the neck, J Pediatr 35:451, 1949.

43. Sullivan CR, Bruver AJ, and Harris LE: Hypermobility of the cervical spine in children: a pitfall in the diagnosis of cervical dislocation, Am J Surg 95:636, 1958.

44. Suss RA, Zimmerman RD, and Leeds NE: Pseudospread of the atlas: false sign of Jefferson fracture in young children, AJR 140:1079, 1983.

45. Swischuk LE: Anterior displacement of C2 in children: physiologic or pathologic? Radiology 122:759, 1977.

46. Taylor AR: The mechanism of injury to the spinal cord in the neck without damage to the vertebral column, J Bone Joint Surg 33B:543, 1951.

47. Towbin A: Spinal cord and brain stem injury at birth, Arch Pathol Lab Med 77:620, 1964.

48. Reference deleted in galleys.

49. Walsh JW, Stevens DB, and Young AB: Traumatic para-
    plegia in children without contiguous spinal fracture or
    dislocation, Neurosurg 12:439, 1983.
50. Winter RB: Spinal Injury. In Moe JH et al, editors:
    Scoliosis and other spinal deformities, Philadelphia, 1978,
    WB Saunders Co.
51. Wolman L: The neuropathology of traumatic paraplegia,
    Paraplegia 1:233, 1964.
52. Yates PO: Birth trauma to vertebral arteries, Arch Dis Child
    34:436, 1959.
53. Zaborowski Z: Extrafetal development of the axis on the
    basis of roentgenoanthropometric measurements, Folia
    Morphol (Warsz) 37:167, 1978.

14

Eye Injuries

Marvin L. Sears

The purpose of this chapter is to present to the nonspecialist physician confronted with an ocular emergency essential diagnostic and therapeutic measures to be taken in commonly occurring ocular injuries. In almost all instances only temporizing measures will be performed until an experienced ophthalmologist can see the patient. From the point of view of primary care, however, the answers to two key questions are required: What are the features of the ocular examination essential to the evaluation of the degree of the injury? What are the limits to which the general physician may extend without jeopardizing the patient?

GENERAL COMMENTS

Although the eye is well protected from injury by the bony rim of the orbit and the eyelids, sharp or blunt instruments may severely damage the eye, although little evidence of the seriousness of the injury is apparent. Furthermore, the eye is small, and many of its structures are avascular and susceptible to injury, whereas others are richly vascularized and prone to severe hemorrhage. Thus the response to injury, as well as the noxious agent itself, may result in damage of a severe nature after apparently mild insults and within short periods of time. The complexities of the ocular injury and response require rapid attention, immediate triage, and the exercise of swift, expert clinical judgment in management.

In the pursuit of an appropriate course of therapy it is necessary for the observer to retain a high index of suspicion that the superficial manifestations of injury may not be the only ones. Thus a patient with a corneal abrasion may have a retinal hemorrhage or tear; one with an ecchymotic lid may have a dislocated lens, edematous retina, or-

bital fracture, and so on. Foreign bodies must be detected and, when indicated, removed.

Furthermore, when vision is lost it must be decided whether the cause is intraocular or whether a lesion in the optic nerve or visual pathway is responsible.

In the evaluation of trauma to the orbit, lids, or eye the following steps must be taken:

1. A history of present and preexisting eye disorders must be taken. The nature of the instrument, object, or chemical producing the injury should be determined and obtained, if possible.
2. Particular attention must be given to possible drug allergies, contraindications to anesthesia, and the adequacy of previous tetanus immunization. Any previous treatment and medications received for the injury should be recorded in the history.
3. Visual acuity must be determined for each eye separately with the patient's corrective lenses in place, if possible. Visual fields can be determined by confrontation using the fingers or a gauze square.
4. Cautious inspection of the orbital rims and lids by palpation and inspection must be done. The presence of foreign material, crepitus, and hemorrhage should be noted. Any lid lesion may be associated with penetration of the globe. On occasion the penetration may be so subtle as to require exploratory intervention in the operating room.
5. The lacrimal puncta and canaliculi must be inspected.
6. After orbital trauma it is important to measure the position of the eyes with respect to the lateral orbital rims using an exophthal-

mometer. Sometimes inspection is useful, that is, standing behind the patient and sighting over the brow.

7. The extraocular movements should be examined. They can be recorded as indicated. (The patient is looking at you.)

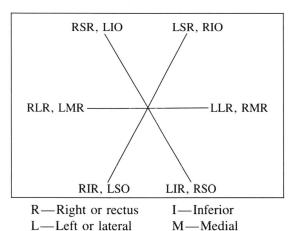

R—Right or rectus   I—Inferior
L—Left or lateral   M—Medial
S—Superior   O—Oblique

8. The pupils must be examined and the results recorded: Round? Regular? Equal reaction to light and near objects?
9. The cornea should be inspected under magnification, and if necessary, a topical anesthetic in liquid form can be applied to facilitate the examination. Staining the cornea with a strip of fluorescein is usually advisable.
10. The anterior chamber should be checked for blood (hyphema) or pus (hypopyon), or for abnormal movement of the iris (iridodialysis—tear of the iris root), or for iridodoneses (abnormal shakiness) usually associated with a dislocated lens.
11. The intraocular pressure should be estimated if possible with a tonometer (if the cornea is intact and no obvious laceration of the globe is seen).
12. If visual acuity has been recorded, pupils examined, and no signs related to head injury are present, the pupils usually should be dilated with a solution of 2.5% phenylephrine applied topically to permit adequate visualization of the fundus with an ophthalmoscope. Opacities in and the general clarity of the media should be recorded. The color, cup, and outline of the disc should be recorded, and a view of the vessels should be established and described. The macula should be inspected.
13. It is probably useful to photograph all injuries.
14. Whenever a possibility of a bony fracture and the presence of a foreign body exists, x-ray films or a computed tomographic (CT) scan must be obtained.

EVALUATION OF PAIN IN AND AROUND THE EYE

Pain of sudden onset in the region of the orbit and eye may take one of several forms. It may be sharp, lancinating, and in particular, related to eye movement. This suggests that an external problem exists either under the lids or on the cornea and could indicate the presence of a foreign body in the cul-de-sac or cornea, a corneal abrasion or infiltrate, or an ulcer related to an infection. A dull deep ache may suggest elevated intraocular pressure or, if the pain increases on eye movement, may suggest the presence of an optic neuritis. A brow ache implies ciliary spasm and may be associated with any severe irritation of the uveal tract. The uvea is innervated by large numbers of pain fibers, and any prolapse of uveal tissue or inflammation within the uvea (uveitis) or any irritating stimulus that gives rise to smooth muscle contraction may also be associated with brow pain. Ciliary spasm is common after corneal injuries, contusion injuries, and intraocular inflammation or after the instillation of cholinomimetic medication (exposure to war gases). The eyes are infrequently the cause of headache. Some aching and asthenopic symptoms may be associated with mild headache on a rare occasion. Pain localized to the temporal fossa may be of a deep and boring nature. In this instance one should suspect the sphenoid sinus as point of origin and not the eye or orbit. Tenderness in the area of the temporal fossa may be associated with any vasculitis. Throbbing in this area may be of vascular origin and is commonly seen in patients with migraine attacks. Unrelenting deep pain may occur as a result of intraocular or orbital infection, either of posttraumatic or postsurgical origin. If pain is accompanied by a Horner's syndrome, a diagnosis of Raeder's paratrigeminal syndrome can be made. Horton's headache, or cluster headache, may on occasion be associated with dilated pupils, but pain is not localized to the eye or orbit.

Photophobia associated with intense pain may

be caused by many types of ocular insults but is particularly severe with corneal lesions. Occasionally these lesions are so fine as to escape careful examination. Improved diagnosis results when fluorescein is applied to the cornea to detect any slight denudation of even a few corneal epithelial cells.

A topical anesthetic agent frequently will distinguish external afflictions from the others mentioned. Since these agents are respiratory poisons and in addition will make the cornea anesthetic, they become hazardous with chronic use and should be applied only for diagnostic purposes, during removal of a corneal foreign body, or to facilitate examination of the eye and under the surface of the eyelids.

TECHNIQUE OF EXAMINATION

Patients with a good deal of lid swelling associated either with contusion or laceration may present a major obstacle to the examiner in the attempt to learn the extent of the ocular injury. If the eye has been penetrated or lacerated, pressure on the globe must be prevented at all costs. Retraction of the lid by an inexperienced examiner, or with the use of excessive force, can accentuate the hazard presented by the injury. It may be necessary to defer a more complete examination to the time when the patient is anesthetized and prepared for surgery lest additional irreparable damage be done. Uncooperative or struggling patients or those in great pain may need to be wrapped or held or restrained suitably. However, the lid squeezing that occurs during these battles can raise intraocular pressure to 60 mm Hg or higher and can cause extrusion of the ocular contents through a perforation site. It may be necessary to postpone the completion of the examination to the time when the patient is anesthetized. During induction it is advisable to cover the eye with a metal shield that rests on the bony parts of the orbit to protect the eye and to eliminate further damage to the eye.

EVERSION OF THE LID

Foreign material of either metallic or chemical nature, or sometimes a contact lens, may lodge either in the upper or lower cul-de-sacs or in the corner of the cul-de-sacs, called the fornices. Whereas the lower lids may be easily retracted simply by using one's thumb and the lower fornices examined as the patient looks upward, the exam-

ination of the upper fornices is another matter.

For eversion of the upper lid there are two movements, one for single eversion and a second for double eversion. For single eversion a small retractor, a cotton swab, the end of a handlight, or even a finger may be used. The upper lid is grasped by the lashes and lid margin and is pulled downward *while the patient is continuously looking downward*. The blunt instrument is then placed with slight pressure at the upper end of the upper tarsus on the skin side at the place where the upper edge makes itself evident through the skin. The lid margin is then flipped upward as the instrument aids in folding the skin at the level of the upper tarsus. The tarsal conjunctiva is then exposed, and the foreign body or other material may be easily removed. Indeed, when the patient believes that something is on the cornea and the cornea is seen to be clear on thorough examination, usually some abnormality is found on the tarsal conjunctiva (Fig. 14-1).

For thorough removal of a chemical or other material from the upper cul-de-sac, double eversion is essential. This is best conducted with a small vein retractor. The movement is the same as that just described, except that the vein retractor is placed on the skin side of the upper edge of the tarsus. After single eversion is accomplished, the handle of the vein retractor is moved toward the patient's forehead and is pulled gently upward. This maneuver effectively rolls the lid almost completely onto the retractor, thereby exposing the upper conjunctiva and fornices in their entirety. In the case of chemical burns, particularly alkali, caustic soda, lime, and so forth, it is imperative that all particulate matter be removed by irrigation or manually by debridement.

EXAMINATION OF THE FUNDUS

For serious-minded evaluation of the fundus in children it is almost always necessary to dilate the pupil. Pupillary dilation is contraindicated only when it is essential that the natural size of the pupil be used in evaluating changing states of consciousness in a patient with a head injury. Otherwise, mydriasis can always be performed but should be done with a quality and quantity of medication that will not produce toxicity. Safe mydriasis in children can be achieved with 0.1% tropicamide; a 0.5% solution of tropicamide may be used together with 1% hydroxyamphetamine or with two to three

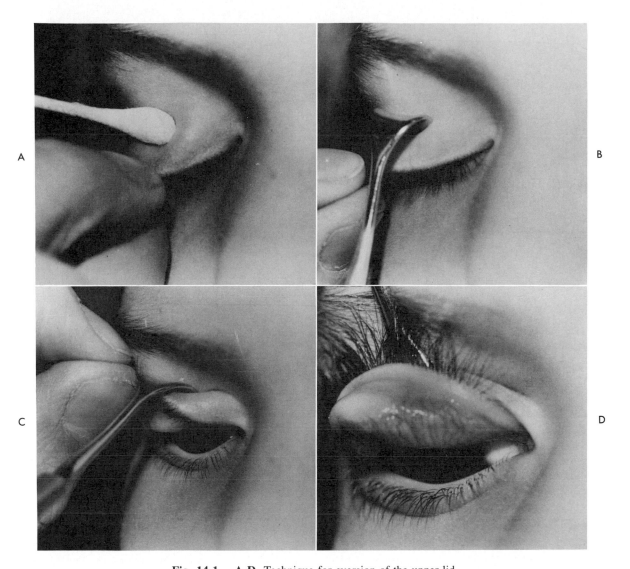

Fig. 14-1   A-D, Technique for eversion of the upper lid.

microdrops of a 2.5% solution of phenylephrine. An equally appropriate alternative is the use of cyclopentolate or 0.1% to 0.2% solution of cyclopentolate together with either a 1% solution of hydroxyamphetamine or a 2.5% solution of phenylephrine. Concentrations of tropicamide or cyclopentolate greater than 1% are excessive and should be avoided. They may produce extreme central nervous stimulation in young patients. Atropine drops should always be avoided because of the hazard of systemic atropine poisoning should the drops be carelessly administered. Homatropine solutions in 2% and 5% concentrations are useful when it is desirable to produce mydriasis for periods of 1 to 2 days.

EVALUATION OF ACUTE LOSS OF VISION

In instances of acute vision loss (see box on p. 250) an immediate determination must be made whether the lesion is bilateral or unilateral. The patient's distance vision should be checked with corrective lenses in place. If a distance visual acuity chart is not available, reading vision should be checked. Ordinary newspaper print held about two thirds of a meter from the eye subtends a visual angle corresponding to 20/50 Snellen acuity. Each eye should be checked separately. The next step is to estimate the degree of transparency of the ocular media. If the examiner can easily see fundal detail but the patient is experiencing a major drop in visual acuity, then clearly the lesion must be either

CAUSES OF VISUAL LOSS AFTER TRAUMA

Problems in the ocular media

1. Lids (swollen) covering globe
2. Exudate or other material covering cornea
3. Corneal distortion
4. Intraocular hemorrhage
5. Dislocated or cataract as crystalline lens

Problems in choroid or retina

1. Retinal hemorrhage, tear, or detachment
2. Choroidal ruptures

Problems in visual pathways

1. Optic nerve tears, avulsions, compression, and so forth
2. Hemorrhage in chiasms or postchiasmal trunks
3. Cortical blindness: hemorrhage or anoxia hysteria, malingering, or both

at the retinal level in the optic nerve or within the cerebrum, and it is not related to any intraocular cause, such as sudden intraocular hemorrhage. If the fundus is normal, then another list of diagnostic possibilities must be considered. It is important to recognize that visual loss related to a vascular lesion close to the eye may occur in spite of a normal appearing fundus. For example, in retrobulbar neuritis, the fundus may be completely and absolutely normal with a drastic reduction in acuity. Temporal arteritis may occur rarely in teenagers. Whereas about one half of the patients have ischemic papilledema and another 10% or so have a frank occlusion of central retinal artery, a very large number of patients show no fundal abnormality whatsoever. In this regard it should be mentioned that involvement of the temporal artery may or may not be obvious. In the absence of obvious signs, such as tenderness and redness, a key diagnostic feature is the *incompressibility* of the artery indicating an infiltration within the arterial wall substance. Other lesions that may cause sudden visual loss together with a normal fundus are the following:

1. Hemorrhage into a pituitary tumor
2. Optic nerve tumor or inflammation
3. Parasellar lesions
4. Supraclinoid aneurysm
5. Third ventricle hydrocephalus
6. Carotid (or branches) arterial thrombosis
7. Fracture of the anterior cranial fossa
8. Basofrontal tumor skull
9. Chiasmal arachnoiditis
10. Pseudotumor cerebri

The diagnosis of a frank occlusion of the central retinal artery is an emergency in youths. It may occur as part of a hematologic disorder, such as polycythemia (Fig. 14-2). The breathing time of the retina is greatly limited by the reduction in blood flow. Ganglion cell death begins within minutes. Fundal examination is most important and should be conducted by someone who can detect the vascular abnormality. A determination must be made as to whether the phenomenon is embolic or thrombotic; the former carries a dire prognosis in older patients. Emboli may appear as white or yellowish shiny spots within the central artery or its branches. In the presence of these, one approach is to encourage the emboli to move downstream to a more peripheral position so that the circulation to the macular area is not compromised. Such movement can be effected by digital massage of the globe and by procedures that will increase the vascular perfusion pressure to the eye, either by placing the patient in a Trendelenburg position or by producing vasodilation of the retinal vessels. The latter may be accomplished to a moderate degree by rebreathing into a paper bag under careful control or by increasing the carbon dioxide content of the inspired air under more controlled conditions. Finally, and more drastically, the aqueous humor within the anterior chamber may be removed through a slit-like corneal incision (paracentesis). These procedures also may be of value in cases of thrombosis for which no embolization is detected. In the instances of embolic phenomena, anticoagulant therapy or fibrinolytic therapy may be considered, although there is but little evidence to indicate any beneficial effects.

If retinal edema and a cherry red spot are present, it is unlikely that the aforementioned therapy will be helpful. The hazards of entering the anterior chamber through the cornea are such that these procedures should be reserved for an experienced person or an ophthalmologist. In any case of acute visual loss, an ophthalmologist should be called so that the patient's visual acuity and field and fundus may be thoroughly evaluated. While waiting for the ophthalmologist the general physician can institute measures such as placing the patient in the Trendelenburg position, instructing the patient to breathe in carbon dioxide, administering digital ocular massage, and perhaps, administering acet-

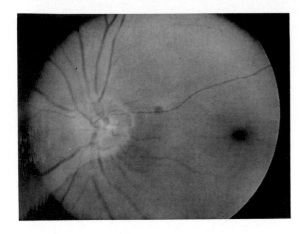

Fig. 14-2   Advanced central retinal artery occlusion secondary to polycythemia.

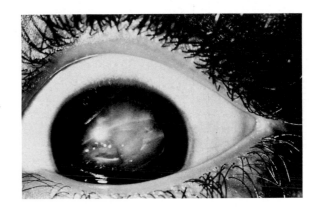

Fig. 14-3   Contusion cataract. Note split in lens capsule.

azolamide (30 mg/kg intravenously for children), a carbonic anhydrase inhibitor that will reduce intraocular pressure.

Contusion of the orbit and eye may result in manifold injuries. Cutaneous hematomas and ecchymoses may occur quite often, but any and every ocular structure also may be involved. The bony parts may be fractured, the globe may be seriously displaced or may actually rupture, traumatic cataract may occur (Fig. 14-3), or hemorrhage from any site within the eye or orbit or along the optic nerve may affect vision. Commonly in contusion injuries the macula may be the site of hemorrhage, swelling, or both. A thorough evaluation of the ocular structures is required to institute proper treatment and to discuss the prognosis with the parents and patient.

The differential diagnosis of orbital swelling in the emergency room includes not only mechanical trauma but also, in the absence of a clear-cut history, the possibility that orbital swelling is related to blood dyscrasia, infection, or tumor. Hemophilia and other hematologic disorders may be manifested by swollen orbits after very mild trauma. Patients with undetected insect bites or with cellulitis from a tiny sty may have orbital edema. Orbital swelling may occur in young patients in association with subperiosteal extension of an ethmoiditis into the orbit. Rapidly growing tumors, particularly rhabdomyosarcoma, may mimic sudden onset of orbital swelling occuring after trauma. Similarly, hemorrhage into certain tumors, such as orbital xanthogranulomas, may give rise to sudden swelling.

CONTUSIONS OF THE ORBIT

Orbital contusions produce a black eye. The picture of ecchymosis of the eyelids is well known but will need to be examined further to be certain that other orbital and ocular damage has not occurred. A black eye may be characterized by swelling of the lids and hemorrhage into them that may extend below (over the malar eminence laterally into the temporal fossa) and above into the subcutaneous area beyond the eyebrow. The hemorrhage may extend across the bridge of the nose.

The ecchymosis appears within hours and may be associated with conjunctival hemorrhage. Blood extending to the lids from an orbital fracture appears intially at the medial borders of the lower lids and may be sharply delimited to the area outlined by the orbital rims and by the orbital septa. With extensive injury, however, the septa may be violated and hemorrhage may extend into the lids themselves. Hemorrhage in both these instances occurs within hours. Seepage of blood into previously normal skin at the inferomesial border of the orbits days after injury should suggest a basal fracture in the anterior fossa. Other clinical signs of skull fracture should be sought and appropriate x-ray films obtained to ascertain the nature of the fracture and to decide whether therapy should be instituted.

ORBITAL FRACTURES

Orbital fractures occur frequently after automobile accidents, athletic events, pugilism, and accidents in the home or at work. Inspection and palpation will frequently reveal asymmetries or discontinuities. Lid crepitus indicates fracture into a paranasal sinus. Local altered sensation may indicate involvement of the supraorbital rim of the inferior orbital fissure. Many maxillofacial fractures are associated with head injuries. Therapeutic priorities must be established according to the seriousness of the several separate wounds.

Superior orbital fractures may involve the orbital rim, the roof, or the frontal sinus. The anterior cranial fossa may be involved. Neurologic involvement may include herniation of cerebral tissues and contusion of the brain. The eye may be displaced, and palpable deformities of the superior orbital rim may occur along with ptosis, involvement of the superior rectus, supraorbital anesthesia, and perhaps fracture of the trochlea. Optic nerve injuries are not uncommon.

Inferior orbital fractures also may show discontinuities in the rim. The floor and antrum may be involved. Comminution often occurs. In severe injuries the body of zygoma yields its attachment to the maxillary bone at its suture line with loss of the anterolateral wall of the antrum.

Blowout Fracture

Blowout fractures ordinarily occur in the region of the floor of the orbit. On occasion the medial wall of the orbit also may blow out into the eth-

moid. The injury usually results from a round object or fist that has a diameter larger than that of the orbital opening.

Pressure within the orbit during the contusion impact is raised sufficiently, so the thin floor of the orbit or medial wall will blow out into the antral sinus. There are four cardinal signs of a simple classic orbital blowout fracture include the following:

1. Enophthalmos
2. Loss of sensation over the malar eminence and cheek
3. Inability to look up on the affected side and, depending on the visual acuity, diplopia
4. Positive traction test

A positive traction test is particularly essential in the diagnosis, but it is difficult to establish with any degree of certainty unless the patient's cooperation is carefully solicited. The conjunctival cul-de-sac must be anesthetized with 0.5% tetracaine or with a 4% solution of cocaine. When the conjunctiva has been anesthetized satisfactorily, a firm grip of the episcleral tissues with a mouse-toothed forceps is obtained several millimeters below the limbus at the 6 o'clock position. As this is done, the patient is instructed to look upward. The globe, grasped through the conjunctiva and episcleral tissues, is then gently moved upward. A positive traction test is indicated by the inability to move the eye upward. This restricted movement is a consequence of the tissue and muscles at the inferior aspect of the eye being trapped within the fracture site. Ordinary x-ray films may be unrevealing or difficult to interpret for several reasons, among which is soft tissue swelling. Often the clinical signs may be more important in making the decision to repair the fracture. In any event, such a decision must involve the ophthalmologist because he or she will be responsible for management of any postoperative sequelae. These may include permanent restrictions of the movement of the globe, displacements of the globe, unsightly cosmetic defects, and of course, the most annoying functional consequence, diplopia in any of the cardinal positions of gaze.

The proper indications for the repair of an orbital floor fracture are to prevent diplopia and significant cosmetic defects. Sometimes serious ocular injury coexists. In that event surgical repair of the blowout fracture is rarely justifiable. On other occasions the blowout fracture is a small part of a serious injury to the life and limb of the patient. In this situation management of the serious head injury is obviously the first priority. Surgery for an orbital blowout fracture never should be considered an emergency. In most instances surgery can be easily delayed until the orbital swelling is reduced so that exploration may be facilitated. Often diplopia is not noted at first in patients with extensive defects of the floor because the inferior oblique and rectus muscles can move quite freely. Later, however, scarring will trap these muscles. Therefore, initially an attempt should be made to repair the floor of the orbit. On the other hand the patient who does have diplopia and a positive traction test usually has a less extensive orbital fracture site, often hinged, in which the muscles have become incarcerated. Under these conditions surgical exploration is required to prevent postoperative diplopia.

Lateral Orbital Fractures

An important associated fracture is discontinuity of the zygoma. The zygomatic bone forms the roof of the maxillary sinus, the lateral portion of the inferior orbital rim, and a good deal of the lateral wall of the orbit. With orbital fracture of the zygoma, the lateral canthal ligament may be involved because its insertion is on the zygoma. (This is particularly true in fracture-dislocations of the zygoma.) Notching of the orbital rim may be palpated, and extensive fractures of the floor may be noted readily or they may be subtle. X-ray examination should include a Waters view and a Cald-

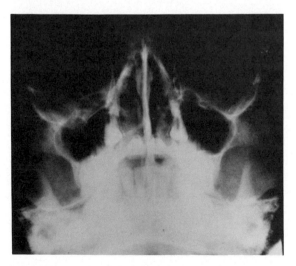

Fig. 14-4 Classic, but not always usual, picture of orbital floor fracture, with herniation of soft tissue into right antrum.

well view. When fracture of the zygomatic arch is present, a vertical submental view is important. With the occurrence of dislocation, reduction of the fracture-dislocation is necessary. In this case an oral approach is useful. If the zygomatic arch is involved in the fracture, an incision can be made in the scalp in the hairline above the ear, an elevator can be passed beneath superficial fascia of the temporalis muscle and directly beneath the zygomatic arch to the medial surface of the bone. The fracture can then be reduced by applying external pressure.

A comment should be made about the use of x-ray films in fractures of the orbit. Fractures may not be diagnosed by standard x-ray techniques, even though they may be suggested by some clinical signs mentioned previously. The percentage of accurate diagnoses of fracture of the orbit will increase if the x-ray technique is of high quality. Ordinary plain views may not be abnormal (Fig. 14-4). With improved tomographic techniques a fracture of even the medial wall of the orbit in difficult cases can be readily diagnosed.

Surgical Repair of a Blowout Fracture: Orbital Approach

Three types of skin incisions are available: last margin, lower lid fold, or inferior orbital rim. Without a doubt the first is preferred because it leaves the least residue. However, it requires the most care in handling the orbicularis and in dissecting the periosteum from the floor of the orbit without violating the inferior orbital septum.

Once the periosteum is elevated, slow, steady, and careful dissection—usually blunt—suffices to expose the fracture site. Excessive pressure must not be put on the globe. If necessary, a thin Silastic implant or Supramid can be used to reconstruct the floor after the incarcerated orbital contents are freed. The floor periosteum is sewn back to the orbital rim periosteum and the overlying tissues closed. Before closure it is essential to be certain that the globe moves freely, corroborating the fracture reduction.

On occasion a Caldwell-Luc approach with evacuation of the antrum and gentle packing may be required.

HEMORRHAGE

After contusion, bleeding into the anterior chamber may occur as a result of iridodialysis or, more commonly, from the face of the ciliary body.

Hyphema

Bleeding into the anterior chamber of the eye may occur with severe or even with mild trauma. After contusion hyphema may give rise to a diffuse haze in the anterior chamber or to an actual blood level (Fig. 14-5). This primary hyphema will frequently disappear without therapy. The patient must be referred to an ophthalmologist, however, because dire consequences may occur (Figs. 14-6 to 14-8). Three to five days after primary hyphema occurs, 20% of the patients may develop a secondary, total, or blackball hyphema. Rebleeding probably occurs from lysis of the clot at the site of the original injury. The treatment of this condition is complex and requires the attention of the ophthalmologist, since in half the cases the eye is lost because of a lack of proper attention.

The primary hyphema should be treated with an antifibrinolytic agent and appropriate sedentary activity. If the cornea is intact and hence less sus-

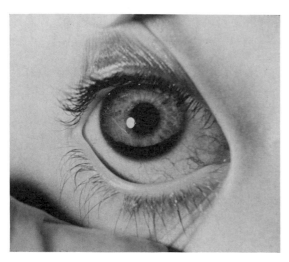

Fig. 14-5   Primary hyphema.

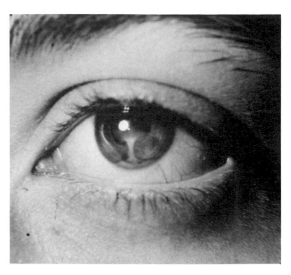

Fig. 14-6   Fibrosis of chamber angle and crystalline lens and secondary glaucoma after hyphema.

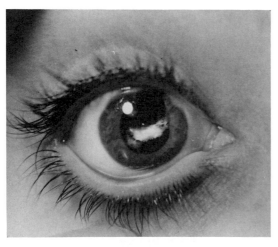

Fig. 14-7   Cataract and cyclitic membrane.

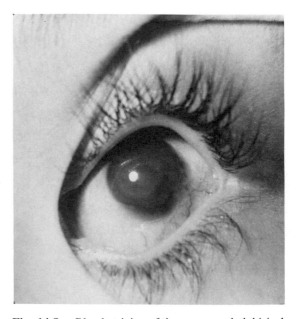

Fig. 14-8   Blood staining of the cornea and phthisical shrunken eye after contusion hyphema.

ceptible to infection, topical steroids may be very useful because of their antifibrinolytic activity. They will therefore effectively reduce the frequency of secondary hyphema. If the cornea is abraded, then the use of epsilon amino caproic acid, a newer antifibrinolytic agent, should be considered. The value of mydriatic or miotic drops has not been established. Follow-up care must be given by an ophthalmologist.

Vitreous Hemorrhage

This condition is very common after contusion injury. The patient should follow a sedentary regime with head elevated so that the blood will sink. Retinal tears, choroidal ruptures, and the condition of the macula can then be determined. The incidence of retinal tears or dialyses after contusion may be as high as 20%. Consultation with an ophthalmologist is essential.

CATARACT AND PAPILLEDEMA

On occasion severe ocular contusion will split the anterior lens capsule and cause opacification of the crystalline lens (Fig. 14-3). Dislocations may occur (Fig. 14-9). If the intraocular pressure is acutely lowered, swelling of the optic nerve head may be related to hypotony.

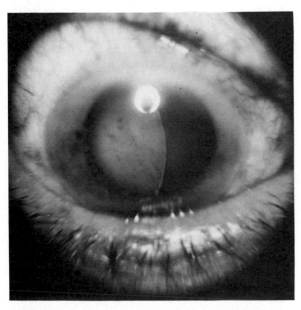

Fig. 14-9 Contusion trauma may cause dislocation of the lens.

PENETRATING INJURIES
Lid Laceration

Proper debridement, search for and removal of foreign material, and control of bleeding should precede the repair of lid lacerations. Before repair the cornea must be protected from inadvertent surgical instrumentation.

The aim in repair of lid lacerations is to prevent a contraction deformity. A key feature is apposition of the grey line so that squamification of the conjunctiva does not occur. In full-thickness vertical lacerations, the grey line should be apposed first, then the last line. The tarsoconjunctival layers can then be sutured and the knots buried. If the muscle and skin layers are closely separated with fine suture material, lid contraction and notching can be prevented. If the lacerations are extensive with wide debridement and excision necessary, then Z-plasty may be helpful. With lacerations involving the medial or lateral canthi, it is essential that these be reattached or resutured. As much tarsus as possible should be preserved, especially near the lid margin. Sliding tarsal or skin flaps can be useful but require the experienced surgeon.

Occasionally, human or dog bites are the cause of lid lacerations. Prophylaxis against rabies must be considered. Antiserum should be administered and the animal sequestered and observed. If rabid, a full course of treatment must be administered to the patient. Of course, tetanus toxoid and systemic penicillin must be considered.

Lacerations of the conjunctiva frequently do not require closure; however, underlying scleral perforation may need to be excluded by careful examination or exploration (Fig. 14-10).

Corneal lacerations frequently are closed by prolapse of the iris. A characteristic teardrop distortion of the pupil may occur (Fig. 14-11). Once the diagnosis of a perforated cornea or sclera is made, first aid therapy consists of protecting the eye with a shield (Fig. 14-12) and administering tetanus toxoid, if necessary, and sedation and analgesia. Broad-spectrum antibiotics are useful. The patient should be prepared for general anesthesia. If the patient is cooperative, a brief but thorough examination of the fellow eye should be attempted, as well as a search for a foreign body in the involved eye.

Direct suturing under the surgical microscope must be performed (Figs. 14-13 and 14-14). The posterior aspects of the wounds must be free of

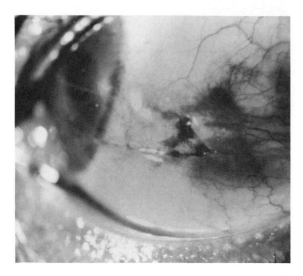

Fig. 14-10 Even a small conjunctival laceration should usually indicate the need for further exploration to rule out a penetrating injury of the globe.

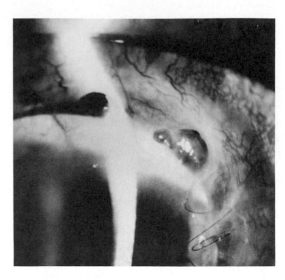

Fig. 14-11 Iris prolapse after trauma plugs a cataract incision.

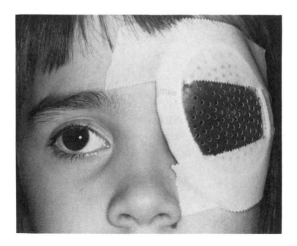

Fig. 14-12 An appropriate patch with shield to protect the ocular structures.

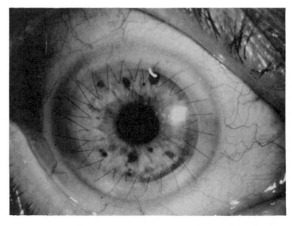

Fig. 14-13 10-0 monofilament nylon is used to close corneal wounds.

extraneous material so that they will heal without loss of the anterior or posterior chambers of the eye. Prolapsed tissue may need to be excised. The pupil should be widely dilated with long-acting drops to prevent seclusion of the pupil.

Lacrimal Apparatus

Fracture of the middle third of the face or occasionally fractures of the nose will compromise the drainage of tears and produce epiphora, an extremely annoying complication. Efforts should be made to repair defects to the lacrimal system (Fig. 14-15).

If the upper canaliculus alone is affected, there is little likelihood of epiphora. Occasionally with damage of the lower canaliculus, no epiphora results as long as the lacrimal sac is not involved. However, discontinuities to the lower canaliculus should always be repaired. A Worst pigtail probe is extremely valuable in these procedures. With the use of this probe, suture material and then soft silicone rubber can be threaded to reestablish the canalicular continuity, after which suturing of the lacerated ends of the canaliculi can be performed. The stent should be left in place for an appropriate period of time, usually several weeks. Primary repairs are not always successful. Later a conjunctivorhinostomy or other procedure may be necessary to eliminate epiphora.

With extensive fractures the continuity of the nasolacrimal duct should be checked with a large blunt probe. In some instances it may be necessary to introduce the probe from the inferior meatus.

Corneal Abrasions and Foreign Bodies

The cornea is one of the most densely innervated structures in the human body, and therefore the protection offered by its innervational anatomy makes the cornea the site of severe pain even with slight injury. A foreign body sensation may be produced by a tiny abrasion. Even with good illumination, the lesion may be missed for several reasons. The patient may be difficult to examine, or even in a cooperative patient the abrasion may be difficult to see. Fluorescein dye is therefore useful in diagnosis. A drop of sterile saline should be placed on a fluorostrip and touched to the conjunctiva. Excess dye can be removed with gentle irrigation. The examination is facilitated by the prior application of 1% tetracaine or 0.5% proparacaine. Wherever there has been epithelial denudation or loss or damage, a fluorescent stain will be seen. These corneal epithelial lesions may be produced by injury with or without foreign body, by contact lenses, or by infections, particularly the herpes simplex virus. Frequently a foreign body

on the upper palpebral conjunctiva may give rise to a corneal erosion, and equally as frequently a corneal epithelial defect will have the effect of making the patient believe that a foreign body is present under the eyelid.

After adequate examination with either magnification or fluorescein staining, the foreign body should be removed by means of a 25-gauge needle. It can be held with a syringe or other suitable handle. If the foreign body is situated on top of the epithelium, gentle removal with a cotton swab may be effective. If the lesion is in the visual axis, or if there is any doubt about the depth of the lesion, an ophthalmologist should be called to institute appropriate therapy.

After this mechanical debridement, the patient usually should be treated topically with a cycloplegic and an antibiotic, and a semipressure patch should be applied to the forehead and cheek. Under no circumstances should topical anesthesia be used for therapy. Cycloplegic drops are useful in alleviating brow pain caused by ciliary spasm associated with corneal irritation. Topical application of 10% or 30% sulfacetamide or 0.5% to 1% solution of chloramphenicol (Chloromycetin) is useful. Ointments should be avoided.

Foreign Bodies in the Orbit or Eye

Detection of perforation in tissue dictates the need to exclude the presence of one or more foreign

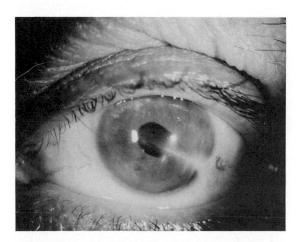

Fig. 14-14   Monofilament sutures are essential in the repair of corneal lacerations.

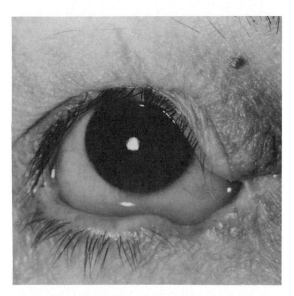

Fig. 14-15   Neglected canalicular repair results in pain and discomfort and serious complications for the patient.

bodies. Many foreign bodies will penetrate the globe at high speed and therefore cause little external reaction. Consequently, even in the absence of external hyperemia, it must be presumed that any patient whose eye is considered to have sustained a penetrating eye injury harbors a foreign body. Appropriate methods of diagnosis may re-quire x-ray studies, electronic, bright light, or ultrasonic methods of detection, CT scans (Figs. 14-16 and 14-17) and, of course, direct visualization (Fig. 14-18). The diagnosis of intraocular foreign body demands immediate attention because many are contaminated. With delay the likelihood of endophthalmitis increases. While cultures are pending, prophylactic antibiotics can be given in these ways: intraocular, gentamicin (Garamycin) 0.1 mg (100 μg) and cefazolin 2.25 mg; topical, gentamicin 10 mg/ml and cefazolin 50 mg/ml; and single subconjunctival injection of gentamicin 40 mg combined with systemic therapy of cefazolin (Ancef or Kefzol) 1000 mg every 6 to 8 hours or gentamicin (Garamycin) 80 mg every 6 to 8 hours. Furthermore, surgical intervention is not a matter to be taken lightly. The decision to remove the foreign body and the method of removal must be made by the ophthalmologist. Even with magnetic foreign bodies, the hazards to the vitreous body, lens, and retina are great. Removal is attended by frequent complications, some of which occur operatively and others postoperatively. The decision to remove foreign material depends on (1) accurate localization, (2) determination of the quality, number, and size of the material, (3) available skills, equipment, and service, and (4) associated injuries.

The hazards created by the removal of foreign bodies, even when these are magnetic, require the services of an ophthalmologist. In the best of circumstances, when the crystalline lens has been in-

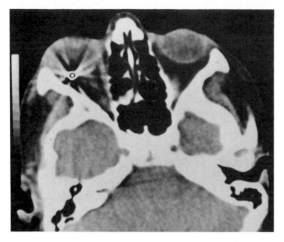

Fig. 14-16 CT scan showing posteriorly located intraocular foreign body.

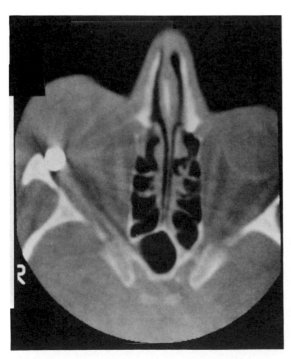

Fig. 14-17 CT scan reveals a bullet fragment in the orbit.

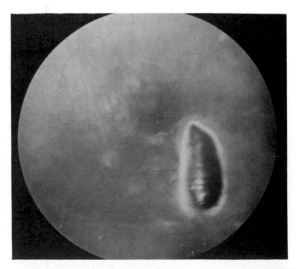

Fig. 14-18 Intraocular foreign body has come to rest on the retina.

volved, the prognosis for useful visual acuity can be as low as 50%. In cases without lens injury the prognosis for a reasonable outcome is still guarded because any penetration of the vitreous cavity may cause retinal deterioration months or years after an apparently successful surgical procedure.

The primary physician should take a careful history, determine the patient's visual acuity, and note the degree of integrity of the ocular structures with as little manipulation as possible. Usually the key to the mode of procedure will be ophthalmoscopy. Here a trained ophthalmologist is almost always required. Among questions that should be asked are the following:

1. Are there any antecedent ocular diseases or problems?
2. How, when, and where did the injury occur?
3. Is any material (for example, hammer or dart) that might have been at the scene available?
4. Tetanus immunization? When? Allergies to antitoxin?

If it can be ensured that the globe is intact, then a scout film of the orbit can be obtained. The uninvolved eye must be examined to establish baseline findings in the rare event that sympathetic ophthalmia occurs. Therapeutic decisions in that condition will depend heavily on the prior state of each eye.

Sympathetic Ophthalmia

This inflammatory response of the uveal tract occurs very rarely after penetrating injuries of the eye. The injured, sympathogenic or exciting eye develops a granulomatous uveitis that usually precedes a similar reaction in the second, noninjured, sympathizing eye. Although there are exceptions, the ophthalmia develops within 2 weeks to 3 months after injury. The inflammatory reaction can be suppressed (or even masted) by steroids. Sometimes the inflammatory lesions are so severe in the sympathizing eye that the sympathogenic eye may eventually have better vision. In this condition the primary physician should obtain baseline information for both eyes in the event that a decision must be made about removal of the offending eye. Furthermore, in the initial examination it is desirable not to manipulate prolapsed uveal tissue because the damage to the eye and the alteration of the uvea, as by cautery or mechanical stimulation, may enhance the changes of the development of sympathetic ophthalmia.

The lesion is rare. It may represent an autoimmune response to some as yet undetected and altered uveal protein.

Occult Ocular Perforation

Even apparently tiny lid perforations or lacerations may be associated with an underlying ocular penetration. The injuries are most commonly caused by sharp pointed or tapered instruments such as knives, picks, wires, and scissors. The conjunctiva in these cases may be normal if the object has been directed posteriorly. Thus a complete ocular examination is useful. Although the wounds created may be self-sealing, evaluation of damage to intraocular structures still must be made to protect the retina and other structures susceptible to injury from the sequelae of hemorrhage, tear, and detachment of retina. If intraocular penetration cannot be excluded because of the patient's age and lack of cooperation, an adequate examination should be conducted with the patient under sedation.

CHEMICAL INJURIES

Alkali burns, especially, and acid burns require emergency attention. All the damage caused by inorganic acids, organic acids, and anhydrides will occur within a few hours. Thereafter little or no further penetration or progression occurs. Alkali precipitate tissue progressively for many hours and even days. Alkaline burns are the most severe chemical ocular injuries. The entire anterior segment of the globe may become disorganized. Alkali binds reversibly to tissue protein, and the destruction continues. Furthermore, cell membranes are essentially saponified and destroyed allowing easy penetration. Lime (CaO) or caustic soda or lye (NaOH or KOH) are the most common offenders.

The mainstay of therapy in these conditions is instant attention to the cornea and cul-de-sac. Double lid eversion coupled with copious lavage is essential. The conjunctival fornices will require debridement to remove foreign material. Sedation and analgesia may be employed so that the work can be conducted more effectively. Early and continuous treatment for 20 to 30 minutes with irrigation by normal saline or a balanced salt solution is required. It should be remembered that water is almost a universal solvent, and it is usually available. It should be used until a more physiologic solution can be obtained. The ophthalmologist may decide to perform paracentesis or to employ other mea-

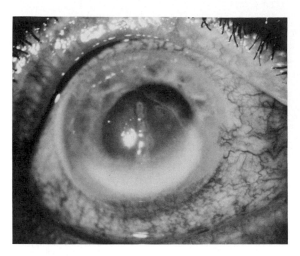

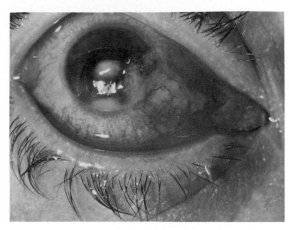

Fig. 14-19 Serious corneal ulcer and scarring may result from chronic use of local anesthetics.

Fig. 14-20 Corneal ulcer frequently is accompanied by hypopyon, pus in the anterior chamber.

sures to reestablish the normal pH of the cul-de-sac and aqueous humor. Mydriasis to prevent iris adhesions to the lens and cornea and cycloplegia to reduce ciliary spasm and cyclitis are additional measures. Antibiotics must be administered. Loss of cutaneous substance may require debridement and immediate grafting.

Lacrimators

Agents used to control riotous crowds irritate the mucous membranes, particularly the cornea and conjunctiva. Alpha-chloroacetophenone, or Mace, is among the most commonly used of the tear gases. These agents do not constitute the hazard that the offensive vesicants do. The latter include mustard gas, nitrogen mustard, and lewisite and cause severe corneal damage and damage to other ocular structures (Figs. 14-19 and 14-20). The lacrimators, on the other hand, produce copious tearing, and the irritation is short lived. There is immediate ocular hyperemia and blepharospasm and uncontrolled tear formation. No permanent effects occur unless the concentration of the gas is very high and the gas is confined. Early copious lavage is important, and oral analgesics may help.

Permanent damage from these irritants result from the instruments used to propel them. When the sprays, shells, bombs, or tear-gas pens are held too close to the eye, they may produce severe contusions or even ocular penetrations. Most commonly, corneal abrasions may occur, and these should be treated as previously indicated.

THERMAL BURNS

Usually, thermal burns do not affect the globe but can cause partial or full-thickness skin loss in the eyelids. In many instances the involvement of the face and skin of the lids are part of a systemic problem. Usually the responsibility for the management of the patient lies with the general surgeon. First, it is necessary to combat shock by the replacement of fluid. Local attention is required to prevent sepis and to restore covering to the burned areas. In cases in which partial thickness is lost, a sterile dressing may suffice. In full-thickness burns of the lids, skin grafting together with full debridement is usually indicated. It will be necessary to protect the cornea with a bandage lens or moist chamber dressing. Occasionally, it will be advisable to create a conjunctival flap surgically.

Complications from cicatrix formation in the lids and cul-de-sacs can be devastating for ocular function. Therefore an early effective plan for conjunctival mucous membrane or skin grafting must be developed. Corneal lesions must be treated with appropriate mydriasis and antibiotics. Steroids usually should be avoided because of the possibility of opportuntistic infections during the chronic use of these drops.

SOLAR RETINITIS

Eclipse blindness or foveomacular retinitis is a lesion that characteristically occurs in young military recruits. Occasionally, sun gazing may be a function of incomplete ocular protection during the viewing of an eclipse or may be associated directly or indirectly with the use of drugs, but more often it is regarded as a manifestation of malingering in connection with military induction or duty. In the acute stage a white or yellow foveal exudate occurs deep within the retina. Later, with resolution, a foveal cyst or hole may form. The foveal ''reflex'' remains absent, and pigmentary changes occur in the perifoveal area. Thorough evaluation of the lesion requires a complete evaluation of visual acuity with several tests of macular function. Therapy in the acute stages with systemic or orbital corticosteroids is not of proven value but may be tried.

As regards the observation of a solar eclipse, at least two recommendations for safe watching can be made: (1) observe the eclipse on a television screen, and (2) allow the light from the sun to pass through a pinhole in one piece of cardboard and focus the image on a second black piece of card board held at a distance beneath the first.

ELECTRIC CATARACTS

Contact of electric current to the head may result in an electric cataract. Full development may take several months or years.

ULTRAVIOLET INJURY

A common painful and therefore incapacitating keratitis occurs after exposure to home sunlamps, to the sun at high altitudes (snow blindness), and in industry, after exposure to welder's arc. The action spectrum of the keratitis caused by ultraviolet light peaks at 288 msec. Stippling and edema of the cornea result in a cumulative manner within 8 to 24 hours. Cold compresses, cycloplegia, and patching are useful to control symptoms, along with analgesia. After 24 hours of therapy the corneal epithelium repairs itself, and the eye recovers completely.

IONIZING RADIATION

Soft x-rays (25 to 75 kV) produce effects that may take months to manifest themselves in the eye (for example, telangiectatic changes of a superficial nature and perhaps keratitis). X-rays in the dose range of 100 kV or more, as well as alpha radiation, will produce a cataract at 150 V as threshold to the lens epithelium. Several months may elapse before visual symptoms occur. The cataract may be seen in the equatorial area and may eventually be found in the posterior subcapsular region.

ATOMIC BOMB

Injuries from nuclear explosions are of three types: mechanical, thermal, and abiotic. The eyes show a keratoconjunctivitis. Later posterior subcapsular cataracts may develop. Changes in the fundus may be similar to those of eclipse blindness. Hemorrhage and exudates in the fundus are usually a result of sickness from total body radiation and are secondary to depression of the bone marrow.

ACUTE RED EYE

In children even mild trauma may call attention to an eye that has been previously irritated. Whereas glaucoma should always be suspected in an acutely red eye in adults, in children the likelihood of an acute glaucoma or an activation of a chronic glaucoma occurring is indeed rare. The glaucoma eye in children usually is seen as a larger than normal cornea, and it may show considerable tearing, falsely suggesting a lacrimal problem. Lesions producing red eye in children are more commonly either conjunctivitis, scleritis, or iridocyclitis. In conjunctivitis, hyperemia is limited to the superficial conjunctival tissue that covers the sclera. The causes may be bacterial, viral, allergic, or on a rare occasion, fungal. Overlooked viral causes are cat scratch fever and infectious mononucleosis. Each of these conditions is usually associated with an enlarged preauricular lymph node, and there may be lacrimal gland swelling. In conjunctivitis the tissues under the conjunctiva are usually white, but in episcleritis or scleritis the tissues are red and will usually not blanch after the administration of topical adrenergic agents. In addition, the scleritis often may be localized to one particular quadrant. Nodules may even be present. When a diffuse brawny scleritis occurs, an underlying collagen vascular disease should be suspected. In iridocyclitis the external hyperemia is invariably circumcorneal. The pupil may be held irregular by synechiae. In the presence of hyperemia without interstitial edema, one should consider the possibility of a vascular or hematologic lesion. The former would be a traumatic carotid cavernous fistula (Figs. 14-21 and 14-22) and the latter would include conditions like polycythemia.

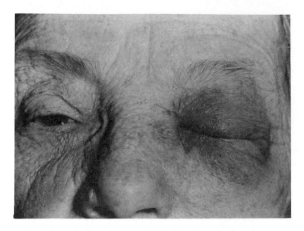

Fig. 14-21   Ecchymosis into the lids from orbital and preorbital hemorrhage associated with carotid cavernous fistula of a traumatic origin.

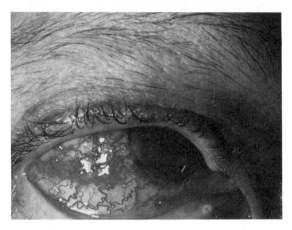

Fig. 14-22   Note the dilated veins and cavernous sinus thrombosis, sequelae to traumatic carotid cavernous fistula.

LOST CONTACT LENS

External irritation from a contact lens may cause corneal abrasion. Often the lens may be displaced into the upper or lower conjunctival fornices. The diagnosis is made simply by the maneuver of double lid eversion (in the case of the upper lid), or by careful examination of the inferior cul-de-sac when the lower conjunctiva harbors the contact lens.

CONSIDERATIONS IN THE USE OF TOPICAL THERAPEUTIC AGENTS

Except under the supervision of an ophthalmologist it is judicious to avoid the use of steroid medication, whether in the form of solution or oint-

ment, or whether on the skin of the lids or in the conjunctival cul-de-sacs. The risks far outweigh the rewards, especially in the presence of superficial wounds or injuries. Steroids will promote, accelerate, or enhance the occurrence of herpetic and fungal infections. In addition, of course, bacterial infections may supervene. Topical anesthesia should be used only for diagnostic purposes to facilitate examination of the patient with intense pain or photophobia. These agents should never be used therapeutically. Ointments are frequently prescribed because they may produce a soothing effect, particularly if the surface of the cornea is eroded for any reason. It is difficult to examine the patient after application of ointment, however, and furthermore the use of ointment in the presence of perforating wound will cause lipoidal matter to enter the eye. In some instances corneal erosion results because ointments retard reepithelialization.

OPHTHALMIA NEONATORUM

The term ophthalmia neonatorum is used to describe any conjunctivitis occurring within the first 10 days of life. Causes included *Diplococcus pneumoniae, Neisseria gonorrhea, Haemophilus* and chlamydial organisms. The routine use of 1% silver nitrate (Credé prophylaxis) has customarily eliminated gonococcal inflammation. When it occurs, however, immediate therapy with systemic penicillin or derivatives is indicated. Local cleansing and mydriasis may be useful. The lesion is important because it can cause corneal ulceration, perforation, scarring, and blindness (Fig. 14-23).

THE EYE IN HEAD INJURIES

The subject of head trauma is vast and has been adequately summarized elsewhere in this volume. An attempt will be made here to give a concise interpretation of some ocular findings in head injuries.

Birth Injuries

Certain ocular findings may indicate or support the conclusion that intracranial damage is present. Normal pupils are 2 to 4 mm in diameter. Light reaction may be sluggish. Dilatation of one pupil may not be localizing; however, the presence of pupillary dilatation, unilateral or bilateral, may indicate the presence of subtentorial hemorrhage. Occasionally the pupil may be small. Miosis may be

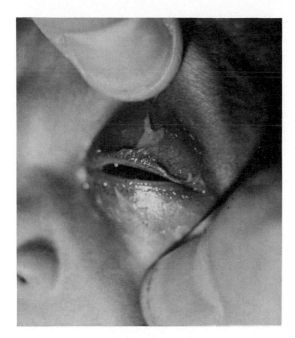

Fig. 14-23 Ophthalmia neonatorum: purulent conjunctivitis in the newborn.

present as part of Horner's syndrome and may indicate birth damage to the brachial plexus. If the complete Horner's syndrome is present, the spinal roots may well have been damaged. Birth injury to the brachial plexus may give anomalous pigmentation (depigmentation) of the iris.

Paralysis of abduction, indicating involvement of the sixth cranial nerve, may, when accompanied by facial paralysis, imply peripheral injury, as by forceps. Isolated third nerve involvement may be a result of a tentorial tear with consequent damage to the nerve before it enters the cavernous sinus.

The second cranial nerve, or optic nerve, may be involved in birth injuries.

Papilledema

Choked disc, or papilledema, refers to swelling of the head of the optic nerve from increased intracranial pressure. Early diagnosis, although desirable, is not easy without an experienced eye. Under ordinary circumstances the nasal margin of the disc may be blurred. In early papilledema the superior and inferior margins may become blurred and then the temporal border may become indistinct. The cup of the nerve head may be absent. An apparent forward protrusion of the disc occurs, but it may be difficult to appreciate without binocular viewing. Usually there is an absence of disc

hemorrhage unless there is associated hypertension. Sometimes one can see concentric ridges about the disc extending into the surrounding retina. These "highlights" may reflect early papilledema and retinal edema. If retinal venous pulsations are present, the pressure in the CSF is less than 180 cm H_2O. Absent venous pulsations are the rule in papilledema, but of course, venous pulsations are absent frequently in the normal eye. In late stages the diagnosis of papilledema presents no problem. In children with head trauma and consequent subdural hematomas or subarachnoid hemorrhage, papilledema does not occur for many hours, and in many instances not at all in the acute phase. Therefore the absence of papilledema should not speak against these diagnoses. The presence of retinal and especially preretinal hemorrhages is an important sign. Papilledema is only a late development. Optic atrophy may occur unilaterally as a result of orbital fracture or dislocation of the eye. When bilateral optic atrophy occurs, asphyxia is usually the cause, and other cerebral damage can be found.

Defects in the visual pathways are difficult, if not impossible, to detect. They may result from cardiac anomalies or from any factor predisposing to cerebral swelling and secondary vascular compression or from cerebral hemorrhage alone. Extensive bilateral defects may go unnoticed for months, whereas isolated homonymous defects may exist for years without detection.

Ocular lesions include retinal hemorrhages (Fig. 14-24). These are common and usually without sequelae. It is thought that macular hemorrhages may account for some instances of otherwise unexplained amblyopia. Corneal opacities may occur as a result of rupture of Descemet's membrane. These opacities must be differentiated from congenital glaucoma. Exophthalmos, as an extension of intracranial hemorrhage, may rarely occur.

Lesions in Infants and Young Children

The most important lesion to consider is subdural hematoma. Many of the signs and symptoms are nonspecific. In infants subdural hematomas are usually bilateral. More than half the patients have intraocular hemorrhage. They may be massive. Papilledema is not a frequent sign. Sixth nerve palsies are, of course, common. Although retinal hemorrhages are not always found in children suffering subdural hematomas, a preretinal hemorrhage usually indicates an intracranial hemorrhage.

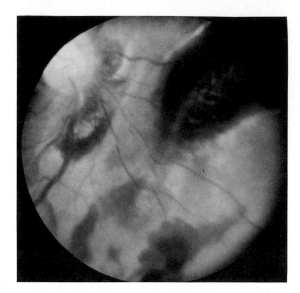

Fig. 14-24 Serious retina and choroidal hemorrhages and surrounding edema limit the visual prognosis in this patient.

The optic nerve may suffer avulsion or transection as a result of head injury. The fundus will be abnormal. There may be indirect injury to the optic nerve. In other words, there may be no obvious ophthalmoscopic evidence of nerve injury, yet a traumatic loss of vision occurs. There are anatomic considerations that can be taken into account to explain such loss of vision. For example, the course of the optic nerve is lengthy. From chiasm to eyeball 5 cm of nerve is vulnerable to injury. Considerable controversy exists as to whether there is any gain in decompressing the nerve in instances of otherwise unexplained visual loss. Intervention is considered in those patients who have retained vision after trauma but who then show progressive decreases. Sporadic case reports are anecdotal at best. In rare instances unroofing the canal or perhaps releasing the sheath of the nerve may prove valuable. Rapid decisions will need to be made within the first few days after a demonstrable decrease in visual acuity or in response to light.

THE EYE IN BODILY INJURY

Fractures of long bones may give rise to fat emboli that may reach the retinal circulation. These emboli appear ophthalmoscopically as hard yellow-white exudates.

Compression of the thorax, abdomen, or both may occur abruptly. The rapid sudden elevation of venous pressure in the head and neck produces retinal exudates and hemorrhages that may be numerous and extensive. A similar syndromic picture may occur in traumatic asphyxia or compression cyanosis. The prognosis for vision in these conditions is generally good.

OXYGEN TOXICITY

Once oxygen was identified as a cause of retrolental fibroplasia the decreased use of oxygen resulted in considerably fewer numbers of reported cases. The disease still occurs, however, and may go unrecognized until the child grows older and a retinal scar is noted.

Controversy exists about the precise role of oxygen and how its use in infants with respiratory distress should be monitored. Hemoglobin saturation and PO_2 levels are linearly related below 80% saturation when cyanosis occurs. Above 90% saturation, however, the S-shaped dissociation curve relating PO_2 and hemoglobin saturation flattens so that further arterial saturation increases significantly only as PO_2 rises. Therefore a pink infant at 90% saturation with an arterial PO_2 of 60 to 100 mm Hg shows little clinical change with large increases in PO_2. It was therefore thought that monitoring PO_2 levels would prevent retinal damage. A recent study has shown that the occurrence of retrolental fibroplasia was unrelated to arterial oxygen tension as determined by intermittent sampling of the umbilical artery. It is clear that the importance of the association between PO_2 levels and disease can be established only by a controlled prospective study. In the meantime a low birth weight and total time in oxygen appear to be the major etiologic factors. Not yet excluded are rates of change of ambient levels of oxygen and other suceptibility factors related to the developing retinal vascularization. In short, monitoring by ophthalmoscopy of those low–birth weight infants requiring prolonged exposure to oxygen would appear to be a practical solution for the moment. When possible, environmental oxygen saturation should be kept below 40%. Short periods of exposure to oxygen at concentrations over 40% are apparently not harmful. PO_2 monitoring can be helpful in preventing overoxygenation.

BATTERED BABY SYNDROME

Physical abuse of children is no more recent a crime than the abuse of adults, but recently in our child-oriented culture it has been given new importance. The idea that children, and even babies, might bear injury at the whim of their parents is difficult to accept, but the action is even more difficult to tolerate.

For the sake of instituting appropriate therapy and in consideration of the future welfare of the infant, an infant with ocular trauma should be dealt with as a battered child until proven otherwise. A history should be obtained and evidence of other general body manifestations recorded. Usually the child is under 3 years of age. Low IQs, illegitimacy, poverty, and marital and psychiatric disorders are frequently found among the parents. Cutaneous ecchymoses, ocular bleeding in all forms, dislocated lens, retinal and optic nerve hemorrhages, and papilledema should be noted. Proper referral to pediatricians, social workers, and therapists should be made.

BIBLIOGRAPHY

Callahan A: Reconstructive surgery of the eyelids and ocular adnexa, Birmingham, Ala, 1966, Aesculapium Publishing Co.

Deutsch TA and Feller DB, editors: Paton and Goldberg's management of ocular injuries, ed 2, Philadelphia, 1985, WB Saunders Co.

Emery JM, von Noorden GK, and Schlernitzauer DA: Management of orbital floor fractures, Am J Ophthalmol 74:299, 1972.

Epstein DL and Paton D: Keratitis from misuse of corneal anesthetics, N Engl J Med 279:396, 1968.

Nicholson DKH and Guzak SV Jr: Visual loss complicating repair of orbital floor fractures, Arch Ophthalmol 86:369, 1971.

15

Cardiothoracic Injuries

H. Biemann Othersen, Jr.

Thoracic injuries in children are age old. A book published 160 years ago[27] graphically illustrates the many accidents that befall children. Fig. 15-1, an illustration from that book, shows a child's chest being crushed under the wheels of a heavy cart. Whereas some of the accidents depicted are no longer seen (Fig. 15-2), general patterns of injury remain unchanged. Automobiles, minibikes, snowmobiles, and even skateboards have been "improved" to travel faster, and at their high speeds intrathoracic damage can occur from compressive or decelerative forces even in the absence of rib fractures or external evidence of injury. Such is the price of improved technology.

Since small children are usually unable to explain their symptoms to physicians, the pediatric specialist has a greater responsibility for diagnosis than other specialists. In 1774 an English physician, Hugh Downman, described in a didactic poem the child's dependence on others for diagnosis and therapy. Part of the poem as reprinted here from Ruhrah[173] should be read by medical students and all physicians who treat sick children.

Because the child, with reason unendow'd
And power of speech, by words to express his grief
Nature permits not; some believe the source
of anguish and affections is conceal'ed
From every eye, and deem assistance vain . . .
. . . Yet nature, in thy child, tho' not in words
Speaks plain to those who in her language vers'd
Justly interpret

The mechanism of injury should be investigated in each instance of trauma. A detailed history may indicate the preventable features of an accident, and by identifying the circumstances probable injuries may be predicted. An earlier attempt at instructing children to be aware of the many perils surrounding them is *The Book of Accidents; De-*

signed for Young Children.[27] Throughout the book a father admonishes his children concerning various injuries that may befall them (Fig. 15-3). The accompanying description to Fig. 15-1 was intended to be read to children, and it is brutally frank.

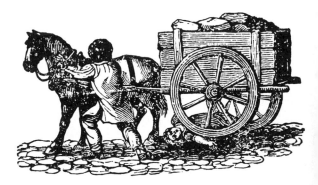

Fig. 15-1 Illustration from *Book of Accidents; Designed for Young Children*, 1830, an early attempt at accident prevention.

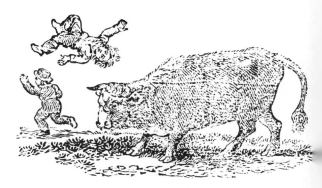

Fig. 15-2 From *Book of Accidents; Designed for Young Children*, 1830, one of few accidents described that are no longer relevant.

Careless children, in spite of warning, often run across the street when carts and carriages are near, and are knocked down and run over. Children have been so very careless at times, that it appeared as if they wanted to see how near they could get to carriages and not be run over. Here is a miserable little girl who attempted to cross the street as a cartman was passing with a heavy load. The horse has knocked her down, and she now lays under the wheel, where she will be crushed to death in spite of the efforts of the man to stop his horse. Children should be particularly careful when crossing the streets in winter, as sleighs are then running to and fro, with great rapidity, and sometimes being without jingles, the little boys and girls know not their approach until their danger stares them in the face, and escape is impossible. Children should always cross the streets after the carriages have passed.

ANATOMY

The child must be considered as a distinct entity and not as a "small adult." For instance, in indi-

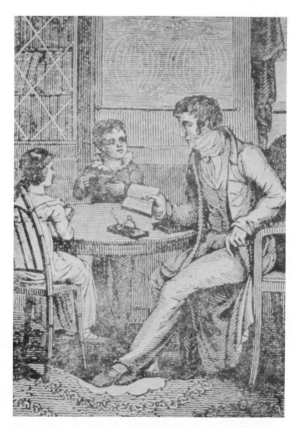

Fig. 15-3   Frontispiece of *Book of Accidents; Designed for Young Children,* 1830, an early attempt to aid parents in instruction of children regarding safety hazards.

viduals under 2 years of age, the cricoid ring represents the smallest cross-sectional diameter of the airway. As age increases the measurements begin to approach those of the adult, in whom the airway is narrowest at the glottis (Fig. 15-4).[166] These differences and their significance must be common knowledge to the physician treating children with thoracic trauma. The small structures of children along with minimal tolerances do not allow time for slow and deliberate contemplation. Therapy must be speedy and specific, and the child will usually reward the efforts with a rapid response.

Today, television offers an excellent source for instruction. Educational programs, especially on television, are expensive and time consuming but so is the treatment of injured children. It is in the area of prevention that innovative ideas and devices will save more lives and suffering than many complicated schemes of therapy.

Statistics now show that thoracic trauma is second only to head injuries as a cause of death in traffic fatalities.[19,106] In the United States 40% of the deaths of children are the result of accidents. In addition to the 13,000 children killed annually, an estimated 100,000 are disabled. Cardiothoracic injuries play a significant part in this carnage.

In this revised chapter, I consider individually the anatomic organs in the thorax and neck and further divide the discussion into injuries of a blunt or penetrating nature produced by external forces that may abrade, contuse, perforate, or severely compress the chest and its contents. Also included are internal injuries that may result from ingestion or inhalation of chemicals, foreign bodies, fumes, or from diagnostic or therapeutic maneuvers, such as those in which tubes are passed down the trachea or esophagus.

BLUNT INJURIES

Penetrating thoracic trauma is relatively rare in young children. In a series of 199 patients compiled by Sinclair and Moore,[185] blunt trauma far exceeded other types of injury occurring in children under 13 years of age. The sources of blunt trauma in children and adolescents are illustrated in Fig. 15-5. In children older than 13 years of age, penetrating injury is more frequent and follows the adult pattern.

The resilient chest wall of the child allows severe intrathoracic injury to occur without detectable damage. A paradox has been noted in patients with

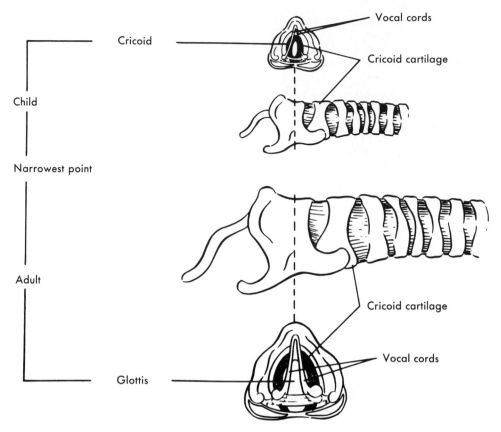

Fig. 15-4   Anatomic comparison of the upper airway of a child and an adult. (From Othersen HB: Ann Surg 189:601, 1979.)

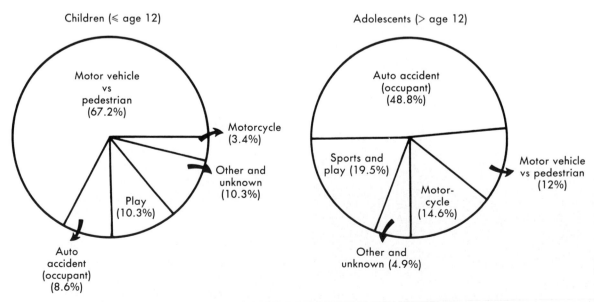

Fig. 15-5   Sources of blunt trauma in children and adolescents. (From Sinclair MC and Moore TC: J Pediatr Surg 9:155, 1974.)

closed chest injuries,[4] namely that the mortality is higher in patients without rib fractures. This discrepancy has been thought to be the result of the severe pulmonary contusion occurring in young children with pliable chest walls. In addition, Alfano and Hale[4] perceived that their patients with fractured ribs were more likely to have localized pulmonary contusion, whereas those without fractured ribs had diffuse pulmonary parenchymal injury. In fact it has been postulated by some[106] that fractures of the sternum or ribs expend a portion of the force applied to the chest wall, and thus injury to the underlying lung is reduced. Rib fractures may also raise suspicion of child abuse.[182]

Burford and Burbank[31] in 1945 first described the "traumatic wet lung syndrome" and attributed to this problem the high mortality of chest injury. Even with a clearer understanding of the part played by pulmonary contusion, the mortality of children with blunt thoracic injury was unchanged until the rapid methods of blood gas determinations were available and until volume respirators had been adapted for use in children.

It must be remembered that severe trauma usually produces multiple injuries and that the thorax is only one part of the problem. Rarely does one isolated injury, such as flail chest, exist without the underlying components, such as pulmonary contusion, pneumothorax, and so on. Therapy must be properly directed at maintenance of the airway and satisfactory ventilation along with optimal tissue perfusion.[82]

TRAUMATIC ASPHYXIA

Traumatic asphyxia is included as a separate entity because pulmonary contusion is only one part of the syndrome. Ollivier[140] in 1837 described victims crushed to death in mob violence, thereby first recording the features seen in traumatic asphyxia. A more complete description of the syndrome was given by Perthes in 1900.[159] The subject was reviewed in 1969,[212] but it was not until 1971 that the topic, specifically as applied to children, was described.[81]

The clinical features of traumatic asphyxia are cyanosis of the face and neck, petechiae in the head and neck and over a V-shaped area of the chest just below the neck, subconjunctival hemorrhages, and mental dullness. Mucosal petechiae and epistaxis may be present as well as hypopyrexia, hemoptysis, tachypnea, and lung contusion. The syn-

drome can be life threatening, and in severe cases spinal cord motor paralysis results.[101] This syndrome occurs when a child with a lung full of air and the glottis closed sustains sudden compression of the thorax. Apparently a brief moment of realization of impending disaster causes the victim to take a deep breath and brace the body to receive the injury. A sudden compression of the chest then raises the pressure in the superior vena cava and, in the absence of valves, the pressure is transmitted to the chest, lungs, neck, head, and brain. The compressing force may be a wheel of an automobile passing directly over the chest of the child or the feet of a trampling mob. Often children are lying on soft ground when the compression occurs and their resilient chest walls allow severe compression of the thorax without rib or sternal fractures.

The mechanism of this syndrome was evaluated in experimental animals.[212] Four events were necessary for the production of traumatic asphyxia: deep inspiration, closure of the glottis, tensing of the thoracoabdominal muscles, and compression of the thorax or upper abdomen. When the above events occurred in proper sequence, a sudden and marked rise in the superior vena caval pressure resulted.

The treatment of this problem consists of dealing with its individual components. Pneumothorax or hemothorax are managed by the insertion of intercostal drainage tubes. Pulmonary contusion is detected by frequent monitoring of arterial blood gases. At the first indication of a falling Po_2 or rising Pco_2 endotracheal intubation with positive pressure ventilation and slight positive end-expiratory pressure (PEEP) are indicated. Tracheostomy is rarely required because respirator support can usually be discontinued in 2 to 3 days. The neurologic signs usually clear rapidly with bed rest and elevation of the patient's head. A more detailed description of the treatment of pulmonary contusion follows in that section of this chapter.

CHEST WALL
Flail Chest

Since the chest wall of small children is pliable, fractures of the rib or sternum are not as easily produced as they are in adults. Occasionally a segment of the thorax may be rendered unstable by multiple rib fractures, and respiration is impaired. Clinically, flail chest can be suspected by observing the child's respiratory motions for evidence of uneven expansion of the chest wall. With suspicion aroused, measurement of arterial blood gases is imperative. The tendency for an elevated PCO_2 and a decreased PO_2, especially with even mild respiratory distress, indicate the need for endotracheal intubation and respiratory support. An evaluation of the severity of the injury can then be made, and if ventilation is required for longer than 5 to 7 days tracheostomy may be indicated. Most textbooks continue to show details of the external stabilization of the chest wall. These measures are not very effective in children. Wires passed through the muscles of the thorax or towel clips applied to the ribs and sternum and used for traction are generally unsatisfactory in children. Internal stabilization with a volume respirator is now the standard therapy. Only under extreme emergency situations when no endotracheal tubes or respirators are available should external stabilization be attempted. Any improvisation that will prevent the paradoxic motion of the chest wall will be helpful until the child can be intubated and assisted by a respirator. Often a bulky dressing and tape will provide temporary stabilization. Schweich and Fleisher[182] have recently reviewed rib fractures in children.

Avery et al.[15] in 1958 first described in detail the use of internal stabilization by positive pressure volume respirators in the management of patients with unstable chest walls. These authors called the principle "internal pneumatic stabilization." They reported that Versailes of Holland in 1542 was the first to use a volume respirator by employing a bellows to insufflate gases into the trachea. The techniques worked out by Avery and his group were quite detailed, and their recommendations are still valid today. They preferred uncuffed tracheostomy tubes and compensated for leak by increasing the volume of air inspired. That principle needs constant emphasis today to prevent the dangers of cuffed tubes. They also recommended slight hyperventilation to wash carbon dioxide from the lungs, thereby lowering the PCO_2 of the circulating blood. As a result the respiratory center was not stimulated and active respirations ceased. Alkalotic apnea was thus produced. With cessation of breathing, negative intrathoracic pressure was not produced, and paradoxic motion of the chest wall ceased. The overriding and grinding of broken rib ends were eliminated and patients made more comfortable. These principles of therapy are applicable today.

The initial volume respirators used for children were not much more than variable displacement pistons. A high degree of sophistication has now been gained, and new respirators are extremely versatile. In spite of the ease with which these patients are now managed, Duff et al.[52] in a review of flail chest believed that internal splinting by mechanical ventilation had displaced older methods but had not been shown to decrease mortality. In 1971 Levy[118] reviewed crushing injuries in children at the Charity Hospital in New Orleans. In a series of 51 young patients 80% were injured by motor vehicles. The author emphasized the importance of early blood gas determinations and recommended endotracheal intubation and mechanical ventilation by a respirator whenever the first indication of a rising PCO_2 or failing PO_2 occurred. Of the children in his series who were supported by respirators, only one required assistance for longer than 4 days.

Treatment of flail chest is as follows:
1. Establish a good airway immediately. If necessary, insert an endotracheal tube rather than attempt emergency tracheostomy.
2. Evaluate and treat other injuries and insert an intercostal pleural catheter if pneumothorax or hemothorax is present.
3. If arterial blood gas determinations indicate a trend toward diminishing PO_2 or rising PCO_2 begin respiratory assistance with a volume-cycled respirator. If respiratory support is required for longer than 5 to 7 days, a tracheostomy may be indicated.

INTERCOSTAL HERNIA

Even in the absence of rib or sternal fractures the intercostal muscles or pleura of small children may be torn by severe nonpenetrating compression injury. Traumatic intercostal hernia has been reported following blunt injury[175] and further described[190] in a 5-year-old boy 3 days following blunt injury. In that patient the lesion disappeared 2 weeks after onset with spontaneous healing.

Intercostal hernias characteristically appear as intercostal bulges that enlarge on expiration and disappear on inspiration. When large they may cause paradoxic respiration and dyspnea. Small hernias should produce no problems. The treatment involves surgical repair by closure of the defect with the use of surrounding muscle or fascia. Synthetic material should rarely be necessary.

PLEURAL INJURIES
Hemothorax and Pneumothorax

Any collection of blood within the pleural cavity is termed "hemothorax." Although massive pleural bleeding is more likely to result from penetrating injuries, hemothorax may result from blunt compression with rupture of the pulmonary parenchyma. A fractured rib may lacerate either the lung or the intercostal or internal mammary blood vessels. Unless a large artery is involved the bleeding is usually self-limited and ceases with tamponade by the lung or by the accumulating volume of blood itself.[136] The intrapleural blood may be accompanied by variable amounts of air, thus producing a hemopneumothorax.

Moderate quantities of blood may collect in the pleural space without producing symptoms, but large accumulations may compress the ipsilateral lung and then cause a shift in the mediastinum along with a compromise of the contralateral lung. At that time respiratory distress becomes obvious. Usually, intrapleural blood does not clot, presumably because of its defibrination by the action of the lung and diaphragm. For some unknown reason this process does not always occur, and rapid clotting may develop and make evacuation of the blood difficult.

Although blunt compression usually produces a mixture of blood and air in the pleural space, laceration of the lung, trachea, or bronchi may produce only pneumothorax. Mediastinal air from tracheal or bronchial rents may dissect into the pleural cavity with pneumothorax. A collapse of one lung produces respiratory distress but is usually not life threatening. Bilateral or tension pneumothorax creates a critical emergency. Tension pneumothorax occurs when air from a pulmonary leak accumulates in the pleural cavity and, without a means of escape, compresses not only the ipsilateral lung but with increasing pressure produces mediastinal shift with compromise of the contralateral lung. Lacerations of the bronchi or trachea may release large amounts of air but may not produce tension pneumothorax because the air can escape back into the brnchial tree through the rent. Pneumomediastinum from any cause may progress to bilateral pneumothorax. This condition occurs as a common complication of tracheostomy. Tracheostomy tubes do not fit tightly into the trachea, and there is always leakage of air; if skin closure is tight the air cannot escape and dissects down into the medias-

tinum and thence into one or both pleural cavities with the production of pneumothorax.

Treatment

The immediate goal of treatment of either hemothorax or pneumothorax following blunt injury to the chest is the prompt and complete expansion of the lung. The insertion of an intercostal tube connected to an underwater drainage apparatus is the safest way to accomplish that objective. Simple thoracentesis for removal of blood or air is not recommended because blunt injury usually produces pulmonary contusion. A sudden reaccumulation of either blood or air may coincide with the development of interstitial edema and cause sudden deterioration of the patient's condition. Any concern about the bacterial contamination of a blood-filled pleural cavity by the introduction of a catheter is outweighed by the need for complete expansion of the lung and the establishment of a "safety vent."

In small children the technique for intercostal tube placement is identical whether blood or fluid is to be removed. In the treatment of pneumothorax placement of a catheter directly through the thin anterior chest wall is not recommended in small children because leakage of air commonly occurs around the catheter.

Technique of Intercostal Tube Placement

After preparation of the skin with an antiseptic, an entry site in the skin is chosen at a point one or two interspaces below the proposed entrance into the pleural cavity. Usually the point of penetration into the pleural cavity is guided by the chest x-ray film, but if none is available, the skin incision is usually placed over the seventh to the tenth ribs and the pleural cavity entered in the fifth through seventh interspaces. After infiltration with local anesthetic, a small incision is made that will just accommodate the proposed tube. With a hemostat a tunnel is made upward two interspaces but not into the pleural cavity. The hemostat is then withdrawn and the chest tube grasped and inserted through the tunnel and plunged into the pleural cavity. Care is taken to avoid the intercostal vessels, which lie just below the ribs. As a substitute for the above technique, a trocar and metal cannula can be used to penetrate the pleural cavity and the chest tube inserted through the cannula. Recently, polyvinyl tubes in various sizes and with an intrinsic trocar are available. It is preferable to bend the tip of the trocar slightly so as to facilitate penetration of the interspace after the subcutaneous tunnel has been traversed. Before placement of the tube additional holes are made as required by the size of the chest cavity, and a small mark or nick is made in the wall of the tube 3 to 4 cm from the proximal hole. This mark then is used for orientation once the tube is in the chest, and the mark is positioned at the skin level. The tube is connected to the underwater drainage apparatus with a negative pressure of only 3 to 5 cm of water. This slight negative pressure helps to keep a constant flow of air and fluid from the pleural cavity. If the catheter does not fit snugly in the skin incision, a suture is taken to close the gap and this suture tied to the chest tube and the catheter further secured with tape (Fig. 15-6).

If, in spite of the intercostal drainage tube, the pneumothorax does not resolve and air continues to leak from the underwater seal, one of three conditions usually exists: a large bronchopleural fistula from a bronchopulmonary laceration is present; the chest tube may have entered the lung itself, particularly when the lung is stiff and nonpliable;[213] there may be a leak around the chest tube, with air sucked into the pleural cavity on inspiration. The latter condition should be eliminated by carefully inspecting the entrance of the tube into the skin. Fluid placed around the tube may help discover whether an air leak is occurring, and if so, nonabsorbable sutures are used to close the skin tightly around the tube. If air continues to escape in large quantities and a bronchopleural fistula is suspected, or if hemothorax does not resolve and blood continues to drain, open thoracotomy through the posterolateral approach is indicated for direct control.

Undrained or rapidly clotting blood in the pleural space may form a fibrin peel over visceral and parietal pleural surfaces. To prevent subsequent fibrous tissue organization and fibrothorax, thoracotomy for decortication is indicated. A delay of 3 to 5 weeks allows the clot to liquefy, and if the blood does not resolve or cannot be removed by needle, decortication is performed. By that time the peel is organized enough for removal but yet is not too tightly adherent. The technique of decortication consists of thoracotomy through the fifth or sixth interspace with dissection between the lung and the visceral membrane. By blunt dissection the peel is completely removed from the entire lung and diaphragm. In adults it may not be necessary to remove the membrane from the parietal pleura, but in children beginning scoliotic contracture is a definite indication for excision of the parietal peel. Enzymatic debridement as recommended by Tillett and Sherry[202] in 1947 is not indicated in small children because of the excessive febrile response to the enzymes and the large outpouring of fluid into the pleural cavity.

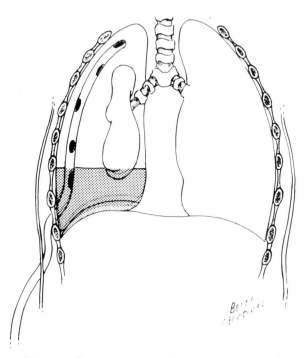

Fig. 15-6   Chest tube placement. Note oblique path of tube through chest wall.

LUNG

Pulmonary Contusion

The term "pulmonary contusion" is used to describe a blunt parenchymal injury that produces edema, hemorrhage, or desquamative alveolitis. These three pathologic changes may be present alone or in combination. Other terms used to describe this condition are "traumatic wet lung," "traumatic lung," "wet lung," "congestive atelectasis," or "blast lung." Similar clinical and pathologic pulmonary findings are found in the entities called "shock lung," "pump lung," and "fat embolization."[209] These latter conditions are often termed "traumatic lung," the name used to describe pulmonary changes that occur as a result of trauma to other parts of the body. The current terminology is "adult respiratory distress syndrome" (ARDS).

The pathophysiology of all of these conditions appears similar except for the initiating agent. To prevent confusion it is best to reserve the name "pulmonary contusion" for the injury produced by compression of the chest by blunt force and in which the lung is not directly lacerated. When other etiologic agents are involved, specific terms such as "shock lung," "pump lung" (postperfusion), or "fat embolization" should be used. Pulmonary changes, both anatomically and physiologically similar to pulmonary contusion, have been produced in dogs simply by the infusion of stored bank blood.[68] The changes could be modified but not eliminated by filtration of the blood. Thus there appears to be a toxic factor in the serum in addition to the deleterious effects of microaggregated blood debris.

Identical clinical, radiographic, and pathologic changes in the lungs may be produced by a variety of causes, and more than one etiologic agent may be acting simultaneously.

The clinical picture, as the pathologic changes, in all of these syndromes usually begins in a similar manner. Pulmonary contusion is commonly produced by blunt trauma to the chest, but it may be masked by more obvious injuries, such as hemopneumothorax or flail chest. Alfano and Hale[4] described a series of patients who were felt to have insignificant chest trauma and in whom the initial chest x-ray film was normal. Subsequently, severe pulmonary contusion developed over the ensuing 2 or 3 days, and some patients died of hypoxia. The appearance of the injured child likewise can be deceptive. With a resilient chest wall, rib fractures may be absent and the initial chest x-ray film may appear normal. Sudden compression of the thorax and the underlying pulmonary parenchyma is analogous to the injury produced by the pressure wave of an explosive blast. Before 1940 it was thought that blast lung was caused by the alternating pressure and suction wave set up by the detonation of a high explosive.[217] In fact the suction component was believed to be the most important. Zuckerman[216] found that by protecting the chests of rabbits with a sponge jacket he could prevent the usual pulmonary injuries produced by explosive blasts. Pulmonary contusion has been created in animals by diverse techniques. Border et al.[28] studied the mechanism of pulmonary trauma by dropping a weight onto the chest wall of dogs. Interestingly, they found that mortality in the dogs was decreased when the endotracheal tube was clamped, simulating a Valsalva maneuver. If the endotracheal tube were opened at the time of chest wall compression, mortality was then increased. They postulated that the lung full of air might serve as a cushion to protect against the blow.

Pathology

Microscopically the changes found in pulmonary contusion vary in degree and in distribution depending on the severity of the injury. Minimal damage produces only focal areas of interstitial edema, whereas severe injury causes a rapid intraalveolar extravasation of blood with consolidation of the lungs.[106] Webster and Blum[209] described the changes in the capillary endothelium of the lung that influenced the fluid membrane in the alveoli. They compiled a list of factors that determined the amount of fluid produced. After injury the pulmonary parenchyma may develop one or all of the following changes: the lower respiratory tract may be filled with fluid; the alveolar spaces may contain numerous red blood cells; the alveolar epithelial cells could become swollen and shoved into the alveolar spaces, producing desquamative alveolitis. By electron microscopic analysis these investigators demonstrated that the early lesion of pulmonary contusion is swelling of the endothelial cells followed by a widening of the canals between these capillary cells. Thus plasma is able to pass into the basement membrane and eventually into the alveolar spaces. This swelling of the basement membrane produces edema of the alveolar epithelium with desquamation into the alveolar spaces. The normal alveolar fluid circulation is then impaired as the circulating canals become blocked and a diminished secretion of surfactant results. The problem is that these changes are nonspecific and can occur in many different types of pulmonary lesions. Oxygen in high concentrations can produce identical changes.[209]

One of the few benefits of war is the improvement in therapy of traumatic injuries. Out of World War I and the work of Graham and Bell[73] came a better understanding of empyema. At that time surgeons described "acute massive collapse" of the lung after severe trauma, and most believed that the atelectasis was produced by a reflex diaphragmatic arrest or bronchiolar spasm. It was not until 25 years later during World War II that Burford and Burbank[31] described similar pulmonary lesions in their patients and coined the term "traumatic wet lung." They emphasized that the lung reacts to trauma just as uniquely as the brain or any other organ. As treatment for the massive outpouring of fluid and secretions from the lungs they urged meticulous attention to bronchopulmonary toilet by aspiration and by the relief of the chest wall pain with intercostal nerve block. With chest pain reduced, patients could breathe better and cough more effectively to clear their own lungs. This observation greatly improved the clinical management of patients with pulmonary contusion.

Clinical Picture

Initially the clinical and radiographic appearance of the child with pulmonary contusion may be misleading. Some patients are asymptomatic and have normal chest x-ray films or minimal patchy consolidation. Mild tachypnea and tachycardia and a few loose rales may be the only premonitory signs. In more severe cases, blood-tinged sputum is the harbinger of severe respiratory distress. After Alfano and Hale[4] stressed the insidiousness of pulmonary contusion, surgeons looked for means of detecting this problem earlier. With the development of rapid and accurate blood gas determinations, it is now recognized that changes in arterial blood gas values may precede clinical and radiographic signs of pulmonary contusion. Initial and serial blood gas determinations are recommended for all patients with pulmonary injury.[190] The percentage of oxygen in the inspired air must be known to interpret the results. The partial pressure of oxygen in the blood should be equal to the barometric pressure minus the partial pressure of water multiplied by the percentage of inspired oxygen and minus the partial pressure of carbon dioxide. The equation can be written as follows:

$$PaO_2 = (PB - PH_2O \times FIO_2 - PaCO_2$$

In estimating the severity of injury Fulton[67] uses the following percentage difference:

$$PO_2 \, (\%) \text{ as } \frac{(PO_2 \text{ expected} - PO_2 \text{ measured})}{PO_2 \text{ expected}} \times 100$$

A further refinement of evaluation is the alveolar-arterial difference in O_2, and this difference can be followed more accurately than PaO_2 alone.[214]

1. On 100% O_2 for 15 minutes (most accurate with respirator)

$$PAO_2 = PB - PH_2O - PaCO_2$$

2. On less than 100% O_2

$$PAO_2 - FIO_2 \times (PB - PH_2O) - PaCO_2$$

3. Derivation of A-aDO$_2$

$$A\text{-}aDO_2 = PAO_2 - PaO_2$$

Where PB represents barometric pressure 760 mm Hg at sea level, PH_2O is partial pressure water 47 mm Hg, PAO_2 is alveolar O_2 tension, PaO_2 is arterial O_2 tension, $PaCO_2$ is arterial CO_2 tension, and $A\text{-}aDO_2$ is the difference between alveolar and arterial PO_2.

The normal arterial oxygen (PaO_2) in children should be 70 to 100 mm of mercury. A slightly low or decreasing PaO_2 and an elevated or increasing $PaCO_2$ on the initial sample is indicative of pulmonary injury, and most likely endotracheal intubation or tracheostomy will be required. Even when the $PaCO_2$ has returned to normal, an abnormal alveolar-arterial oxygen tension difference ($A\text{-}aDO_2$) with the patient in a high concentration of inspired oxygen usually indicates a pulmonary complication or the continuation and progression of pulmonary contusion. This finding should alert the physician to investigate completely the status of the respiratory system.[167] The value of initial and serial blood gas determinations cannot be overemphasized, and no child who has sustained thoracic or multiple injuries should be treated without the benefit of these laboratory determinations.[25]

Treatment

The best treatment starts with early recognition. The goal of therapy is to restore and maintain adequate oxygenation.[106] Depending on the severity of injury and the rapidity of onset of symptoms, patients may be divided into three groups—minimal, moderate, and severe. General measures are of value in all three groups. Moderate elevation of the patient's head and careful limitation of intravenous fluids are helpful adjuncts. It has been shown that in dogs the intravenous infusion of isotonic sodium chloride in amounts and at rates of injection that had little effect on the lungs of normal animals produced pulmonary edema in even the slightly traumatized lung.[45] For that reason intravenous fluid administration should be carefully monitored and should be given only in amounts necessary to restore blood volume and to maintain adequate urine output. Skillman et al.[186] described the improvement of patients given concentrated salt-poor albumin and an intravenous diuretic, ethacrynic acid. An initial dose for children would be salt-poor albumin 0.5 g/kg and ethacrynic acid or furosemide 1 mg/kg. These drugs are given immediately after injury and daily or more often as determined by the response. Good tracheobronchial care to include tracheal suction and physical therapy are essential. Ultrasonic nebulization may help decrease the viscosity of secretions, and with adequate relief of pain by narcotics or intercostal nerve blocks tracheal secretions can be coughed up. Because the superimposition of infection on pulmonary contusion can be disastrous, broad-spectrum antibiotics are given. A suitable combination of antibiotics for children is penicillin G, 100,000 units/kg/day and gentamycin 3 to 5 mg/kg/day. Both of these antibiotics can be given intravenously every 8 hours. Sputum cultures are obtained before the administration of antibiotics. The role of steroids in initial therapy continues to be controversial.[106] The exact mechanism of the benefits of steroids is still unknown. Humidified oxygen is supplied in concentrations necessary only to keep the arterial blood at 90% saturation.

Pulmonary consolidation in patients with minimal pulmonary contusion should clear rapidly within 48 to 72 hours. Figs. 15-7, 15-8, and 15-9 demonstrate the radiographic appearance of severe pulmonary contusion along with computed tomography (CT). Those who fall within the category of moderate injury are usually manifest by copious secretions that eventually become blood tinged. When clinical symptoms appear early or when blood gas determinations first indicate a departure from normal, endotracheal intubation should be conducted with careful tracheal and bronchial toilet. If the clinical and radiographic picture then indicates a rapidly advancing extensive pulmonic consolidation, then it is evident that the intubation and mechanical ventilaton will be required for longer than 48 hours. An elective tracheostomy may then be indicated. Ventilation with a volume cycled respirator is initiated with increasing concentration of inspired oxygen as necessary to maintain PaO_2 at 70 to 100 mm Hg. If increasing FIO_2 does not accomplish the desired result the pressure of the inspired gases is gradually increased until adequate oxygenation is established. A nasogastric tube is placed to suction to prevent aspiration of gastric contents.

It is important to remember that endotracheal tubes should not fit too tightly in the trachea. Compensation for leak around the tube can be made simply by increasing the tidal volume. *Cuffed tubes*

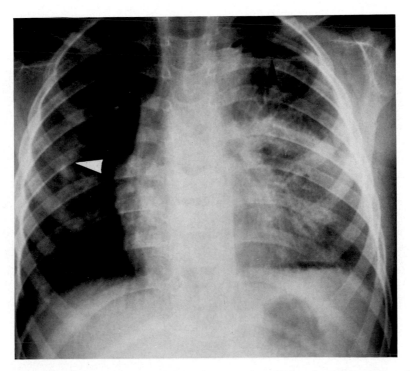

Fig. 15-7   Child with blunt trauma in motor vehicle accident. White arrow shows early pulmonary contusion. Black arrow demonstrates pneumothorax in apex on left.

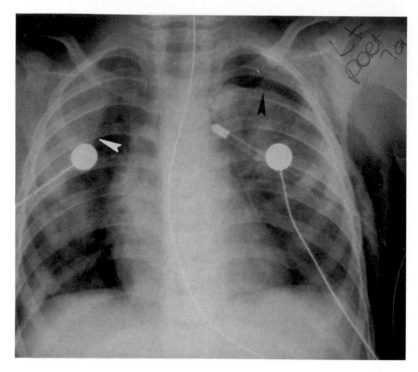

Fig. 15-8   Progressing pulmonary contusion *(white arrow)* and pneumothorax persisting *(black arrow)* in spite of chest tube.

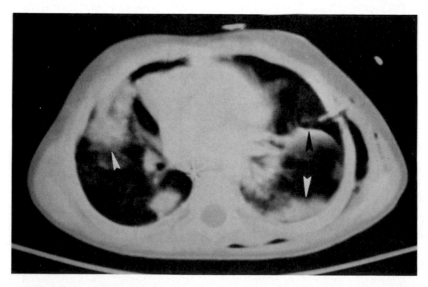

Fig. 15-9   Computerized tomographic (CT) view of chest with contusion *(white arrows)* and pneumothorax *(black arrow)*.

are unnecessary in children. If intubation will be required for longer than 48 to 72 hours, or if mechanical ventilation is required, tracheostomy should be considered. It is much better to begin the above therapy early rather than to await diffuse pulmonic consolidation.

Since arterial blood gas determinations are essential to the therapy of pulmonary contusion, it is desirable to have an indwelling arterial cannula for sampling of blood. In most children percutaneous puncture of the radial artery can be performed easily with a 20 gauge or 22 gauge Jelco-type needle (plastic cannula). Before placement the radial artery should be compressed to check for adequacy of the blood supply to the hand via the ulnar collaterals. A Doppler flowmeter is helpful in this maneuver. The temporal artery is no longer used because of the danger of retrograde cerebral embolization.[164]

Patients who show initial response to treatment and then develop progressive deterioration of the arterial Po_2 and widening of the alveolar-arterial oxygen tension gradient (A-aDo_2) should be suspected as having developed complications from infection (pneumonia) or embolization of fat or clot. Furthermore, even with prompt treatment some patients rapidly progress to complete consolidation. Until recently there has been no therapy available for these children. The membrane oxygenator now offers some hope,[93] although extracorporeal membrane oxygenation (ECMO) is currently primarily indicated and useful in neonates. It has been established that the lungs will improve if given time to recover while oxygenation is furnished through the membrane oxygenator.[106] Further development in this area has occurred with technical refinements of the oxygenator. Older children still do not respond to this therapy as well as infants with meconium aspiration.[157]

Bronchopulmonary Laceration

Large lacerations of the lung or tracheobronchial tree can occur with closed injury of the chest. Usually a massive pneumothorax is produced and after insertion of a drainage tube, air continues to leak profusely. Often the diagnosis is missed initially and complete transection of a bronchus may be undetected. Larizadeh,[113] in reporting the cases of two young boys with bronchial rupture, noted that the first successful repair of bronchial rupture due to penetrating wound was performed by Sanger in 1945, but it was not until 1949 that Griffith repaired

a bronchus that had been completely severed 8 months previously by blunt injury. Other reports can be found of complete transection of a bronchus with late repair. There is disagreement regarding the manner in which bronchial disruption occurs. In fact the exact pathogenesis probably depends on the manner of injury.

Various theories have been proposed and are summarized as follows[113]:

1. A simple shearing force acts on the lung and bronchi, such as would occur with rapid deceleration.
2. A bursting force results from an increase in intraluminal tracheobronchial pressure, as would occur with compression of the chest when the glottis is closed. Some experimental evidence in dogs indicates that rupture of alveoli occur before that of the trachea or bronchi.[38]
3. A sudden compression of the anteroposterior diameter of the chest leads to lateral widening and distraction of the carinal region. This force would be accentuated with the glottis closed and the lungs inflated.[38]
4. A compression of the semirigid bronchus against the spine produces rupture, but the more elastic structures such as blood vessels and lungs remain intact.[117]

All of the proposed modes of injury probably operate under different circumstances. The most likely explanation for tracheal disruption is that of increased intraluminal pressure with a bursting injury or a shearing force. When the injury includes only a segmental bronchus[162] or separation of apex of the upper lobe,[153] shearing forces or direct compression must be suspected. Actual torsion of a lobe without transection has been reported.[183]

Early detection and repair of bronchial injuries are essential, since atelectasis and infection commonly occur when bronchial strictures form. With complete transection of a bronchus, a fibrin clot may form and prevent further leakage of air. The bronchial ends then heal by granulation, and stenosis and obstruction gradually develop.

Aids to early diagnosis of tracheobronchial disruption are: (1) an abnormal outline of air in the trachea or bronchi with extensive mediastinal emphysema, (2) air in the deep cervical fascia as seen on lateral films of the neck (a distinct radiolucent shadow is found along the anterior aspect of the spine),[56] and (3) fracture of the upper three ribs. As many as 91% of all patients with bronchial ruptures and broken ribs had broken one or all three of the first three ribs on the side of the bronchial rupture.[32] A recent review of rib fractures in children showed no correlation between first and second rib and the severity of intrathoracic injuries.[185] Auscultation of the heart reveals a crunching sound with each heart beat (Hamman's sign).

With suspicion raised by any of the preceding findings, bronchoscopy may be necessary for confirmation. The procedure should be performed in the operating room with instruments and facilities available for immediate thoracotomy. If the diagnosis is not made early and stenosis develops, atelectasis may occur without suppuration, and late bronchoplasty is successful in restoring pulmonary function. Experimental work in rabbits has shown that complete ligation of a main bronchus produced atelectasis without suppuration when no communication persisted.[201] Even with a diagnosis of tracheobronchial disruption and with the child's condition stable, deliberate delay until acute edema and the inflammation have subsided has been recommended.[135] In these instances bronchoscopy and endotracheal suction must be performed to maintain ventilation of the lungs until elective repair can be accomplished.

Treatment

Rupture of the trachea or bronchi requires immediate placement of an intercostal chest catheter for drainage of air. If an uncontrolled air leak continues, and if the diagnosis of tracheobronchial disruption is established, thoracotomy is indicated. The preferred definitive therapy for tracheal and bronchial injuries is primary suture of the laceration.[55] Operation should be performed through the right fourth intercostal space for lacerations of the trachea or right bronchus, but with left bronchial injury, left thoracotomy is required.[78] The anesthesiologist should be prepared to insert a long endotracheal tube beyond the area of injury, and sterile endotracheal tubes should be available in the surgical field for ventilation of the distal lung if complete transection has occurred. Double-lumen tubes, such as Carlen's tube, are extremely difficult to insert in small children and are not recommended. The lacerations are repaired by debridement and primary anastomosis with interrupted absorbable sutures and careful mucosal approximation. Some believe that the sutures should pass through the wall and catch but not penetrate the mucosa.

If these injuries are detected late and stricture and stenosis have led to atelectasis, bronchoplasty should be considered if suppuration has not occurred. Extensive infection of the lungs will require pulmonary resection. Ingenious techniques for salvage of pulmonary tissue have been described, such as the implantation of the main bronchus higher on the trachea.[46]

Traumatic Lung Cyst

Acute cystic lesions in the lung may occur almost immediately following blunt trauma to the chest. These cystic lesions have been described as occurring as early as 20 minutes following injury.[156] They probably occur as a result of laceration of the pulmonary parenchyma with hematoma and entry of air from ruptured bronchioles and alveoli.[58] Most case reports have not been associated with chest wall injury and thus have been in children with elastic thoracic cages. The roentgenographic findings can be variable ranging from simple air cysts, resembling a poststaphylococcal pneumatocele, to multiple cysts with air-fluid levels resembling an abscess. Occasionally, surrounding hemorrhage and hematoma may obscure the cyst for a few days. The cyst need not be located in the area of external trauma and may be the result of a contrecoup injury.[60] A common location is the left retrocardiac region, and it may be confused with a congenital cyst or hiatal hernia.[99]

These lesions usually resolve slowly and require only symptomatic therapy and possibly the administration of antibiotics for infection. Resection or drainage are usually not necessary.

Smoke Inhalation

Severe injury to the trachea, bronchi, and lungs can result from inhalation of irritating and noxious gases. This topic will be covered in the section on burn injury, but because of the implications regarding airway management, it is discussed here.

Diagnosis

The early recognition of inhalation injuries to the respiratory tract is often difficult. History of a burn sustained in a closed space with dense smoke should be suspicious enough to warrant hospitalization for observation. The child in a burning house is a prime candidate for inhalation injury even if there is no thermal injury. Burns of the face, singed nasal hair, or cough with carbonaceous particles in the sputum are obvious evidences of respiratory injury. As in pulmonary contusion, the chest film may be clear initially. Bronchospasm, cyanosis, restlessness, hoarseness, or cough occur after 24 to 36 hours, and pulmonary edema may progress to bronchopneumonic changes.

The three criteria most important in making the diagnosis of respiratory injury are: flame burns involving the face or singed nasal hairs; burns sustained in a closed space; and entrapment in a closed space with smoke.[197] Arterial blood gas determinations are performed initially. Chest x-ray films may be normal. Recently, xenon perfusion ventilation lung scan has been helpful in the early diagnosis of inhalation injury.[2] Until these techniques are readily available for all children a detailed history and clinical suspicion of injury should be the most reliable diagnostic measures. Stone et al.,[197] in an investigation of pulmonary burns in rats, found that smoke and humidity were as important in the production of pulmonary burns as was temperature. Inhaled steam produced severe respiratory burns.

Polk and Stone[163] have described the following useful staging of respiratory burns:

Stage one—Bronchospasms, cyanosis, restlessness, hoarseness, cough, and negative chest x-ray film

Stage two—Pulmonary edema with the characteristic x-ray changes and frothy sputum

Stage three—Bronchopneumonic stage occurring 3 to 10 days after injury

Treatment

Smoke inhalation resembles pulmonary contusion, and treatment is similar. Arterial blood gas determinations are essential and initially only slight elevation of the $PaCO_2$ may be noted. Soon a decrease in PaO_2 occurs. The child should be placed in an atmosphere of humidified oxygen and the tracheobronchial tree cleared by aspiration with direct catheterization of the trachea if necessary. Corticosteroids (prednisone 2 to 4 mg/kg/day) for 24 to 48 hours may be helpful.[126] As in pulmonary contusion, humidified oxygen is supplied in concentrations sufficient to maintain the PaO_2 at 70 to 100 mm Hg.[189] If improvement does not occur, endotracheal intubation or tracheostomy is indicated. Again, care must be taken to select an endotracheal tube that is not too tight, since the damaged tracheal mucosa will swell and produce severe tracheitis in the subglottic region.

Hydrocarbon Ingestion

Ingestion of hydrocarbon compounds such as kerosene or cleaning fluids can result in severe pneumonia and death. This condition has been known for many years, and controversy continues regarding the best method of therapy.[206] Richardson and Pratt-Thomas,[170] in their studies of experimental animals, believed that the primary injurious effect of the hydrocarbons was inhalation or aspiration during ingestion and vomiting. They did demonstrate the harmful effects of oil compounds when injected intravenously but did not feel that absorption from the gastrointestinal tract was significant in producing symptoms. However, it is known clinically that coma and death have occurred in patients who did not aspirate or vomit. An extensive survey conducted by the American Academy of Pediatrics did not reach any firm conclusions regarding the best method of therapy, although the study did point out that aspiration was the chief source of harm to the lungs and that vomiting produced more aspiration than gastric lavage.[6] This report is contradicted by a newer study showing that vomiting induced by ipecac produces less pulmonary aspiration than attempts at gastric lavage.[138] There is still disagreement as to whether removal of the hydrocarbon from the stomach is important. If the amount ingested was small and the danger of aspiration while trying to recover it is great, it should be left undisturbed to pass through the gastrointestinal tract. Two well-controlled experimental and clinical studies of hydrocarbon aspiration demonstrate no benefit to be derived from treatment with antibiotics and steroids.[125,195]

Accordingly the best advice is to leave the gastric contents undisturbed if the amount of hydrocarbon ingested was 1 oz or less; if a large amount is believed to be in the stomach, careful gastric lavage or vomiting induced by ipecac should be the treatment. Antibiotics and steroids have not been shown to be helpful.

Penetrating Injuries

Penetrating injuries to the chest and its contents are rare in preadolescents, and thereafter the adult pattern is followed. Principles of management are similar to those described for adults by Beale et al.[16] An outline of their management is as follows:

1. A history of injury is obtained simultaneously with rapid and complete physical examination with the patient completely disrobed. An

airway is established by endotracheal intubation if necessary, and a large-bore needle inserted in the vein.

2. Sucking wounds of the chest are closed with a pressure dressing of Vaseline gauze or temporary sutures.

3. A urinary catheter is inserted to follow urine output, and a central venous line is inserted if possible.

4. If any significant degree of pneumothorax or hemothorax is present, intercostal tube thoracostomy is instituted immediately. For emergency insertion, a tube as large as possible that will fit through the interspace is inserted (as previously described in the section on pneumothorax), but the chest is entered through the fourth or fifth intercostal space. This high insertion is performed to prevent injury to a high-lying diaphragm and spleen or liver.

5. If the condition is stabilized the chest wounds are sutured electively.

6. Penetrating thoracic injury alone is not considered an indication for thoracotomy. After pulmonary reexpansion and replacement of circulating blood volume, and relief of cardiac tamponade, if present, reevaluation is made. Specific indications such as continued bleeding, persistent air leaks, or esophageal injury necessitate a thoracotomy.

7. Early delayed thoracotomy for evacuation of clots may be indicated for removal of large quantities of unevacuated blood. Thoracotomy is performed after the patient is stabilized but before a peel has developed.

These principles have been applied to penetrating injuries in children who were casualties of the war in Viet Nam, and excellent results were obtained.[18]

Prevention of Bronchopulmonary Injuries

Since most blunt thoracic injuries are sustained as the result of automobile accidents, the wearing of seatbelts by all children should be advocated. Constant education of children and their parents is essential. Knowledge and dissemination of the information regarding infant and child restraints should be made available to the parents of all children.[51] Very often programs aimed at the children will be more fruitful, and in the process parents may wear the seat belts more often also. There are now child-restraint laws in all 50 states.

Inhalation or aspiration injuries are usually the result of carelessness with dangerous material such as kerosene stored in containers formerly used for food or beverages. All harmful substances should be kept out of the reach of small children. Especially dangerous are furniture polishes containing hydrocarbons and fuels such as kerosene. Kerosene is clear and colorless and easily mistaken for water.

CARDIAC
Blunt Injury

The heart lies in a protected position behind the sternum and within the costal cage. Ordinarily, overt injury to the heart and pericardium is relatively rare in children, but cardiac contusion is frequently unrecognized as a component of severe blunt trauma to the chest. As passengers in automobiles children are not injured by the steering wheel but may strike the back of a seat or the dashboard and sustain thoracic compression to which the heart is as susceptible as other intrathoracic organs. One of the earliest reports of blunt cardiac injury was made by Akenside[3] in 1763. He described a 14-year-old waiter who was carrying a plate under his left arm. A blow by his master forced the edge of the plate between the ribs. He became violently ill, and his condition gradually deteriorated over a period of 6 months. After death, examination showed "on the left ventricle of the heart near its apex, there was a livid spot, almost as large as a half-crown piece, bruised and jelly-like; the part underneath being mortified quite to the cavity of the ventricle." This injury was the result of direct cardiac contusion, but severe thoracic compression can produce similar findings or even laceration of the pericardium, myocardium, the cardiac valves, or coronary arteries. Liedtke and DeMuth[119] in a collective review of nonpenetrating cardiac injuries presented the following classification:

1. Pericardium
   a. Disruption
   b. Hemopericardium and tamponade
   c. Pericarditis
2. Myocardium
   a. Contusion
   b. Rupture
   c. Septal perforation
   d. Late aneurysm
3. Valves, chordae tendinae, and papillary muscles

4. Coronary arteries
   a. Contusion and thrombosis
   b. Laceration

The shearing forces acting upon viscera such as the heart during high-speed deceleration can be calculated. An additional "hydraulic ram" effect of intravascular blood has been described.[115,194] Bright and Beck[30] in 1935 reviewed their clinical cases of blunt cardiac injury and described experimental studies on dogs. They produced direct injury to the canine myocardium and with distant compression of the vascular tree could not produce rupture of the heart, although the right arterial pressure rose markedly.

Automobile and motorcycle accidents account for most of the blunt injuries to the heart and great vessels in children.[37] Numerous case reports attest to the ease with which myocardial injury can occur. O'Reilly et al.[141] described a 12-year-old girl who fell while riding a bicycle and was struck in the precordium by the handle bar. She subsequently developed a pseudoaneurysm of the left ventricle, and cardiopulmonary bypass was required for repair. Moraes et al.[134] have reported the traumatic rupture of the ventricular septum in young children involved in automobile accidents.

As in pulmonary contusion, it has been observed[10,30,53] that cardiac injury is less severe in patients with fracture of the sternum or ribs than in those with an intact costal cage.

Diagnosis

Myocardial contusion is rarely obvious on initial examination unless complications such as arrhythmia or pericardial tamponade exist. Twelve-lead electrocardiography[119] has been found to be the most reliable means of demonstrating cardiac contusion. During the first 24 to 48 hours after injury, one third of the patients with nonpenetrating myocardial trauma will develop S-T segment and T-wave changes similar to those of myocardial ischemia and infarction. These changes may last as long as a month. If they persist longer, myocardial scarring or ventricular aneurysm should be suspected. Echocardiography can demonstrate cardiac structure as well as function. Serum enzyme changes are not specific for myocardial injury because significant elevations of serum glutamic oxaloacetic transaminase (SGOT) and lactic dehydrogenase (LDH) occur also in hemorrhagic shock. Fracture of the sternum or soft tissue injury to the precordium should suggest cardiac injury even if the silhouette appears normal on the chest x-ray film. It has been suggested that the diagnosis of acute hemopericardium can be made by x-ray films even with small amounts of blood in the pericardial sac.[191] The lucent epicardial fat line may be seen separated from the pericardium by a layer of blood. The presence of blood or fluid in the pericardial sac can be confirmed by echocardiography with ultrasound.[192] Since cardiac contusion can mimic myocardial infarction with similar pathologic changes and complications, ventricular aneurysms should be suspected in young patients who have sustained severe thoracic injuries.[191] The anterior descending branch of the left coronary artery may be directly contused and become thrombosed with resulting myocardial infarction.[155] Findings identical to those in the postpericardiotomy syndrome can follow blunt trauma to the chest.[181]

An unusual cause of mediastinal widening following blunt injury to the precordium was reported to be an intrapericardial hematoma.[72] Simple evacuation was effective. In any severe deceleration injury mediastinal widening should immediately raise the suspicion of aortic rupture. Depression of the left main stem bronchus or deviation of the trachea to the right are suspicious roentgenographic findings.[108] Definitive diagnosis is made by retrograde aortography. Repair of aortic rupture can be accomplished safely using a bypass shunt without extracorporeal circulation.[107]

Treatment

Cardiac contusion, like myocardial infarction, is treated initially with bedrest for 2 to 4 weeks. Patients should be observed carefully because rupture of a damaged myocardium can occur during the second week after injury. With signs of cardiac tamponade manifested by depressed arterial blood pressure, distended neck veins, elevated central venous pressure, muffled heart sounds, pericardial friction rub, and enlarged cardiac shadow, operative repair is indicated. Interim pericardiocentesis is of doubtful benefit. The absence of extracorporeal-assist devices should not discourage operation, since direct repair of a myocardial wound is possible. The bleeding point can be controlled with a finger or the atrium may be clamped to allow placement of sutures. (The technique of approach and myocardial suture is described in the section on penetrating injury.) Blunt injury with septal perforations, or injuries of the valves, chordae tendinae, or papillary muscles are best treated by early referral to centers where cardiopulmonary bypass is available for operative repair.

Penetrating Injuries

Cardiac wounds had been viewed as uniformly fatal until 1829, when Baron Larrey,[114] Napoleon's surgeon, treated a wounded heart by decompression and drainage and later demonstrated by experiments on dogs that these injuries were not always fatal. In 1884 Rose[171] coined the term "heart tamponade." In 1895 Cappelan[36] sutured a wound in the human heart, but the patient survived only 2½ days. In 1897 Rehn[168] sutured an actively bleeding wound in the right ventricle with recovery of the patient. In the United States the first successful cardiac suture was performed by Dr. Luther Hill in Montgomery, Alabama in 1902.[91]

In 1926 Beck[17] reviewed his cases and recognized the following three periods in the history of penetrating cardiac injury:

1. The period of mysticism, which considered heart wounds necessarily fatal
2. The period of observation and experiment
3. The period of suture, beginning in 1882

Beck described surgical approaches to the heart and favored median sternotomy to the level of the second or third interspace where the sternum was transected. He advised placing an apical traction suture in the heart. He held the suture with the middle finger and thumb and used his index finger to control bleeding. Sutures were then placed for closure of the wound. A technique to aid in closure of ventricular wounds is to insert a balloon catheter through the laceration, inflate the balloon, and pull it back to seal the opening. Sutures are placed and tied as the catheter is removed with the balloon deflated.

Several extensive reviews of penetrating wounds of the heart have been made.[123,199] The present trend is toward aggressive treatment of cardiac wounds with early surgical repair. Pericardiocentesis is recommended only to permit a short period of stabilization before operative control. If pericardiocentesis is performed, it is best done with electrocardiographic monitoring (Fig. 15-10).[24] Small wounds in the pericardium and heart made by knives, icepicks, or small caliber bullets do not usually cause death by external hemorrhage but rather through accumulation of blood in the pericardial sac and compression of the heart. It is now known that restricted ventricular filling is the principal effect of compression and not, as was previously thought, interference with return of blood from the vena cava to the right atrium. The pericardium is relatively nonelastic, and a small amount of blood (100 cc or less) may increase the intrapericardial pressure to the point at which death results from tamponade. With slow accumulation of blood or fluid the pericardial sac distends slowly, and its capacity may be markedly increased. The clinical features of cardiac tamponade include pallor, restlessness, air hunger, and sighing. Superficial veins are distended, and the neck veins show paradoxic filling during inspiration. Pulse pressure narrows, and systolic blood pressure is paradoxic. The pulse is rapid and thready. Pericardiocentesis is performed initially, and if bleeding does not recur, thoracotomy is not indicated.

Pericardial tamponade may also be produced by erosion of central venous catheters through the cardiac wall. This form of injury may become more frequent as central venous catheters are used for monitoring of venous pressure or for infusion of hyperalimentation fluids. In addition to the danger of hemopericardium produced by the erosion, tamponade may be caused by the infusion of the fluid directly into the pericardium. In small children the dangers inherent in movement of catheters placed in the neck veins have been documented.[64] It was found that 2 to 6 cm of movement of the catheter tip could occur when the catheter was placed in the neck and the child allowed to move the head

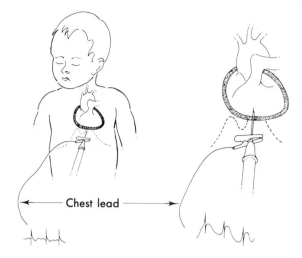

Fig. 15-10   Attachment of a chest lead to the pericardial needle. When the endocardium is contacted there is elevation of the ST segment, "the current of injury."

without restriction. Present techniques of tunneling the catheter to exit on the anterior chest wall may solve this problem.

An unusual sequel of penetrating wounds of the heart is the embolization of a bullet to a peripheral artery. The missile may enter the heart or its great vessels and be carried to any distant blood vessel.[205] I have treated a 6-year-old boy with a small caliber bullet wound traversing the thoracic spinal cord and producing paraplegia. The bullet then entered the thoracic aorta with minimal hemorrhage and was carried to the left femoral artery, from which it was removed.

Prevention

As with blunt pulmonary injury, cardiac contusion is less likely when children are properly restrained by seat belts in automobiles.

A good detailed history of injury will usually point to cardiac contusion as a possibility. The danger is in overlooking this aspect of the injured child. Electrocardiographic evaluation should be made of all children with blunt thoracic trauma.

DIAPHRAGM

The diaphragm serves as the upper limit for the peritoneal cavity and may be subject to extreme forces during abdominal compression. Just as compression of the chest may produce a syndrome known as traumatic asphyxia, severe abdominal compression causes stress at either end of the peritoneal cavity. A perineal blowout or rupture of the diaphragm may occur. Ordinarily the left diaphragm is the most susceptible to rupture. On the right the liver tends to protect the diaphragmatic leaf.

As early as 1579 the great French surgeon, Ambrose Pare, described the characteristic signs of diaphragmatic injury in a patient who had recovered from a gunshot wound only to die later of incarcerated bowel in an unrepaired diaphragmatic hernia.[154] Now most diaphragmatic ruptures are caused by automobile accidents.[128] The typical injury to the diaphragm occurs when a young child is struck and the wheel of a vehicle passes over the abdomen.[11] Among the damage produced by such an injury is a bursting laceration of the diaphragm. Penetrating injuries of the diaphragm are unusual in small children and rarely seen until they become teenagers and receive stab and gunshot wounds.[100]

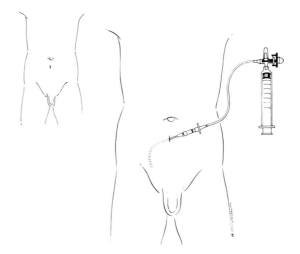

Fig. 15-11 Technique of peritoneography. A plastic cannula needle is inserted into the midline. Attachment of an extension stopcock allows the patient to lie on the abdomen. Contrast is injected, and with the head down it travels along the wall to diaphragm; with head up, to the inguinal region.

Diagnosis

Diaphragmatic rupture is evident when x-ray films of the chest show herniation of abdominal contents. A high central venous pressure in the presence of shock may indicate mediastinal compression by a diaphragmatic hernia.[65] Peritoneal lavage has been inadequate in diagnosing acute diaphragmatic rupture and is not recommended.[66] In suspicious cases contrast GI studies may be confirmatory. Perhaps in the future the accurate and detailed information obtained by positive contrast peritoneography may be helpful in doubtful cases.[145,211]

One area in which positive contrast peritoneography has been invaluable is the delineation of diaphragmatic defects and the differentiation of paralysis from eventration. Injury to the phrenic nerve during thoracotomy for division of a patent ductus arteriosus has produced paralysis of the diaphragm.[187] An elevated diaphragm especially on the right may be confused with an abdominal or thoracic mass. Peritoneography is simple and accurate. With a Jelco-type needle the abdomen is entered in the midline just below the umbilicus. The stylette is removed and the catheter secured and attached to a stopcock and syringe (Fig. 15-11). With the patient prone and the head down 30 to 45 degrees the contrast material is injected (2 to

3 ml/kg of 25% diatrizoate sodium) and films taken. The diaphragmatic outline is usually clear and precise.

Treatment

Acute diaphragmatic rupture should usually be approached by an abdominal incision. The entire chest is prepared and included in the operative field so that thoracic extension is possible if required. The abdominal approach has several advantages. Concomitant injuries, such as ruptured spleen, can be readily observed and treated. Both diaphragmatic leaves can be seen through the abdomen, whereas the thoracic approach allows inspection of only one diaphragm.

The technique of repair of the diaphragm is to close the muscle in two layers with interrupted sutures of nonabsorbable material. In some cases in which there has been loss of tissue and some tension, the sutures may be passed through small pledgets of Dacron or Teflon, which act as bolsters to prevent the sutures from pulling through the tissue. When large defects in the diaphragm preclude direct closure, Marlex mesh, Teflon, or Dacron-reinforced Silastic may be used to fill the defect.

If the initial rupture is not detected a period of time may pass before a loop of intestine becomes incarcerated in the defect, and strangulation may occur. Three phases of traumatic rupture of the diaphragm have been observed: acute, quiescent, and strangulation.[49,131,200] When a child is seen with an old diaphragmatic rupture and incarcerated intestine, significant adhesions in the abdomen may make approach through a thoracotomy advisable. The repair is then easily accomplished.

In correction of paralysis either the abdominal or thoracic approach can be used. The diaphragm is plicated with Dacron or nylon sutures tied over bolsters. A small Dacron or nylon vascular prosthesis is held on each side of the folded diaphragm and sutures passed through the prosthesis and the muscles, thus preventing the sutures from tearing through the muscle.

LARYNX AND TRACHEA

External

External trauma to the larynx and trachea in childhood is unusual, but the use of minibikes and motorcycles by young children is changing existing patterns of injury. A minibike is lower than a motorcycle, and the rider's neck is unprotected with

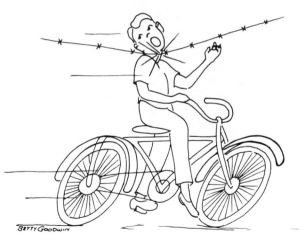

Fig. 15-12 Child on a bicycle or minibike may run into a wire or cable. The speed of a minibike increases the injury.

the chin slightly elevated and the neck in extension.[5] A wire or cable may be undetected and subsequently compress the larynx and trachea against the cervical vertebrae (Fig. 15-12). The trachea, recurrent laryngeal nerves, and the esophagus may be transected without laceration of the skin.[71]

Diagnosis

The history of the mechanism of injury is of paramount importance. In the "padded dash syndrome" the passenger in the right front seat is thrown forward with the head encountering the windshield. This contact produces cervical extension, and the neck forcefully strikes the padded dashboard (Fig. 15-13). Severe fracture of the larynx, cricoid, or tracheal rings may occur with barely detectable contusion of the skin.[12]

Children with blunt injury to the airway usually have severe respiratory distress. If there is any air exchange, it is preferable to perform an immediate tracheostomy rather than endotracheal intubation. Since fragments of the trachea may be torn, mucosal flaps can be dislodged during attempts at tube insertion and produce complete respiratory obstruction. If complete airway obstruction is present initially, endotracheal intubation should be tried. If unsuccessful, transtracheal ventilation through a needle inserted directly into the trachea may allow minimal oxygenation until a standard tracheostomy can be performed.[188] Once tracheostomy has been established below the level of injury, the emergency is over.

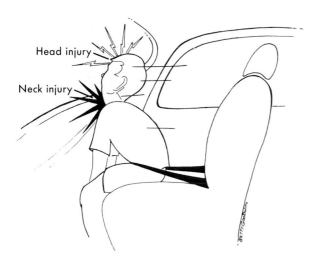

Fig. 15-13 Mechanism of head and neck injury. With a padded dash, external skin injury is minimal.

Treatment

Repair may be immediate or delayed, and if the patient is stable it can be accomplished within hours after injury. Otherwise, a delay of 5 to 6 days will allow partial resolution of edema or hemorrhage and also permits stabilization of other injuries. Treatment depends on the types of injury, that is, the mechanism and anatomic structures that are damaged. Definite patterns of laryngotracheal

trauma have been described.[86,95,158] Operative correction is accomplished through a transverse or vertical neck incision with laryngofissure and direct exposure of all injuries. Absorbable sutures of 5-0 and 6-0 size are used internally and careful anatomic apposition of tissues made with the aid of the operating microscope. Some form of endotracheal support must be used to keep the mucosa flat against the walls of the larynx and trachea. Foam rubber or Silastic are acceptable materials for a stent, and Evans[59] has described an internal stent made from Silastic sheeting. I prefer the method described by Birck.[23] His stent was fashioned from a Portex (polyvinyl) endotracheal tube with a flattened keel proximally to prevent pressure on the vocal cords (Fig. 15-14). No attempt should be made to visualize the recurrent laryngeal nerves during operative repair. If the cords are immobile then the nerves may be intact but contused, and attempts to locate them may result in further injury. As the tracheal injury heals a stricture may develop. The treatment of these chronic strictures will be covered later in this chapter.

Airway disruption is not limited to the cervical region. The thoracic trachea or bronchi may be lacerated through a variety of mechanisms.[109] Some of the theories are outlined in the portion of this chapter dealing with bronchopulmonary lacerations. The reader is referred to that section for description of clinical features and therapy.

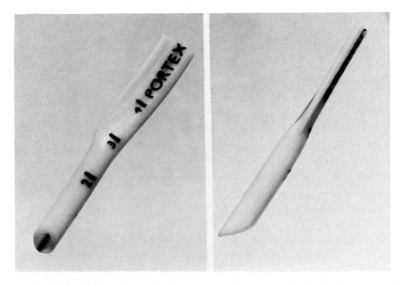

Fig. 15-14 Stent made from appropriate size of Portex endotracheal tube (opaque variety). The flattened keel is molded by heat and fits between the cords.

Internal

In 1962 Burke[32] reported a tenfold increase in the incidence of bronchial injury from external trauma. Now there is occurring a similar epidemic of laryngeal and tracheal injuries due to internal injury.[142] Iatrogenic subglottic stenosis is becoming a common occurrence. Premature infants and other children, previously unsalvagable, are surviving after endotracheal intubation and respiratory support only to develop tracheal necrosis and subsequent stenosis. Even with short-term intubation, a cuffed tube, a tight fit, underlying laryngotracheal inflammation, or the piston-like motion imparted by a respirator all may produce rapid necrosis of the tracheal mucosa and subsequent insidious stenosis. Anatomic differences between small children and adults contribute to the tendency toward tracheal injury in children. In adults the narrowest point of the airway is at the glottis, and a tube that passes through the cords will fit well within the remainder of the trachea. In small children the cricoid ring is the narrowest point of the airway, and a tube that easily traverses the vocal cords may be too tight in the subglottic area.[166] Calibration of the airway during pediatric autopsies revealed the glottis in small children to be larger than the tracheal origin by an average of 4F (French gauge).[34]

Diagnosis

When an endotracheal tube has been used in a patient for longer than 24 hours and that child at any time subsequently develops respiratory distress with suprasternal retraction, the diagnosis of tracheal stenosis should be strongly considered. Anteroposterior and lateral films of the neck are helpful in evaluating the airway, but airway fluoroscopy is usually required. Definite confirmation is made by rigid bronchoscopy or with the new flexible scopes.

Treatment

If a diagnosis is made during the stage of acute tracheal inflammation, treatment with antibiotics, steroids, and gentle dilation may be possible without a tracheostomy. With severe encroachment on the lumen or with a fibrotic stricture, tracheostomy usually is required before the initiation of therapy. Many internal stents have been used in the past,[179] and ingenious techniques have been tried and discarded. All methods of therapy for subglottic stenosis have had some limited success. Resection and direct anastomosis is appealing,[70] but this procedure in itself may lead to subsequent stenosis. In addition, the danger of injury to the recurrent laryngeal nerves is great. Other techniques that have been advocated for the treatment of this condition are repeated dilations,[180] internal stenting,[23] and intralesional injection of steroids.[26,39] In the past I had preferred a modification consisting of dilation and endoscopic resection of the stricture with intralesional injection of steroids and then insertion of an endotracheal stent.[147,148] This technique required a specially designed needle and syringe for injection of the scar through the bronchoscope. The stent was made according to the technique described by Birck.[23] A Portex endotracheal tube of the proper size is selected and measured so that it projects just above the vocal cords and the distal end lies just above the tracheostomy stoma. The tube is then removed and cut at the measured location. A Kelly clamp, the serrations on the blade of which have been ground smooth, is then applied to the tube to form the keel. The clamp is applied only to the first detente in the ratchet. The extent of the keel is determined by the length necessary to pass through the cords. The clamped tube is then placed in a steam autoclave and is heated to a temperature of 240° F and immediately exhausted. After cooling in water the clamp is removed from the molded stent. The lumen of the stent is packed with petrolatum gauze to prevent aspiration of secretions through the tube. A monofilament nylon suture is placed anteriorly near the tip of the tube, and the stent is inserted through the larynx. The retaining suture is retrieved through the tracheostomy stoma, threaded on a needle, and brought out through the trachea and into an incision in the anterior neck. Previously, I had brought the suture out through the skin and tied it over a button, but granulation tissue ingrowth through this suture now has led to its placement subcutaneously and threaded through a portion of Silastic tubing and tied (Fig. 15-15). At the time of removal of the stent a small incision is made in the neck and the suture cut with removal of the Silastic tubing. With direct laryngoscopy the stent can then be extracted. Various treatment regimes for tracheal stenosis follow.

Early Stenosis

Early stenosis is usually encountered in small infants shortly after long-term intubation. Endoscopy shows an acute inflammatory reaction with granulation tissue and encroachment of the lumen.

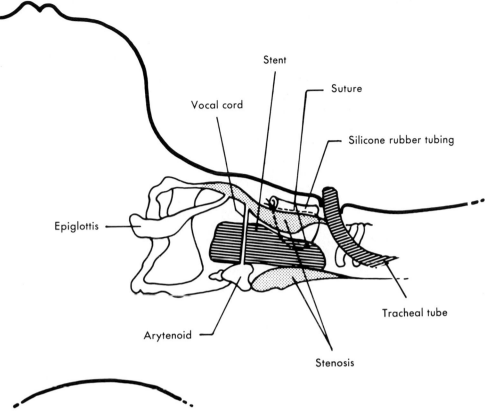

Vocal cord

Stent

Suture

Silicone rubber tubing

Epiglottis

Tracheal tube

Arytenoid

Stenosis

Fig. 15-15   Endotracheal stent fixed into position.

This type of tracheal stenosis usually requires removal of the granulation and gentle dilation. In the past treatment has been performed with metal or Teflon dilators inserted through the larynx. Unfortunately there was not only a dilating force imparted to the trachea but also a shearing force to the tracheal mucosa. A newer technique[146] for dilation is to insert an angioplasty balloon in its deflated state, and when it is positioned in the stenotic area it is inflated to its predetermined pressure so that the desired diameter of the balloon is reached. Thus the full size of the dilator does not pass through the cords, and only the radially dilating forces are applied with no shearing action on the mucosa. When an adequate lumen has been reached a soft Portex endotracheal tube is inserted to maintain the lumen. With the child intubated and the head restrained the child is sedated for 72 hours. During that time dexamethasone 0.8 mg/kg/day is given intravenously. At the end of 72 hours the patient is extubated by using an extubation protocol that consists of sedation with seco-

barbital; albumin 0.5 g/kg intravenously 1 hour before extubation; and furosemide (Lasix) 1 mg/kg intravenously 30 minutes before extubation. After removal of the tube the patient inhales nebulized racemic epinephrine 0.5 cc diluted to 2 cc of saline.

Chronic Strictures

With fibrotic but not calcific strictures, repeated balloon tracheoplasty may be successful. The dilations may be combined with the insertion of stent described by Birck.[23] However, with severe well-established strictures an open tracheoplasty is necessary. Some authors describe success with tracheal resection in children,[9,84] but most prefer cartilage tracheoplasty.[92,121] The trachea is exposed through a transverse cervical incision and the area of stenosis localized. Evans[59] has previously described a castellated incision that on closure allows expansion of the lumen, but cartilage inserted into the trachea works well with long areas of complete rings.[35] With so many various methods of therapy for tracheal strictures in children, it is apparent that none are universally applicable and successful. A clearer understanding of the pathophysiology may lead to better therapy.[132]

In summary:

1. If the tracheal stenotic lesion is detected early, as in a patient recently extubated and found to have internal ulceration and granulation, balloon tracheoplasty followed by insertion of a temporary stent in the form of a soft (opaque) polyvinyl endotracheal tube may be utilized for 72 hours. During that time high doses of steroids (triamcinolone 0.8 mg/kg/day) are administered. After 72 hours the extubation protocol is used and the tube removed.

2. If the stricture is older but yet not severely fibrotic or calcific, balloon dilation can be followed by insertion of an endotracheal stent as described by Birck and with the administration of steroids for 4 to 6 weeks.

3. If the stricture is long standing with severe fibrosis, calcification, or both, open tracheoplasty with insertion of a portion of cartilage or resection of the stricture will be necessary.

Prevention

Most internal tracheal injuries are preventable by adherence to proper techniques of insertion and care of endotracheal tubes. These tubes should not fit tightly. A rough guide to the proper size is the external naris of the child (Figs. 15-16 and 15-17). Any tube that will pass through the nose without deforming the naris is usually accepted by the trachea. Rubber endotracheal tubes are contraindicated, since they produce too much local reaction, but the polyvinyl (Portex) tubes have been satisfactory. Polyvinyl tends to soften slightly at body temperatures and thus will conform to the larynx and trachea. Endotracheal tubes of the Cole type are easier to insert in emergencies, but there is a tendency to advance the tube until the expanded portion impinges on the cord. Severe damage to the glottis with necrosis can result from prolonged pressure. A more serious injury is that produced by the inflated cuff of an endotracheal or tracheostomy tube.[42] The site of necrosis is often too low in the trachea to be relieved by tracheostomy, and treatment is difficult.[76,77] Although low-pressure cuffs have been developed to help eliminate this problem,[79] there are practically no indications for the use of cuffed tubes in children. Even with the

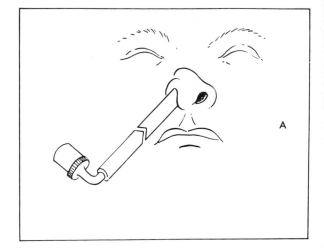

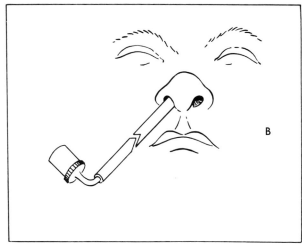

Fig. 15-16   A, Endotracheal tube is too large. Note distortion of naris by tube. **B,** Endotracheal tube is just right. (From Otherson HB: Ann Surg 189:601, 1979.)

tube attached to a respirator, a slight air leak around the tube is desirable because it indicates that the tube does not fit too tightly. Compensation for this small leak can be made by increasing the tidal volume of the respirator. As an aid to tube insertion to the proper length, some endotracheal tubes have internal and external diameters stamped on them as well as calibrations for length (Fig. 15-17). I have summarized the techniques for endotracheal intubation and tracheostomy and illustrated those procedures that may lead to tracheal injury and stenosis.[143]

In infants under 6 months of age, endotracheal intubation is much easier to maintain than is tracheostomy. It is relatively simple to restrain the

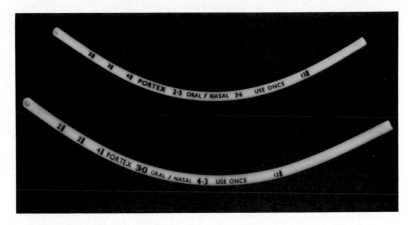

Fig. 15-17   Endotracheal tube of polyvinyl with length and diameter indicated. (From Am Surg 43:108, 1977.)

head of these small infants, thus preventing the shearing action produced by motion of the tube in the trachea. Sedation and muscle relaxants may be required.

Tracheostomy Indications

Voluminous literature reflects the continuing arguments concerning prolonged endotracheal intubation versus tracheostomy in children.* Since there are complications of tracheostomy especially in very small infants,[196] I have proposed the following recommendations[149]:

1. In infants up to 3 and even 6 months of age, prolonged endotracheal intubation is well tolerated and probably can be managed more effectively than tracheostomy.
2. With severe inflammatory glottic and tracheal disease, endotracheal intubation should be performed only long enough for tracheostomy to be conducted. Edema in the area of the cricoid may cause pressure against the tube, and necrosis results.
3. If endotracheal intubation is required for longer than 7 to 10 days in a child over 6 months of age, tracheostomy should be considered.
4. When respirator support is necessary for longer than 5 to 7 days in a child over 6 months of age, tracheostomy should be considered.

Tracheostomy Techniques

Tracheostomy (or tracheotomy, the older term) was described as early as 124 BC but was probably

---

*References 50, 61, 89, 102, 198, 203.

first performed in a patient in 1546.[165] Since that time the details of technique have been changed or modified,[137,177] and the following is my current procedure[143]:

1. An endotracheal tube or bronchoscope is inserted if possible to allow the procedure to be performed without undue haste. When intubation is impossible a cricothyroidotomy with a scalpel or with a plastic cannula needle is done (Fig. 15-18). These manuevers will allow a small airway to be established until tracheostomy can be performed. This technique (cricothyroidotomy) is reserved for dire emergencies.
2. A transverse neck incision is made between the larynx and suprasternal notch, and the strap muscles are separated in the midline.
3. The trachea is identified by repeated palpation so that dissection proceeds directly down to the anterior tracheal wall.
4. The pretracheal fascia is incised and dissected only slightly laterally to insert a small retractor on either side.
5. A linear incision is made through tracheal rings two and three (and four if necessary). No tracheal tissue is excised (Fig. 15-19, A).
6. Hemostasis is carefully secured with electrocautery, especially the small tracheal vessels.
7. A silk suture is placed on either side of the tracheal incision (Fig. 15-19, B).
8. Retraction of the silk sutures allows insertion of the tracheostomy tube without inverting any tissue. The tube should not fit tightly.
9. The skin incision is not closed. Air escapes

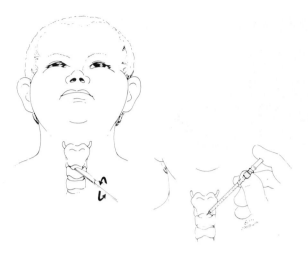

Fig. 15-18   Emergency cricothyroidotomy techniques with either a knife or a plastic cannula needle.

from the trachea around the tube and must be allowed to exit through the wound. Otherwise, the air dissects into the mediastinum and ruptures the pleura producing pneumothorax.

In addition to a knowledge of the proper technique of tracheostomy, tubes must be available in all sizes. There are three types of tracheostomy tubes for children (Fig. 15-20):

1. *Metal tubes*—These tubes are made of silver or stainless steel and can be obtained in Jackson or Holinger design. The Holinger tube is curved more suitably for children. The advantages of these tubes are the full ranges of sizes available and the lack of tissue reaction. They have thin walls and inner cannulae for cleaning. Disadvantages are the rigidity of the tubes and consequent damage from impingement of the tip. Without special inner cannulae, attachment to a respirator is difficult. We do not use metal tubes now.

2. *Silastic*—These tubes are made of silicone rubber and have the advantage of an almost complete lack of tissue reaction but yet are not as rigid as the metal tubes. However, the greater wall thickness required reduces the effective internal diameter. Connection to a respirator requires special adapters. These tubes are of Aberdeen design.

3. *Shiley*—These tubes are constructed of polyvinyl material and are available in a full range of sizes beginning at 00. The internal and external diameters are marked on the wings. These plastic tubes are pliable and come supplied with obturators. A 15-mm adaptor is an integral part of the tube, and this projection facilitates respirator attachment and also

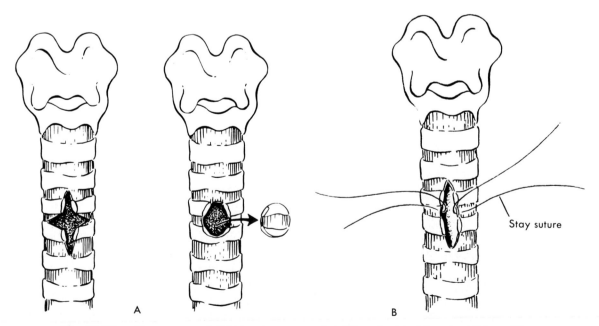

A   B   Stay suture

Fig. 15-19   Nonrecommended (**A**) and recommended (**B**) tracheal incisions in children. (From Othersen HB: Ann Surg 189:601, 1979.)

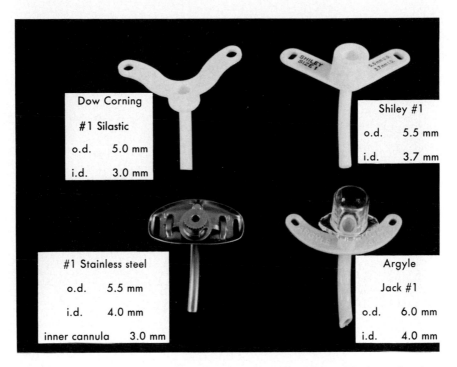

Fig. 15-20 Various types of tracheostomy tubes available for children. The internal and external diameters vary according to thickness of the walls of the tubes.

helps prevent occlusion of the tube ostium by neck tissues. This tube is a current choice for small children.

4. *Silicone rubber tubes*—These tubes are made of silicone rubber (other than the Dow Corning brand [Silastic]) and have very low tissue reactivity. Whereas polyvinyl tubes gradually leach out their plasticizers and need to be changed every 6 to 8 weeks, silicone rubber tubes remain pliable. These tubes are of the Dover design and manufactured by Argyle. They have a built-in 15-mm adapter. The advantage over the Shiley tube is that, in children who must be attached to respirators for ventilatory support, the connection between the 15-mm adapter and the tube is flexible and allows considerable movement of the ventilator tubing without dislodging or displacing the tracheostomy tube. Thus these tubes are preferred for small infants and for any child attached to a ventilator. Because of their flexibility these tubes are more difficult to reinsert if they should become dislodged. Accordingly, a Shiley tube of a similar or smaller size should be available at the bedside of all patients with tracheostomy.

Tracheostomy Care

Of equal importance to technique is the postoperative care of a tracheostomy.[1] Meticulous adherence to aseptic techniques of suctioning is mandatory. During hospitalization the parents should be taught to care for the tracheostomy, since children are often sent home to allow more time for tracheal enlargement before removal of the tracheostomy tube. During that time the primary care must be furnished by parents. Before the child is discharged from the hospital, the parents are taught to change the tracheostomy tube daily so that they become proficient at this task. The primary purpose of this instruction is to impress on the parents the necessity for removing the tube should an obstruction to the airway occur. Occasionally a small thrombus will become attached to the end of the tracheostomy tube and cannot be dislodged with suction. If the parents feel comfortable in changing the tube, they will be able to remove the obstructed tube and replace it with a new one. This course of action is much preferable to rushing a cyanotic child to an emergency room. The parents should be furnished with extra tubes and sterile suction catheters and a portable suction machine. A spare tracheostomy tube of the same size as that in the

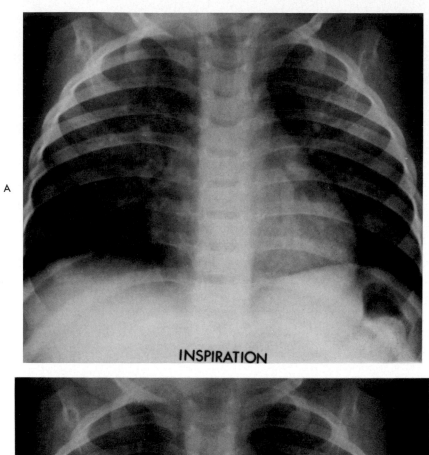

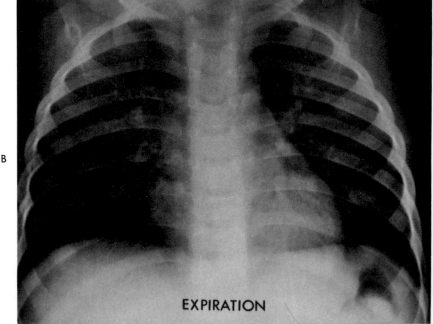

Fig. 15-21   A, Inspiratory chest film of a small child with suspected foreign body (peanut). **B,** Expiratory film of same patient. Child was uncooperative, and emphysema usually seen on expiratory films could not be demonstrated.

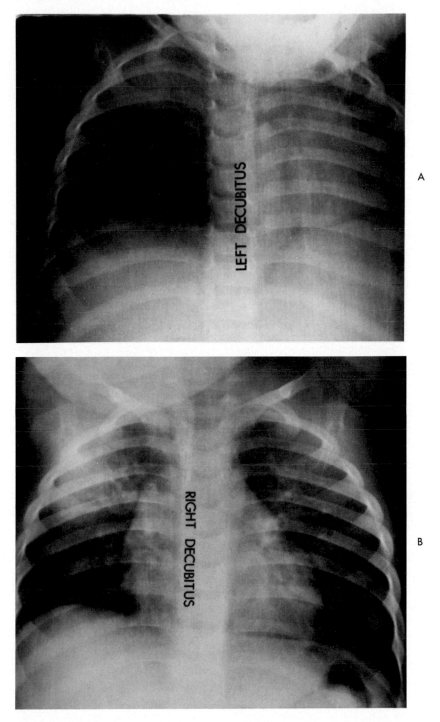

Fig. 15-22   **A,** Left lateral decubitus. Note emptying of the dependent left lung. **B,** Right lateral decubitus. Note right upper lobe emptying but middle and lower lobes do not. Peanut was found in the right intermediate bronchus.

patient should be kept readily accessible and taped to the patient's bed in a package that has been opened so that the tube can be quickly removed in an emergency.

Tracheobronchial Foreign Bodies
Diagnosis

Foreign bodies lodged in the trachea or bronchi are most strongly suspected by a good history. There is no problem with radiopaque objects because they are easily seen on chest x-ray films. Food such as peanuts or vegetable seeds will not be visible on chest films and can be diagnosed definitely only by bronchoscopy. Fluoroscopy may show mediastinal shift toward the involved side. Inspiratory and expiratory chest films often show air trapping and increased lucency of the involved lung after expiration (Fig. 15-21). Small children too young to cooperate can be evaluated by decubitus views (Fig. 15-22). If the history of aspiration is definite and if the child has significant symptoms of coughing and sputtering, bronchoscopy is definitely indicated. Bronchoscopes with telescopic magnification make identification of foreign bodies precise and simple.

Treatment

Bronchoscopic removal of aspirated foreign bodies is still the standard therapy and generally is a safe procedure. The telescopic bronchoscopes allow clear visualization of the foreign body and removal under direct vision. If the object is too large to be pulled back into the bronchoscope, it must be firmly grasped and brought out with the bronchoscope. It is in these situations that dangerous problems may arise. The foreign body may be released in the trachea and may fall down into the other bronchus, thereby producing respiratory obstruction, or it may be dislodged by the vocal cords and produce complete laryngeal obstruction. With sharp metal objects it may be necessary to perform a tracheostomy, and when the foreign body has been pulled up into the proximal trachea, the tracheostomy tube is inserted and the foreign body removed without fear of dislodgement or tracheal obstruction.

A technique for removal of aspirated foreign body by the inhalation of bronchodilators and postural drainage has been presented.[33,43] Seventy-five children were treated by bronchoscopy at the Children's Hospital in Denver, while 24 pediatric patients at the Colorado General Hospital were treated initially by postural drainage and bronchodilators. Peanuts and food were the major offenders, composing 80% of the foreign bodies, and 20% were toys or nonvegetable matter. Of the children treated by bronchoscopic removal, 12 developed complications, 8 of which were pneumonia not present before endoscopy. Of the 24 children treated by postural drainage, there were two serious complications of cardiorespiratory arrest. In these cases the foreign body had lodged in the main stem bronchus with complete obstruction to the lung, and when the object was dislodged it obstructed the opposite bronchus or trachea and hypoxia resulted. These authors now propose that if the foreign body is lodged in the main bronchus, 100% oxygen is inhaled before each treatment and isoproterenol and postural drainage attempted for 4 days. If unsuccessful, bronchoscopy is performed. If the foreign body was in a segmental bronchus, bronchoscopy was not advised and the postural drainage adhered to for as long as 7 days and 70 treatments.

Bronchial foreign bodies usually do not require removal immediately after admission. There will be some exceptions, but endoscopic extraction with the patient under general anesthesia should be accomplished the day following admission. With presently available bronchoscopes and the use of ancillary measures such as balloon catheters passed beyond the object and then inflated, most foreign bodies can be safely removed through the endoscope. Large foreign bodies in the main bronchi or trachea can be potentially lethal when removal is attempted either by bronchoscopy or by postural drainage. The removal of foreign bodies from the segmental bronchi by nonoperative means has considerable appeal, but caution should be exercised in applying this technique to large foreign bodies in the main bronchi or trachea. In those situations endoscopic removal offers greater control and safety.

ESOPHAGUS
External Injury
Blunt trauma

The esophagus in the thorax is deeply situated and protected so that blunt injury is rare. In the neck it is more vulnerable. It may be trapped between an external compressing force and the vertebrae. Not uncommonly, children on motorcycles or snowmobiles encounter an unexpected wire stretched across their paths. Contact in the neck can produce transection of both trachea and esophagus without skin laceration (see Fig. 15-12).

Penetrating trauma

Penetrating injuries to the esophagus are usually produced by gunshot or stab wounds. The deep location of the esophagus conceals external evidence of injury and the possibility of esophageal penetration must be suspected and confirmed. Suspicion is raised by subcutaneous emphysema in the neck or air in the mediastinum or pleura. The ingestion or injection of a water-soluble contrast material into the esophagus will radiographically confirm a leak.

Treatment. If the patient's condition is unstable and the injury has produced a communication between the esophagus and pleural cavity, a pleural catheter should be inserted to underwater drainage (Fig. 15-23).[144] As soon as the condition is stabilized, direct repair is accomplished with two layers of sutures and a drain placed near but not adjacent to the suture line. The closure is reinforced with adjacent tissue or pleura.

Perforations that cannot be closed primarily can be handled in a variety of ways. Small perforations can be managed with a pleural patch.[174] These methods will be discussed in the following section on treatment of internal disruptions.

Internal

Ingestion of lye or other caustic agents

In spite of extensive attempts at public education, strong caustic agents are still available in most homes and easily accessible to ingestion by curious children. The resulting injuries are as catastrophic as a major thermal burn and represent not only an immediate threat to survival but also a severe chronic disability. The magnitude of the problem is reflected in the extensive experimental and clinical investigations.

Experimental

Since the early 1950s evidence has accumulated that cortisone inhibits fibrous tissue proliferation and prevents excessive scarring. Rosenberg et al.[172] demonstrated that large doses of cortisone administered to rabbits after chemical (sodium hydroxide) burns of the esophagus diminished the tendency to fibrous stricture formation. However, there was a high mortality from suppurative infection. Other investigators[98,210] showed a marked inhibition of inflammatory response and granulation with the use of cortisone. Spain et al.[193] reported that when the administration of cortisone was delayed for 48 hours after injury there was no difference from the control in the amount of granulation produced. Uniformity of experimental burns was difficult to achieve, and Bosher and his team[29] developed a standardized method of producing caustic burns in dogs. They performed laparotomy and occluded the cardioesophageal junction after which 10% lye solution was introduced into the esophagus and allowed to remain in contact for 60 seconds. The lye was then neutralized with 0.1 N hydrochloric acid and flushed with water. Subsequent investigators have confirmed the necessity of using 10% sodium

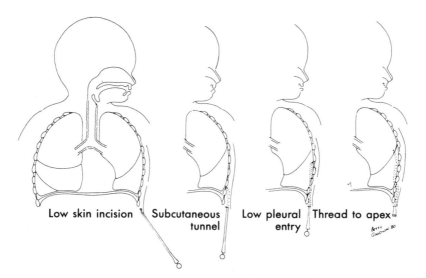

Low skin incision   Subcutaneous tunnel   Low pleural entry   Thread to apex

Fig. 15-23   Correct technique of tube thoracostomy.

hydroxide solution with a contact time of 60 seconds. In 1963 Haller and Bachman[80] described a method of producing standardized caustic burns of the esophagus in cats. They felt that the cat's esophagus anatomically resembled that of the child more closely than did other experimental animals except primates. Four different experimental groups of cats were used to determine the effect of steroid alone, steroid with antibiotics, bougie dilations combined with antibiotics, and bougie dilations combined with steroids and antibiotics. They found that the group treated with steroids (prednisolone) and antibiotics produced the best results in the prevention of stricture. They could demonstrate no improvement by the addition of bougienage. In 1966 Fell and co-workers[63] showed in cats that intraluminal splinting for at least 15 days after caustic burns protected against stricture. This approach was confirmed by Reyes et al.[169] who produced lye burns in cats and compared a corticosteroid-treated group (methylprednisolone 5 mg/kg) with groups treated by intraluminal splinting for 2 or 3 weeks. There was a significant reduction in the strictures of animals treated with an intraluminal splint for 3 weeks. As a logical sequel to the treatment of keloids with the injection of triamcinolone acetonide as described by Ketchum and his group[105] and later confirmed by other plastic surgeons,[74] Ashcraft and Holder[13] treated esophageal strictures with the intralesional injection of triamcinolone. They found that the treatment of very short strictures resulted in variable benefits in dogs. In 1967 Knox et al.[110] compared in dogs the treatment of esophageal burns by low doses of prednisolone alone with prednisolone in combination with bougienage. The best results were obtained in animals treated by a combination of low-dose steroids (prednisolone 0.1 mg/kg/day) and bougienage begun on the seventh or tenth postburn day. This study was contrary to the previously reported findings of Haller and Bachman[80] that the addition of bougienage did not decrease the incidence of stricture in cats.

Davis et al.[47] used a different approach to the problem. After developing a standardized method of producing burns in dogs, they could prevent esophageal strictures by injections of beta-aminopropionitrile (BAPN), a lathrogenic agent that specifically inhibits intermolecular covalent cross-bonding in newly synthesized collagen. They further extended the study by waiting 4 weeks after the esophageal burn to allow a stricture to develop. The lesion was then treated for 6 weeks with BAPN. Mechanical bougienage was used to dilate the stricture daily. The BAPN-treated group was compared with a group treated with prednisolone (0.1 mg/kg/day) combined with daily dilations. The BAPN-treated group showed much superior results. However, systemically induced lathyrism was produced in all animals.

In 1972 this same group of investigators[48] summarized the morphologic aspects of experimental lye strictures in dogs and found that full-thickness injury is necessary for the development of severe stenosis. However, they indicated that full-thickness esophageal injury did not guarantee the development of a stricture.

All of the above experimental work has demonstrated that esophageal strictures can be produced in a variety of experimental animals by the application of 10% sodium hydroxide for a period of 60 seconds. A review of the photographs of strictures in most of the animals reveals that the narrowing is a total reduction and constriction of the entire wall rather than excessive formation of scar tissue. The appearance of the esophagus resembles that of an hourglass. These experimental strictures are thus dissimilar to that seen in humans. In children with chronic strictures the esophageal wall may be greatly increased in thickness by scar tissue. The confusing picture is further compounded by the fact that many experimental models do not permit reproducible strictures in all animals. An esophageal burn that appears severe on endoscopic evaluation and that would seem to represent a full-thickness burn may not develop a stricture regardless of the therapy used. Furthermore, in most experimental studies corticosteroids are used in various dosages and for varying periods of time.

A summary of the experimental evidence to date can be made as follows:

1. Strictures of the esophagus can be produced in a variety of experimental animals—the rat,[129] rabbit,[111] dog,[48] and cat.[80]
2. Transmural full-thickness burns of the esophagus are necessary to produce severe strictures.
3. Stricture formation may not occur even with full-thickness burns.
4. Corticosteroids administered shortly after the burn and given in doses of approximately 0.5 to 1 mg/kg/day will decrease the incidence of stricture but may not prevent stenosis in severe full-thickness injuries. Higher dosages may be necessary initially.

5. Intraluminal splinting for 3 weeks will probably prevent stricture, but the esophagus will remain only as wide as the diameter of the splint.

6. Antibiotics are essential to prevent infectious complications when steroid therapy is used.

7. Benefits from the intralesional injection of steroids into esophageal scars have not been conclusively demonstrated.

8. Systemically induced lathyrism will alleviate early and established strictures.

9. Bougienage combined with steroid administration may help prevent esophageal strictures, but this treatment carries considerable risk of perforation.

Clinical management of acute burns

Strong alkalis are present in most households and are used as drain cleaners. These agents are often kept under the sink and are easily available for ingestion by curious children. Especially dangerous are the caustic solutions that are kept in old soft drink or other beverage containers. Some products are available as crystalline granules. This form fortunately is not as easily swallowed because the particles adhere to the oral mucosa and can be spit out when symptoms occur. Liquid caustic agents easily enter the esophagus to produce deep burns. The most severe injuries are produced at the sites of anatomic or physiologic constriction—the cricopharyngeus, the aortic arch region, or the esophagogastric junction. In contrast to strong acids, which produce a coagulation necrosis and pass into the stomach, strong caustic agents, such as lye, injure the esophagus by liquefaction necrosis. The caustic agents are usually 10% concentrations of sodium or potassium hydroxide. Krey[111] showed in rabbits that the depth of necrosis depended on the concentration of the caustic agent. A commercial preparation (Liquid Plumr) initially had a 30% solution of sodium hydroxide and has been shown in the cat to produce full-thickness injury of the esophagus with only a 3-second exposure.[116] The concentration of that product has now been reduced to 10%.

Based on their classical experimental studies with cats, Haller and his associates[83] at Johns Hopkins treated all of their suspected esophageal burns in the following manner: esophagoscopy for diagnosis, prednisone 2 mg/kg/day, and ampicillin for 10 days. As many as 285 children with possible caustic burns were treated, and of those patients 235 had immediate esophagoscopy. Significant esophageal burns were present in 69 children, who were treated with steroids and antibiotics; eight of these (12%) developed strictures. No children required esophageal replacement, since the strictures responded to prolonged dilations. Griffin,[75] in a review of the management of esophageal lye burns at Columbus Children's Hospital, used slightly higher doses of prednisolone, which varied from 60 mg/day for 4 days for a child 1 to 4 years of age, followed by 40 mg/day for the next 4 days. Thereafter 10 mg/day was given until the esophagus was healed.

Yarington and his associates[215] classified esophageal burns by the depth noted at esophagoscopy. They used three categories—superficial, transmucosal, and full thickness. Others have designated them as first, second, and third degree. The superficial burns were found to have hyperemia with patchy areas of exudate and no bleeding or circumferential burns. The transmucosal or second-degree burns had all of the previous findings plus erosion of mucosa with exudate and pseudomembrane formation, granulation tissue, and frank ulceration. The full-thickness or third-degree burns had all of the findings of the other two categories plus obstruction of the lumen with inflammatory reaction, lack of peristalsis, loss of muscle tone, persistent narrowing, and failure of mucosal regeneration. The most severe form of full-thickness burn also had mediastinitis with perforation. The depth of burn is difficult to determine by initial endoscopic evaluation, but serial esophagoscopy is required. The findings may be altered by therapy, thereby rendering the exact classification difficult. Muscular integrity cannot be evaluated by endoscopic examination alone, but requires radiographic determinations. Yarington also noted in his series of 70 patients that 14 had burns due to Clorox. In my experience and that of others[161] Clorox produces only mild erythema of the esophagus and rarely can be implicated in the production of caustic strictures. On the other hand, some laundry detergents still contain large amounts of phosphates that act as strong caustic agents to produce severe burns.[62,124] Webb and his group[208] studied 68 patients, of whom only 17 were over 20 years of age. Children in the series were treated with immediate esophagoscopy, and if burns were present, 1.5 mg/kg/day of prednisone was administered along with penicillin and streptomycin for 2 weeks. Dilations were never started until at least 2 weeks after injury.

Of 13 patients with first-degree burns, none required dilation and not one developed stricture. Of the burns, 21 were classified as second degree; 18 patients received antibiotics and steroids. Five developed minimal stricture, and these were felt to have more extensive second-degree burns, and in two the burns were circumferential. Only one required a single dilation, and all have remained asymptomatic. Eight patients were placed in the category of third-degree burns. Six received antibiotics and steroids, and two received antibiotics only. All developed severe strictures, and three required colon interposition. This group of investigators did not advocate the early dilation of the esophagus, as advised by Saltzer,[176] since contracture and symptoms of obstruction did not develop until the end of the second week. Hanckel[85] agreed that a 2-week interval should elapse before beginning dilations. Ashcraft and Simon[14] reviewed the pathogenesis of caustic esophageal injury and current concepts of treatment. Their experience with liquid lye preparations indicated that severe circumferential esophageal burns result from ingestion. Their patients were treated with steroids and antibiotics, and 11 developed complete esophageal obstruction requiring colon replacement. Only one child did not develop stricture in spite of definite esophageal injury. They concluded that the efficacy of steroids in the treatment of caustic injury to the esophagus was still in doubt.

My approach to the management of children with acute esophageal burns is as follows:

1. All children with suspected caustic ingestion should have esophagoscopy performed while under general anesthesia within the first 12 hours after admission. If the child is admitted late at night, steroids and antibiotics are begun and esophagoscopy performed early the next morning. If no burns are found, the antibiotics and steroids are discontinued. It is important that steroids be started early after the burn.
2. With the child under general anesthesia, esophagoscopy is performed only to the level of definite burn injury. Once the diagnosis of esophageal burn is established, the procedure is terminated.
3. Corticosteroids (prednisone or prednisolone) in the dose of 4 to 6 mg/kg/day are given for the first week and the dosage schedule tapered—prednisone 4 to 6 mg/kg/day for first week, 3 mg/kg/day for second week, 2 mg/kg/day until healing occurs.
4. Esophagoscopy is repeated in 10 to 14 days to assess the degree of healing. Again the esophagoscope is not advanced beyond the first area of injury. Steroids are continued in the dose of 2 mg/kg/day until complete healing occurs.
5. Antibiotics (ampicillin) in the dose of 50 to 100 mg/kg/day are administered as long as the steroids are given.
6. Dilations are not begun until there is evidence of definite stricture, usually approximately 2 weeks after burn. If dilations are required, endoscopic esophagoplasty with balloon dilation is the treatment of choice.
7. All medications are given by mouth if tolerated and, in addition, antacids are administered to prevent hyperacidity and steroid-induced ulcers.

With this regimen of therapy patients with mild to moderate esophageal burns usually heal without stricture. Severe full-thickness injury of the entire esophageal wall also will heal except for the areas of maximal burn, usually located at the level of the aortic arch. Commonly a section of the esophagus 4 to 6 cm in length reveals persistent granulation tissue and contracts to form a chronic stricture. Some burns are deep enough to develop tracheoesophageal fistula.[7] In patients with marked swelling and edema in the hypopharynx, tracheostomy may be required for resolving respiratory distress. These patients are particularly susceptible to develop tracheoesophageal fistulae, since the tip of the tracheostomy tube may produce pressure on the posterior tracheal wall and, especially if there is an indwelling esophageal tube or stent, pressure necrosis of the wall between the esophagus and trachea may occur.

It is still unclear exactly what benefits are derived from the early administration of steroids in the treatment of acute caustic burns of the esophagus. In experimental animals steroids must be given early and in adequate doses to be effective. Further experimental study has demonstrated increased collagenolytic activity as a result of steroid administration.[97] In addition, local atrophy that has been associated with triamcinolone injection may actually be beneficial when that steroid is used therapeutically.[54] On the other hand, there are complications associated with this regimen of high-dosage steroid administration. Stress ulceration frequently occurs and may lead to perforation. Long-term effects of steroids may include skeletal growth changes.

Prevention

The best treatment for esophageal burns is prevention. Parents should be instructed to keep all toxic products out of the reach of children. When caustic solutions have been made, they should never be placed in bottles ordinarily used for beverages. Childproof caps are required on toxic products available commercially. Most of these strong caustic agents are sold as drain cleaners, with advertisements describing rapid dissolution of the occluding material in drain pipes. Consumer Reports[41] evaluated these products and could find no advantage over the mechanical methods of freeing an occluded drain pipe. The "metal snake" or the standard rubber plunger were more effective in dislodging the offending bolus than were any of the chemicals. Perhaps it is time for these products to be abandoned either by the public or by legislation.

Foreign Bodies

It is not surprising to find a variety of foreign bodies lodged in the esophagus, since small children and infants put everything they encounter into their mouths. Most objects that can be swallowed will pass into the stomach and thence through the intestines without difficulty. Some articles, because of their size, configuration, or sharp edges, become stuck, especially in midesophagus at the level of the aortic arch.

If the foreign body is radiopaque, a chest film that includes the neck should demonstrate it. If it is not seen or if the object is nonradiopaque, a barium swallow should be conducted. Fig. 15-24 is an x-ray film of a 10-month-old child who had "congestion" for 1 month. He then developed asthma-like wheezing, and during an examination by his pediatrician he stopped breathing. An endotracheal tube was passed, and the child was resuscitated. Spot films show a radiopaque object in the esophagus with extensive edema occluding the tracheal air column (Fig. 15-25). A 2-cm square, flat portion of bone was removed from the esophagus, and an endotracheal tube was required for 48 hours until edema had subsided. That foreign body probably had been present for 1 month before removal. The x-ray films were deceptive because the bone fragment was thin and was always viewed on end. Esophageal foreign bodies, because of their size or from subsequent edema, can produce encroachment on the tracheal lumen and cause wheezing symptoms that are similar to those found in tracheal foreign bodies.

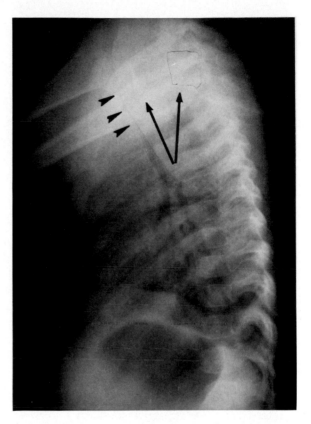

Fig. 15-24   Lateral view of chest and neck. Arrowheads point to narrowed tracheal air column. Anterior long arrow shows foreign body on end, and posterior arrow points to outline of approximate size of the flat bone in the esophagus.

Treatment

If the impacted object is smooth, such as a coin, it will usually pass. The child may be given atropine and a small amount of viscous Xylocaine by mouth to relieve spasm and lubricate the mucosa. The patient is then encouraged to walk around. These simple maneuvers will often allow the object to pass into the stomach. Once in the stomach the foreign body should traverse the remainder of the GI tract. If the object remains impacted a Foley catheter can be passed into the esophagus beyond the foreign body and the balloon inflated with a radiopaque liquid. The balloon is then pulled back under fluoroscopic control and the offending object can often be dislodged and retrieved. Occasionally a bolus of food, usually meat, becomes obstructed proximal to a stricture or in a dyskinetic esophagus. The instillation of a small amount of meat tenderizer (Papain) may aid in dislodgement.

If lesser methods fail, esophagoscopy with the

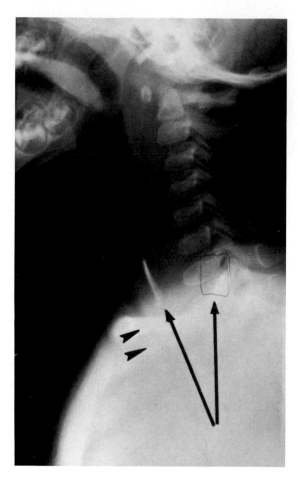

Fig. 15-25   Close-up view of the area described in Fig. 15-24.

child under general endotracheal anesthesia is indicated. Visualization of foreign bodies is usually not difficult with the telescopic endoscopes. Copious irrigation through a side arm of the scope distends the esophagus and permits visualization of an object hidden in edematous mucosal folds. When removing foreign bodies a large esophagoscope is passed to dilate the esophageal lumen proximal to the offending object. Under direct vision the foreign body is pulled up into the tip of the scope, and both the scope and the foreign body are withdrawn together. Irrigation during withdrawal helps to distend the esophagus to facilitate passage of the foreign body. Rarely will it be necessary to perform direct esophagotomy and removal of the object.

Esophageal Perforation

Perforations of the esophagus may occur after internal instrumentation, especially during endos-

copy for acute burns or as a consequence of dilation of tight strictures. The esophagus proximal to an obstruction is dilated and is easily perforated. For that reason antegrade dilation is much more hazardous than the retrograde method.[22] Even when the retrograde Tucker dilators are pulled through with a string, a tight stricture may split with laceration of the entire esophageal wall. Balloon esophagoplasty eliminates the shearing force of antegrade or retrograde techniques and is conducted under fluoroscopic control. Sharp foreign bodies may lacerate the esophagus either during ingestion or while attempting removal.

Since early recognition of a perforation is essential for successful therapy, any suspicion of esophageal injury should be investigated by a chest x-ray film and further evaluated by soluble contrast material injected through a tube that has been passed into the esophagus.

Most esophageal perforations require immediate thoracotomy for primary repair and drainage. A small leak localized to the mediastinum and without pleural involvement may be treated with antibiotics and aspiration of the proximal esophagus with a sump catheter. In adults, but rarely indicated in children, intubation of the esophagus with a tube (Celestin tube) may allow a critically ill patient to be improved before thoracotomy.[20]

Large rents in the esophagus may be difficult to close especially when the wall is edematous and friable. Some helpful adjuncts to surgical closure when the perforation is in the lower third of the esophagus include the following:

1. An onlay gastric patch with a portion of stomach pulled up through the esophageal hiatus[88]
2. A vascularized pedicle of pericardium[204]
3. A flap of intact omentum[133]
4. A pleural flap[174]

When the perforation is in the upper esophagus and if direct closure is impossible, a cervical esophagostomy and closure of the distal esophagus may be necessary. This operation requires subsequent esophageal replacement by stomach or intestines. Attempts at interposition of intestines or stomach in the treatment of acute perforation are not recommended, since local inflammatory reaction is great and the intestines are unprepared.

An unusual form of esophageal perforation has been described.[40,104,167] A blast of air distends and ruptures the esophagus. This injury may be sustained when a small child bites an inflated inner tube and pneumatic rupture of the esophagus occurs usually into the left chest just above the diaphragm. Cole and Burcher,[40] in describing one gastric and one esophageal rupture, postulated that when there is a sudden rapid rise in pressure in the mouth, reflex closure of the glottis occurs and the cricopharyngeus opens. The cardia fails to relax, and the esophagus distends and ruptures at its weakest point (the left lateral wall just above the diaphragm). A slow rise in pressure allows the cardia to relax, and the stomach distends. If the pylorus does not open, gastric perforation may occur. This theory is substantiated by a case report in which gastric perforation occurred as a result of pneumatic distention in a child with tracheoesophageal fistula.[152]

Chronic Strictures and Scars

In spite of adequate and aggressive therapy of acute esophageal injury, many full-thickness burns develop chronic granulations and eventually tough scar and stricture. In the past various forms of bougienage have been the mainstay of conservative therapy.[44,96] In small children repeated dilations have been performed in the retrograde manner with Tucker dilators.[22] Newer procedures have been proposed,[120,127] but the one we prefer now is balloon esophagoplasty.[146] With that procedure angioplasty-type balloons are passed either endoscopically under direct vision or with fluroscopic guidance. When performed in combination with fluroscopy the balloon is inflated with a contrast material and the dilation observed. A contrast esophagogram is always obtained before and after the dilation. If the stricture is severe a gastrostomy should be performed for feeding, and a small silicone rubber tube can be passed through the esophagus and out the gastrostomy and through the nose. This tube acts as a guide until the lumen has been sufficiently enlarged.

The best approach is to conserve the esophagus if at all possible. Conduits fashioned from stomach or intestine are no substitute for the esophagus and are only second best. In the past when the stricture has been short (less than 4 cm) and the remainder of the esophagus has been adequate, I attempted repeated dilations and steroid injections every 6 weeks. This method had been previously reported in animals and children.[94] I have used special needles and syringes with the local injection of triamcinolone. However, long-term results with this technique have been disappointing. In evaluating results, the strictures formed as a result of anas-tomoses in children with esophageal atresia respond readily to balloon esophagoplasty. However, longer and more dense strictures as a result of caustic burns either require very long-term treatment or open esophagoplasty.[146]

Replacement Operations

Considerable effort has been expended to devise suitable substitutes for the esophagus. Initially, skin tubes were fashioned that could reach from the cervical esophagus, subcutaneously over the thorax, to the stomach. These tubes were unsightly and functionally inadequate. Furthermore, the stomach has been mobilized and advanced for direct anastomosis with the cervical esophagus. This arrangement in small children is unsatisfactory because the dilated stomach in the thoracic cavity can produce respiratory distress. The history of the surgical treatment of esophageal strictures has been extensively reviewed by Meade.[130]

The following four surgical procedures are currently used for replacement of the esophagus:
1. Colon interposition[69,151,207]
2. Gastric tube[8,57]
3. Small intestinal interposition[160]
4. Colic patch esophagoplasty[90]

Of these four procedures only one, the colic patch esophagoplasty, is new. The other methods, including skin tubes and total transposition of the stomach, were described in an article by Ochsner and Owens[139] in 1934.

The small intestine offers the advantage of a size comparable to that of the esophagus, but it has a considerable disadvantage. The vascular supply of the small intestine does not allow a straight tube to be brought from the stomach to the neck. The vascular arcades can be manipulated, but there is usually considerable redundancy of the intestine. In addition, the peristaltic activity is slow and segmenting, causing food to be transmitted slowly into the stomach. The gastric tube seems to offer no advantages over the colon, although its use has been more popular in recent years. Long-term follow-up will determine whether its functional capacity is adequate to permit normal growth and development. Before use of the colic patch the most satisfactory esophageal replacement was the colon. Right, transverse, or left colon may be used in either an antegrade or retrograde fashion. The colonic segment may be placed either substernally or in the posterior mediastinum. The colon acts primarily as a conduit, and functional evaluation has

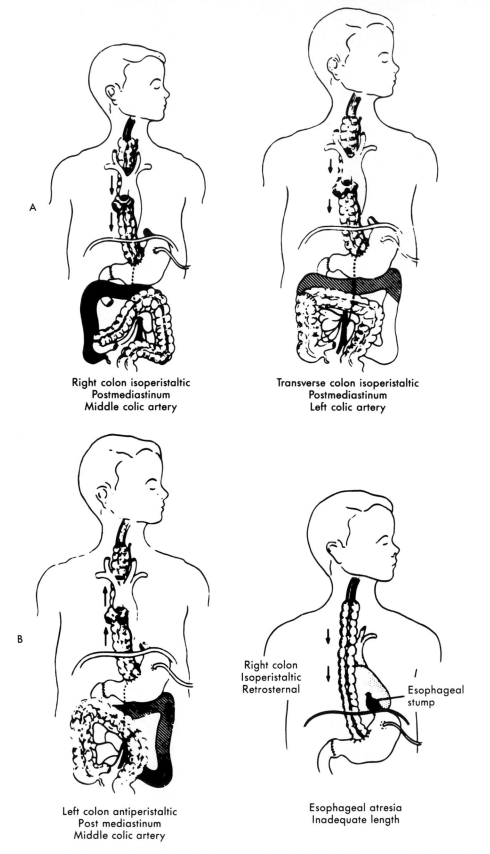

Right colon isoperistaltic
Postmediastinum
Middle colic artery

Transverse colon isoperistaltic
Postmediastinum
Left colic artery

Left colon antiperistaltic
Post mediastinum
Middle colic artery

Right colon
Isoperistaltic
Retrosternal

Esophageal
stump

Esophageal atresia
Inadequate length

Fig. 15-26   **A,** Two methods of colonic interposition in isoperistaltic manner. **B,** Two other techniques of colonic interposition.

demonstrated that it is important to obtain a patent anastomoses without redundancy of the colon.[178] The segment of colon used and the direction of its peristalsis is relatively unimportant (Fig. 15-26).[150] The technique has been described in detail and various modifications and refinements offered.[122,207] The important features of this operation in children are the following:

1. The operative procedure should be performed as a single stage without preliminary exteriorization of the colon or esophagus in the neck.

2. The proximal anastomosis is best performed in the neck, and the distal anastomosis may be performed either in the abdomen directly to the stomach or in the chest to *normal* esophagus above the diaphragm. Retention of the gastroesophageal junction may help to prevent esophagogastric reflux, but the distal esophagus should be normal if that technique is used.

3. A good vascular pedicle must be obtained, and the colonic segment should be stretched taut between the proximal and distal esophagus to prevent redundancy. The colon either dilates or grows faster than the child's length, since redundancy occurs frequently.

4. It is probably preferable to place the colon in the posterior mediastinum with resection of the scarred esophagus. Placement in the substernal position avoids thoracotomy, but in small children there is very little room at the thoracic inlet and the colon is compressed behind the sternum. If a substernal route is taken, care must be exercised to remove some of the sternum to prevent compression of the colonic segment. The stenotic esophagus is excised because if it is closed and left in place it may fill with secretions and rupture. There is also a chance of carcinoma developing in a retained scarred esophagus.[103] In children with a long life expectancy, malignancy may develop 15 to 20 years after therapy.

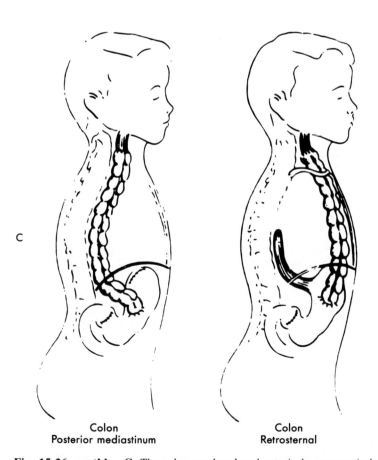

Colon
Posterior mediastinum

Colon
Retrosternal

Fig. 15-26, cont'd   C, The colon can be placed anteriorly or posteriorly.

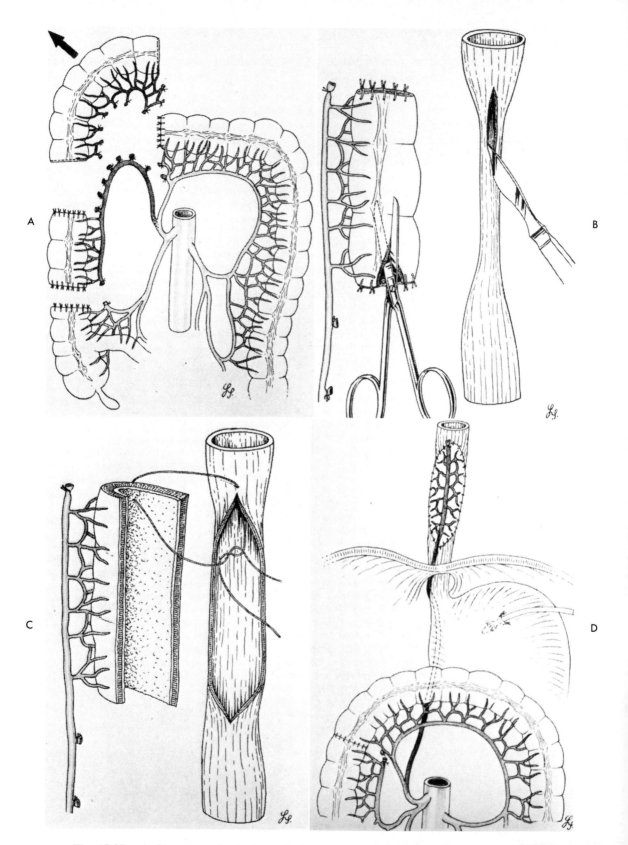

Fig. 15-27 **A,** First stage of colonic patch: freeing up a vascularized segment of colon. **B,** The vascularized segment of colon is incised longitudinally. The esophageal stricture is incised throughout its length. **C,** The vascularized patch is trimmed to fit the defect created in the esophagus. **D,** The completed colonic patch. (From Hecker WC and Hollmann G: Prog Ped Surg 8:81, 1975.)

The current operation of choice for esophageal strictures less than 10 cm in length is the colic patch esophagoplasty.[90] The stricture is incised longitudinally and the patch sewn into the defect (Fig. 15-27). This procedure offers promise of preserving the esophagus.

Results

There has been considerable progress in the treatment of esophageal injuries in children during the last century. There are techniques to prevent injury and to treat the injury shortly after its occurrence. For esophageal strictures that do not involve the entire esophagus, the colic patch, as originally described by Hecker and Hallman[90] in 1974, is preferred. Balloon esophagoplasty of early strictures, particularly postanastomotic ones, has been satisfactory.[146]

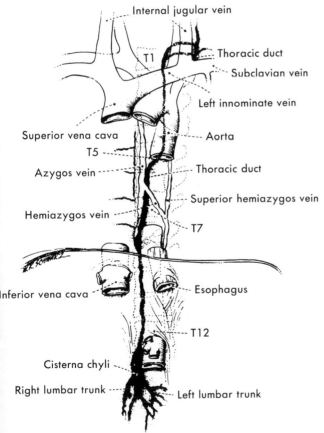

Fig. 15-28   Anatomy of thoracic duct. (Reprinted with permission from The Society of Thoracic Surgeons; The Annals of Thoracic Surgery, vol 12, 1971, 527.)

THORACIC DUCT INJURIES

The thoracic duct is situated deep within the thorax and is well protected from external trauma. However, its location in the chest renders it vulnerable to injury during operations that involve mobilization of the aortic arch, the left subclavian artery, or the esophagus.

Anatomy

Channels from the cisterna chyli converge to form the thoracic duct. Above the diaphragm this duct lies to the right of the midline and aorta, anterior to the vertebrae, and posterior to the esophagus. At the level of the fifth thoracic vertebra, the duct crosses to the left and ascends behind the aortic arch and assumes a position to the left of the esophagus. It then lies behind the left subclavian artery and in the base of the neck turns to the left anterior to the vertebral artery and enters the venous system at or near the confluence of the left subclavian and left internal jugular veins (Fig. 15-28).

Injuries to the thoracic duct permit leakage of chyle with resultant chylothorax. Bessone et al.,[21] in an excellent review, classified chylothorax as congenital, traumatic-postoperative, traumatic-nonsurgical, and nontraumatic.

Traumatic Chylothorax
Postoperative

In children, operations that occasionally produce injury to the thoracic duct are those procedures for repair of coarctation of the aorta, vascular rings, and patent ductus arteriosus or the formation of a Blalock-Taussig shunt. Mobilization of the esophagus in its middle third may also result in injury to the thoracic duct.

Nonsurgical

Although penetrating injuries of the neck or chest may injure the thoracic duct (Fig. 15-29), rupture has also been described as resulting from crushing or blast injuries.

Diagnosis

In the postoperative variety of chylothorax, effusion is usually not manifest for 1 to 2 weeks. Thoracentesis produces a milky fluid that does not clot. Posttraumatic effusion usually is slightly bloody. Free fat is present in the fluid.

Treatment

Before 1948 it was believed that an obstructed thoracic duct resulted in death. Surgeons described

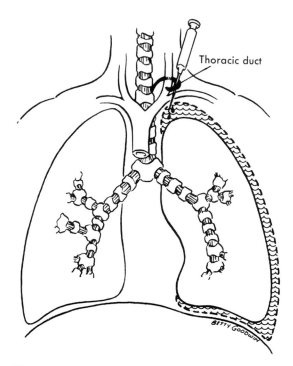

Fig. 15-29 Traumatic chylothorax. Needle aspiration of veins in the left neck may lacerate the thoracic duct and produce chylothorax. (From Welch KJ, editor: Complications of pediatric surgery, Philadelphia, 1981, WB Saunders Co.)

attempts at anastomosis of the divided duct to a vein. In 1948 Lampson[112] reported a successful transthoracic ligation of the thoracic duct. Since that time the definitive therapy has been ligation with nonabsorbable sutures.

Postoperative chylothorax should be treated initially by pleural drainage via an intercostal thoracostomy tube. All feedings are discontinued. Some investigators recommend oral administration of medium chain triglycerides.[82] Others prefer total parenteral alimentation for 3 to 4 weeks.

If after approximately 1 month of nonoperative therapy a chyle leak continues, thoracotomy should be performed on the side of effusion except when the effusion is bilateral. In the latter condition right thoracotomy permits ligation just above the diaphragm. The leak may be difficult to find; aids to its localization are the injection of blue dye (sky blue) around the esophageal hiatus, the administration of a fatty meal preoperatively, the filling of the pleural cavity with saline, and subcutaneous injection of Evans blue dye into the thigh before operation. When the leak is found, nonabsorbable

ligatures are placed on each side of the rent. Parietal pleurectomy will produce adhesions and may prevent further leakage. Adequate tube drainage is mandatory. If the leak cannot be found, a technique of closure of the mediastinal pleura over gelfoam bolsters has been described.[184]

REFERENCES

1. Aberdeen E: Mechanical pulmonary ventilation in infants, Proc Roy Soc Med 58:900, 1965.
2. Agee RN et al: Use of xenon-133 in early diagnosis of inhalation injury, J Trauma 16:218, 1976.
3. Akenside A: An account of a blow upon the heart and its effects, Philos Trans R Soc 1764.
4. Alfano GS and Hale HW Jr: Pulmonary contusion, J Trauma 5:647, 1965.
5. Alonso WA, Caruso VG, and Roncace EA: Minibikes, a new factor in laryngotracheal trauma, Ann Otol Rhinol Laryngol 82:800, 1973.
6. American Academy of Pediatrics—Report of Subcommittee on Accidental Poisoning: Cooperative kerosene poisoning study: evaluation of gastric lavage and other factors in the treatment of accidental ingestion of petroleum distillate products, Pediatrics 29:648, 1962.
7. Amoury RA et al: Tracheoesophageal fistula after lye ingestion, J Pediatr Surg 10:273, 1975.
8. Anderson KD and Randolph JG: The gastric tube for esophageal replacement in children, J Thorac Cardiovasc Surg 66:333, 1973.
9. Angerpointer TA et al: Resection of an intrathoracic tracheal stenosis in a child, Prog Pediatr Surg 21:64, 1987.
10. Arenberg H: Traumatic heart disease: a clinical study of 250 cases of nonpenetrating chest injuries and their relation to cardiac disability, Ann Intern Med 19:326, 1943.
11. Asburg GF: Rupture of the diaphragm from blunt trauma, Arch Surg 97:801, 1968.
12. Ashbaugh DG and Gordon JH: Traumatic avulsion of the trachea associated with cricoid fracture, J Thorac Cardiovasc Surg 69:800, 1975.
13. Ashcraft KW and Holder TM: The experimental treatment of esophageal strictures by intralesional steroid injections, J Thorac Cardiovasc Surg 58:685, 1969.
14. Ashcraft KW and Simon JL: Accidental caustic injection in childhood, a review: pathogenesis and concepts of treatment, Tex Med 68:86, 1972.
15. Avery EE, Morch ET, and Benson DW: Critically crushed chests, J Thorac Surg 32:291, 1956.
16. Beale AC Jr et al: Considerations in the management of penetrating thoracic trauma, J Trauma 8:408, 1968.
17. Beck CS: Wounds of the heart—the technique of suture, Arch Surg 13:205, 1926.
18. Bellinger SB: Penetrating chest injuries in children, Ann Thorac Surg 14:635, 1972.
19. Bender TM et al: Pediatric chest trauma, J Thorac Imaging 2:60, 1987.
20. Berger RL and Donato AT: Treatment of esophageal disruption by intubation, Ann Thorac Surg 13:27, 1972.
21. Bessone LN, Ferguson TB, and Burford TH: Chylothorax, Ann Thorac Surg 12:527, 1971.
22. Bill AH Jr, Mebust WK, and Sauvage LR: Elevation of

techniques of esophageal dilation in relation to the danger of perforation, J Thorac Cardiovasc Surg 45:510, 1963.

23. Birck HG: Endoscopic repair of laryngeal stenosis, Trans Am Acad Ophthal Otol 74:140, 1970.

24. Bishop LH Jr, Estes EH Jr, and McIntosh HD: The electrocardiogram as a safeguard in pericardiocentesis, JAMA 162:264, 1956.

25. Blair E: Pulmonary barriers to oxygen transport in chest, Am Surg 42:55, 1976.

26. Bonchek LI: Successful treatment of postintubation subglottic stenosis with intralesional steroid injections, Ann Thorac Surg 15:84, 1972.

27. Book of accidents; designed for young children, New Haven, Conn, 1830, S Babcock.

28. Border JR, Hokinson BR, and Schenk WG Jr: Mechanisms of pulmonary trauma—an experimental study, J Trauma 8:47, 1968.

29. Bosher LH, Burford TH, and Ackerman L: The pathology of experimentally produced lye burns and strictures of the esophagus, J Thorac Surg 21:483, 1951.

30. Bright EF and Beck CS: Nonpenetrating wounds of the heart: a clinical and experimental study, Am Heart J 10:293, 1935

31. Burford TH and Burbank B: Traumatic wet lung, J Thorac Surg 14:415, 1945.

32. Burke JF: Early diagnosis of traumatic rupture of the bronchus, JAMA 181:682, 1962.

33. Burrington JD and Cotton EK: Removal of foreign bodies from the tracheobronchial tree, J Pediatr Surg 7:119, 1972.

34. Butz RO Jr: Length and cross-section growth patterns in the human trachea, Pediatrics 42:336, 1968.

35. Campbell DN and Lilly JR: Surgery for total congenital tracheal stenosis, J Pediatr Surg 2:934, 1986.

36. Cappelen A: Vulnus cordis sutur af hjertet, Norsk Mag f Laequevidensk 11:285, 1896; cited by Lyons C and Perkins R: Am Surg 23:507, 1957.

37. Castagna J and Nelson RJ: Blunt injuries to branches of the aortic arch, J Thorac Cardiovasc Surg 69:521, 1975.

38. Chesterman JT and Satsangi PN: Rupture of the trachea and bronchi by closed injury, Thorax 21:21, 1966.

39. Cobb WB and Sudderth JF: Intralesional steroids in laryngeal stenosis, Arch Otolaryngol 96:52, 1972.

40. Cole DS and Burcher SK: Accidental pneumatic rupture of oesophagus and stomach, Lancet 1:24, 1961.

41. Consumer Reports 41:592, 1976.

42. Cooper JD and Grillo HC: Experimental production and prevention of injury due to cuffed tracheal tubes, Surg Gynecol Obstet 129:1235, 1969.

43. Cotton EK et al: Removal of aspirated foreign bodies by inhalation and postural drainage, Clin Pediatr 12:270, 1973.

44. Cotton R and Fearon B: Esophageal strictures in infants and children, Can J Otolaryngol 1:224, 1972.

45. Daniel RA Jr and Cate WR Jr: "Wet lung"—an experimental study, Ann Surg 127:836, 1948.

46. Danis RK and Schweiss JF: Late repair of bronchial rupture in a child by bronchial replantation, J Pediatr Surg 11:235, 1976.

47. Davis WM, Madden JW, and Peacock EE: Prevention of esophageal stenosis with induced lathyrism, Surg Forum 22:193, 1971.

48. Davis WM, Madden JW, and Peacock EE Jr: A new approach to the control of esophageal stenosis, Ann Surg 176:469, 1972.

49. Deforges G et al: Traumatic rupture of the diaphragm, J Thorac Surg 34:779, 1957.

50. Dixon TC et al: A report of 342 cases of prolonged endotracheal intubation, Med J Aust 2:529, 1968.

51. "Don't risk your child's life!": Physicians for Automotive Safety in Cooperation with the New Jersey State Department of Health, ed 8, 1975,

52. Duff JH et al: Flain chest: a clinical review and physiological study, J Trauma 8:63, 1968.

53. Dunseth W and Ferguson TB: Acquired cardiac septal defect due to thoracic trauma, J Trauma 5:142, 1965.

54. Dymet PG: Local atrophy following triamcinolone injection, Pediatrics 46:136, 1970.

55. Ecker RR et al: Injuries of the trachea and bronchi, Ann Thorac Surg 11:289, 1971.

56. Eijgelaar A and Homan van der Heide JN: A reliable early symptom of bronchial or tracheal rupture, Thorax 25:120, 1970.

57. Ein SH et al: A further look at the gastric tube as an esophageal replacement in infants and children, J Pediatr Surg 8:859, 1973.

58. Ellis R: Traumatic lung cysts, JAMA 236:1976, 1976.

59. Evans JNG: Laryngeal disorders in children. In Wilkinson AW, editor: Recent advance in pediatric surgery, Edinburgh, 1975, Churchill Livingstone.

60. Fagan CJ: Traumatic lung cyst, Am J Roentgenol Radium Ther Nucl Med 97:186, 1966.

61. Fearon B et al: Airway problems in children following prolonged endotracheal intubation, An Otol Rhinol Laryngol 75:975, 1966.

62. Feldman M, Iben AB, and Hurley EJ: Corrosive injury to oropharynx and esophagus, 85 consecutive cases, Calif Med 6:118, 1973.

63. Fell SC et al: The effect of intraluminal splinting in the prevention of caustic stricture of the esophagus, J Thorac Cardiovasc Surg 52:675, 1966.

64. Fischer GW and Scherz RG: Neck vein catheters and pericardial tamponade, Pediatrics 52:868, 1973.

65. Freeark RJ et al. Rupture of the diaphragm caused by blunt trauma, J Trauma 16:531, 1976.

66. Freeman T and Fischer RP: The inadequacy of peritoneal lavage in diagnosing acute diaphragmatic rupture, J Trauma 16:538, 1976.

67. Fulton RL, Peter ET, and Wilson JN: The pathophysiology and treatment of pulmonary contusions, J Trauma 10:719, 1970.

68. Geelhoed GW and Bennett SH: "Shock lung" resulting from perfusion of canine lungs with stored bank blood, Am Surg 41:671, 1975.

69. German JC and Waterson DJ: Colon interposition for the replacement of the esophagus in children, J Pediatr Surg 11:227, 1976.

70. Gerwat J and Bryce DP: The management of subglottic laryngeal stenosis by resection and direct anastomosis, Laryngoscope 84:940, 1974.

71. Gill AJ: Rupture of the cervical trachea and esophagus, Arch Otolaryngol 90:95, 1969.

72. Goldberg LR and Spraygregen S: Traumatic intrapericardial hematoma: an unusual cause of mediastinal widening, Angiology 25:495, 1974.

73. Graham EA and Bell RD: Open pneumothorax: its relation to the treatment of empyema, Am J Med Sci 156:839, 1918.
74. Griffin BH, Monroe CW, and McKinney P: A follow-up study on the treatment of keloids with triamcinolone, Plast Reconstr Surg 46:145, 1970.
75. Griffin CS: Management of children with suspected esophageal burns, Postgrad Med 35:611, 1964.
76. Grillo HC: Surgical approaches to the trachea, Surg Gynecol Obstet 192:347, 1969.
77. Grillo HC: The management of tracheal stenosis following assisted respiration, J Thorac Cardiovasc Surg 57:52, 1969.
78. Grillo HC, editor: Current problems in surgery, Chicago, 1970, Year Book Medical Publishers.
79. Grillo HC et al: A low-pressure cuff for tracheostomy tubes to minimize tracheal injury, J Thorac Cardiovasc Surg 62:898, 1961.
80. Haller JA Jr and Bachman K: The comparative effect of current therapy of experimental caustic burns of the esophagus, Pediatrics 34:236, 1964.
81. Haller JA Jr and Donahoo JS: Traumatic asphyxia in children: pathophysiology and management, J Trauma 11:453, 1971.
82. Haller JA Jr and Shermeta DW: Major thoracic trauma in children, Pediatr Clin North Am 22:341, 1975.
83. Haller JA Jr et al: Pathophysiology and management of acute corrosive burns of esophagus: results of treatment in 285 children, J Pediatr Surg 6:578, 1971.
84. Halsband H: Long-distance resection of the trachea with primary anastomosis in small chilren, Prog Pediatr Surg 21:76, 1987.
85. Hanckel RW Jr: Some observations concerning the Salzer method of treatment of lye burns of the esophagus, South Med J 39:263, 1946.
86. Harris HH: Symposium on trauma in otolaryngology. IV. Management of injuries to the larynx and trachea, Laryngoscope 82:1924, 1972.
87. Hashim SA et al: Treatment of chyluria and chylothorax with medium-chain triglyceride. N Engl J Med 270:756, 1964.
88. Hatafuku T and Thal AP: The use of the onlay gastric patch with experimental perforations of the distal esophagus, Surgery 56:556, 1964.
89. Hatch DJ: Prolonged nasotracheal intubation in infants and children, Lancet 1:1272, 1968.
90. Hecker WC and Hollmann G: Correction of long segment oesophageal stenoses by a colonic patch. In Rickham PP, Hecker WC, and Prevot J, editors: Progress in pediatric surgery, vol 8, Baltimore, 1974, University Park Press.
91. Hill LL: Report of case of successful suturing of heart, and table of 37 other cases of suturing by different operators with various terminations and conclusions drawn, Med Record p 846, November 1902; cited by Sugg WL and Ecker RR: J Thorac Cardiovasc Surg 56:531, 1968.
92. Hof E: Surgical correction of laryngotracheal stenoses in children, Prog Pediatr Surg 21:20, 1987.
93. Holdefer WF, Dowling EA, and Kirklin JW: Hemodynamic, metabolic, and organ function studies in animals subjected to prolonged venoarterial bypass with the Bramson membrane lung, J Thorac Cardiovasc Surg 61:217, 1971.
94. Holder TM, Ashcraft KW, and Leape L: The treatment of patients with esophageal strictures by local steroid injection, J Pediatr Surg 4:646, 1969.
95. Holinger PH and Schild JA: Pharyngeal, laryngeal, and tracheal injuries in the pediatric age group, Ann Otol Rhinol Laryngol 81:538, 1972.
96. Holinger PH et al: The conservative and surgical management of benign strictures of the esophagus, J Thorac Surg 28:345, 1954.
97. Houck JC and Patel YM: Proposed mode of action of corticosteroids on the connective tissue, Nature 206:158, 1965.
98. Howes EL et al: Retardation of wound healing by cortisone, Surgery 28:177, 1950.
99. Hyde I: Traumatic paramediastinal air cysts, Br J Radiol 44:389, 1971.
100. Johnson CF, Reyes HM, and Repologe R: Diaphragmatic hernia from penetrating thoracoabdominal injury in an infant, J Pediatr Surg 5:572, 1970.
101. Jones MJ and James EC: The management of traumatic asphyxia: case report and literature review, J Trauma 16:235, 1976.
102. Joshi VV et al: Acute lesions induced by endotracheal intubation, Am J Dis Child 124:646, 1972.
103. Joske RA and Benedict EB: The role of benign esophageal obstruction in the development of carcinoma of the esophagus, Gastroenterology 36:749, 1959.
104. Kerr HH, Sloan H, and O'Brien CE: Rupture of the esophagus by compressed air, Surgery 33:417, 1953.
105. Ketchum LD et al: The treatment of hypertropic scar, keloid and scar contracture by triamcinolone acetonide, Plast Reconstr Surg 38:209, 1966.
106. Kirsch MM, Pellegrini RV, and Sloan HE: Treatment of blunt chest trauma, Surg Ann 4:51, 1972.
107. Kirsh MM et al: Repair of acute traumatic rupture of the aorta without extracorporeal circulation, Ann Thorac Surg 10:227, 1970.
108. Kirsh MM et al: Roentgenographic evaluation of traumatic rupture of the aorta, Surg Gynecol Obstet 131:900, 1970.
109. Kirsh MM et al: Management of tracheobronchial disruption secondary to nonpenetrating trauma, Ann Thorac Surg 22:93, 1976.
110. Knox WG et al: Bouginage and steroids used singly or in combination in experimental corrosive esophagitis, Ann Surg 166:930, 1967.
111. Krey H: On the treatment of corrosive lesions in the oesophagus: an experimental study, Acta Otolaryngol [Suppl] (Stockh) 102:1, 1952.
112. Lampson RS: Traumatic chylothorax—a review of the literature and report of a case treated by mediastinal ligation of the thoracic duct, J Thorac Surg 17:778, 1948.
113. Larizadeh R: Rupture of the bronchus, Thorax 21:28, 1966.
114. Larrey DJ: Clin Chir Paris 2:284, 1829; cited by Sugg WL et al: J Thorac Cardiovasc Surg 56:531, 1973.
115. Lasky II, Nahum AM, and Siegel AW: Cardiac injuries incurred by drivers in automobile accidents, J Forensic Sci 14:13, 1969.
116. Leape LL et al: Hazard to health—liquid lye, N Engl J Med 284:578, 1971.
117. Lee SS and Hong PW: Rupture of the bronchus, Arch Surg 95:123, 1967.

118. Levy JL Jr: Management of crushing chest injuries in children, South Med J 65:1040, 1972.

119. Liedtke AJ and DeMuth WE Jr: Nonpenetrating cardiac injuries: a collective review, Am Heart J 86:687, 1973.

120. Lilly JO and McCaffery TD: Esophageal stricture dilation: a new method adapted to the fiberoptic esophagoscope, Am Dig Dis 15:1137, 1971.

121. Lobe TE, Hayden CK, and Nicholas D: Successful management of congenital tracheal stenosis in infancy, J Pediatr Surg 22:1137, 1987.

122. Lynn HB: Simple method of enlongating a colonic segment for esophageal replacement, J Pediatr Surg 8:391, 1973.

123. Lyons C and Perkins R: Cardiac stab wounds, Am Surg 23:507, 1957.

124. Management of lye burns of the esophagus, Med Lett Drugs Ther 6:18, 1972.

125. Marks MI et al: Adrenocorticosteroid treatment of hydrocarbon pneumonia in children—a cooperative study, J Pediatr 81:366, 1972.

126. Martin JE: Respiratory burns, Ill Med J 147:345, 1975.

127. Mazure PA, Chiocca JC, and Sferco AG: New device for progressive dilation of benign esophageal stricture, Gut 13:153, 1972.

128. McCune RP, Roda CP, and Eckert C: Rupture of the diaphragm caused by blunt trauma, J Trauma 16:531, 1976.

129. McNeill RA and Welbourn RB: Prevention of corrosive stricture of the oesophagus in the rat, J Laryngol Otol 80:346, 1966.

130. Meade RH: The surgical treatment of stricture of the esophagus. In Meade RH, editor: A history of thoracic surgery, Springfield, Ill, 1961, Charles C. Thomas.

131. Meyers NA: Traumatic rupture of the diaphragm in children, Aust N Z J Surg 34:123, 1964.

132. Minnigerode B and Richter HB: Pathophysiology of subglottic tracheal stenosis in childhood, Prog Pediatr Surg 21:7, 1987.

133. Moore TC and Goldstein J: Use of intact omentum for closure of full-thickness esophageal defects, Surgery 45:899, 1959.

134. Moraes CR et al: Ventricular septal defect following nonpenetrating trauma: case report and review of the surgical literature, Angiology 24:222, 1973.

135. Myers WO, Leape LL, and Holder TM: Bronchial rupture on a child with subsequent stenosis, resection, and anastomosis, Ann Thorac Surg 12:442, 1971.

136. Naclerio EA: Chest injuries: physiologic principles and emergency management, New York, 1971, Grune & Stratton.

137. Nelson TG: Tracheotomy: a clinical and experimental study, Am Surg 23:660, 1957.

138. Ng RC, Darwish H, and Stewart DA: Emergency treatment of petroleum distillate and turpentine ingestine, Can Med Assoc J 111:537, 1974.

139. Ochsner A and Owens N: Anterothoracic oesophagoplasty for impermeable stricture of the oesophagus, Ann Surg 100:1055, 1934.

140. Ollivier d-A: Relation medicale des evenements survenus an Champ-de-Mars le 17 juin, 1937. Ann d'hyg 18:485, 1937; cited by Williams JS: Ann Surg 167:384, 1968.

141. O'Reilly RJ, Kazenelson G, and Spellberg RD: Traumatic pseudoaneurysm of the left ventricle, Am J Dis Child 120:252, 1970.

142. Othersen HB: Subglottic stenosis: a new epidemic in children, Contemp Surg 12:9, 1978.

143. Othersen HB: Intubation injuries of the trachea in children: management and prevention, Ann Surg 189:601, 1979.

144. Othersen HB: Trachea, lungs, pleural cavity. In Welch KG, editor: Complications of pediatric surgery prevention and management, Philadelphia, 1982, WB Saunders Co.

145. Othersen HB and Lorenzo RL: Diaphragmatic paralysis and eventration: newer approaches to diagnosis and operative correction (in press).

146. Othersen HB et al: Endoscopic tracheoplasty and esophagoplasty in children: a new technique utilizing balloon catheters (unpublished data).

147. Othersen HB Jr: Steroid therapy for tracheal stenosis in children, Ann Thorac Surg 17:254, 1974.

148. Othersen HB Jr: The technique of intraluminal stenting and steroid administration in the treatment of tracheal stenosis in children, J Pediatr Surg 9:683, 1974.

149. Othersen HB Jr: The prevention and treatment of tracheal injuries in children, Am Surg 43:108, 1977.

150. Othersen HB Jr and Clatworthy HW Jr: Functional evaluation of esophageal replacement in children, J Thorac Cardiovasc Surg 53:55, 1967.

151. Othersen HB Jr and Gregorie HB Jr: Esophagectomy for benign lesions, J SC Med Assoc 58:441, 1962.

152. Othersen HB Jr and Gregorie HB Jr: Pneumatic rupture of the stomach in a newborn infant with esophageal atresia and tracheoesophageal fistula, Surgery 53:362, 1963.

153. Papamichael EE and Fotiou G: Rupture of the thoracic trachea with avulsion of the apex of the right upper lobe, J Thorac Cardiovasc Surg 50:742, 1965.

154. Pare A: The works of that famous chirugeon Ambrose Pare. Translated out of Latin and compared with the French by Thomas Johnson, London, 1634, L Cotes & R Young; cited by McCune RP, Roda CP, and Eckert C: J Trauma 16:531, 1976.

155. Parmley LF, Manion WC, and Mattingly TW: Nonpenetrating traumatic injury of the heart, Circulation 18:371, 1958.

156. Pearl M, Milstein M, and Rook GD: Pseudocyst of the lung due to traumatic nonpenetrating injury, J Pediatr Surg 8:967, 1973.

157. Peirce EC II et al: Techniques of extended perfusion using a membrane lung, Ann Thorac Surg 12:451, 1971.

158. Pennington CL: External trauma of larynx and trachea: immediate treatment and management, Ann Otol Rhinol Laryngol 81:546, 1972.

159. Perthes G: Ueber "Drunkstrauung." Deutsche Ztsch f Chir LV, 1900; cited by Williams JS: Ann Surg 167:384, 1968.

160. Petrow BA: Retrosternal artificial esophagus from jejunum and colon, Surgery 45:890, 1959.

161. Pike DG et al: A reevaluation of the dangers of clorox injestion, J Pediatr 63:303, 1963.

162. Polin SG and Spiegel P: Rupture of a segmental bronchus, Ann Thorac Surg 6:384, 1968.

163. Polk HC and Stone HH, editors: Contemporary burn management, Boston, 1971, Little, Brown & Co.

164. Prian GW: New proximal approach works well in temporal artery catherization, JAMA 235:2693, 1976.

165. Priest RE: History of tracheotomy, Ann Otol Rhinol Laryngol 61:1039, 1952.
166. Proctor DF: The air passages. In The biologic basis of pediatric research, vol 1, New York, 1968, McGraw Hill Book Co.
167. Randolph H, Melick DW, and Grant AR: Perforation of the esophagus from external trauma or blast injuries, Dis Chest 51:121, 1967.
168. Rehn L: Uber penetrirende herzwanden and herznaht. Arch f Klin Chir 55:315, 1897; cited by Sugg WL and Ecker RR: J Thorac Cardiovasc Surg 56:531, 1968.
169. Reyes HM et al: Experimental treatment of corrosive esophageal burns, J Pediatr Surg 9:317, 1974.
170. Richardson JA and Pratt-Thomas HR: Toxic effects of varying doses of kerosene administered by different routes, Am J Med Sci 221:531, 1951.
171. Rose E: Herztamponade (ein beitrag zur herzchirugie) Deutsche Ztsch f Chir 20:329, 1884; cited by Lyons C and Perkins R: Am Surg 23:507, 1957.
172. Rosenberg N et al: Prevention of experimental esophageal stricture by cortisone. II. Control of suppurative complications by penicillin. Arch Surg 66:593, 1953.
173. Ruhrah J: Pediatrics of the past, New York, 1925, Paul B Hoeber.
174. Saad SA and Othersen HB: Esophageal perforation in an infant: repair with a pleural flap, South Med J 72:1596, 1979.
175. Salter DG and Hopton DS: Traumatic intercostal hernia without penetrating injury in a child: case report, Br J Surg 56:550, 1969.
176. Salzer H: Early treatment of corrosive esophagitis, Wien Klin Wochenschr 33:307, 1920; cited by Webb WW et al: Ann Thorac Surg 9:95, 1970.
177. Sampson PC: Tracheostomy, Hosp Med 1:2, 1964.
178. Schiller M, Frye TR, and Boles ET Jr: Evaluation of colonic replacement of the esophagus in children, J Pediatr Surg 6:753, 1971.
179. Schmiegelow E: Stenosis of the larynx: a new method of surgical treatment, Arch Otolaryngol 9:473, 1929.
180. Schofield J: Conservative treatment of subglottic stenosis of the larynx, Arch Otolaryngol 95:457, 1972.
181. Schramel R et al: Traumatic pericarditis, J Cardiovasc Surg 6:244, 1965.
182. Schweich P and Fleisher G: Rib fractures in children, Pediatr Emerg Care 1:187, 1985.
183. Selmonosky CA, Flege JB Jr, and Ehrenhaft JL: Torsion of a lobe of the lung due to blunt thoracic trauma, Ann Thorac Surg 4:166, 1967.
184. Shumacker HB Jr and Moore TC: Surgical management of traumatic chylothorax, Surg Gynecol Obstet 93:46, 1951.
185. Sinclair MC and Moore TC: Major surgery for abdominal and thoracic trauma in childhood and adolescence, J Pediatr Surg 9:155, 1974.
186. Skillman JJ, Parikh BM, and Tanenbaum BJ: Pulmonary arteriovenous admixture—improvement with albumin and diuresis, Am J Surg 119:440, 1970.
187. Smith CD et al: Diaphragmatic paralysis and eventration in infants, J Thorac Cardiovasc Surg 91:490, 1986.
188. Smith RB, Myers EN, and Sherman H: Transtracheal ventilation in paediatric patients, Br J Anesth 46:313, 1974.
189. Smith RD, Miller SH, and Graham WP III: Inhalation injury in burned patients, Pa Med 78:66, 1975.
190. Smith W and Stempel D: Spontaneous healing of traumatic intercostal pulmonary hernia, Am J Dis Child 126:354, 1973.
191. Soulen RL and Freeman E: Radiologic evaluation of traumatic heart disease, Radiol Clin North Am 9:285, 1971.
192. Soulen RL, Lapayowker MS, and Gimenez JL: Echocardiography in diagnosis of pericardial effusion, Radiology 86:1047, 1966.
193. Spain DM, Malomut N, and Haber A: The effect of cortisone on the formation of granulation tissue in mice, Am J Pathol 26:710, 1950.
194. Stapp JP: Gravitational stress in aerospace medicine, Boston, Little, Brown & Company.
195. Steele RW, Conklin RH, and Mark HM: Corticosteroids and antibiotics for treatment of fulminant hydrocarbon aspiration, JAMA 219:1434, 1972.
196. Stemmer EA et al: Fatal complications of tracheotomy, Am J Surg 131:288, 1976.
197. Stone HH et al: Respiratory burns: a correlation of clinical and laboratory results, Ann Surg 165:157, 1967.
198. Striker TW, Stool S, and Downes JJ: Prolonged nasotracheal intubation in infants and children, Arch Otolaryngol 85:210, 1967.
199. Sugg WL et al: Penetrating wounds of the heart: an analysis of 459 cases, J Thorac Cardiovasc Surg 56:531, 1973.
200. Sutherland HD: Indirect traumatic rupture of the diaphragm, Post Grad Med J 34:210, 1958.
201. Tannenberg J and Pinner M: Atelectasis and bronchiectasis, J Thoracic Surg 11:571, 1942.
202. Tillett WS and Sherry S: The effect in patients of streptococcal fibrinolysin (streptokinase) and streptococcal deoxyribonuclease on fibrinous, purulent, and sanguineous pleural exudations, J Clin Invest 28:173, 1949.
203. VerMeulen V and Birck H: Prolonged intubation vs tracheotomy in children, Arch Otolaryngol 87:152, 1968.
204. Vidine B and Levy MJ: Use of pericardium for esophagoplasty in congenital esophageal stenosis, Surgery 68:389, 1970.
205. Ward PA and Suzuki A: Gunshot wound of the heart with peripheral embolization: a case report with review of the literature, J Thorac Cardiovasc Surg 68:440, 1974.
206. Waring JI: Pneumonia in kerosene poisoning, Am J Med Sci 185:325, 1933.
207. Waterson DJ: Reconstruction of the esophagus. In Mustard WT et al, editors: Pediatric surgery, vol 1, ed 2, Chicago, 1969, Year Book Medical Publishers.
208. Webb WR et al: An evaluation of the steroids and antibiotics in caustic burns of the esophagus, Ann Thorac Surg 9:95, 1970.
209. Webster I and Blum LJ: Traumatic lung, Forensic Sci 1:167, 1972.
210. Weisskopf A: Effects of cortisone on experimental lye burn of the esophagus, Ann Otol Rhinol Laryngol 61:681, 1952.
211. White JJ, Oh KS, and Haller JA Jr: Positive-contrast peritoneography for accurate delineation of diaphragmatic abnormalities, Surgery 76:398, 1974.
212. Williams JS, Minken SL, and Adams JT: Traumatic asphyxia—reappraised, Ann Surg 167:384, 1968.

213. Wilson AJ and Kraus HG: Lung perforation during chest tube placement in stiff lung syndrome, J Pediatr Surg 9:213, 1974.

214. Wise AJ et al: The importance of serial blood gas determinations in blunt chest trauma, J Thorac Cardiovasc Surg 56:520, 1968.

215. Yarington CT, Bales GA, and Frazer JP: A study of the management of caustic esophageal trauma, Ann Otol Rhinol Laryngol 73:1130, 1964.

216. Zuckerman S: Experimental study of blast injuries to the lungs, Lancet 2:219, 1940.

217. Zuckerman S: Discussion on the problem of blast injuries, Proc R Soc Med 34:171, 1941.

16

Abdomen

HEPATIC, BILIARY TREE, AND PANCREATIC INJURY

Donald R. Cooney and Deborah F. Billmire

LIVER
Incidence and Associated Injuries

The liver is the second most commonly injured intraabdominal organ in pediatric patients. Hepatic injuries are detected in 16% to 31% of the cases of abdominal trauma in childhood. This incidence has been reported by institutions favoring operative therapy and also by centers that have adopted a more selective approach, including nonoperative management.[16,54,65,74] The majority of liver injuries in younger children are caused by blunt trauma. In contrast, a greater percentage of the hepatic lacerations seen in adolescent patients residing in urban centers result from penetrating injuries to the abdomen.[72] On rare occasions, birth trauma may result in liver lacerations in the newborn.[5,68] Additional injuries are detected in approximately two thirds of the children who have sustained significant liver trauma. The most frequently associated injuries are to the head and chest. Splenic lacerations, renal trauma, and long bone fractures are also common associated findings.

Recent Advances in Management

During the 1960s and early 1970s most liver injuries were considered to be associated with a very high mortality. Before the routine use of noninvasive diagnostic techniques such as nuclear scanning, ultrasound examination, and CT scanning many less extensive hepatic injuries were simply not recognized. This diagnostic shortcoming led to the false impression that most liver trauma should be treated surgically to prevent the reported high mortality. In addition, clinical reports of liver injuries diagnosed at laparotomy disclosed that

over 60% of these lacerations had spontaneously stopped bleeding by the time of exploration.[40,72] These factors led to a reevaluation of the clinical approach regarding the diagnosis and management of hepatic trauma not only in children but also in adults.[11,25,48,77] Today the trauma surgeon must be able to diagnose all forms of intraabdominal trauma and is required to exercise prudent judgment regarding appropriate management based on the severity and extent of each organ injury. Pediatric surgeons who accept responsibility for multiply injured children should be prepared to diagnose and manage both major and minor hepatic injuries. In addition, surgeons should have a comprehensive understanding of the alternative surgical procedures to be applied to each operative situation and should also be familiar with the concepts of selective and nonoperative management.

Diagnosis

Hepatic injury should be considered in all cases of abdominal trauma. The majority of children will have abdominal tenderness; however, significant injuries are frequently encountered in patients who have surprisingly benign abdominal findings.[54] The common association of liver lacerations with closed head trauma, musculoskeletal, and chest injuries may make the physical examination unreliable. Reported experiences of hepatic trauma during the early 1970s revealed that patients with liver injuries often presented with severe hypotension and gross abdominal distention requiring urgent laparotomy.[40] Today, however, superior diagnostic techniques that provide much better anatomic detail have more accurately defined the true spectrum of these injuries. Clinicians now appreciate that these high-risk patients probably represent only a small fraction of the total number of children who will be admitted with hepatic lacerations.

Several physical findings should increase the index of suspicion for liver laceration: upper abdominal wall contusions, right upper quadrant tenderness, hypoactive bowel sounds, shoulder pain, and a right upper quadrant mass. Suggestive x-ray findings are nonspecific but include right-sided rib fractures, right pleural effusion, elevated right hemidiaphragm, adynamic ileus, and irregularity of the liver contour.[40] Oldham and co-workers[53] advocated the measurement of hepatic enzymes as a screening procedure to identify children with he-

patic injury. In this series from the Children's Hospital in Cincinnati, 95 patients sustained abdominal trauma, and 94 of the children were studied by CT scan. STAT liver enzymes were obtained from all these patients during their initial evaluation in the emergency room. All of the patients sustaining a liver laceration had both SGOT levels greater than 200 IU and SGPT levels greater than 100 IU. Although 38% of children with enzymes elevated to these levels did not have a liver injury, this study suggests that all children with elevations in this range should be scanned to prevent missing a significant hepatic injury. Measurement of "liver" enzymes appears to be an excellent screening test for hepatic trauma in children and may be particularly

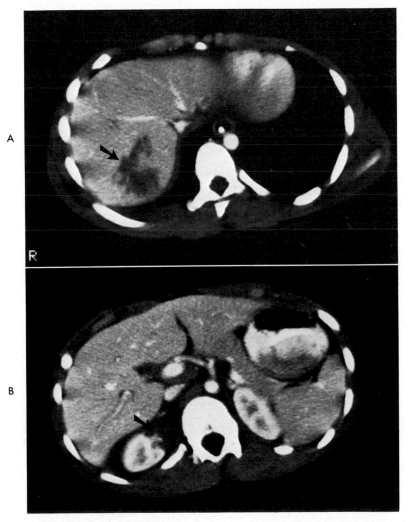

Fig. 16-1   CT scan of a 10-year-old boy struck by a car while on his bicycle. **A,** Large contusion in the posterior superior right lobe of the liver *(arrow)*. **B,** Area of hypoperfusion in the superior medial aspect of the right kidney *(arrow)* representing renal contusion and edema.

useful in selecting those patients who wil benefit most from CT scanning.

Radiologic techniques most useful in detecting hepatic injury include nuclear scanning, ultrasound, and CT scanning. Of these, CT scanning is clearly the most sensitive and provides more comprehensive information about other intraperitoneal and retroperitoneal organs (Fig. 16-1).[38,39,41] A preponderance of right lobe injuries has consistently been observed in reported series of blunt hepatic trauma. Lacerations along the attachment of the falciform ligament between the lateral and medial segments of the left lobe are also very common. A recently reported confirmatory analysis of CT-detected injuries disclosed that right lobe trauma constitutes over 80% of the cases. The posterior segment of the right lobe is the most frequently injured area of the liver.[69]

Several classification systems have been proposed to allow for comparative evaluation of morbidity and mortality following hepatic injury. These systems may be useful in planning therapy and predicting outcome. Most of the classification sys-

tems follow a pattern similar to that described by Moore,[51] which is outlined in Table 16-1.

Initial Management

As in all cases of abdominal trauma the initial priorities in the emergency room consist of primary attention to ventilation, circulation, and establishment of adequate intravenous access. Avoidance of lower extremity intravenous lines is suggested in these cases, since possible coexistent caval or hepatic venous injuries may result in the potential loss of resuscitation fluids into the peritoneal cavity.[13]

The majority of children with liver trauma will be hemodynamically stable on arrival in the emergency room. However, if the patient exhibits cardiovascular instability and has obvious abdominal distension, exploratory laparotomy should be undertaken immediately after paracentesis documentation of the hemoperitoneum. If the child is stable, it is advisable to proceed with noninvasive radiographic confirmation of the hepatic injury and a careful evaluation of all organ systems. Because

Table 16-1   Classification of hepatic injuries

Class	Liver injury		Expected frequency (%)	Management options in children
I	Capsular avulsion Parenchymal fracture	1 cm deep	15	1. Selective nonoperative approach possible
II	Parenchymal fracture Subcapsular hematoma Peripheral penetrating wound	1-3 cm deep 10 cm diameter	55	2. Operation involves: a. Control of hemorrhage (hemostatic agents, simple suturing)
III	Parenchymal fracture Subcapsular hematoma Central penetrating wound	3 cm deep 10 cm diameter	25	b. Debridement c. Drainage
IV	Lobar tissue destruction Massive central hematoma		3	1. Need for operation depends on status of hemorrhage; operation usually required 2. Operation involves: a. Control of hemorrhage b. Debridement c. Drainage d. Lobar resection ? e. Packing ?
V	Retrohepatic vena cava injury Extensive bilobar disruption		2	Operation required Vascular repair Lobar resection ? Packing ? Drainage

Modified after Moore EE: Am J Surg 148:713, 1984.

of the concern of persistent hemorrhage, exploration was previously recommended for the majority of patients with liver injury. However, clinical experiences at many children's centers support a more selective approach, including nonoperative management under carefully controlled intensive care conditions. This precedent was first suggested by Richie and Fonkalsrud[60] in 1972 for a subgroup of patients with contained intracapsular hematomas. The growing acceptance of nonoperative management for pediatric splenic injuries and the increasing finding of unsuspected hepatic injuries in stable trauma patients undergoing scintigraphy or CT scanning gave birth to the concept of selective nonoperative management of children with hepatic injury. In 1983 Karp et al.[39] reported a series of 17 consecutive patients with CT documented hepatic trauma who were managed nonoperatively with good results. Several additional reports confirming the successful use of selective nonoperative management of liver injuries in children have since appeared in the literature.[16,29,54]

Adherence to a strict protocol for nonoperative management cannot be overemphasized. These patients require close monitoring in an intensive care setting by surgeons experienced in trauma care. A prerequisite is 24-hour-a-day immediate accessibility to the operating room. Reliable intravenous access must be maintained, and a nasogastric tube should be placed to manage the accompanying paralytic ileus. Serial hematocrits and physical examinations should be performed at frequent intervals. The onset of hemodynamic instability, signs of increasing peritoneal irritation, or transfusion requirements greater than 30 to 40 cc/kg (one third to one half of estimated blood volume) are indications for exploratory laparotomy. Applying these criteria will permit 43% to 88% of these children to be managed successfully without operation.[26,54]

A single report by Bass et al.[2] from the Children's Hospital National Medical Center warned of possible increased morbidity with the use of nonoperative management for pediatric liver injuries. This series consisted of seven children, four of whom required transfusions in excess of 40 cc/kg. These patients would have failed to meet the Buffalo criteria for continued nonoperative management, as outlined and adopted by other pediatric trauma centers. The surgeon must be willing to interrupt the conservative management for a more traditional surgical approach if the child's condition

does not meet the established criteria for nonoperative management.

Operative Management

Certainly, there is a subset of patients with hepatic injury that require immediate laparotomy for control of hemorrhage. When mortality results from hepatic injury, it is almost always caused by uncontrolled bleeding. In approximately 2% to 5% of patients, there is an associated injury to the retrohepatic vena cava or hepatic veins that carries a mortality in excess of 50%. Children who remain hemodynamically unstable after 20 to 30 cc/kg of initial fluid resuscitation should be taken directly to the operating room for exploratory laparotomy.

In the operating room preparation and draping of the field should include the thorax in the event that the incision has to be extended into a median sternotomy to obtain vascular control. The peritoneal cavity should be entered through a midline incision. This approach is faster than the traditional transverse pediatric incision and allows for excellent exposure of the entire peritoneal cavity. Visible bleeding from anterior lacerations and fractures should initially be controlled by direct compression. If both the spleen and liver are lacerated and bleeding significantly, it is advisable that the second assistant hold compression on the liver while the surgeon and first assistant quickly remove the spleen so that all attention can be directed to the liver. Control of hemorrhage should be followed by debridement of devitalized tissue and direct suture ligation of bleeding vessels. Occasionally, hemostatic agents such as topical thrombin or microfibrillar collagen may be very useful in controlling minor hemorrhage. Most grade I and grade II injuries will be effectively controlled by these techniques. Contained subcapsular hematomas should be left undisturbed. "Unroofing" these lesions will only initiate bleeding and will not benefit the patient in any way.

Although drainage of hepatic injuries has long been considered standard practice, the comparative data of Fischer et al.[23] suggests that for minor, nonbursting hepatic injuries, drainage may not always be indicated. If drains are employed, suction sump catheters brought out through a separate dependent exit site are most appropriate. These catheters should be removed once they have stopped draining and usually after a postoperative CT scan confirms that no large fluid collections remain.

Extensive hepatic injuries consisting of deep parenchymal penetration or those characterized as a "bursting" type of laceration that continue to bleed despite simple maneuvers will require more aggressive therapy. Formal hepatic lobectomy in the trauma setting carries a mortality of approximately 70%.[52] Major liver resections should be considered as the last resort and only for extensive devitalizing injuries. The concept of aggressive debridement and limited resection has become the preferred mode of therapy.[52]

When bleeding cannot be controlled by direct pressure, compression of the portal triad (Pringle maneuver) should be carried out as a temporizing measure to provide relative hemostatis and improve exposure. Although back bleeding from the vena cava will continue, this maneuver is most effective when used in combination with direct compression of the affected lobe. In Pachter and co-workers'[57] series of 75 patients, this technique was helpful in gaining temporary hemostasis in over 85% of patients with extensive lacerations. The hepatic wound may have to be extended carefully by blunt fracture technique to gain exposure to bleeding vessels and lacerated bile ducts to facilitate precise ligation.[55,57] The resulting open hepatic defect can either be left open to provide free drainage or, if minor bleeding persists, it can be closed over a "pack" of omentum attached to its vascular pedicle, as described by Stone and Lamb.[73]

If bleeding persists despite these efforts, selective ligation of the hepatic artery may be considered as the next step.[51] Although a high success rate has been reported by some authors, others have raised concerns that the resulting decrease in perfusion and oxygenation may increase the subsequent risk of perihepatic postoperative infection.[1,24] Perioperative prophylactic antibiotics are considered prudent management in this situation.

Failure to achieve hemostasis despite all of the above measures may be because of the development of a progressive coagulopathy from the combined effects of hypothermia, acidosis, and depletion of coagulation factors from massive transfusion. The resulting diffuse ooze from all raw surfaces is not amenable to specific surgical therapy. Under these life-threatening circumstances, packing of the hepatic wound with gauze or laparotomy pads with a plan to return to the operating room for inspection and removal of the packs should be considered. This technique has been successful in controlling hemorrhage in over 90% of patients in a recently reported experience.[21] Removal of the packs should be carried out after correction of any coagulopathy and stabilization of hemodynamic parameters. Packs should be removed in the operating room, allowing for reinspection of the wound, further debridement of necrotic tissue, ligation of bleeding vessels, and placement of drains.

Patients with grade V injuries involving the vena cava or hepatic veins represent a small but lethal subgroup. These injuries usually present with massive bleeding and hypotension, but there may be an initial brief period of stability followed by abrupt deterioration.[13] The usual laceration is a posterolateral deep stellate fracture extending through the coronary ligament with avulsion of the hepatic veins. This extensive injury should be suspected not only in cases of massive hemoperitoneum but also when disruption of the coronary ligament is found on palpation of the dome of the liver or when brisk bleeding results from attempts at downward traction on the liver. When this injury exists, initial efforts should be directed at restoring the blood volume before reexposure of the injury. The liver should first be compressed superiorly against the diaphragm during occlusion of the porta hepatis. Once the blood volume is adequately restored, an attempt should be made to visualize the injury. Usually some degree of unavoidable hemorrhage will occur during exposure and repair of the veins. If vascular control cannot be achieved on the first attempt, the liver should again be compressed. The midline laparotomy should be extended as a median sternotomy and an incision should be made through the central tendon of the diaphragm to gain access to the suprahepatic vena cava and hepatic veins. In most instances this will allow more adequate exposure and direct control of the injury. This technique was used by Coln et al.[13] in treating four children, resulting in survival in each case. Intracaval shunts were not used in any of their cases. In fact, these authors suggested they were neither indicated nor necessary in children because of the additional time and blood loss involved in their insertion. The concept of the intracaval shunt as described by Schrock et al.[64] in 1968 was actually first used clinically in a child without success. The technique involves insertion of a chest tube or vascular cannula of appropriate size through a purse string in the right atrial appendage down into the suprarenal cava (Fig. 16-2). Although this maneuver has rarely been successful, its occasional use

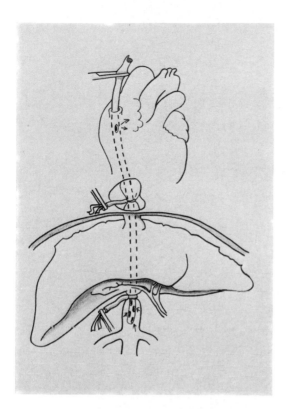

Fig. 16-2 Intracaval shunt, as described by Schrock.[64] Chest tube inserted via right atrial appendage to suprarenal IVC via combined median sternotomy, laparotomy approach. Additional holes must be cut in the portion of the tube within the atrium to allow flow through the shunt.

in properly selected patients may be lifesaving.[78] It should also be noted that in life-threatening situations surgeons at the Children's Hospital of Buffalo have simply ligated one of the hepatic veins when venous repair would have been technically very difficult and too time consuming. Two children treated at our hospital have survived when one of the hepatic veins was ligated in this desperate situation without subsequent lobe resection or complication.

Nonoperative Management and Postoperative Care

Children who remain stable during nonoperative management may be advanced to a diet as tolerated when their ileus resolves. Monitoring in the intensive care unit should continue for a period of 48 to 72 hours, after which further hemodynamic changes are unlikely. The patient may then be

transferred to the surgical ward for continued bedrest. A repeat CT scan should be obtained at 10 to 14 days to assess the healing or progression of the injury. Karp et al.[39] noted a predictable series of changes after hepatic trauma (Fig. 16-3). The first stage of healing, which should be apparent at 10 to 14 days after injury, is characterized by the absorption of intraperitoneal blood. At this point most children may be discharged from the hospital on limited activity with frequent and careful outpatient follow-up. The second stage of healing is characterized by coalescence of the lacerations into a larger single cavity of low density. The third and final stage is recognized by an increasing density in the area of the injury and a shrinking in size of the wound. Complete resolution occurs 2 to 6 months following the injury, depending on the size and complexity of the initial lesion. CT scans can be repeated at 6- to 8-week intervals on an outpatient basis until complete healing is documented and should serve as a guide to recommend resumption of physical activities. It is also important to note that the same CT patterns of healing are seen in children whose hepatic injuries are treated surgically and would support a similar plan of postoperative management in this group of children.[39]

Nonoperative management of subcapsular hematomas has raised concern regarding the possibility of subsequent episodes of rebleeding or infection. Delayed rupture, although uncommon, has been reported to occur as late as 6 weeks after the injury, indicating the need for limited activity and careful radiographic and clinical follow-up.[11] In the absence of hemodynamic instability, delayed hemorrhage can be successfully managed nonoperatively.[16] Infection has also been described in children with subcapsular hematomas. Two children in another series developed an hepatic abscess at 6 and 28 days after injury.[25] Late infection has not been reported from other pediatric trauma centers, supporting the concept of conservative management of subcapsular hematomas. The observations of Geis et al.,[25] however, again emphasize the need for careful monitoring until the injury resolves radiographically.

Hemobilia

Hemobilia is a rare complication of hepatic injury. It results from injury to a hepatic arterial branch with subsequent pseudoaneurysm formation. Rupture of the pseudoaneurysm into the biliary tree produces the classic triad of colicky ab-

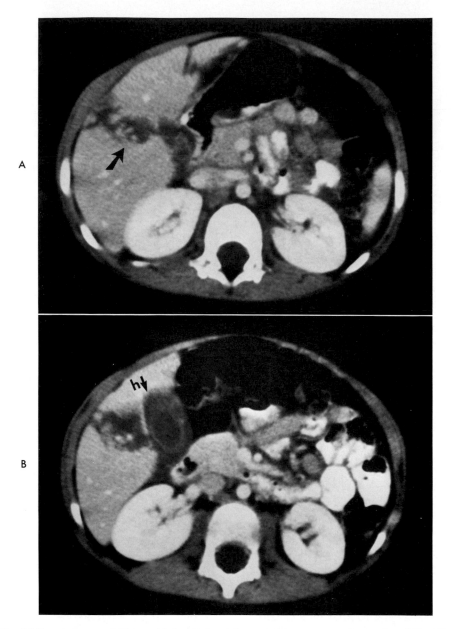

Fig. 16-3 A 4-year-old boy with handlebar injury to right upper quadrant. **A** and **B,** CT scans at time of injury reveal a large liver laceration *(arrow)* through the anterior segment of the right lobe extending through the gallbladder fossa with surrounding hematoma *(arrow h)*.

dominal pain, jaundice, and gastrointestinal hemorrhage. These bleeding episodes may occur days to months following the injury without any warning and may be life threatening. Mortality is reported to be as high as 25%. To date, most cases of hemobilia in childhood have followed surgical management of the primary liver injury.[33,42,44,72] Not unexpectantly, in the last few years hemobilia has

also been reported following nonoperative therapy in two children.[44,54]

Although spontaneous healing of the underlying arterial lesion has been documented, the risk of unpredictable acute life-threatening hemorrhage makes expectant management of hemobilia unacceptable.[33,54] Surgical options for treatment have included selective hepatic artery ligation, lobec-

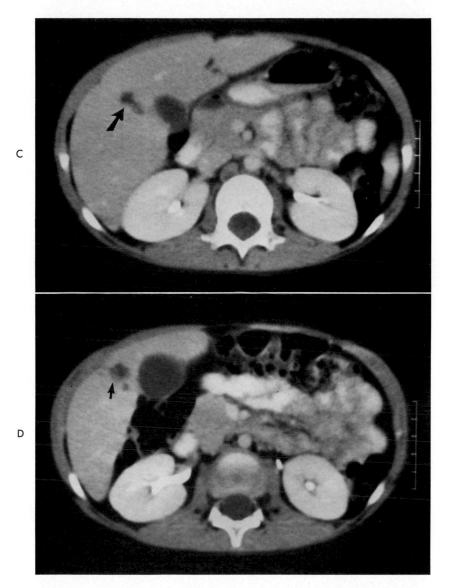

Fig. 16-3, cont'd   C and **D,** Same area 11 days after injury with significant healing, resorption of hematoma, and reduction in fracture size *(arrows).*

Continued.

tomy, and hepatotomy with direct ligation of the involved vessel. The increasing use of therapeutic angiography has led to successful embolization of this lesion in several cases.[8,42,44] If this relatively less aggressive treatment modality continues to be used successfully for pediatric patients, it may eliminate the need for more radical and sometimes difficult surgery.

EXTRAHEPATIC BILIARY TREE
Incidence and Associated Injuries

Injuries to the gallbladder, extrahepatic biliary tract, or both are uncommon. The overall incidence of these injuries in both children and adults who are explored for abdominal trauma is approximately 2%.[65,67] The vast majority of these injuries are caused by blunt trauma, and many authors have

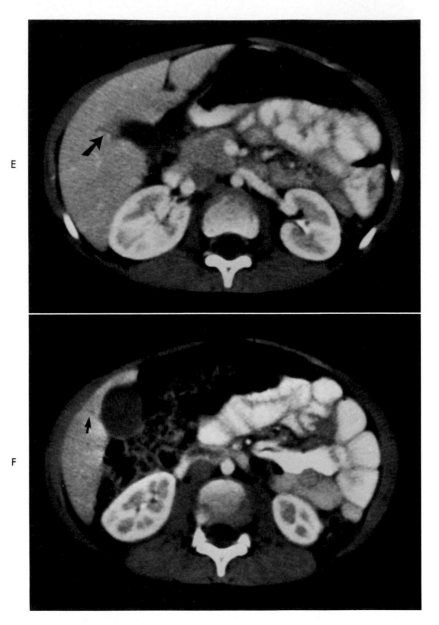

Fig. 16-3, cont'd   **E** and **F,** Three months after injury, only a small scar remains *(arrows)*.

speculated on the specific mechanisms involved. Distention combined with rapid increase in intraluminal pressure at the time of impact and shearing forces against relatively fixed structures have both been proposed as important contributing factors.

Isolated extrahepatic biliary injuries are extremely unusual. Nearly all patients sustain injuries to several additional abdominal organs. The most common associated injuries include trauma to the liver, duodenum, pancreas, and colon. Penetrating injuries to the bile ducts have often been associated

with trauma to neighboring vascular structures.[20] It is significant to note that blunt injury to the extrahepatic biliary tree has never been reported in association with hepatic artery or portal vein injury.[43]

Diagnosis

Early diagnosis of extrahepatic biliary tract injury is almost universally made during laparotomy for other injuries. Signs and symptoms related to the biliary injury are minimal, and even peritoneal lavage fluid will often fail to contain bile when this injury is present.[59] In the absence of other indications for surgery the diagnosis will frequently be delayed for days to weeks, resulting in the gradual development of bile peritonitis.

Early diagnosis at the time of initial laparotomy depends on a high index of suspicion and careful exploration. In Michelassi and Ranson's[49] collective review of blunt biliary tract trauma, 12% of these injuries were overlooked at initial laparotomy. Hematoma or contusion along the course of the biliary tree and bile staining of the retroperitoneum or lesser sac are signs of potential injury. In this situation a Kocher maneuver and opening of the lesser sac should be performed to improve exposure. If there is any doubt about the integrity of the ductal system, an intraoperative cholangiogram should be performed. The gallbladder should be preserved until completion of the cholangiogram in the event it is needed to be used as a diverting conduit or patch graft for a more significant major ductal injury.[20]

Operative Management

Approximately 80% of all extrahepatic biliary tract injuries include the gallbladder.[43] These range from simple contusions to perforation, laceration, and complete avulsion of the gallbladder from its liver bed. Although these injuries have been previously managed either by cholecystostomy or repair of the gallbladder, the current recommendation for any significant injury to the gallbladder is cholecystectomy. Minor contusions should be managed expectantly without increased concern of delayed complications.[67]

Injury to the ductal system is more challenging in the acute situation and is also controversial. The spectrum of injuries range from minor tangential tears to complete avulsion of the common duct. Most authors are in agreement that partial thickness or tangential injuries should be managed by primary repair with fine absorbable suture and T-tube drainage.* Complete transection of the duct most often occurs at the site where the bile duct enters the pancreas. Clinical experience in adults suggests that a high incidence of anastomic strictures may be expected following primary repair.[10,43] Reconstruction with a Roux-en-Y-jejunal loop is recommended as the preferred procedure. Published reports describing these injuries in children are in-

---

*References 10,20,32,43,49,59.

sufficient to draw any conclusions. Because of the even smaller size of the structures in pediatric patients, the authors suggest that the same general principles should be applied. In hemodynamically unstable patients with multiple-organ system trauma and a major biliary injury, end-tube hepatodochostomy or choledochostomy may be used as a temporizing measure with a plan for later reconstruction.

Postoperative Management

Repair of biliary tract injuries is associated with a low incidence of morbidity in the early postoperative period. Commitment to long-term, careful follow-up, however, is important because strictures and cholangitis may occur many months later.

Missed Diagnosis

A second category of patients exists in which the injury was not initially detected during nonoperative management or was unrecognized at the time of the initial exploratory laparotomy.[32,49,54] These patients develop bile peritonitis characterized by the gradual onset of abdominal distention, low grade fever, jaundice, and malnutrition. This symptom complex may be seen at any time from a few days to several weeks following the episode of abdominal trauma. Paracentesis will reveal bile-stained ascites, and nuclear image display and analysis (IDA) scan may demonstrate free intraperitoneal leakage of the isotope.[70] The increasing use of endoscopic retrograde choledochopancreatograph (ERCP) in children may also be a helpful adjunct in diagnosing this injury. At exploration, findings may include free biliary ascites or a loculated pseudocyst.[49] Operative therapy should be determined by the site and nature of the injury and should follow the general guidelines for acute injuries previously described. An operative cholangiogram should always be performed at the conclusion of any reparative operative procedure on the biliary tract to ensure that all injuries have been adequately treated.

PANCREAS

Incidence and Associated Injuries

Pancreatic injury is estimated to occur in 1% to 10% of children sustaining blunt abdominal trauma.[63,65] The actual incidence of pancreatic injuries in pediatric patients has been difficult to determine because of the lack of a reliable method of diagnosis short of laparotomy. The majority of reported experiences have originated from clinical reports of patients whose injuries were found at laparotomy.[28,47,63,71] During the last few years the increased use of ultrasound examination and CT scanning has identified a group of children with confirmed pancreatic injuries who have not undergone operation as part of their treatment (Fig. 16-4).[17,27] The true incidence of pancreatic injuries in children should soon be more accurately determined as ultrasound evaluation and CT scanning become routine at pediatric trauma centers.[34]

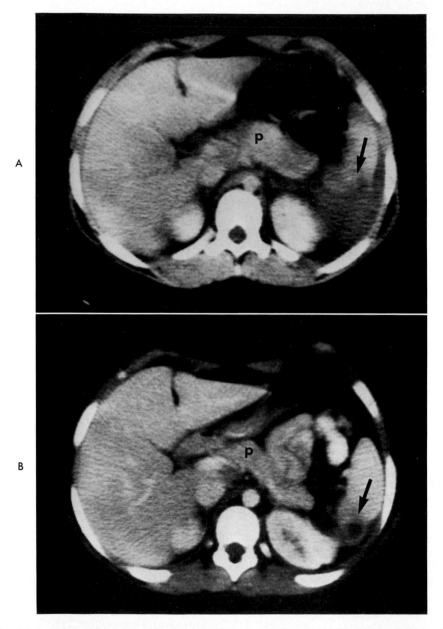

Fig. 16-4   This 12-year-old girl was a non-belted passenger in a high-speed collision. **A,** CT scan at time of injury reveals pancreatic (p) enlargement with variable mottled enhancement after intravenous contrast representing edema and contusion. In addition, rupture and contusion of the inferior splenic pole are present (arrow). **B,** Follow-up 2 months later shows a normal sized pancreas (p) with uniform enhancement after intravenous contast. A small low-density area persists in the spleen at the site of hematoma formation (arrow).

As in all other forms of trauma, pancreatic injury is more common in males. Between 56% to 91% of these injuries occur in boys. Blunt trauma is the most common form of injury. Handlebar injuries, motor vehicle accidents, child abuse, and falls account for the majority of cases. In a review of 51 children, Graham et al.[28] noted that as the age of the injured child increased there tended to be a greater percentage of male patients and penetrating injuries (Table 16-2).

The pattern of injury appears to depend on the type and degree of the force applied to the abdomen. Direct blows to the upper abdomen from handlebar impingements or severe child abuse compress the body of the pancreas between the causative agent and the unyielding vertebral column.

Table 16-2   Pancreatic injuries in children: comparison of age and sex

Age (yr)	Total number of patients	Sex		Type of injury	
		Male	Female	Penetrating	Blunt
2 - 7	18	11	7	2	16
8 - 12	8	8	0	0	8
13 - 16	25	19	6	17	8
TOTAL	51	38	13	19	32

From Graham JM et al: Surgical management of acute pancreatic injuries in children, J Pediatr Surg 13:694, 1978.

Table 16-3   Classification of pancreatic injuries

Class	Extent of injury	Treatment options
I	Contusion, peripheral laceration, intact ductal system	1. Nonoperative management 2. Debridement and drainage
II	Distal laceration, transection, disruption, suspected ductal disruption: no duodenal injury	Distal gland resection and drainage
III	Proximal laceration, transection, disruption, suspected ductal injury: no duodenal injury	1. Distal gland resection 2. GI diversion 3. Drainage
IV	Severe combined pancreaticoduodenal disruption	Pancreaticoduodenectomy and drainage

Modified after Lucas CE: Diagnosis and treatment of pancreatic and duodenal injury, Surg Clin North Am 57:57, 1977.

Table 16-4   Pancreatic injuries and associated trauma

Associated injuries	Number of children	Type of injury	
		Penetrating	Blunt
Kidney	17	10	7
Vascular	16	13	3
Liver	16	8	8
Stomach	16	16	0
Small bowel	16	12	4
Spleen	14	4	10
Lung	14	8	6
Major fracture	11	0	11
Brain	10	0	10
Other	8	2	6
Duodenum	7	3	4
Colon	6	3	3

From Graham JM et al: Surgical management of acute pancreatic injuries in children, J Pediatr Surg 13:694, 1978.

The severity of injury varies from simple contusion to complete transection of the gland. When forces are directed against the head of the pancreas, coexisting injuries to the duodenum ranging from intramural hematoma to perforation are commonly diagnosed.[35] A classification system for pancreatic injuries based on severity was developed by Lucas[46] in 1977. This system facilitates a comparison of possible treatment modalities and expected prognosis based on severity of injury (Table 16-3).

Associated injuries frequently occur in blunt trauma. Injuries to adjacent solid organs such as the spleen and liver are very common. Closed head trauma and major fractures are often diagnosed. Penetrating injuries of the abdomen result in the highest incidence of associated injuries (Table 16-4). Stone's experience indicated that an average of 4.1 additional organ injuries should be expected when the child's pancreatic trauma was sustained as the result of a penetrating abdominal wound.[71] The vascular system along with the genitourinary and gastrointestinal tracts are the most frequently involved organ systems in patients with penetrating pancreatic trauma.

Morbidity and Mortality

Mortality in patients with pancreatic trauma is directly influenced by the presence, type, and extent of other associated injuries both in children and adults. Jones'[36] widely quoted review of pancreatic trauma in adults included 500 patients with pancreatic injury confirmed at laparotomy. These authors report an overall mortality of 22% for penetrating injuries and a 19% death rate for blunt trauma. It is significant to note that a more detailed analysis of these patients reveals that no deaths occurred in patients with isolated pancreatic injuries. In addition, only 3% of the mortality in patients who died from multiple-organ trauma was the result of complications arising directly from the actual pancreatic injury. Mortality rates due to pancreatic trauma in pediatric patients follow a similar pattern. However, the overall mortality appears to be significantly lower in children, considering the fact that in a collected series of 156 children there were 12 deaths (7.6%) and only two patients (1.3%) died as a result of actual pancreatic injury (Table 16-5).

Diagnosis

The possibility of a pancreatic injury should be considered in all cases of upper abdominal trauma. Due to the retroperitoneal location of the pancreas, the initial physical findings may be misleading even in cases of severe combined pancreatoduodenal injury. Frequently, repeated physical examinations are essential for any child whose history suggests a potential pancreatic injury. Most patients develop some clinical evidence of injury within 24 to 48 hours. However, the clinician should always be cognizant of the fact that posttraumatic pseudocysts have been described as occurring months following what is recalled as a very minor injury to the upper abdomen. Depressed levels of consciousness resulting from closed head injuries, associated musculoskeletal injuries, or both that cause significant pain may make abdominal examinations difficult or unreliable.

The serum amylase should always be measured. The level is elevated in 60% to 100% of patients with blunt pancreatic trauma but is abnormal in only 0% to 16% of penetrating pancreatic injuries. Unfortunately, the finding of hyperamylasemia in trauma is not specific for pancreatic injury. It may also occur with salivary gland trauma, bowel perforation or infarction, and hepatic injury. The most common causes of nontraumatic hyperamylasemia include renal failure, peptic ulcer disease, parotitis,

Table 16-5 Comparison of mortality in children with pancreatic injury

Series	Number of patients	Total number of deaths	Deaths due to the actual pancreatic injury
Stone,[71] 1972	54	5 (9%)	2
Meier et al.,[47] 1978	16	3 (19%)	0
Graham et al.,[28] 1978	51	4 (7.8%)	0
Dahman and Stephens,[17] 1981	6	0	0
Salonen and Aarnio,[63] 1985	8	0	0
Gorenstein et al.,[27] 1987	21	0	0
TOTAL	156	12 (7.6%)	2 (1.3%)

salpingitis, ruptured ectopic pregnancy, and opiate administration.[19] In an effort to increase the specificity of amylase analysis for trauma victims, serum fractionation into isoamylase subgroups has been suggested.[6] Unfortunately, Bouwman and coauthors[6] conclude that isoenzymes may not always be useful in discriminating pancreatic injuries from other conditions.

Plain abdominal x-ray films may occasionally be helpful. The findings of pain-induced scoliosis, obliteration of the right psoas margin, or retroperitoneal air suggest the diagnosis of pancreatic trauma or associated duodenal perforation.[46] Ultrasound and CT scan evaluation of the abdomen have been advocated by several pediatric trauma centers as useful modalities during the admission evaluation.[27,75] Experience indicates that these diagnostic techniques are capable of defining edema, hematoma, and even severe lacerations of the pancreas.[63] More recently, a number of authors have recommended that a wider application of ultrasound be employed in the postinjury period to provide for more accurate assessment of the progression of the injury and to check for the formation of a pancreatic pseudocyst.[31,37,66]

Initial Management

Once the diagnosis of pancreatic injury has been established the choice between operative and nonoperative management must be made. This decision applies mainly to blunt injuries, since essentially all patients with penetrating abdominal trauma will require laparotomy. For the patient with stable vital signs who has no signs of peritonitis, a conservative plan may initially be undertaken. This mode of therapy is acceptable only after confirmation of the absence of associated duodenal perforation or laceration by upper GI contrast examination. The essential elements of nonoperative management include a period of nasogastric decompression, intravenous support, and frequent reevaluations of the patient's clinical status. For the majority of patients with simple contusion, conservative management should result in resolution of symptoms within 2 or 3 weeks.[19] A prolonged clinical course characterized by fever, ileus, pain, and persistent hyperamylasemia is suggestive of a complication of a pancreatic injury, such as pseudocyst formation or major ductal injury. Ultrasound or CT scan reevaluation in these cases is absolutely essential to better define the nature and extent of the problem.

The development of severe peritoneal irritation or a worsening clinical condition mandates operative intervention. Exploration should be carried out through a generous midline incision. Operative therapy begins with careful and complete inspection of the pancreatic injury. Adequate assessment requires performance of a Kocher maneuver and mobilization of the hepatic flexure of the colon to visualize the pancreatic head and second and third portions of the duodenum. The lesser sac should be widely opened by dividing the gastrocolic ligament to permit complete visualization and palpation of the entire body and tail of the pancreas. It is useful to categorize the injury by the Lucas classification to provide a basis for determining the most appropriate treatment and to estimate the expected morbidity.

Simple contusions or superficial lacerations of the pancreas (Lucas class I) should be treated by debridement of any devitalized tissue and drainage. Controversy persists over the choice of sump or penrose drains. Proponents of sump drainage cite lower infection rates and better fluid evacuation,[12] whereas those who favor simple penrose drainage warn of the possible complications of erosion into bowel or vascular structures occasionally reported with sump catheters.

Injuries of the distal gland characterized by major ductal disruption or complete transection of the pancreas to the left of the superior mesenteric vessels (Lucas class II) are best managed by resection of the distal gland. Experience in children indicates that distal pancreatectomy is well tolerated. Many series of reported cases have emphasized that very low morbidity should be expected in children.[27,28,47,63,71] The spleen can be preserved in many cases of distal pancreatectomy, as emphasized by Robey et al.[62] However, in the face of an associated splenic injury or multiple-organ injuries, and in the relatively unstable patient, a more expeditious distal pancreatectomy-splenectomy is preferred. Closure of the distal pancreatic resection line should be achieved by direct suture ligation of the transected ductal orifice and suture closure of the capsule, which is fashioned in a bevelled-fishmouth configuration. Good results have also been achieved with the use of the auto-stapling device, but it may be difficult to use when the gland is edematous.[56] The pancreatic bed should always be drained in all cases of resection.

A class III pancreatic injury includes a proximal laceration or parenchymal disruption with suspected ductal injury. This is a much more serious injury because surgical intervention usually requires consideration of partial pancreatectomy and diversion of gastric secretions. Intraoperative decisions depend on the diagnosis and management of any ductal injury. Some authors recommend either intraoperative pancreatography via cannulation of the ampulla of Vater to document ductal integrity or alternatively the liberal use of partial pancreatectomy when a major ductal disruption exists.[4,45] Other authors caution that the duodenotomy required to carry out the pancreatogram creates an additional and possibly unnecessary duodenal suture line with the attendant risks of leak or fistula formation. The criteria recommended by Berni et al.[4] for intraoperative pancreatography include direct visualization of an obvious ductal injury, transection of the pancreas, parenchymal lacerations involving greater than 50% of the gland, a deep perforation of the central portion of the gland, and severe gland contusion. In the absence of these criteria, our preference for isolated proximal injuries is meticulous debridement, resection of devitalized tissue, and drainage without intraoperative pancreatogram. Reconstruction with a Roux-en-Y loop of jejunum anastomozed to the injured area of the gland has been proposed as an alternate form of management for patients with suspected or confirmed proximal duct injuries. Unfortunately, this operation appears to be associated with a high rate of anastomic leak and abscess formation.[4]

Exclusion of the pancreas and duodenum from proximal gastric secretions in the setting of severe combined pancreatoduodenal injury has been recommended. The Berne[3] "diverticulization" procedure accomplishes this by suture closure of the duodenal injury, closure of the proximal duodenum and gastric antrectomy with end-to-side gastrojejunostomy, tube duodenostomy, and generous drainage of the pancreatic bed (Fig. 16-5). Vagotomy and T-tube biliary drainage may be used to complement this procedure. In Berne's experience this procedure reduced the mortality for adult patients with severe combined pancreatoduodenal injury from 33% to 16%.

A less extensive procedure for diversion of gastric secretions for these injuries has been proposed by Vaughn et al.[76] This procedure, termed "pyloric exclusion," involves gastrostomy on the greater curvature, allowing closure of the pylorus with absorbable chromic catgut followed by side-to-side gastrojejunostomy (Fig. 16-6). Vaughn and co-workers reported that this operation in 75 adult patients resulted in an overall mortality of 19%.

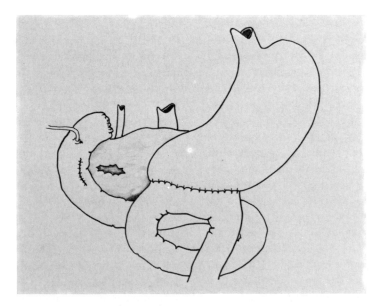

Fig. 16-5   Berne diverticulization procedure for severe combined pancreatoduodenal trauma. Essential features are primary closure of the duodenal injury with tube duodenostomy, antrectomy with side-side gastrojejunostomy, and drainage of the injury. Vagotomy and T-tube biliary drainage are variably included.

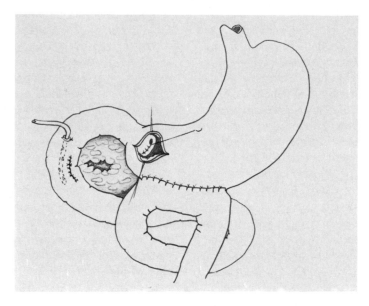

Fig. 16-6   Vaughn exclusion procedure for severe combined pancreatoduodenal injury. Included are primary closure of the duodenal injury with tube duodenostomy, gastrotomy with suture closure of the pylorus and side-side gastrojejunostomy, and drainage of the site of injury.

Functional patency of the pylorus was subsequently reestablished by reabsorption of the pyloric suture line and was documented in all 25 patients in whom it was studied.

Although both the Berne and Vaughn procedures have been alluded to in several review articles on pancreatic trauma in childhood, actual use of these more extensive procedures has not been described in children. The authors have used the pyloric exclusion operation on one occasion with success. Concern must be raised regarding the long-term consequences of unprotected gastrojejunostomy in patients expected to have an extended life span. The incidence of marginal ulceration was 4% after only 2 years of follow-up in these adult patients. The rationale for the use of gastrojejunostomy was to allow the earlier institution of enteric feedings. An alternative to be considered would be pyloric closure with gastrostomy drainage and nutritional support via needle-catheter jejunostomy or total parenteral nutrition.

Finally, there is a small percentage of patients with such extensive combined pancreatic and duodenal trauma (Lucas class IV) that pancreatoduodenectomy may be required. The overall mortality for adults undergoing a Whipple procedure in the trauma setting is approximately 26%.[36] Although experiences with pancreatoduodenectomies

in children are limited, Graham and co-workers[28] series included two children who underwent pancreatoduodenectomy for trauma without complication.

Delayed Complications and Management

Late complications of pancreatic injury are usually secondary to major ductal injury and can be considered under four groups: pancreatic fistula, pseudocyst formation, pancreatic ascites, and recurrent attacks of pancreatitis. Endoscopic retrograde cannulation of the pancreatic duct (ERCP) has become commonplace in the management of adult pancreatic disease and is being reported with increasing frequency in children during the past decade.[15,22,30] This technique provides detailed anatomic information regarding the integrity and patency of the pancreatic duct and may be helpful in planning operative management. Although overall complication rates are low in experienced hands, ERCP has been known to induce pancreatitis with pancreatic necrosis and carries the potential risk of introducing infection in the pancreatic pseudocyst.[61] Therefore ERCP should be restricted to subsets of patients in whom clinical management will actually be altered by the endoscopic findings. This procedure should be undertaken only before the anticipated operation.

Pancreatic fistulas

The presence of a minor fistula after laparotomy for pancreatic injury is not uncommon. The vast majority of these close spontaneously within 3 weeks if the patient is kept NPO and maintained on total parenteral nutrition. The failure of a fistula to close with conservative management is suggestive of an unrecognized major ductal injury or an obstruction that will require operative repair or partial pancreatic resection.[28]

Pseudocysts

Pseudocyst formation is known to occur as a sequela of both conservative and operative management of pancreatic injuries.[17,27,50,58] The diagnosis of pseudocyst should be suspected in patients with recurrent epigastric pain and vomiting after a history of epigastric trauma. Hyperamylasemia is seen in 88% of these children, and a palpable mass can be detected in 64%.[14] Since the use of ultrasound for monitoring pancreatic injuries has gained widespread acceptance, both the incidence of peripancreatic fluid collections and pseudocysts and their spontaneous resolution have been observed with increasing frequency. The interval between injury and pseudocyst formation is highly variable, with a range of 15 to 712 days, as was noted in the large collective review by Cooney and Grosfeld.[14] In a more recent group of children with documented blunt injury to the pancreas that was followed with serial ultrasound examinations, 10 of 21 patients developed pancreatic pseudocysts with an onset of 3 to 30 days following the injury.[27]

Spontaneous resolution of posttraumatic pseudocysts during conservative treatment, which consists of nasogastric decompression and parenteral nutritional support, is also being documented with increasing frequency. Collected data from six pediatric centers, in which at least some of the patients were initially treated conservatively, reveal an overall rate of spontaneous resolution of 45% (Table 16-6). Controversy persists in both the adult and pediatric surgical literature over the appropriateness of conservative management and the timing of surgical intervention. Risks of conservative management include rupture or infection of the pseudocyst and hemorrhage from erosion of the cyst into a major vascular structure or the gastrointestinal tract. The data of Bradley et al.[7] regarding the natural history of pseudocyst evolution in adults suggest that spontaneous resolution is usually an early event occurring within 4 to 7 weeks after recognition of pseudocyst formation. The occurrence of complications during expectant therapy is usually a late event, occurring an average of 13.5 weeks after diagnosis of the pseudocyst. These two observations have led to the recommendation that early nonoperative therapy should be undertaken for a period of 4 to 6 weeks to allow for spontaneous resolution, which is frequently observed in these cases. In addition, the first few weeks of nonoperative management allow for thickening of the fibrous capsule in those pseudocysts, which will ultimately require operative internal drainage.[7] Problems with early operative intervention are mainly related to the friability of the cyst wall,

Table 16-6 Results of conservative management of traumatic pancreatic pseudocysts in children

Series	Number of patients	Spontaneous resolution	Operative management
Kagan et al.,[37] 1980	3	1	2 Cyst-gastrostomy
Slovis et al.,[66] 1980	3	2	1 Unspecified drainage
Dahman and Stephens,[17] 1981	6	1	3 External drainage
			1 Cyst-gastrostomy
			1 Multiple procedure
Harkanyi et al.,[31] 1981	2	1	1 Cyst-gastrostomy
Gorenstein et al.,[27] 1987	10	6	1 Distal resection
			1 External drainage
			1 Cyst-gastrostomy
			1 Percutaneous drainage
Millar et al.,[50] 1988	14	6	7 Cyst-gastrostomy
			1 Roux-en-Y
TOTAL	38	17 (45%)	21 (55%)

which may necessitate external drainage with its attendant high recurrence rate and prolonged fistula drainage. On the other hand, prolongation of the expectant therapy beyond 6 to 8 weeks exposes the child to a greater risk of serious complications from the pseudocyst itself. In a recent report from the Hospital for Sick Children in Toronto, several pseudocysts were successfully drained by percutaneous needle aspiration.[9] In this series of 13 children, six pseudocysts resolved without operation, whereas seven required a drainage procedure. Two of the seven patients underwent a traditional operative

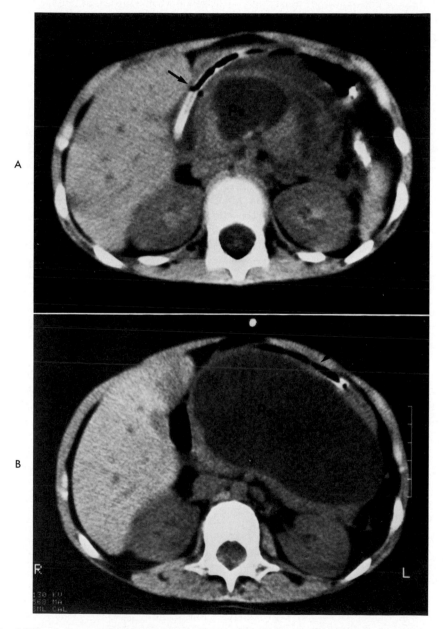

Fig. 16-7   A 5-year-old girl who sustained a handlebar injury to the epigastrium. Initial CT scan, done elsewhere, was reported to show pancreatic contusion. **A,** CT scan 6 days after injury demonstrates psuedocyst formation *(Ps)* with anterior displacement of the stomach, seen with a decompressing nasogastric tube *(arrow)*. **B,** Patient treated with nasogastric decompression and intravenous hyperalimentation but continued to show progressive enlargement of her pseudocyst on follow-up studies. At 6 weeks after injury she underwent cyst-gastrostomy with excellent results.

cystenterostomy; the other five were drained percutaneously using ultrasound guidance. These pseudocysts had been present for an average of 26 days. This alternative may be an attractive and useful treatment option if increasing clinical experience documents its safety and efficacy.

Our current recommendations for posttraumatic pseudocyst management consist of an initial trial of nasogastric suction and total parenteral alimentation. Daily physical examinations should be aimed at detecting an increasing cyst size or progression of abdominal tenderness. Serum amylase levels should be monitored frequently, and an abdominal ultrasound examination should be obtained weekly. An improving clinical course characterized by decreasing pain, mass, and a stable or decreasing serum amylase are indications for continued conservative management. Increasing pain or size of the pseudocyst suggests the need for operative intervention (Fig. 16-7). The development of hemorrhage or infection is also an obvious indication for surgery.

ERCP is not indicated for simple unilocular cysts, as it will not alter the intraoperative management. In contrast, ERCP may be helpful in selected cases of complex multicystic lesions with suspected multiple areas of ductal stricture or injury. Intraoperative cystograms performed by injection of contrast directly into the largest cyst cavity may be helpful. This is especially true when the surgeon is uncertain whether all cysts communicate and will be drained by a single drainage procedure. This technique may alert the surgeon to a more complex anatomic arrangement and prevent incomplete drainage of multilocular cysts. Although the type of drainage procedure will be dictated by the anatomic location of the cyst, internal drainage is the treatment of choice whenever feasible. External drainage is required when the cyst is infected or thin walled. Unfortunately, external drainage is associated with recurrence rates of 22% to 24%, and many cases of prolonged fistula drainage have been reported following this form of therapy.[14] Most pseudocysts can be effectively managed by cyst-gastrostomy with very low morbidity and a recurrence rate of less than 5%.[14] This operation is preferred when the cyst lies dorsal and adherent to the posterior wall of the stomach. In circumstances in which the cyst is not adherent to the gastric wall, internal drainage can be accomplished by anastomosis to a Roux-en-Y loop of jejunum. Limited distal pancreatic resection may

occasionally be indicated for cysts located in the tail of the gland but will usually require splenectomy.

Pancreatic ascites

Pancreatic ascites is a rare complication of trauma in childhood.[18] It results from major ductal disruption without local inflammatory containment of the pancreatic leak. Patients present with the gradual development of gross abdominal distention. Diagnosis is confirmed by paracentesis. Ascitic fluid has a markedly elevated amylase level and a protein content greater than 2.5 g/dl. An ultrasound examination or CT scan should be obtained. These studies may be helpful in identifying and locating areas of injury to the gland. To achieve the best operative result the area of disruption must be localized and inspected very carefully. ERCP has been shown to be helpful in this setting in both adults and children. A preoperative "road-map" should be obtained to direct the surgeon to specific operative therapy based on the known area of injury. Intraoperative pancreatograms may also be necessary. In the past, treatment by simple drainage was carried out with some degree of success but usually required extended hospitalization because of prolonged drainage.[22] Resection or internal drainage is preferred when technically feasible.

Recurrent pancreatitis

The development of multiple bouts of recurrent pancreatitis after a traumatic injury may also be seen as a consequence of injury to the ductal system. ERCP again may be helpful in this setting. Sequelae such as stricture with distal dilatation or contained leaks have been demonstrated.[15,27] Specific operative therapy should be undertaken based on the anatomic findings as discussed previously.

REFERENCES

1. Aaron WS, Fulton RL, and Mays ET: Selective ligation of the hepatic artery for trauma of the liver, Surg Gynecol Obstet 141:187, 1975.
2. Bass BL et al: Hazards of nonoperative therapy of hepatic injury in children, J Trauma 24:978, 1984.
3. Berne CJ et al: Duodenal "diverticulization" for duodenal and pancreatic injury, Am J Surg 127:503, 1974.
4. Berni GA et al: Role of intraoperative pancreatography in patients with injury to the pancreas, Am J Surg 143:602, 1982.
5. Blocker SH and Ternberg JL: Traumatic liver laceration in the newborn: repair with fibrin glue, J Pediatr Surg 21:369, 1986.
6. Bouwman DL, Weaver DW, and Walt AJ: Serum amylase

and its isoenzymes: a clarification of their implications in trauma, J Trauma 24:573, 1984.

7. Bradley EL III, Clements JL Jr, and Gonzalez AC: The natural history of pancreatic pseudocysts: a unified concept of management, Am J Surg 137:135, 1979.

8. Brunelle F et al: Emergency embolization in posttraumatic hemobilia in a child, J Pediatr Surg 20:172, 1985.

9. Burnweit CA, Filler RM, and Wesson DE: Percutaneous drainage of traumatic pancreatic pseudocysts in children. Ninth Annual Pediatric Surgical Resident's Conference, Nov 4-6, 1988, Boston.

10. Busuttil RW et al: Management of blunt and penetrating injuries to the porta hepatis, Ann Surg 191:641, 1980.

11. Cheatham JE Jr et al: Nonoperative management of subcapsular hematomas of the liver, Am J Surg 140:852, 1980.

12. Cogbill TH, Moore EE, and Kashuk JL: Changing trends in the management of pancreatic trauma, Arch Surg 117:722, 1982.

13. Coln D, Crighton J, and Schorn L: Successful management of hepatic vein injury from blunt trauma in children, Am J Surg 140:858, 1980.

14. Cooney DR and Grosfeld JL: Operative management of pancreatic pseudocysts in infants and children: a review of 75 cases, Ann Surg 182:590, 1975.

15. Cotton PB and Laage NJ: Endoscopic retrograde cholangiopancreatography in children, Arch Dis Child 57:131, 1982.

16. Cywes S, Rode H, and Millar AJW: Blunt liver trauma in children: nonoperative management, J Pediatr Surg 20:14, 1985.

17. Dahman B and Stephens CA: Pseudocysts of the pancreas after blunt abdominal trauma in children, J Pediatr Surg 16:17, 1981.

18. Donald JW, Ozment ED, and Smith CB: Pancreatic ascites in childhood, South Med J 75:1419, 1982.

19. Eichelberger MR, Hoelzer DJ, and Koop CE: Acute pancreatitis: the difficulties of diagnosis and therapy, J Pediatr Surg 17:244, 1982.

20. Feliciano DV et al: Management of traumatic injuries to the extrahepatic biliary ducts, Am J Surg 150:705, 1985.

21. Feliciano DV et al: Packing for control of hepatic hemorrhage, J Trauma 26:738, 1986.

22. Filston HC et al: Improved management of pancreatic lesions in children aided by ERCP, J Pediatr Surg 15:121, 1980.

23. Fischer DP, O'Farrell KA, and Perry JF Jr: The value of peritoneal drains in the treatment of liver injuries, J Trauma 18:393, 1978.

24. Flint LM and Polk HC: Selective hepatic artery ligation: limitations and failures, J Trauma 19:319, 1979.

25. Geis WP et al: The fate of unruptured intrahepatic hematomas, Surgery 90:689, 1981.

26. Giacomantonio M, Filler RM, and Rich RH: Blunt hepatic trauma in children: experience with operative and nonoperative management, J Pediatr Surg 19:519, 1984.

27. Gorenstein A et al: Blunt injury to the pancreas in children: selective management based on ultrasound, J Pediatr Surg 22:1110, 1987.

28. Graham JM et al: Surgical management of acute pancreatic injuries in children, J Pediatr Surg 13:693, 1978.

29. Grisoni ER et al: Nonoperative management of liver injuries following blunt abdominal trauma in children, J Pediatr Surg 19:515, 1984.

30. Hall RI, Lavelle MI, and Venables CW: Use of ERCP to identify the site of traumatic injuries of the main pancreatic duct in children, Br J Surg 73:411, 1986.

31. Harkanyi Z et al: Gray-scale echography of traumatic pancreatic cysts in children, Pediatr Radiol 11:81, 1981.

32. Hartman SW and Greaney EM Jr: Traumatic injuries to the biliary system in children, Am J Surg 108:150, 1964.

33. Hendren WH et al: Traumatic hemobilia: nonoperative management with healing documented by serial angiography, Ann Surg 174:991, 1971.

34. Jeffrey RB Jr, Federle MP, and Crass RA: Computed tomography of pancreatic trauma, Radiology 147:491, 1983.

35. Jewett TC Jr et al: Intramural hematoma of the duodenum, Arch Surg 123:54, 1988.

36. Jones RC: Management of pancreatic trauma, Am J Surg 150:698, 1985.

37. Kagan RJ, Reyes HM, and Asokan S: Pseudocysts of the pancreas in childhood, Arch Surg 116:1200, 1981.

38. Karp MP et al: The role of computed tomography in the evaluation of blunt abdominal trauma in children, J Pediatr Surg 16:316, 1981.

39. Karp MP et al: The nonoperative management of pediatric hepatic trauma, J Pediatr Surg 18:512, 1983.

40. Kaufman JM and Burrington JD: Liver trauma in children, J Pediatr Surg 6:585, 1971.

41. Kaufman RA et al: Upper abdominal trauma in children: imaging evaluation, AJR 142:449, 1984.

42. Keller FS et al: Percutaneous angiographic embolization: a procedure of increasing usefulness, Am J Surg 142:5, 1981.

43. Kitahama A et al: The extrahepatic biliary tract injury, Ann Surg 196:536, 1982.

44. Lackgren G et al: Hemobilia in childhood, J Pediatr Surg 23:105, 1988.

45. Laraja RD et al: Intraoperative endoscopic retrograde cholangiopancreatography (ERCP) in penetrating trauma of the pancreas, J Trauma 26:1146, 1986.

46. Lucas CE: Diagnosis and treatment of pancreatic and duodenal injury, Surg Clin North Am 57:49, 1977.

47. Meier D et al: Blunt trauma to the pancreas in children, South Med J 71:895, 1978.

48. Meyer AA et al: Selective nonoperative management of blunt liver injury using computed tomography, Arch Surg 120:550, 1985.

49. Michelassi F and Ranson JHC: Bile duct disruption by blunt trauma, J Trauma 25:454, 1985.

50. Millar AJW et al: Management of pancreatic pseudocysts in children, J Pediatr Surg 23:122, 1988.

51. Moore EE: Critical decisions in the management of hepatic trauma, Am J Surg 148:712, 1984.

52. Moore FA, Moore EE, and Seagraves A: Nonresectional management of major hepatic trauma, Am J Surg 150:725, 1985.

53. Oldham KT et al: Blunt hepatic injury and elevated hepatic enzymes: a clinical correlation in children, J Pediatr Surg 19:457, 1984.

54. Oldham KT et al: Blunt liver injury in childhood: evolution of therapy and current perspective, Surgery 100:542, 1986.

55. Pachter HL and Spencer FC: Recent concepts in the treatment of hepatic trauma, Ann Surg 190:423, 1979.

56. Pachter HL et al: Simplified distal pancreatectomy with the auto suture stapler: preliminary clinical observations, Surgery 85:166, 1979.

57. Pachter HL et al: Experience with the finger fracture technique to achieve intrahepatic hemostasis in 75 patients with severe injuries to the liver, Ann Surg 197:771, 1983.

58. Pokorny WJ, Raffensperger JG, and Harberg FJ: Pancreatic pseudocysts in children, Surg Gynecol Obstet 151:182, 1980.

59. Posner MC and Moore EE: Extrahepatic biliary tract injury: operative management plan, J Trauma 25:833, 1985.

60. Richie JP and Fonkalsrud EW: Subcapsular hematoma of the liver, Arch Surg 104:781, 1972.

61. Riemann JF and Koch H: Endoscopy of the biliary tract and the pancreas in children, Endoscopy 10:166, 1978.

62. Robey E, Mullen JT, and Schwab EW: Blunt transection of the pancreas treated by distal pancreatectomy, splenic salvage and hyperalimentation, Ann Surg 196:695, 1982.

63. Salonen IS and Aarnio P: Treatment of acute pancreatic injuries in childhood, Ann Chir Gynaecol 74:167, 1985.

64. Schrock T, Balisdell FW, and Matthewson C Jr: Management of blunt trauma to the liver and hepatic veins, Arch Surg 96:698, 1968.

65. Sinclair MC and Moore TC: Major surgery for abdominal and thoracic trauma in childhood and adolescence, J Pediatr Surg 9:155, 1974.

66. Slovis TL, Von Berg VJ, and Mikelic V: Sonography in the diagnosis and management of pancreatic pseudocysts and effusions in childhood, Radiology 135:153, 1980.

67. Soderstrom CA et al: Gallbladder injuries resulting from blunt abdominal trauma, Ann Surg 193:60, 1981.

68. Sokol DM, Tompkins D, and Izant RJ Jr: Rupture of the spleen and liver in the newborn: a report of the first survivor and a review of the literature, J Pediatr Surg 9:227, 1974.

69. Stalker HP, Kaufman RA, and Towbin R: Patterns of liver injury in childhood: CT analysis, AJR 147:1199, 1986.

70. Sty JR, Starshak RJ, and Hubbard AM: Radionuclide hepatobiliary imaging in the detection of traumatic biliary tract disease in children, Pediatr Radiol 12:115, 1982.

71. Stone HH: Pancreatic and duodenal trauma in children, J Pediatr Surg 7:670, 1972.

72. Stone HH and Ansley JD: Management of liver trauma in children, J Pediatr Surg 12:3, 1977.

73. Stone HH and Lamb JM: Use of pedicled omentum as an autogenous pack for control of hemorrhage in major injuries of the liver, Surg Gynecol Obstet 141:92, 1975.

74. Suson EM, Klotz D Jr, and Kottmeier PK: Liver trauma in children, J Pediatr Surg 10:411, 1975.

75. Touloukian RJ: Protocol for the nonoperative treatment of obstructing intramural duodenal hematoma during childhood, Am J Surg 145:330, 1983.

76. Vaughn GD III et al: The use of pyloric exclusion in the management of severe duodenal injuries, Am J Surg 134:785, 1977.

77. Vock P, Kehrer B, and Tschaeppeler H: Blunt liver trauma in children: the role of computed tomography in diagnosis and treatment, J Pediatr Surg 21:413, 1986.

78. Walt AJ: The mythology of hepatic trauma—or Babel revisited, Am J Surg 135:12, 1978.

SPLENIC INJURY

Robert J. Touloukian

Injuries of the spleen demand excision of the gland. No evil effects follow its removal while the danger of hemorrhage is effectively stopped.

E.T. KOCHER, 1911

Kocher[33] and other equally influential surgeons dominated the philosophy of treating splenic injury during the first half of the twentieth century. A complete reversal of this longstanding approach came about during the past 2 decades with periodic observations that children developed overwhelming postsplenectomy infection (OPSI) following splenectomy for trauma, oftentimes years following operation, and coincidental evidence that the injured spleen may be preserved by nonoperative management in patients having spontaneous cessation of hemorrhage, and, in others, by direct operative control of the bleeding.

The spleen is the most commonly injured intraabdominal organ in children and is therefore the most likely cause of intraabdominal bleeding, but an accurate diagnosis followed by appropriate resuscitative measures are essential before selecting the appropriate method of splenic preservation.

ETIOLOGY AND CLINICAL PRESENTATION

Splenic injury in childhood characteristically occurs following blunt trauma to the upper abdomen or lower thorax but is rarely accompanied by rib

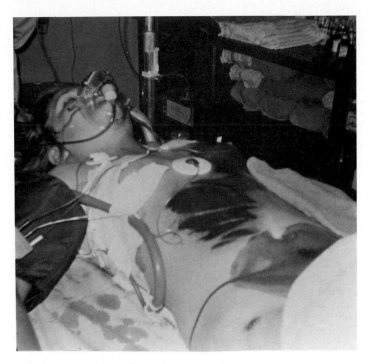

Fig. 16-8   This 14-year-old girl was struck by a car while riding her bike and then dragged about 150 feet, sustaining road burns across the abdomen and left chest. She had a tension hemopneumothorax on the right and a ruptured spleen.

fractures, a fairly frequent finding in adults. Bruises or ecchymoses overlying the lower chest wall or left upper quadrant should suggest the possibility of splenic injury (Fig. 16-8). Approximately one half of these injuries occur during play or athletic activities, whereas the remainder result from vehicular trauma, with the child an innocent bystander in the great majority of cases.[58,59] Abuse or neglect is important to consider in children under 4 years of age when a reliable history is unavailable.[57] Irritation of the left hemidiaphragm and referred pain to the shoulder occurs in about 40% of children with splenic injury, but signs of intraabdominal bleeding, hypotension, and abdominal distention occur in only one fourth of cases seen in our emergency room. An early episode of syncope or faintness may be neurogenic in origin and not necessarily the result of acute blood loss. Referred pain to the left shoulder occurs in less than half of children with splenic injury. Children with splenic injury normally have left upper quadrant tenderness, but a palpable enlarged spleen is both difficult to detect and unusual during the early hours following injury (Fig. 16-9). The initial physical findings may be confused with an abdominal wall con-

tusion, but progressively severe abdominal pain, persistent or spreading tenderness, and muscle spasm follow shortly thereafter.

Nearly one half of all children with a splenic injury have at least one other major associated cranial, thoracic, or musculoskeletal injury.[58,59] Multiple injuries following vehicular trauma are more common in smaller children than in adults, with a combination of serious head and splenic injuries a frequently encountered association. Hepatic, duodenal, and pancreatic injuries must also be suspected, but bowel perforation plus splenic rupture is a rare combination. An elevated serum amylase is found in about one third of children with splenic injury because of contusion to the tail of the pancreas, but pancreatic duct injury or pseudocyst formation is unusual.

DIAGNOSIS

Abdominal films are rarely diagnostic but may be useful in directing attention to the spleen (Fig. 16-10, *A*). Medial displacement of the splenic flexure of the colon or the gastric air bubble (Fig. 16-10, *B*) and splenic enlargement (Fig. 16-10, *C*) are

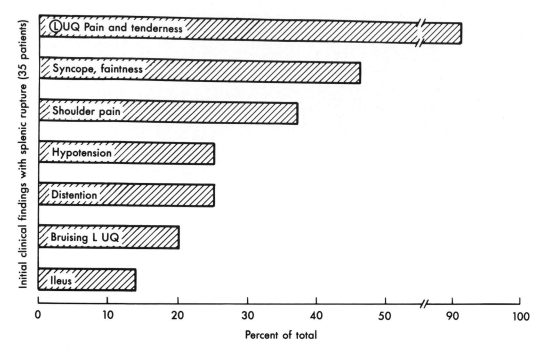

Fig. 16-9   The most frequent clinical findings in children with splenic injury based on a retrospective review of 35 cases at Yale–New Haven Hospital.

observed in about 25% of children with documented splenic rupture.[58,59] Elevation of the hemidiaphragm, loss of the psoas margin, and evidence of peritoneal fluid are seen in about 15% of cases.[58]

Nuclear Scan

The technetium (Tc 99m) sulfur colloid scan and computed tomography (CT) remain the simplest, most available, and reliable diagnostic tests to confirm suspected isolated splenic injury. The study should be obtained even when the level of suspicion is low and the patient's condition stable.

The technique uses the reticuloendothelial function of the spleen in clearing colloidal substances from the blood. Technetium Tc 99m sulfur colloid has a physical half-life of 6 hours and an essentially monoenergetic gamma emission of 140 keV and no beta emission. The technetium Tc 99m sulfur colloid is available commercially and may be administered easily through the intravenous line. The radiation dose estimates for the liver and total body for an average 1 year old is 1.3 rads and 0.007 rad and less for older children and adults. These figures are well within acceptable limits for diagnostic radiography. These scans must be obtained in multiple views including anterior, posterior, and right

and left lateral. Oblique projections are often helpful but may be misleading if other views are not obtained. The scanning time for the four basic views in a cooperative patient is about 30 minutes. Some sedation of the agitated younger child may be necessary to get reliable studies. By far the most common finding is a radiolucent linear defect within the substance of the spleen usually through the hilum, giving the impression of some separation of the splenic pulp. The "double-density" sign if observed when the fragment displaced toward the camera crystal is of greater intensity than the nondisplaced fragment (Fig. 16-11). Gross displacement of the fragments, splenomegaly, and a diffusely mottled unhomogeneous pattern are other abnormalities that are highly suggestive of splenic injury. CT has the advantage of offering more specific information about the characteristics of injury to all solid viscera and the retroperitoneum (Fig. 16-12), but its disadvantages include higher cost, additional irradiation exposure, a motionless patient, and a lack of immediate availability in many centers. The CT scan has supplanted nuclear imaging as the best diagnostic test[27] for multiple trauma, particularly to survey the abdomen in a neurologically unstable child with a head injury.[4]

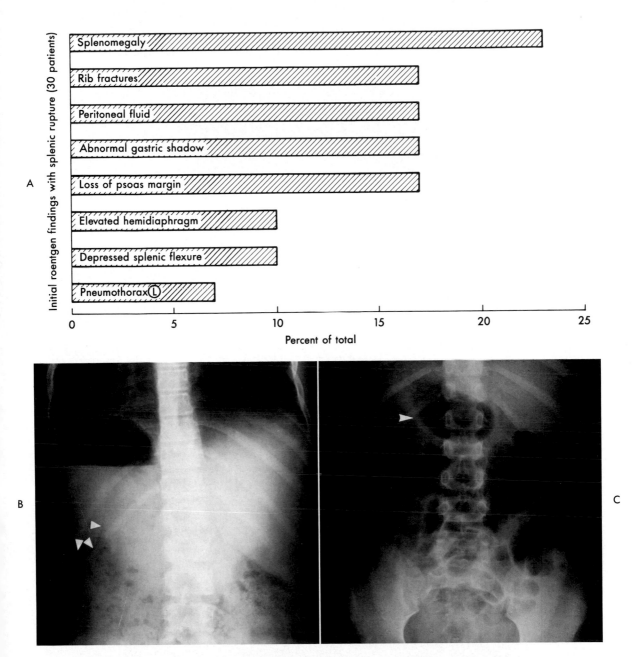

Fig. 16-10 **A,** Common roentgen findings in 30 consecutive children with splenic injury. **B,** Gastric air bubble in an 11-year-old girl is medially displaced by a ruptured spleen. **C,** This 12-year-old boy with a ruptured spleen has downward displacement of the open splenic fat line consistent with splenic enlargement.

INITIAL MANAGEMENT

The first steps in resuscitation are placement of an intravenous line in an upper extremity, volume replacement with crystalloid fluid, blood transfusion as indicated, and insertion of a nasogastric tube to decompress the stomach and prevent acute gastric dilatation with its consequences of forceful vomiting and possible aspiration.

Sequential monitoring of both vital signs and physical findings is essential to detect evidence of instability or deterioration warranting additional fluid, blood, or the need for the operative control

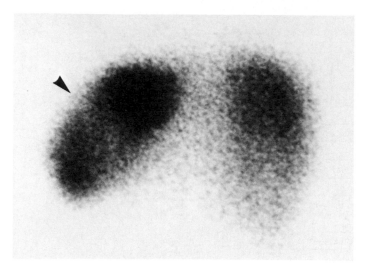

Fig. 16-11   Technetium (Tc 99m) sulfur colloid scan in a 12-year-old boy with a ruptured spleen shows an oblique lucent line *(arrow)* and a "double-density" sign on the left posterior oblique view.

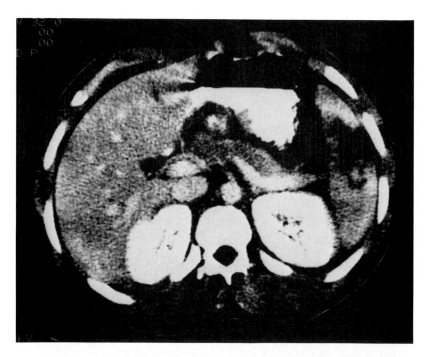

Fig. 16-12   CT scan with intravenous and oral contrast reveals defect in upper pole of spleen extending to outer capsule. Examination of other solid viscera is within normal limits.

of bleeding. The distinction between the *stable* and *unstable* patient is critical in directing treatment and is made on the basis of whether there is deterioration of vital signs or an increasing possibility of coexisting intraabdominal injuries. For these reasons, patients with an apparently stable splenic in-

jury should be monitored in a pediatric intensive care unit.

Pathology

Several patterns of splenic injury (Fig. 16-13) may be classified into three distinct categories: cap-

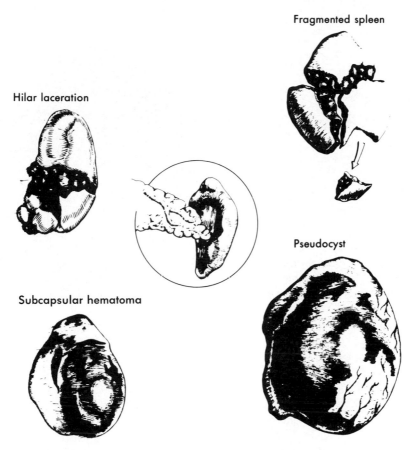

Fig. 16-13   Typical patterns of splenic injury following blunt abdominal trauma. Hilar laceration is far more common than either subcapsular hematoma or splenic fragmentation. Pseudocyst is likely to be a late sequela of subcapsular hematoma.

sular, parenchymal, and hilar (see box at right). Superficial *capsular abrasions* or *avulsions* cause bleeding by tearing or shearing the spleen from its ligamentous attachments. Bleeding is initially brisk but will cease with local pressure or topical coagulants. *Subcapsular hematoma,* with or without laceration of the capsule, occurs less frequently in children than in adults. Only isolated examples of intact or delayed rupture of the spleen have been reported in children,[65] although this entity is reputedly more common in adults. A *linear laceration,* extending downward from the capsule toward the hilum, is the most common splenic injury. Presumably, bleeding occurs from either lacerated hilar vessels or branches passing between splenic segments within the parenchyma. Upadhyaya and Simpson[62] describe a trisegmental blood supply that generally respects the vascular integrity of each segment (Fig. 16-14). The three vascular compo-

---

CLASSIFICATION OF PEDIATRIC SPLENIC INJURY

Capsular

Avulsion, abrasions
Ligamentous disruption
Subcapsular hematoma (intact or "delayed rupture")

Parenchymal

Linear laceration—segmental
Stellate tear—with or without fragmentation
Hematoma—"pseudocyst"

Hilar (extraparenchymal)

Polar vessel
Splenic artery/vein

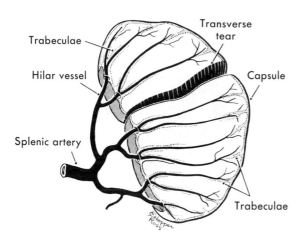

Fig. 16-14 Intrasplenic vascular arrangement is shown with a transverse tear separating the upper polar vessels from lower splenic segments. Note that the splenic artery divides outside the hilus, forming an arcade. (From Upadhyaya P and Simpson JS: Surg Gynecol Obstet 126:781, 1968.)

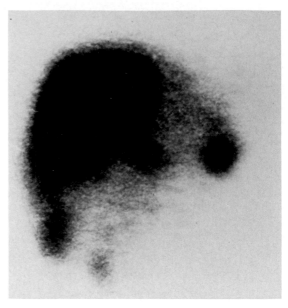

Fig. 16-15 Anterolateral technetium sulfur colloid scan in a 15-year-old boy 8 years following splenectomy for trauma. At least four nodules of splenic tissue are visible below the liver.

nents are large and small arteriovenous communications, an arterial capillary venous circulation, and an arterial capillary-sinus circulation. The arteriovenous anastomoses permit the parenchymal circulation to be bypassed, and bleeding ceases spontaneously in the majority of children within the first 12 to 18 hours as clot forms in the laceration. Presumably, this predisposes then to organization, fibrosis, and complete healing.

Splenic disruption is a consequence of more severe impact resulting in fragmentation of the spleen with pieces lodging throughout the peritoneal cavity and pelvis. Splenectomy may be required to control hemorrhage. "Spontaneous" splenosis from implantation of splenic tissue occurs following complete splenectomy even when visible fragments of splenic debris are irrigated and removed from the operative field. Pearson et al.[45] reported that 13 of 22 children, studied 1 to 10 years after splenectomy for trauma, had a lower percentage of pitted red blood cells in the peripheral circulation than did others having elective splenectomy for a specific hematologic indication, suggesting the presence of splenic activity. In five of these children, a Tc 99m sulfur colloid scan demonstrated multiple nodules of splenic tissue, indicating a totally unanticipated "rebirth" of the spleen (Fig. 16-15). The born-again spleen has been observed in over 50% of postsplenectomy trauma patients, but not in children following elective splenectomy for

hematologic disorders. This phenomenon is presumed to result from regenerated clusters of splenic cells implanted on adjacent tissue rather than enlargement of previously existing accessory spleens.

Pseudocysts of the spleen are likely to be a consequence of an old splenic hematoma from a previous injury or spontaneous bleeding,[32,53] but serial nuclear imaging that would document the evolution of a pseudocyst from a subcapsular hematoma has not been reported. A "binary" spleen sign is characteristic of these lesions.[44] The internal surface of the cyst wall is lined by fibrous septa covered by islands of dysplastic squamous epithelium (Fig. 16-16). The fluid contents are turbid and contain hemoglobin breakdown products, but no epithelial debris, thereby ruling out the possibility of congenital origin.

Sustained hemorrhage is the more likely consequence of parenchymal injury when associated with a torn hilar vessel. The superior polar artery is the most prominent and exposed segmental vessel and requires surgical repair when lacerated. Dearterialization injury, however, more commonly involves the inferior segment. This injury tends not to cause sustained bleeding and generally does not need surgical control. Injuries to the main trunk of

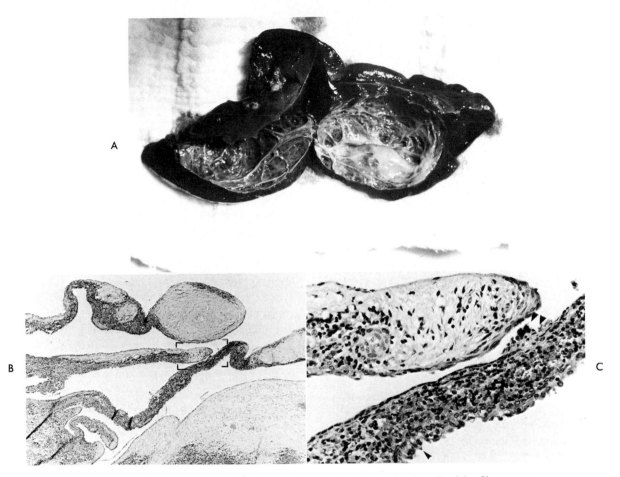

Fig. 16-16   Splenic pseudocyst in a 4-year-old girl. **A,** The cyst wall is lined by fibrous septa resembling chordae tendineac. The frondlike projections forming the wall of the pseudocyst (**B**) are lined by islands of squamous epithelium (**C,** *arrows*).

the splenic artery or vein from blunt injury are rarely encountered but obviously cause major hemorrhage and possible exsanguination unless prompt operative measures are undertaken.

Overwhelming Postsplenectomy Infection

The current interest in splenic preservation stems from King and Shumacker's[31] observations, reported in 1952, that fulminant sepsis followed splenectomy performed in infancy for hereditary spherocytosis. Two of the five affected infants died during the first year after operation.

Additional long-term studies confirm that the risk of overwhelming postsplenectomy infection (OPSI) varies with both the indication for and the age at which splenectomy was performed. Eraklis et al.[20] reviewed the records of 467 patients having splenectomy at the Children's Hospital in Boston

before 1967. The mortality from OPSI performed for accidental injury or idiopathic thrombocytopenic purpura was zero, but it was higher for those with hereditary spherocytosis or aplastic or hypoplastic anemia and considerable for others with serious primary conditions such as Cooley's anemia, Wiskott-Aldrich syndrome, histiocytosis, and lipidosis. An extensive review of the existing literature by Singer[52] in 1973 reported a 1.5% incidence of OPSI with a 50% mortality following splenectomy for trauma. Additional reports were cited by Balfanz and co-workers.[3] Burrington[9] concluded that the relative risk of sepsis increases fiftyfold in the postsplenectomy patient, and the septic child has a 50 times greater risk of dying than does a child with an intact spleen. An inverse relationship of OPSI with the age of the child has been observed. The combined risk of a fatal infection in reports by Eraklis et al.[20] and Horan and Colebatch[25] was 12% for 49 infants under 1 year of age, 6.9% for 245 patients between 1 and 6 years of age, and 3.2% for 315 patients between 6 and 16 years of age.

OPSI follows a fulminant clinical course varying between 12 to 24 hours from the time of onset to death. Signs of disseminated intravascular coagulation (DIC), shock, and adrenal hemorrhage are frequently observed. In about two thirds of cases the organism is *Diplococcus pneumoniae*. *Haemophilus influenzae* (type B) is the next most frequent organism, whereas a small proportion are caused by meningococcus *(Neisseria meningitidis)*, *Escherichia coli,* and *Staphylococcus aureus*.[52] Enormous numbers of these organisms are found in the blood, and often bacteria can be demonstrated in the buffy coat.[43]

The age relationships, clinical syndrome, and bacteriology of OPSI emphasize that the spleen not only serves as a bacterial filter and source of reticuloendothelial phagocytosis but also provides immunologic competence for the younger child. Clinical and experimental studies of serum IgM,[12] properdin,[10] plasma fibronectin,[22] and alternative complement pathway activity[46] are decreased in the immature splenectomized host. Opsonization of circulating bacteria also fails to occur because specific antibody is not present or is present at very low levels.[6,39] The loss of passive acquired immunity from transplacental transfer of IgM during the first 6 months of life increases the likelihood of OPSI during the ensuing 1- to 4-year period when most normal children lack specific circulating antibodies against responsible organisms.[55] Additional depressant effects of splenectomy on pulmonary reticuloendothelial and alveolar macrophages have been described in laboratory subjects.[11,50]

Prophylaxis with antibiotics and immunization have proven only partially protective against acquired infection. Currently available Pneumovax contains antigen for 24 pneumococcal subtypes of the 84 identified, making total protection impossible. There are reports of fatal bacteremia in vaccinated splenectomized and functionally asplenic individuals.[1,40] Additional disadvantages of Pneumovax as a substitute for the intact spleen are the absence of protection rendered against infection by other organisms and the risk of a hyperimmune reaction to the booster, normally required 2 years after initial immunization. The timing of Pneumovax administration also affects immunity. Hebert et al.[23] has demonstrated a lower level of protection in mice challenged with aerosolized pneumococci when pneumococcal vaccine is given after rather than before splenectomy, a situation invariably encountered in splenectomy for trauma. For this reason the vaccine is administered 1 to 2 weeks before elective splenectomy. Recently, we have also immunized children under 6 years of age against *H. influenzae,* type B, because of the prevalence of this organism in the younger age group.

Penicillin is the best antibiotic for long-term prophylaxis, and we continue to advocate 250 mg of oral penicillin V, twice a day, for asplenic and hyposplenic children younger than 6 years of age[43] because of the various side effects of long-term ampicillin administration. Duration of use remains undetermined, since OPSI may develop in adults from atypical serotypes of pneumococcus,[18] but generally prophylaxis is continued only to about 10 years of age. Concerns raised as to the wisdom of prolonged antibiotic coverage are the uncertainties in compliance, inadequate dosage, and the emergence of antibiotic-resistant organisms. Despite these questions the combination of preoperative immunization and long-term antibiotic coverage have become customary and prudent for children undergoing elective splenectomy and when splenic preservation is not possible following injury.

Splenic Preservation

The four available options to preserve splenic tissue are: (1) nonoperative management, (2) splenorrhaphy, (3) segmental resection, and (4) splenectomy with autotransplantation. The trend in treating children with a "stable" splenic injury who have no other obvious associated intraabdominal injuries is to observe the patient in an intensive care unit (ICU) where serial monitoring of vital signs and physical findings is possible.

Douglas and Simpson,[19] in their initial somewhat anecdotal study of "conservative management," reported in 1971 that 25 patients at the Hospital for Sick Children in Toronto had the clinical diagnosis of splenic injury (confirmed by neither nuclear scanning nor angiography). All recovered without operation. During their period of study, only six children deteriorated enough during the course of conservative treatment to require splenectomy. The authors presumed that the spleen spontaneously healed in the remaining patients and that splenectomy would have been unnecessary. The modern protocol for *nonoperative treatment* of the stable patient requires monitoring in the ICU for 1 to 3 days, bed rest for 3 to 5 days, placement of a nasogastric tube until ileus has cleared, and intravenous fluids or blood transfusion as appropriate. In a recently reported 5-year update of Douglas and Simpson's experience at the Hospital for Sick Children, transfusion was reserved for hemodynamic instability or if the Hgb fell below 8.0 g/dl. Almost all cases of isolated splenic injury stabilized with 20 ml/kg of blood replacement.[42] Serial nuclear scans are also obtained. In most cases the child is discharged from the hospital between the seventh and tenth day following injury, with precautions not to participate in any vigorous physical or athletic activity for 4 to 6 weeks. In nearly 300 cases of prospective nonoperative management reported from many institutions,* operative intervention was necessitated because persistent bleeding occurred less than 5% of the time. The principal concern of advocates favoring early operation for even "stable" patients is the risk of delayed rupture of the spleen and the possibility of overlooking a second injury. Neither concern appears substantiated by the growing body of clinical experience. Non-

---

*References 2, 13, 26, 30, 42, 65.

operative management, even in children with infectious mononucleosis,[21] has proven successful.

A second nuclear scan is obtained before discharge from the hospital to detect asymptomatic enlargement of the defect. In 19 consecutive cases of splenic injury treated at our institution[58] the visualized abnormality on the scan was unchanged or smaller in size after 1 week, and all patients went on to full recovery (Fig. 16-17). A significantly increased uptake of technetium sulfur colloid is a unique finding observed in some patients following a major dearterialization injury to one segment (Fig. 16-18, *A*). The significance of splenic hyperfunction is unknown but may reflect compensatory increased blood flow during the reparative phase of healing. Experimental studies show complete regeneration of the residual segments within 2 months of injury (Fig. 16-18, *B*).[60]

Eventual resolution of the initial splenic defect on follow-up scans of recovered patients is a customary finding,[24] but occasionally, longstanding linear defects persist, which are believed to represent scarring and do not interfere with splenic function or increase the risk of reinjury. The possibility of subcapsular hematoma, possibly evolving into a splenic pseudocyst, is a rare event,[13,65] as are reports of an infected splenic hematoma forming an abscess.[49] In a study of spontaneously

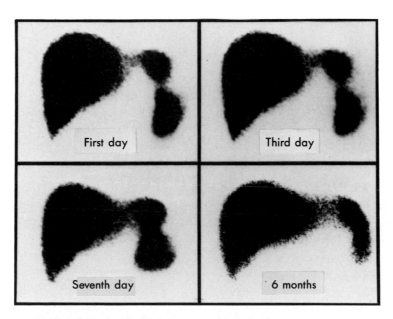

Fig. 16-17 Serial technetium (99m Tc) sulfur colloid scan in an 11-year-old boy beginning on the day of injury following a sledding accident. There is demonstrable "healing" of the spleen within 1 week of injury and return to "normal" 6 months later.

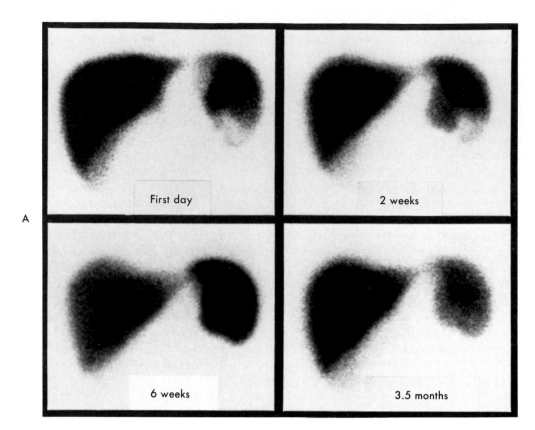

Fig. 16-18   A, Evolution of nuclear scan in a 15 year old with splenic rupture sustained while playing football. At 6 weeks there is a marked amount of colloid shift to the spleen, which is not evident on the previous or subsequent examinations. This finding is occasionally observed following splenic injury and suggests hyperfunctioning of a regenerating spleen during the healing phase.

healing experimental splenic injury to rats, survival, bacterial clearance, and antibody response to pneumococcal polysaccharide challenge were all superior to that seen in the splenectomized subjects. Apparently, healed splenic disruption does not impair clearance of blood-borne encapsulated bacteria.[28] Traumatic asplenia has been reported in adults but is rare.[17]

Operative Intervention

Approximately 25% of all children with splenic injury become clinically unstable following initial resuscitation and require operation.[13,30,65] In most cases, serious multiple injuries are also present. Whether total splenectomy is performed depends on the training, background, and clinical judgment of the surgeon, as well as the operative findings. Splenectomy is appropriate when attempts to control hemorrhage and preserve a portion of spleen are impossible or when the time necessitated for a

splenic preservation procedure would be contraindicated because of other considerations. Before a decision is made to proceed with splenectomy, the spleen must be fully mobilized by dividing all ligamentous attachments and examined, thereby allowing the surgeon to control the hilar blood supply. Bleeding from capsular avulsions or very superficial linear lacerations will stop following topical application of microfibrillar collagen (Avitene).[38]

Control of sustained bleeding can also be achieved by *splenorrhaphy*, using the same principles of debridement: through-and-through suture placement with chromic catgut and coaptation and compression of torn edges, as have been described in the treatment of hepatic or renal injuries. In the King et al.[30] series, splenorrhaphy was successful in 16 of 38 operated patients. Unfortunately the splenic capsule is more fragile than that of other solid viscera. If further tearing ensues, a simple

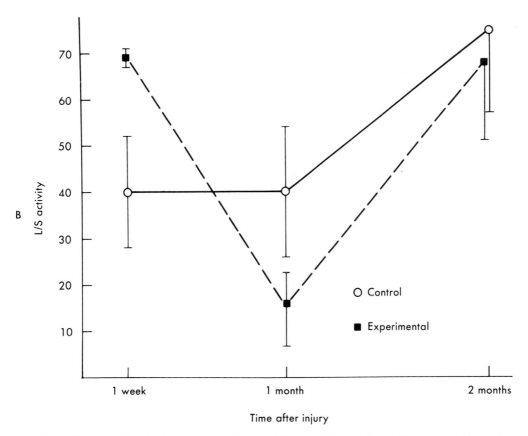

Fig. 16-18, cont'd   B, In experimental dearterialization injury in the suckling rat, splenic nuclear activity initially decreases, then rebounds above control values by 1 month, then returns to normal. (From Touloukian RJ, Dang CV, and Caride VJ: J Pediatr Surg 13:13a, 1978.)

method reported by Buntain and Lynn,[7] of passing several sutures through a kidney biopsy needle and tying the ends on each side of the divided spleen to one another, is another option (Fig. 16-19). Successful splenorrhaphy was performed on 59 children in nine institutions* and remains the simplest and most frequently performed method of operative splenic preservation. Anatomic appearance and splenic function return to normal, since the hilar blood supply is retained and healing proceeds, as would be anticipated, following repair of any visceral injury. Rabbits undergoing repair of experimental splenic injury had normal clearance of pneumococci from the circulation.[14]

Segmental resection of the spleen may become necessary if one pole is devitalized or fragmented or bleeding from a polar vessel cannot be controlled by simple measures. Under these circumstances the arterial branch to the segment is clamped, divided, and tied, leaving a clear zone of demarcation between the violaceous segment to be resected and the adjacent red vascularized spleen. Thereafter the segment is removed by bluntly dissecting the splenic parenchyma with the scalpel handle and securing any crossing vessels as they are encountered. The method is similar to that employed for hepatic resection. With the resection complete, additional bleeding from arterial branches is controlled by simple ligation of the vessel ends, venous tears oversewn with a running silk suture, and sinusoidal ooze compressed and Avitene applied to the entire surface. Further hemostasis may be required. A popular approach is to place interlocking chromic mattress sutures along the whole length of the divided parenchyma and tie under just enough tension to compress the splenic parenchyma gently (Fig. 16-20).[38]

Patients recovered from partial splenectomy

---

*References 8, 15, 26, 35-37, 47, 51, 65.

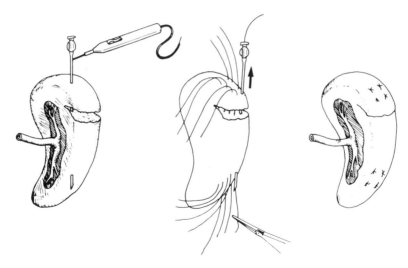

Fig. 16-19   Method splenorrhaphy coapts edges of laceration with sutures passed through vertical axis of spleen to prevent tears of the capsule. (From Buntain WL and Lynn HB: Surgery 86:748, 1979.)

have nearly normal splenic function. Partially splenectomized animals also have higher pneumococcal antibody titers and better bacterial blood stream clearance and survival than others with splenic reimplants,[16] but Okinaga's[39] experiments indicate that partial resections, which leave one third or less of the splenic mass, may not provide adequate protection. If bleeding is sustained after splenorrhaphy or partial splenectomy, splenic artery ligation effectively controls hemorrhage without defunctionalizing the spleen, as reported by Keramidas et al.[29] in two patients who underwent postoperative nuclear imaging. The principal concern of routine splenic artery ligation is that the

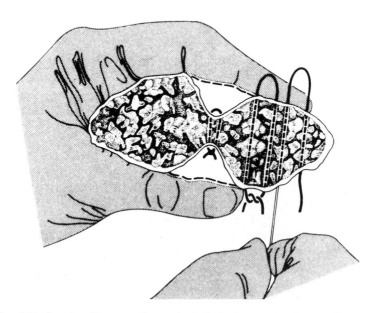

Fig. 16-20   This drawing illustrates the method of placing mattress sutures for hemostasis. For purposes of clarity the sutures are not shown interlocked. Sutures of 3-0 chromic catgut should overlap and be tied with a surgeon's knot. Pledgets beneath the knot are unnecessary if the suture is tied with the correct degree of tension. (From Morgenstern L: Surg Rounds 3:13, 1980.)

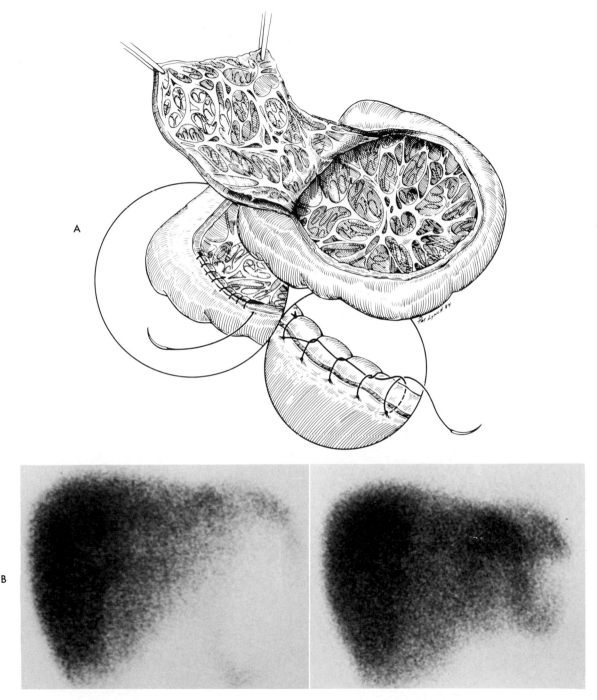

Fig. 16-21   A, The outer pseudocyst wall is excised with the electrocautery and the cuff of the splenic remnant oversewn with a running interlocked suture. **B,** The binary spleen sign is seen on the preoperative technetium sulfur colloid scan in the right anterior oblique projection. **C,** Six months following splenic decapsulation, the spleen is smaller, leaving only a crescent-shaped defect. (From Touloukian RJ and Seashore JH: J Pediatr Surg 22:135, 1987.)

filtration capacity of encapsulated organisms may be reduced.

Total splenectomy with autotransplantation has been the subject of considerably more laboratory than clinical interest. Regeneration of spontaneously implanted splenic tissue explains the relatively low mortality after splenectomy for trauma[45] in comparison to elective splenectomy for hematologic indications, but the likelihood of significant regeneration following operative autotransplantation varies with the size of the graft, the site of implantation, and the age and maturity of the host. The central portion of splenic implants in experimental subjects become necrotic with only peripheral cells revascularizing,[56] whereas homogenates have a good chance for complete survival and regeneration.[34] To enhance the prospect of a good take, a rich capillary bed, as found within the omentum or splenic fossa, is preferable to subcutaneous or subfascial pockets. Serosal or peritoneal grafts will also survive but carry the risk of causing secondary intestinal obstruction.[54] A protocol for splenic replantation after splenectomy has been proposed by Velcek et al.[64] to include only

those individuals who had such extensive injury that other attempts at preservation were impossible. Fifteen to twenty-five, $1.5 \times 1.5 \times 0.2$ cm decapsulated splenic wafers were placed into three omental rows and kept in place with interrupted 4-0 atraumatic catgut sutures placed between the transplants. Three children undergoing replantation were studied during a 3-year follow-up documenting the return of filtration function, normal immunoglobulin (IgM) levels, and antibody response to pneumococcal vaccination. These results were anticipated from studies of numerous parameters of immunity lost after splenectomy.[63] More importantly, animals with replanted splenic fragments challenged with aerosolized pneumococci have a significantly better survival rate than splenectomized animals similarly challenged.[18] The immune response of reimplanted spleen can be accelerated by dietary ascorbic acid.[22] Despite these encouraging reports, postoperative polyvalent pneumococcal vaccination and antibody prophylaxis are still recommended, since patients with "splenosis" have died following overwhelming sepsis,[48] and the total amount of regenerated spleen is limited to

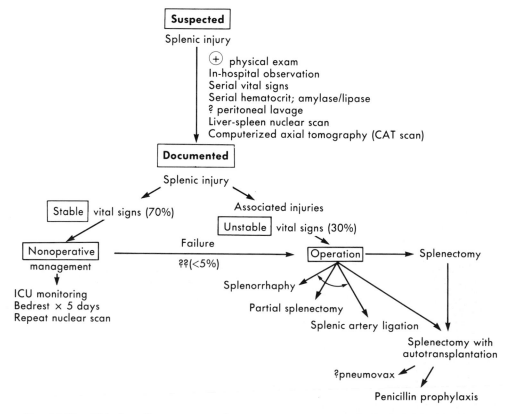

Fig. 16-22 This flow diagram summarizes current management of splenic injury in children.

usually no more than 10% to 30% of the size of an intact spleen.[34,63] Maturity of the host is also an important factor in graft survival. Spleen homogenates implanted in suckling rats uniformly regenerated, whereas regenerated nodules are found only in 10% of adult animals.[34] Our impression is that splenic implantation is the least desirable option for splenic preservation, but together with immunization and antibiotics it may make the difference between survival and death from OPSI. Only long-term follow-up of previously reported cases[5,41] will determine the outlook with this procedure.

Traditional treatment of a splenic pseudocyst is either splenectomy or partial splenectomy with excision of the cyst lining. However, these large unilocular cysts lend themselves to partial splenic decapsulation,[61] which is simpler and safer than other preservation procedures and carries no increased risk of recurrence from leaving a portion of the pseudocyst wall. The operation involves: (1) mobilizing the spleen by dividing the renal, colic, and diaphragmatic attachments; (2) decompressing the liquefied cyst contents through a thoracostomy trochar; (3) excising the outer splenic capsule and achieving hemostasis of the splenic pulp with a running interlocked silk suture; and (4) providing external tube drainage of the left upper quadrant. Postoperative scan has remarkably normal nuclear activity (Fig. 16-21).

The concept of regionalizing trauma care to a center having a pediatric intensive care unit to ensure proper monitoring of the critically ill or injured child, and a surgeon, knowledgeable about the treatment options, has made successful splenic preservation a reality. A flow diagram (Fig. 16-22) summarizes the management of splenic injury in childhood at our institution and emphasizes the concepts outlined and their relevance in various clinical settings.

REFERENCES

1. Applebaum PC et al: Fatal pneumococcal bacteremia in a vaccinated, splenectomized child, N Engl J Med 300:203, 1979.
2. Aronson DZ et al: Nonoperative management of splenic injury: a report of six consecutive cases, Pediatrics 60:482, 1977.
3. Balfanz JR et al: Overwhelming sepsis following splenectomy for trauma, J Pediatr 88:458, 1976.
4. Beaver BL et al: The efficacy of computer tomography in evaluating abdominal injuries in children with major head trauma, J Pediatr Surg 22:1117, 1987.
5. Benjamin JT et al: Alternatives to total splenectomy: two case reports, J Pediatr Surg 13:137, 1978.
6. Biggar WD et al: Impaired phagocytosis of pneumococcus type 3 in splenectomized rats, Proc Soc Exp Biol Med 139:903, 1972.
7. Buntain WL and Lynn HB: Splenorrhaphy: changing concepts for the traumatized spleen, Surgery 86:748, 1979.
8. Burrington JD: Surgical repair of a ruptured spleen in children: report of eight cases, Arch Surg 112:417, 1977.
9. Burrington JD: Preservation of the traumatized spleen in children, Contemp Surg 15:11, 1979.
10. Carlisle HN and Saslaw S: Properdin levels in splenectomized persons, Proc Soc Exp Biol Med 102:150, 1959.
11. Chaudry IH et al: Effect of splenectomy on reticuloendothelial function and survival following sepsis, J Trauma 20:649, 1980.
12. Claret I, Morales L, and Montaner A: Immunological studies in the postsplenectomy syndrome, J Pediatr Surg 10:59, 1975.
13. Cohen RC: Blunt splenic trauma in children: a retrospective study of nonoperative management, Aust Paediatr J 18:211, 1982.
14. Coln D et al: Clearance of pneumococcal organisms after repair of injured spleens, J Pediatr Surg 18:280, 1983.
15. Cooney DR: Splenic and hepatic trauma in children, Surg Clin North Am 61:1165, 1981.
16. Cooney DR et al: Comparative methods of splenic preservation, J Pediatr Surg 16:327, 1981.
17. Dickerman JD: Traumatic asplenia in adults, Arch Surg 116:361, 1981.
18. Dickerman JD et al: The protective effect of intraperitoneal splenic autotransplants in mice exposed to an aerosolized suspension of type III Streptococcus pneumoniae, Blood 54:354, 1979.
19. Douglas GJ and Simpson JS: The conservative management of splenic trauma, J Pediatr Surg 6:565, 1971.
20. Eraklis AJ et al: Hazard of overwhelming infection after splenectomy in childhood, N Engl J Med 276:1225, 1967.
21. Gauderer M, Stellato TA, and Hutton M: Traumatic splenic injury: nonoperative management in three patients with infectious mononucleosis, J Pediatr Surg 24:118, 1989.
22. Hashimoto T et al: Plasma fibronectin levels after splenectomy and splenic autoimplantation in rats with and without dietary ascorbic acid supplementation, J Pediatr Surg 18:805, 1983.
23. Hebert JC et al: Lack of protection by pneumococcal vaccine after splenectomy in mice challenged with aerosolized pneumococci, J Trauma 23:1, 1983.
24. Howman-Giles R et al: Splenic trauma, nonoperative management and long-term follow-up by scintiscan, J Pediatr Surg 13:121, 1978.
25. Horan M and Colebatch JH: Relationship between splenectomy and subsequent infection, Arch Dis Child 37:398, 1962.
26. Joseph TP, Wyllie GG, and Savage JP: The nonoperative management of splenic trauma, Aust NZ J Surg 47:179, 1977.
27. Karp MP et al: The role of computed tomography in the evaluation of blunt abdominal trauma in children, J Pediatr Surg 16:316, 1981.
28. Karp MP et al: Immune consequences of nonoperative treatment of splenic trauma, J Pediatric Surg 24:112, 1989.
29. Keramidas DC et al: Ligation of the splenic artery: effects

on the injured spleen and its function, J Pediatr Surg 15:38, 1980.

30. King DR et al: Selective management of injured spleen, Surgery 90:677, 1981.

31. King H and Shumacker HB: Splenic studies. I. Susceptibility to infection after splenectomy performed in infancy, Ann Surg 136:239, 1952.

32. Kober RS and Kumar APM: Splenic pseudocyst: preoperative diagnosis with ultrasonography, J Pediatr Surg 14:601, 1979.

33. Kocher ET, quoted by Sherman R: Perspectives in management of trauma to the spleen: presidential address to the American Association for the Surgery of Trauma, J Trauma 20:1, 1980.

34. Kovacs KF, Caride VJ, and Touloukian RJ: Regeneration of splenic autotransplants in suckling and adult rats, Arch Surg 116:335, 1981.

35. La Mura J, Chung-Fat SP, and San Filippo A: Splenorrhaphy for the treatment of splenic rupture in infants and children, Surgery 81:497, 1977.

36. Matsuyama S, Suzuki N, and Nagamachi Y: Rupture of the spleen in the newborn: treatment without splenectomy, J Pediatr Surg 11:115, 1976.

37. Mishalany H: Repair of the ruptured spleen, J Pediatr Surg 9:175, 1974.

38. Morgenstern L: Conservation of the injured spleen, Surg Rounds 3:13, 1980.

39. Okinaga K et al: The effect of partial splenectomy on experimental pneumococcal bacteremia in an animal model, J Pediatr Surg 16:717, 1981.

40. Overturf GD, Field R, and Edmonds R: Death from type 6 pneumococcal septicemia in a vaccinated child with sickle cell disease, N Engl J Med 300:143, 1979.

41. Patel J et al: Preservation of splenic function by autotransplantation of traumatized spleen in man, Surgery 90:683, 1981.

42. Pearl RH et al: Splenic injury—a 5-year update, with improved results and changing criteria for conservative management, J Pediatr Surg 24:121, 1989.

43. Pearson HA: The spleen and postsplenectomy infection. Med Times 110:31, 1982.

44. Pearson HA, Touloukian RJ, and Spencer RP: The binary spleen: a radioisotopic scan sign of splenic pseudocyst, J Pediatr 77:216, 1970.

45. Pearson HA et al: The born-again spleen: return of splenic function after splenectomy for trauma, N Engl J Med 298:1389, 1978.

46. Polhill RB Jr and Johnston RB Jr: Diminished alternatives complement pathway (ACP) activity after splenectomy, Pediatr Res 9:333, 1975.

47. Ratner MH et al: Surgical repair of the injured spleen, J Pediatr Surg 12:1019, 1977.

48. Rice HM and James PD: Ectopic splenic tissue failed to prevent fatal pneumococcal septicaemia after splenectomy for trauma, Lancet 1:565, 1980.

49. Sands M, Page D, and Brown RB: Splenic abscess following nonoperative management of splenic rupture, J Pediatr Surg 21:900, 1986.

50. Shennib H, Chen R, and Mulder DS: The effects of splenectomy and splenic implantation on alveolar macrophage function, J Trauma 23:7, 1983.

51. Sherman NJ and Asch M: Conservative surgery for splenic injuries, Pediatrics 61:267, 1978.

52. Singer DB: Postsplenectomy sepsis: perspectives in pediatric pathology, vol 1, Chicago, 1973, Year Book Medical Publishers.

53. Sink JD et al: Removal of splenic cyst with salvage of functional splenic tissue, J Pediatr 100:412, 1982.

54. Stephenson LW, Leonard RP, and Longino LA: Splenosis, South Med J 68:1046, 1975.

55. Sutliff WD and Finland M: Antipneumococcal immunity reactions in individuals of different ages, J Exp Med 55:837, 1932.

56. Tavassoli M, Ratzan RJ, and Crosby WH: Studies on regeneration of heterotopic splenic autotransplants, Blood 41:701, 1973.

57. Touloukian RJ: Abdominal visceral injuries in battered children, Pediatrics 42:642, 1968.

58. Touloukian RJ: Abdominal injuries. In Touloukian RJ, editor: Pediatric trauma, ed 1, New York, 1978, John Wiley & Sons.

59. Touloukian RJ: Splenic preservation in children, World J Surg 9:214, 1985.

60. Touloukian RJ, Dang CV, and Caride VJ: Splenic function following dearterialization injury in the suckling rat, J Pediatr Surg 13:131, 1978.

61. Touloukian RJ and Seashore JH: Partial splenic decapsulation: a simplified operation for splenic pseudocyst, J Pediatr Surg 22:135, 1987.

62. Upadhyaya P and Simpson JS: Splenic trauma in children, Surg Gynecol Obstet 126:781, 1968.

63. Velcek FT et al: Function of the replanted spleen in dogs, J Trauma 22:502, 1982.

64. Velcek FT et al: Posttraumatic splenic replantation in children, J Pediatr Surg 17:879, 1982.

65. Wesson DE et al: Ruptured spleen — when to operate? J Pediatr Surg 16:324, 1981.

GASTRIC AND INTESTINAL INJURY

Kurt D. Newman and Martin R. Eichelberger

INCIDENCE AND ASSOCIATED INJURIES

Trauma to the abdomen causing intestinal or gastric injury is rare in childhood. Nevertheless, many children sustain abdominal injury and require evaluation for potential surgery. Of 2300 consecutive admissions for trauma to Children's Hospital National Medical Center (CHNMC) in the last 3 years, only 2.3% required operative intervention for gastric or intestinal injury. The mechanism of injury in abdominal trauma is classified as blunt and penetrating. Although the operative management of children with blunt and penetrating trauma is similar, the diagnostic approach is different. Knowledge of the mechanism of injury is crucial to appropriate management.

Blunt trauma accounts for 60% of childhood injury at CHNMC. Injury to the stomach or intestine ranks third behind injuries to the liver and spleen. The two most common mechanisms of injury causing intestinal trauma are motor vehicle impact and child abuse. Penetrating injury is much less common in children than in adults, accounting for 3.6% of trauma admissions to CHNMC. The most common anatomic regions in descending order of frequency are the head, chest, back, and extremities; only 11% of penetrating wounds injured an abdominal hollow viscus. Gunshot wounds were twice as common as stab wounds in producing injury to the stomach or intestine; the small bowel is the most frequently injured abdominal organ.

Several social trends have led to an increasing incidence of small bowel injury in children. The compliance of parents with automotive seat belt laws and higher speed limits have enhanced conditions for more frequent injuries. The general availability of weapons within society increases their access to children. Consequently, gunshot and stab wounds to the abdomen in children increased by 300% over the last 3 years in the metropolitan Washington, D.C. area. Unfortunately, child abuse continues unabated, with abdominal injury a result of violent assault.

The first reported American case of intestinal perforation caused by blunt trauma was published by Samuel Annan in 1837. Although many descriptions of adult patients were published in the twentieth century, it was not until the early 1970s that the diagnosis and management of intestinal injury in children were discussed. Schuster et al.[18] in 1966 urged expeditious exploration of the abdomen in children with blunt abdominal trauma in which the diagnosis was unclear. Dickinson et al.[5] reported five children in 1970 who ruptured the gastrointestinal tract as a result of blunt trauma and reported a low mortality rate with early recognition and operation. Richardson et al.[16] emphasized the morbidity of associated injuries, the need for definitive operation, and paracentesis to assist diagnosis in uncertain cases. Kakos and co-workers[11] reported a group of 26 children with small bowel injuries in 1970 and advocated a conservative approach to the management of duodenal hematoma. The successful nonoperative management of intestinal duodenal hematoma in children was confirmed by Wooley and co-workers,[27] Touloukian,[25] and Jewett et al.[10] As nonoperative management of blunt injury to the liver and spleen has become common, Cobb et al.[3] emphasized that, although an intestinal injury in children is rare, the index of suspicion must remain high to prevent an error in diagnosis and treatment (see box below).

The modern management of penetrating injury in children began in 1960 when Shaftan[19] established the morbidity of negative abdominal exploration for stab wounds in adults. Nance and Cohn[14]

INJURY TO THE GASTROINTESTINAL TRACT FROM BLUNT TRAUMA

Dickinson et al.,[5] 1970	5 cases
Richardson et al.,[16] 1971	8 cases
Kakos et al.,[11] 1971	17 cases
Cobb et al.,[3] 1986	12 cases
CHNMC, 1988	45 cases

in 1969 suggested a selective approach to abdominal exploration based on physical examination, which reduced the negative celiotomy rate from 50% to 10%. In adults this rate was reduced to 4% using local wound exploration and peritoneal lavage.[24] At CHNMC we apply this approach using a result of greater than 50,000 red blood cells per high power field, evisceration, presence of bile, stool, or an elevated amylase as an indication for laparotomy.

The injury patterns produced by abdominal trauma depend on the mechanism of injury. A stab wound may produce one or more localized perforations usually of the small intestine, since it composes a large portion of the abdominal cavity. Laceration of a mesenteric vessel can occur, although destruction of surrounding tissue is limited. Gunshot wounds, however, cause more destruction not only to the organ directly affected but also to the adjacent structures as a consequence of dissipation of large amounts of kinetic energy. The extent of bowel injury and specific organ involvement are unpredictable, thus explaining the need for exploratory laparotomy to guarantee proper diagnosis and treatment.

Blunt trauma to the abdomen can produce bowel injury in several ways.[21] The most common mechanism is a result of rapid deceleration forces that can crush the small bowel and mesentery between the spine and the abdominal wall.[26] Children are especially at risk because of their small transverse abdominal diameter. Unfortunately, improper usage of automobile lap belt safety restraints produces injury to the intestine and spine.[2] Consequently, bowel perforation can occur synchronously with vertebral trauma and paralysis.[8] When the bowel is compressed, laceration or transection may occur. Increased abdominal pressure from blunt injury may be transmitted directly to a closed loop of fluid-filled intestine. Perforation occurs in accordance with the law of Laplace, when intraluminal pressure exceeds the tension of the bowel wall. The intestine also sustains injury by shear forces associated with sudden deceleration.[17] Intestinal perforation also occurs at points of fixation to the abdominal cavity, such as the proximal duodenal-jejunal junction (ligament of Treitz) or the distal ileum (ileocecal region).[4] A duodenal hematoma results from a direct blow or deceleration force that produces submucosal bleeding and luminal obstruction.

DIAGNOSIS

The key to successful treatment of intestinal trauma is a high index of suspicion of injury and an expeditious, systematic approach to diagnosis and management. A predetermined approach to diagnosis of intraabdominal injury begins with the mechanism of injury. A stab wound to the abdomen is best managed selectively.[20] Exploratory laparotomy is mandatory in children who manifest unstable vital signs, unexplained blood loss, or evisceration through the wound. In the stable, cooperative child local wound assessment enhanced by local anesthesia is helpful. Absence of fascial penetration permits observation of the child and local wound care. If peritoneal penetration is present, peritoneal lavage (15 cc/kg) helps determine whether intestinal injury occurred. Lavage fluid containing bile, bacteria, or amylase elevation are indications for surgery. Children with peritoneal penetration and a negative lavage do not require exploratory laparotomy. If the child develops peritonitis, exploration is essential. All children who suffer a penetrating gunshot wound to the abdomen require exploratory laparotomy. Abdominal x-ray films occasionally reveal pneumoperitoneum, an objective indication for surgery. Penetrating trauma may cause severe bleeding; all children require adequate cardiovascular resuscitation with crystalloid and blood infusion if necessary before proceeding with laparotomy.

The child involved in a motor vehicle accident either as a pedestrian or passenger has a higher risk for intraabdominal injury. Management of the airway and cardiopulmonary resuscitation take precedence. Gastric dilatation from aerophagia produces abdominal distention, tachycardia, and restlessness. Nasogastric tube decompression of the stomach alleviates discomfort, improves ventilation, and enhances the potential for diagnosis of intraabdominal injury. Children, especially in the younger age group, may develop severe respiratory compromise from pneumoperitoneum associated with proximal bowel injury. Limitation of diaphragmatic excursion from air beneath the diaphragm causes serious respiratory insufficiency; needle aspiration of the pneumoperitoneum is lifesaving.

As part of the secondary survey, observation of abdominal contusion, ecchymosis, or a tire track mark is important, as this may be the key to the diagnosis of intestinal injury (Fig. 16-23). If the

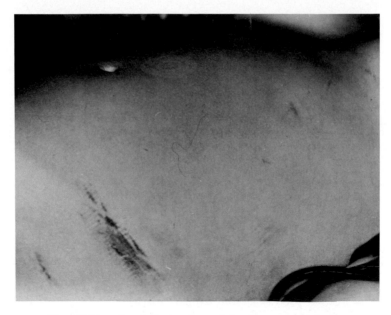

Fig. 16-23   Seat belt abrasions of the abdomen and flank.

child is conscious, the degree of abdominal pain requires assessment; intestinal injury causes muscular guarding, tenderness and rebound, and signs of peritonitis. The unconscious child is difficult to evaluate by physical examination. Unfortunately, a plain film of the abdomen may not show free intraabdominal air even with intestinal perforation. However, lumbar fractures may provide the clue to intestinal injury. When the child is stable, a CT scan of the abdomen may demonstrate pneumoperitoneum, but associated injury to the pancreas, liver, or spleen increases the suspicion of bowel

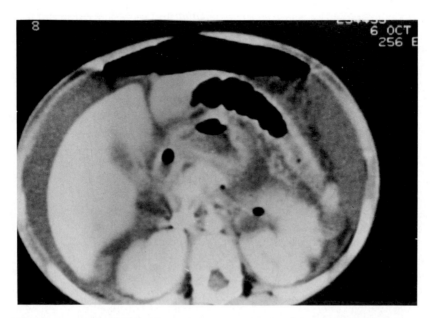

Fig. 16-24   Pneumoperitoneum. CT scan of an 8-year-old child who was a passenger wearing a seat belt that ruptured the jejunum, resulting in free air.

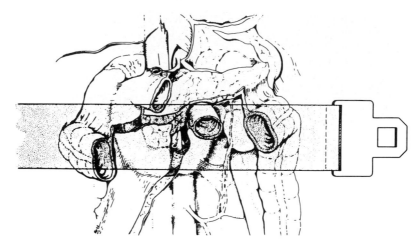

Fig. 16-25   Diagram demonstrating the relative positions of a lap belt and internal organs.

injury (Fig. 16-24).[12] Free peritoneal fluid without evidence of solid organ injury is suggestive of intestinal injury.[23] If no clear diagnosis of intestinal injury is possible, yet there is a high index of suspicion based on mechanism of injury, peritoneal signs, or associated injuries, a peritoneal lavage enhances the ability to decide whether exploratory laparotomy is indicated.

At CHNMC five children demonstrated a "lap belt complex." All were passengers who were restrained by a lap belt and involved in a motor vehicle accident. Abdominal abrasion and contusion were present in association with abdominal tenderness. A lumbosacral fracture was present in all five, with paralysis in three children. Laparotomy revealed a small bowel rupture. The mechanism appears to be a combination of a compressing force of the lap belt and hyperflexion of the lumbosacral spine at the point of lap belt restraint, which functions as a fulcrum (Fig. 16-25). Eight others had fracture of the lumbar spine only. The lap belt complex consists of abdominal abrasion, lumbosacral spine fracture, and hollow viscus perforation.

A CT scan of the abdomen may be normal in spite of intestinal injury. Of 473 consecutive children with injury evaluated by CT scan at CHNMC, only 1.3% had an intestinal injury. The CT scan missed a bowel perforation in two of these children. Treatment delay is frequent if suspicion for the injury is low. Early peritoneal lavage or exploratory laparotomy helps prevent sepsis resulting from delays in surgical management.

In children with abdominal pain and vomiting following blunt abdominal trauma, the possibility of an intramural hematoma of the duodenum is present. The most common cause of this rare injury in children is a direct blow to the abdomen during play or from bicycle trauma; however, child abuse from aggressive assault results in this entity in children under the age of 5 years. Although the plain films are usually normal, an upper GI contrast examination often reveals a "coiled spring" sign with duodenal obstruction; a CT scan can also demonstrate the lesion. Since pancreatitis occurs in a quarter of the children with intramural hematoma of the duodenum, ultrasound is a useful adjunct for evaluation of pancreatic injury.

Diagnosis of rectal injury is difficult. Impalement on a sharp object is a frequent cause of injury. Physical examination is the key to diagnosis, since abdominal signs are usually absent because of the extraperitoneal location of the rectum. Laceration of the anal skin, bleeding per rectum, or an anal hematoma suggest rectal injury. If digital examination and proctoscopy are difficult because of age or pain, examination with the patient under anesthesia permits thorough rectal-perineal inspection to rule out injury.

OPERATIVE APPROACH

Exploratory laparotomy for gastric or intestinal injury is best through a midline abdominal incision from xiphoid to pubis. Iatrogenic injury to the high-riding bladder in young children can occur during entry into the abdominal cavity. Management of life-threatening hemorrhage often from a liver or spleen injury takes precedence. Injury to the mesenteric vessels may cause severe bleeding and require hemostasis before treatment of the viscus injury. The entire stomach, small intestine, and colon require mobilization and visual inspection. If rectal injury is suspected, digital examination and endoscopy precede the exploratory celiotomy.

Stomach

Stomach injury is more common in children than in adults. The stomach is prone to rupture especially when full and particularly when there is a closed pylorus and competent gastroesophageal junction. A bicycle handlebar, seat belt, and nasogastric tube are frequent causes of injury. Overdistention of the stomach during airway management with excessive insufflation also can cause perforation.

Rupture of the stomach from blunt injury usually occurs along the greater curvature. Exposure of the injury is best achieved by dividing the gastrocolic ligament and by freeing the duodenal attachments to the retroperitoneum (Kocher maneuver). Debridement of the edges of the defect and control of bleeding in the submucosa of the stomach wall permit safe closure of the defect. A two-layer closure is best using an inner layer of absorbable sutures and an outer layer of nonabsorbable suture. A nasogastric tube usually provides effective decompression.

Penetrating injury of the stomach by stab wound or gunshot is easy to overlook at exploration. Identification of the entry and exit wound by adequate mobilization of the stomach permits debridement and closure of the defect. Occasionally the stomach can bleed extensively and produce hypotension.

Duodenum

When the diagnosis of intramural hematoma of the duodenum is clear radiologically, nonoperative management is preferable if no perforation is present. Nasogastric suction and parenteral nutrition are employed until the obstruction resolves, usually without surgery. Operation is reserved for those children who develop peritonitis or fail to resolve after 2 to 3 weeks of obstruction.[25] If an intramural hematoma is found in the course of operative management for other indications, evacuation of the hematoma alone suffices.[10,27]

Duodenal injury occurs with blunt trauma or de-

celeration because of the duodenum's fixation to the retroperitoneum.[9] Forceful compression of distended bowel may result in rupture along the mesenteric border. A simple tear of the duodenum is safely repaired by a layered closure after adequate intestinal mobilization. Complete transection requires debridement of devitalized tissue and anastomosis.[6]

Trauma to the duodenum is often associated with pancreatic injury.[7] Simple drainage is sufficient if the pancreatic injury is minimal and if the duct of Wirsung is intact. If the duct is transected distally, resection of the tail of the pancreas with splenic preservation is preferable. This technique was employed successfully at CHNMC in a 14-year-old girl who was struck in the abdomen and developed life-threatening intraabdominal hemorrhage. At laparotomy an epithelial tumor of the distal pancreas required resection with preservation of the spleen.

Resection of the duodenum and head of the pancreas in children is rare.[15] Other techniques have evolved to isolate the pancreas and duodenum when major injury occurs. The goal is to prevent the complication of duodenal fistula, especially if there are other associated vascular or visceral injuries. Diverticulization of the duodenum is one alternative in which the surgeon performs a distal gastrectomy with Billroth II reconstruction, truncal vagotomy, tube decompression of the duodenum, cholecystostomy, and extensive drainage of the pancreatic bed.[1,22] Total parenteral nutrition helps reduce the pancreatic and duodenal secretions.

Other alternatives to pancreaticoduodenectomy are also available. The first is pyloric exclusion to divert the gastrointestinal secretions away from a duodenal wound[13]; the pylorus is oversewn through a gastrotomy employing absorbable sutures that resorb in 2 to 3 weeks to reestablish pyloric integrity. The second, a gastrojejunostomy with or without vagotomy, is used to bypass the duodenum. This allows healing of the duodenum without resection of the antrum. A third alternative employs gastrostomy and jejunostomy to decompress the duodenum. In all cases, when decompression of the biliary tree is necessary, cholecystostomy prevents the potential for common duct stricture secondary to T-tube drainage.

The major complications are duodenal fistula, abscess formation, and pancreatic fistula. Most are managed conservatively with drainage, antibiotics, and total parenteral nutrition. The keys to preventing the high morbidity and mortality of duodenal injuries are to have a high index of suspicion of pancreatic injury when duodenal injury is present and to tailor the operative repair to the specific injury. A conservative management scheme is usually justified.

Jejunum and Ileum

The spectrum of injury to the small intestine in children is wide. Gunshot wounds often produce multiple enterotomies, whereas a stab wound is more localized. Blunt trauma can result in a small mesenteric tear, a linear luminal laceration, or a complete viscus transection (Fig. 16-26).

A small laceration is best treated by debridement of devitalized tissue and transverse closure of the defect in two layers (Fig. 16-27). A more extensive small bowel injury requires segmental resection of intestine to viable tissue with anastomosis. Three children in the last year have been treated at CHNMC with a tear of the proximal jejunum on the mesenteric wall of the bowel from a lap belt injury (Fig. 16-28). These children were treated successfully with segmental resection and anastomosis. Construction of a diverting enterostomy for small bowel injury is rarely required but may be useful with concomitant colon injury or extensive bowel ischemia.

An unusual source of injury to the small bowel is from an ingested foreign body. Most often a sharp object becomes impacted at a site of narrowing of the bowel, such as the pylorus or ileocecal valve, causing erosion, perforation, and peritonitis. A congenital anomaly such as Meckel's diverticulum can also retard the passage of a foreign object and become the site of perforation.

Colon and Rectum

Although the colon is usually spared in blunt trauma, penetrating trauma usually causes injury and perforation. Injury to the colon is best managed by fecal diversion using a colostomy or ileostomy with repair of the injured segment and drainage of the site of injury. Resection of severely injured colon followed by creation of a colostomy and mucous fistula is the safest treatment. Subsequent anastomosis is possible at 6 to 8 weeks following injury. Primary repair of colonic injury is indicated if a sharp, clean injury is present without a delay in treatment, stool contamination, excessive blood loss, or associated severe injury. Diversion of the fecal stream by colostomy is always the safest operative management.

When anorectal trauma occurs usually from impalement, straddle of an object, penetration from a missile, or child abuse the distal rectum should

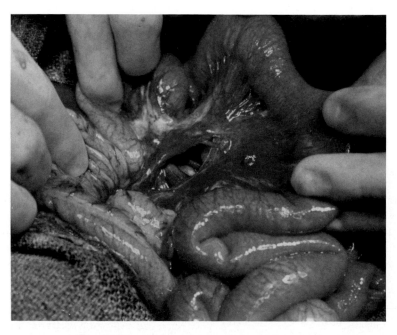

Fig. 16-26   Mesenteric tear due to blunt trauma.

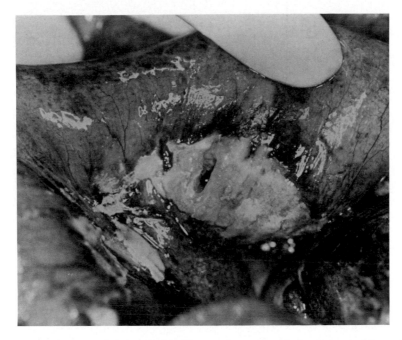

Fig. 16-27   Perforation of the small intestine on the mesenteric border caused by a gunshot wound.

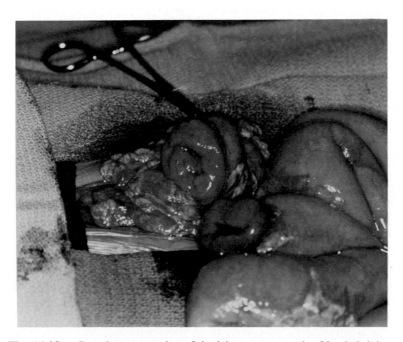

Fig. 16-28   Complete transection of the jejunum as a result of lap belt injury.

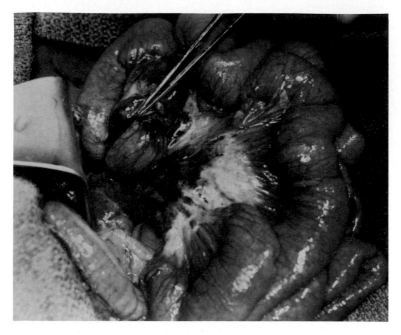

Fig. 16-29   Hematoma at base of the mesentery from injury to mesenteric vein.

be irrigated clean of fecal material. An injury extending above the peritoneal reflection requires laparotomy to ensure safe repair of the rectum. In contrast, injury below the peritoneal reflection permits debridement of devitalized anorectal tissue followed by a primary layered closure; diverting colostomy and mucous fistula ensures diversion of feces away from the injury. Presacral dependent drainage minimizes abscess formation and sepsis.

Mesenteric and Vascular Injury

Both blunt and penetrating injury produce tears in the mesentery that may cause vascular injury. Inspection of the mesentery suggests vascular injury when hematoma is present at the base (Fig. 16-29). Bleeding points in the mesentery are easily controlled by precise ligation. Nevertheless, if a segment of the intestine becomes ischemic, segmental resection and anastomosis of the bowel ends are indicated. A large or expanding hematoma at the base of the mesentery should be explored.

Although infrequent in children, major mesenteric retroperitoneal vascular injury is potentially devastating. If possible, proximal and distal control of the injured vessel before repair permits best treatment. Lateral venorrhaphy is possible with localized injury to the superior mesenteric vein. If vascular anastomosis is not technically possible,

then ligation is indicated. Ligation of the superior mesenteric artery in children rarely results in ischemia because of a rich collateral blood supply and the absence of arteriosclerosis. A second-look operation within 48 hours permits evaluation of bowel viability. Such an approach avoids extensive bowel resection and subsequent short gut syndrome.

AFTERCARE

Following small bowel injury and repair, children require nasogastric decompression and intravenous fluids until resolution of ileus is manifested by passage of flatus or a bowel movement. Parenteral nutrition is a useful adjunct especially in children with associated severe injury, pancreatitis, or prolonged inability to eat. Broad-spectrum antibiotics are employed for 7 to 10 days to lessen the likelihood of intraabdominal abscess; discontinuation is proper when the leukocyte count returns to normal and the child is afebrile. Postoperative complications include atelectasis, pancreatitis, wound infection, development of intraabdominal abscess, and bowel obstruction. Careful physical examination and laboratory evaluation performed daily guarantee prompt identification of these problems. The use of ultrasound and CT scan has helped in the evaluation and localization of intraabdominal abscesses. Percutaneous drainage with radiologic control is often useful in the management of postoperative intraabdominal abscess.

SUMMARY

Management of children with gastric or intestinal injury secondary to trauma is possible by maintaining a high index of suspicion, by recognizing the injury patterns based on the mechanism, and by appropriately applying surgical treatment. Even though gastric and intestinal injury are rare, proper surgical judgment reduces delay in management and resultant sepsis.

REFERENCES

1. Berne CJ et al: Duodenal "diverticulization" for duodenal and pancreatic injury, Am J Surg 127:503, 1974.
2. Christophi FT et al: Seatbelt-induced trauma to the small bowel, World J Surg 9:747, 1985.
3. Cobb LM et al: Intestinal perforation due to blunt trauma in children in an era of increased nonoperative treatment, Trauma 26:461, 1986.
4. Dauterive AH, Flanabaum MD, and Cox EF: Blunt intestinal trauma, a modern day review, Ann Surg 201:198, 1985.
5. Dickinson S, Shaw A, and Santulli T: Rupture of the gastrointestinal tract in children by blunt trauma, Surg Gynecol Obstet 130:655, 1970.
6. Donahue JH, Cross RA, and Tunkey DD: The management of duodenal and other small intestinal trauma, World J Surg 9:904, 1985.
7. Feliciano DV et al: Management of combine pancreatoduodenal injuries, Ann Surg 205:673, 1987.
8. Hudson I and Kavanagh TG: Duodenal transection and vertebral injury occurring in combination in a patient wearing a seat belt, Injury 15:6, 1983.
9. Lucas CE and Lederwood AM: Factors influencing outcome after blunt duodenal injury, J Trauma 15:839, 1975.
10. Jewett TC et al: Intramural hematoma of the duodenum, Arch Surg 123:54, 1988.
11. Kakos GS, Grosfeld JL, and Morse TS: Small bowel injuries in children after blunt abdominal trauma, Ann Surg 174:238, 1971.
12. Kane NM et al: Pediatric abdominal trauma: evaluation by computed tomography, Pediatrics 82:11, 1988.
13. Martin TD et al: Severe duodenal injuries, treatment with pyloric exclusion and gastrojejunostomy, Arch Surg 118:631, 635, 1983.
14. Nance FC and Cohn I: Surgical judgment in the management of stab wounds of the abdomen: a retrospective and prospective analysis based on a study of 600 stabbed patients, Ann Surg 170:569, 1969.
15. Oreskovich MR and Carrico CJ: Pancreaticoduodenectomy for trauma: a viable option? Am J Surg 147:618, 1984.
16. Richardson JD, Belin RP, and Griffin WO: Blunt abdominal trauma, South Med J 64:719, 1971.
17. Ritchie W, Ersek RA, and Simmons RL: Combined visceral and vertebral injuries from lap type seat belts, Surg Gynecol Obstet 131:431, 1970.
18. Schuster SR, Eraklis AJ, and Trump DS: Urgent surgical problems in childhood, Surg Clin North Am 46:76, 1966.
19. Shaftan GW: Indications for operation in abdominal trauma, Am J Surg 99:657, 1960.
20. Shorr RM et al: Selective management of abdominal stab wounds, Arch Surg 123:1141, 1988.
21. Smith WS and Kaufer H: Patterns and mechanisms of lumbar injuries associated with lap seat belts, Bone Joint Surg 51A:239, 1969.
22. Stone HH and Fabian TC: Management of duodenal wounds, J Trauma 19:334, 1979.
23. Taylor GA et al: The role of computed tomography in blunt abdominal trauma in children, J Trauma 28:1660, 1988.
24. Thal E: Evaluation of peritoneal lavage and local exploration in lower chest and abdominal wounds, J Trauma 17:642, 1977.
25. Touloukian RJ: Protocol for the nonoperative treatment of obstructing intramural duodenal hematoma during childhood, Am J Surg 145:330, 1983.
26. Williams RP and Sargent FT: The mechanism of intestinal injury and trauma, J Trauma 3:288, 1963.
27. Woolley MM, Mahour GH, and Sloan T: Duodenal hematoma in infancy and childhood: changing etiology and changing management, Am J Surg 136:8, 1978.

17

Renal Injuries

Terry W. Hensle and Peter Dillon

Renal injury with its subsequent complications remains a major source of morbidity in the pediatric trauma patient. In the active and often violent world of the pediatric patient, urinary tract trauma, of which injury to the kidney predominates, is second in frequency only to central nervous system injury.[9] With increasing attention focused on coordinated pediatric trauma care, the pediatric trauma specialist will be faced with an increasing number of patients with renal injuries. Proper management will depend on a rational approach to the evaluation of these injuries and an understanding of treatment alternatives. Over the last several years the approach to these injuries has been aided by the emergence and availability of the CT scan in evaluating complex injuries.

Just as the management of splenic and hepatic pediatric injuries has become increasingly more conservative and less invasive, very few renal injuries today require emergency operative intervention. Of course, controversies in management still exist, particularly with complex lesions. The current literature is hampered by the lack of prospective randomized studies and represents an amalgam of institutional experiences and biases. We believe that a rational approach to the evaluation and management of pediatric renal injury can be devised and should be adopted by those treating major renal trauma.

ETIOLOGY

By an overwhelming margin, most pediatric renal injuries are caused by blunt or nonpenetrating traumatic forces rather than penetrating injuries. Penetrating trauma in the pediatric population has been documented to be the cause of only 3% to 4% of all pediatric renal injuries.[14] In the case of blunt trauma, over 75% of the injuries result from traffic accidents. The second most common mechanism of renal injury involves a fall from a height, whereas sports-related injuries are third. Preexisting renal anomalies have been documented in up to 10% of injuries.[15] Abnormal kidneys are thought to be more easily injured by lesser degrees of trauma. Renal abnormalities associated with traumatic disruption include ureteropelvic junction obstruction, horseshoe kidney, pelvic kidney, and an unsuspected Wilm's tumor.

Children of all ages are subject to renal trauma; however, the most commonly injured group remains those children over 10 years of age. Males are more commonly injured than are females. A number of different theories have been proposed to explain why more children than adults sustain renal injuries resulting from blunt trauma.[12] Anatomically, the child's kidney is larger than that of the adult in relation to overall body mass. It is more likely to have fetal lobulations and is protected by only a small amount of perirenal fat. The less ossified thoracic cage of the child fails to provide significant protection from external forces, and the vascular pedicle provides the only solid fixation within the retroperitoneum.

Since motor vehicle accidents and falls are the most common causes of pediatric renal trauma, the mechanism of most injuries involves the effects of acceleration-deceleration forces on the various renal substructures. The four major substructures injured include the parenchyma, capsule, collecting system, and major vessels (or pedicle). A force applied to the kidney by a sudden acceleration-deceleration process may cause differential energy transmission through the kidney with resultant shearing, rupture, or compression of the kidney tissues. The fixed vascular pedicle becomes a fulcrum over which the vessels can be stretched or lacerated.

358

CLASSIFICATION

A number of different classification systems have been proposed for describing renal injuries; all greatly depend on the proper interpretation of radiographic modalities. All are based on the anatomic severity of injury to the underlying renal substructures. We classify all renal injuries into one of five general categories (see the box at right and Fig. 17-1).

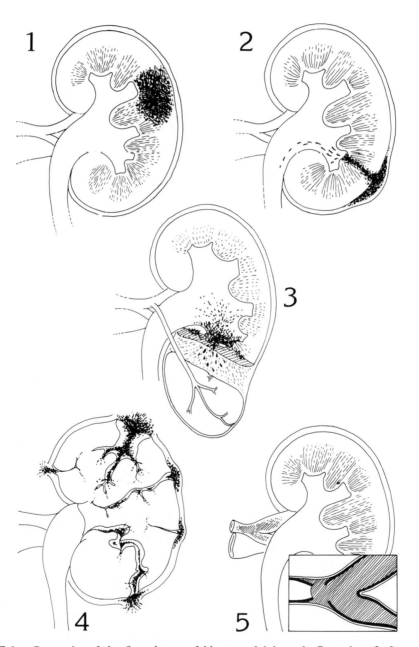

Fig. 17-1   Composite of the five classes of blunt renal injury: *1*, Contusion; *2*, Laceration; *3*, Transection; *4*, Fragmentation; *5*, Pedicle injury.

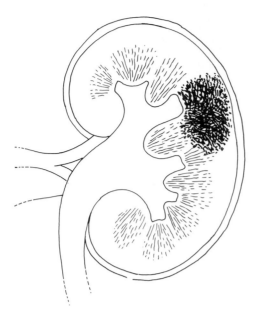

Fig. 17-2 Renal contusion. Renal capsule and collecting system intact.

Contusion

By far the most common renal injury is parenchymal contusion (Fig. 17-2). In most collected series it constitutes 60%-90% of all injuries from blunt trauma.[5,11,12] It usually results from direct injury to the renal parenchyma while the collecting system, vascular system, and capsule remain in-

tact. Hematuria is the most common presenting sign of renal contusion, with escape of red cells from the damaged microvascular system into the tubules. The capsule usually remains intact, and there is no extravasation of blood or urine in the perirenal tissue. Since the overwhelming number of renal injuries result in a contusion, the other injury categories represent a very small population of cases.

Laceration

Disruption of the capsule, collecting system, or both results from a renal laceration. These injuries account for 10% or less of all pediatric renal injuries,[5,6] although they are the second most common type of pediatric renal injury after contusion. With disruption of either the renal capsule or the collecting system, blood or urine may extravasate. This extravasation can form either a urinoma or a hematoma, and these collections can range from very small to very significant (Fig. 17-3).

Transection and Fragmentation

Renal transection represents a more extensive injury than a laceration and can be described as a separation of renal tissue. The spectrum of this type of injury ranges from a solitary through and through laceration of the kidney into two separate pieces (Fig. 17-4) to extensive fragmentation or shattering of the renal parenchyma into multiple pieces (Fig.

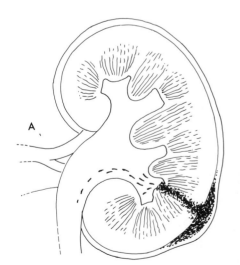
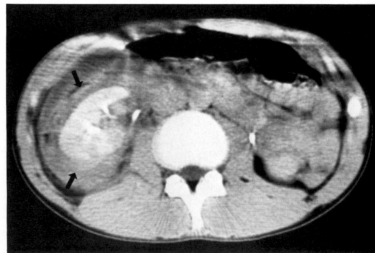

Fig. 17-3 **A,** Renal laceration with potential extravasation of either blood or urine into perinephric space. **B,** CT scan showing small renal laceration without detectable extravasation of contrast and yet a large perinephric hematoma *(arrows).*

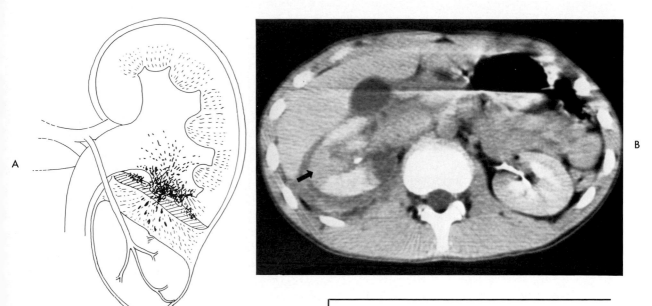

Fig. 17-4 A, Renal transection with separation of renal tissue. Usually a polar lesion with intact vasculature or totally detached. **B,** CT scan showing complete disruption with separation of renal parenchyma *(arrow).*

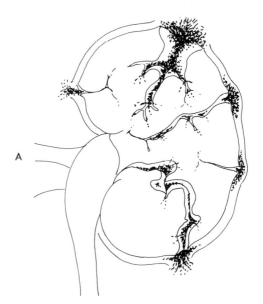

Fig. 17-5 A, Renal fragmentation. Multiple stellate lacerations through renal parenchyma. **B,** CT scan showing a fragmented kidney with marked extravasation of blood and urine *(arrow).*

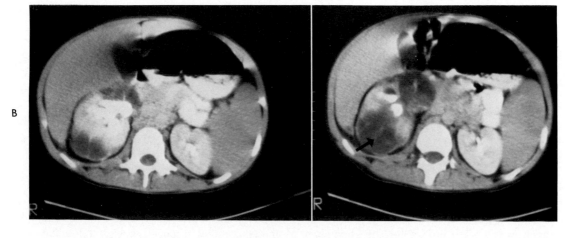

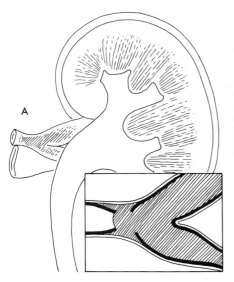
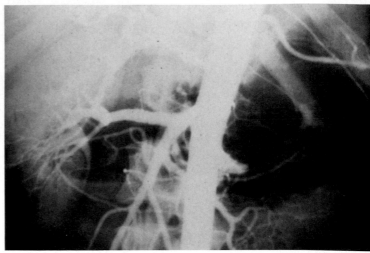

Fig. 17-6 **A,** Renal pedicle injury with intimal disruption and arterial occlusion. **B,** Angiogram showing left renal artery cut off in its proximal position. The IVP demonstrated nonvisualization on the left.

17-5). Isolated traumatic disruption of renal parenchyma usually involves the inferior or superior renal pole.[16,20] These extensive injuries occur in less than 5% of all cases, and the differentiation of these lesions from simple renal lacerations may affect the ultimate course of treatment.

Pedicle Injury

Although renal pedicle or vascular injuries are probably the rarest form of injuries, accounting for about 3% of all renal trauma, they remain the most serious. These injuries result from lateral displacement of the kidney with stretching of the tethered renal vessels (Fig. 17-6). Complete vessel disruption or occlusion results in a totally ischemic kidney, whereas intimal disruption with thrombosis results in progressive ischemia. Such injuries have serious implications in regard to the importance of rapid recognition, evaluation, and management.

ASSOCIATED INJURIES

Depending on the study, associated injuries have been reported to range from 25% to 70% in children with all forms of renal trauma.[1,5,14] The number depends on the population studied. The most common extrarenal injury involves skeletal fractures, and 25% to 35% of children with blunt renal injuries have an associated fracture. Severe head injuries with CNS lesions are the second most common injuries and occur in 20% to 30% of children

with blunt renal trauma. Trauma to other intraabdominal organs has been reported in 10% to 20% of cases, with injury to the spleen and liver representing the third and fourth most commonly associated injuries, respectively. The severity of renal trauma has been directly related to the number and extent of associated lesions. Cass[5] reported that 67% of the children with renal contusion had associated injuries, whereas 100% of the children with renal transection, fragmentation, or pedicle injuries had multisystem trauma. Moreover, those children with the most severe renal injuries, such as fragmentation or pedicle injuries, averaged three extrarenal injuries per patient. The overall mortality in these patients is 10%, with all deaths attributed to associated injuries.

Emergency surgery for associated injuries is necessary in about one third of all patients with renal injuries. In those patients with severe renal injuries, such as renal fragmentation or pedicle injury and associated injuries, the requirement for emergency surgery may approach 100%. This fact reflects the greater degree of trauma associated with these injuries. Hence, the importance of preoperative multisystem assessment of the patient is paramount.

CLINICAL PRESENTATION

The signs and symptoms of renal trauma may often be the same as those for injuries to other intraabdominal organs. Shock, abdominal pain, and generalized tenderness are relatively nonspecific indicators of abdominal trauma, and any one of them may be present in the setting of renal injury. Numerous studies have shown that significant renal injuries produce localized signs during physical examination, for example, localized abdominal tenderness or costovertebral tenderness. Even a palpable flank mass may be present. However, the primary clinical marker of renal injury remains hematuria, either gross or microscopic. Any child with a flank mass, flank pain, or abdominal pain plus hematuria should be considered as having a renal injury until proven otherwise. Unfortunately, in all the major studies no correlation has been found between the degree of injury and the amount of blood in the urine. Renal lacerations and fragmentation injuries may have increasing amounts of hematuria, whereas renal pedicle injuries and subsequent vascular disruption may have little or no hematuria in up to 50% of the cases.

In a study by Karp et al.,[11] patients who were found to have the combination of hematuria, abdominal pain, and tenderness had a significant renal injury in 41% of the cases. In that study the majority of patients with hematuria but with no other physical signs or symptoms had no radiographically demonstrable injury and were thus judged to have renal contusions.

DIAGNOSTIC TECHNIQUES

Fortunately, the kidney lends itself to easy radiographic evaluation, and a number of roentgenographic methods have evolved in trauma management. Initial assessment of pediatric renal trauma must always include a chest roentgenogram and a flat plate of the abdomen. Radiographic findings, such as rib fractures, spinal body fractures, psoas margin obliteration, or an intraabdominal mass effect, may suggest renal injury. Injuries to other organs can also be evaluated.

Intravenous Pyelography

In the past, intravenous pyelography (IVP) was the standard initial radiographic study obtained for the assessment of all renal trauma. More recently, CT scanning has evolved, and with increased availability, has become the study of choice for major abdominal injury including renal injury. The IVP remains a useful tool in the evaluation of asymptomatic hematuria in the setting of minimal trauma. The technique of infusion pyelography using 1 ml of undiluted contrast material per pound of body weight, injected over 1 to 2 minutes yields the best results. The first exposure, following a scout film, should be made at the end of the infusion to obtain a nephrogram. Subsequent exposures should be at 5, 10, and 20 minutes to assess parenchymal and calyceal anatomy. The IVP with infusion technique, however, has been found to stage renal injuries adequately in only 60% to 85% of cases. A major problem in its interpretation of results is that abnormal findings are often nonspecific. These findings include delayed or diminished opacification of the kidney on the side of suspected renal trauma, complete nonvisualization of a traumatized kidney, and extravasation of contrast material.

When applied to injury classification, the nonspecific nature of the IVP is apparent.[2] In the evaluation of renal contusion up to 80% of all IVPs will be normal, whereas 20% will show delayed function or incomplete filling (Fig. 17-7). A renal laceration can exist without demonstrable extravasation of IVP contrast and will have a normal IVP in over half the cases with delayed function or diminished opacification in the remaining patients. In the evaluation of potential fractured or fragmented kidneys the IVP will be abnormal 75% of the time but may show actual contrast extravasation in as few as 5% of the injuries (Fig. 17-8). The majority of the time there will be diminished opacification, and only with pedicle injuries is the IVP more specific; with pedicle injury there is an 85% to 90% nonvisualization rate.

In no cases of renal pathology greater than a contusion is an IVP normal; however, findings such as delayed function or poor visualization are very nonspecific.

CT Scan

Over the last decade CT staging of renal trauma in the pediatric patient has become the method of choice for radiographic assessment, particularly in blunt trauma.[3] CT has distinct advantages over the IVP and is a much more accurate diagnostic procedure. Using CT scanning with intravenous contrast (1 cc per kg body weight) one can define parenchymal lacerations, extravasation, fragmentation, perirenal collections, and most pedicle injuries. CT scanning can differentiate major from minor renal lacerations and allows for a more precise staging of the initial injury. It is currently recommended that CT be used as the initial study, especially if there is any suspicion of an associated abdominal or CNS injury.

The sensitivity and specificity of CT evaluation

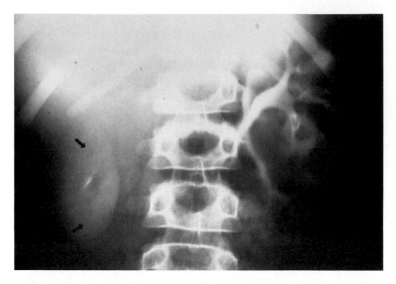

Fig. 17-7   IVP on a 12-year-old boy with a blunt abdominal injury from a sledding accident. The 15-minute film shows only a nephrogram on the affected side *(arrows)*. The patient's IVP was normal 1 week later.

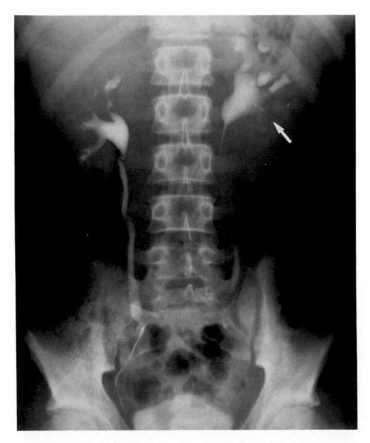

Fig. 17-8   IVP demonstrates nonvisualization of the left lower pole calyx in a 17-year-old male with a renal transection at the lower pole. There is a faint suggestion of extravasation at the lower pole *(arrow)*.

CT SCAN GRADING SCHEME FOR RENAL TRAUMA

Grade I   Small parenchymal injury
           No subcapsular or perirenal fluid
Grade II   Incomplete renal laceration
           Subcapsular or small perinephric collection
Grade III Extensive laceration or fracture
           Large perinephric fluid collection
Grade IV   Multiple fragments (shattered)
Grade V   Vascular injury

From Karp MP et al: J Pediatr Surg 21:617, 1986.

of renal trauma have been reported as high as 100% in those studies confirmed by exploratory laparotomy. It has also been found that its sensitivity exaggerates the traumatic lesions when compared with either IVP or angiography. Karp et al.[11] at the Children's Hospital of Buffalo have devised a grading scheme for renal trauma based on CT evaluation (see box above). A frame of reference such as this gives us the ability to differentiate simple lacerations from complete fractures and fragmentation injuries, thus modifying the subsequent surgical approach to these lesions. It has been clearly shown that extravasation of contrast material is not an absolute indication for operative exploration, whereas fragmentation and complete disruption certainly may be.

The CT scan has also proven to be of value in following renal trauma. The healing patterns of the various grades of injuries can now be predicted and used to guide appropriate therapy. Late follow-up studies can document complete renal healing as well as persistent scar formation or nonfunctioning renal segments.

Most pediatric trauma centers now propose that patients with stable vital signs, hematuria, and evidence of potential multiorgan system injury should be evaluated by CT scan. Those patients, however, with hematuria, stable vital signs, and no other signs of additional organ system injury should still be screened initially with an IVP before proceeding with additional radiographic examinations. In those rare patients who cannot be stabilized despite emergency resuscitative intervention a "one-shot" IVP before proceeding with emergency laparotomy is advisable.

Angiography

Angiography is of limited usefulness in pediatric renal trauma. It is most useful in the evaluation of suspected renal vascular lesions and pedicle injuries. However, the complication rate for angiography in the pediatric patient is much higher than in the adult patient because of the technical problems of vascular access.

Ultrasound

Ultrasound has been proposed as a rapid initial screening procedure in the investigation of children with abdominal trauma.[10] It can provide a rapid overall assessment of liver, spleen, kidneys, and retroperitoneum, as well as determine the presence of hemoperitoneum. It does not require the patient to be sedated and can be performed in a matter of minutes by trained personnel. Ultrasound should not be used as a sole method of evaluation, and it provides no functional information.[17] Current protocols always couple ultrasound examination with either IVP or CT scan (Fig. 17-9), and its exact role in evaluating renal trauma remains to be worked out.

Radioisotope Renal Scanning

Radioisotope renal scanning in the initial evaluation of renal trauma has found limited use. It is helpful in determining the amount and location of vascularized renal parenchyma and in evaluating suspected vascular injuries.[7] Its most important use is in follow-up evaluation of renal injury, particularly in the setting of new-onset hypertension (Fig. 17-10).

Magnetic Resonance Imaging

The use of magnetic resonance imaging (MRI) in evaluating renal trauma is unexplored at this time. Since its use in assessing Wilm's tumors and abdominal neuroblastomas has been quite promising, one can only assume that MRI may someday replace or at least augment the CT scan and angiogram in evaluating renal lesions of all kinds.

THERAPY

The cornerstone in the management of pediatric renal trauma is the preservation of renal tissue and function without endangering the health of the child. Controversy exists as to the proper management of blunt renal trauma, particularly in cases of major injuries, such as polar transection or major

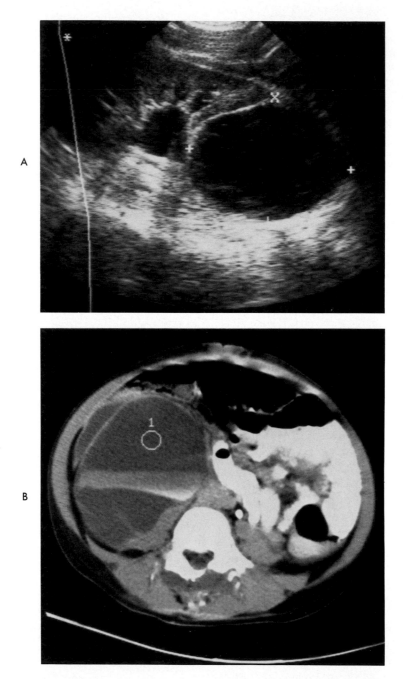

Fig. 17-9 **A,** Renal ultrasonogram showing a dilated renal pelvis and a large perinephric collection. **B,** CT scan showing large perinephric urinoma below kidney of patient shown in **A.**

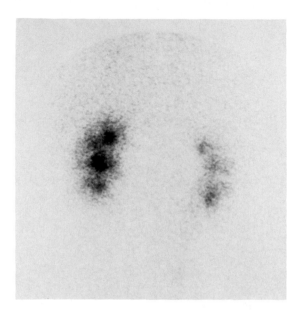

Fig. 17-10   DTPA renal scan showing reduced uptake by the right kidney of a patient 3 months following a renal transection injury that was treated conservatively.

laceration. Just as in the management of blunt hepatic and splenic injury, the pendulum has swung toward nonoperative management for most renal injuries. Since a high percentage of renal injuries heal spontaneously, one might reason that surgical intervention is unnecessary. Moreover, surgical intervention has been associated with a much higher nephrectomy rate than has conservative management.[18] On the other hand, proponents of surgical intervention cite the lower morbidity and shortened hospitalization associated with early renal repair.[4,13] The bias, however, has moved clearly toward conservatism in the management of blunt renal trauma.

Renal contusions and simple lacerations with minor degrees of contrast extravasation are universally treated with conservative management. These lesions involve grade I and grade II injuries on CT scan. These lesions heal spontaneously with few complications or long-term sequelae. Current therapy involves bedrest until gross hematuria clears, with limited activity until the microhematuria disappears. The overall length of convalescence usually ranges from 2 to 6 weeks. There has been no documentation of loss of renal function, hypertension, or hydronephrosis following the conservative management of these lesions. Since renal contusion and minor lacerations compose 70%-85% of all

renal injuries, the majority of patients will not require surgery for their renal injuries.

There is also no question that patients with renal pedicle injury or those with a shattered or fragmented kidney require surgical intervention. In most instances surgery involves nephrectomy, assuming that the other kidney is normal. Numerous authors have documented the dismal results of attempted renal salvage in renal vascular trauma. The current success rate of revascularization of traumatically occluded renal arteries is about 10% or less and should be attempted only in very unusual circumstances.[19] In children, isolated cases of successful revascularization attempts have been reported when branch arteries are involved.[5]

The renal trauma that evokes the greatest controversy regarding management is the grade III injury (see box on p. 365) with either an extensive laceration of the parenchyma or calyx or complete transection of the kidney without extensive fragmentation. The debate centers around conservative nonoperative management of major renal lacerations versus immediate surgical intervention and repair. No precise method of predicting eventual outcome of a severe renal injury has been determined. Scattered reports exist supporting nonoperative management of *severe* renal lacerations.[1,8] If nonoperative management is chosen in this group, up to 50% of these patients will eventually require surgery for a subsequent complication.[1] These complications include persistent or recurrent hemorrhage in the renal parenchyma, parenchymal infarction, or segmental hydronephrosis. Partial nephrectomy is the most common operation performed in these cases (Fig. 17-11). The overall nephrectomy rate with delayed surgery is generally lower than 10%. When immediate surgical intervention is employed, older studies have documented nephrectomy rates as high as 40%.[18] With improvement in surgical technique, including proper vascular control of the pedicle before renal exploration, most series now document a nephrectomy rate of 10% to 20% in cases of immediate surgical repair of major lacerations or transections.[1,6,11] Immediate surgical intervention for these renal injuries may now have a nephrectomy rate that rivals the results for conservative nonoperative management while decreasing the substantial number of delayed operations for subsequent complications.

For 75% to 80% of all pediatric blunt renal trauma, conservative nonoperative management is

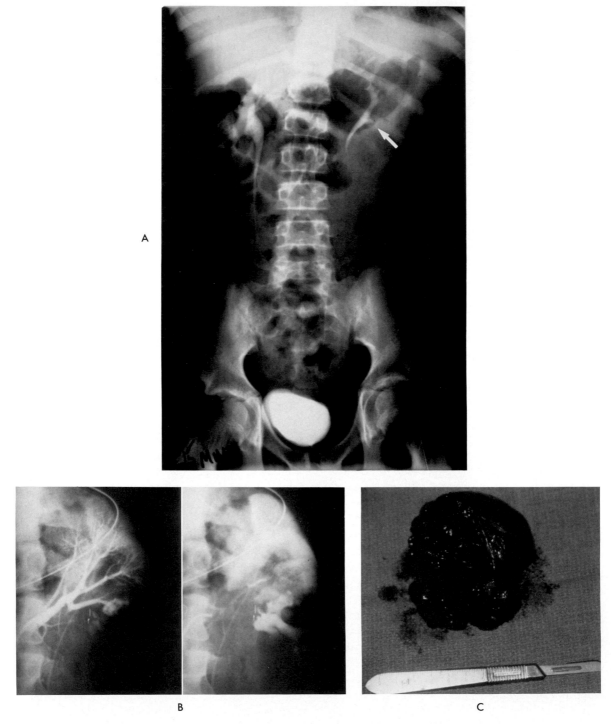

Fig. 17-11 **A,** IVP demonstrating cut off of the left lower pole collecting system *(arrow)* in a 16 year old following a bicycle accident. **B,** Renal arteriogram performed because of continuing rapid blood loss showing massive extravasation of blood from left lower pole; *Left,* Arterial phase; *Right,* venous phase. **C,** Lower pole of left kidney after renal exploration and partial nephrectomy.

the therapy of choice. These injuries include contusions, minor perirenal collections, and uncomplicated lacerations. Most transections, fragmented or shattered kidneys, and all renal pedicle injuries require operative intervention and attempted repair if possible.

COMPLICATIONS

Few long-term follow-up studies exist to judge properly the various forms of therapy chosen. Reported short-term complications include persistent renal hemorrhage, abscess formation, urinoma formation, and ureteral obstruction secondary to clot formation. These problems usually require some form of direct surgical intervention (Fig. 17-12). Percutaneous drainage of perirenal collections and intravascular embolization of persistent renal hemorrhage are viable therapeutic options.[16] Selective embolization for the control of bleeding vessels is particularly successful in the management of persistent, intermittent, or delayed traumatic hematuria. The reported incidence of functionless renal segments after renal trauma is less than 5% of all cases of injury.[16] These can be managed nonoperatively, although a small percentage of them may require removal for the control of subsequent hypertension. Sustained hypertension is a very rare

complication following renal injuries in children. Its overall incidence appears to be 1% to 2% in most large studies.

CONCLUSION

The concepts of evaluation and treatment of most renal injuries in children have evolved along lines similar to those seen in the current management of trauma to other intraabdominal organs. Those children with massive injuries leading to an unstable hemodynamic situation despite aggressive resuscitation require urgent laparotomy for assessment and control of injuries. A "one-shot" IVP is the initial screening test for renal injury in this situation. Those children with a stable hemodynamic pattern and evidence of multisystem trauma require

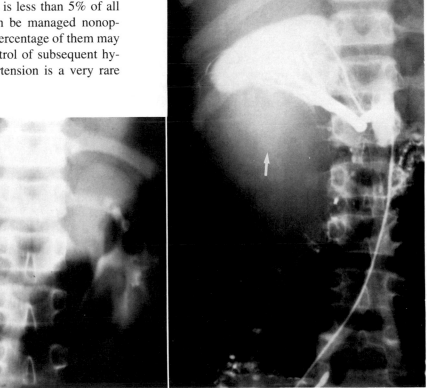

Fig. 17-12 **A,** IVP showing poor visualization of right lower pole *(arrow)* 1 day following blunt renal trauma. **B,** Renal angiogram following 3 weeks of conservative therapy in the same patient. The study shows upward displacement of kidney secondary to a massive urinoma *(arrow)*. A lower pole heminephrectomy was necessary when the patient became septic.

CT scan evaluation and appropriate grading of the renal injury.

Approximately 70% to 80% of all injuries consist of renal contusions or simple lacerations with minimal dye extravasation and can be managed nonoperatively. A small percentage involve complete transections, complex fragmentation, or renal pedicle injuries. These injuries should be managed with surgical intervention with a careful, well-planned approach to renal anatomy. This method will minimize the risk of total renal loss, as well as the potential complications and long-term morbidity.

REFERENCES

1. Ahmed S and Morris LL: Renal parenchymal injuries secondary to blunt abdominal trauma in childhood: a 10-year review, Br J Urol 54:470, 1982.
2. Bergren CT, Chan FN, and Bodzin JH: Intravenous pyelogram results in association with renal pathology and therapy in trauma patients, J Trauma 27:515, 1987.
3. Bretan PN et al: Computerized tomographic staging of renal trauma: 85 consecutive cases, J Urol 136:561, 1986.
4. Cass AS: Immediate radiologic and surgical management of renal injuries, J Trauma 22:361, 1982.
5. Cass AS: Blunt renal trauma in children, J Trauma 23:123, 1983.
6. Cass AS et al: Long-term results of conservative and surgical management of blunt renal lacerations, Br J Urol 59:17, 1987.
7. Chopp RT, Hekmat-Ravan H, and Mendez R: Technetium 99m glucoheptonate renal scan in diagnosis of acute renal injury, Urology 15:201, 1980.
8. Evins S, Thomason WB, and Rosenblum R: Nonoperative management of severe renal laceration, J Urol 123:247, 1980.
9. Feins NR: Multiple trauma, Pediatr Clin North Am 26:759, 1979.
10. Filiautrault D, Longpre D, and Patriquin H: Investigation of childhood blunt abdominal trauma: a practical approach using ultrasound as the initial diagnostic modality, Radiology 165:373, 1987.
11. Karp MP et al: The impact of computed tomography scanning on the child with renal trauma, Pediatr Surg 21:617, 1986.
12. Kuzmarov IW, Morehouse DD, and Gibson S: Blunt renal trauma in the pediatric population: a retrospective study, J Urol 126:648, 1981.
13. McAninch JW and Carroll PR: Renal trauma: kidney preservation through improved vascular control—a refined approach, J Trauma 22:285, 1982.
14. Morse TS: Renal injuries. In Touloukian RJ, editor: Pediatric trauma, New York, 1978, John Wiley & Sons.
15. Morse TS et al: Kidney injuries in children, J Urol 98:539, 1967.
16. Peterson N: Fate of functionless posttraumatic renal segment, Urology 27:237, 1986.
17. Schmoller H, Kunit G, and Frick J: Sonography in blunt renal trauma, Eur Urol 7:11, 1981.
18. Thompson IM et al: Results of nonoperative management of blunt renal trauma, J Urol 118:522, 1977.
19. Turner WW Jr, Snyder WH III, and Fry WJ: Mortality and renal salvage after renovascular trauma, Am J Surg 146:848, 1983.
20. Waxman J, Belman AB, and Kass EJ: Traumatic amputation of the left lower renal pole in children, J Urol 134:114, 1985.

18

Lower Urinary Tract and Perineal Injuries

W. Hardy Hendren and Craig A. Peters

In multiple trauma the urinary tract is second only to the central nervous system in the frequency of injury.[26] Injuries to the lower genitourinary tract and perineum account for about 1% of pediatric trauma center admissions.[18,76,84] Although the etiology of trauma varies widely, injuries resulting from automobile accidents are most common. The possibility of ureteral, bladder, or urethral injury must always be suspected in children with either pelvic or perineal trauma, since clinical evidence of injury is rarely visible.

DIAGNOSIS

Physical examination of the lower abdomen, pelvis, and genitalia should seek signs of specific injuries.[46,76,86] In addition to obvious lacerations or contusions, one should be alert for scrotal swelling and ecchymosis, perineal ecchymosis in a "butterfly" distribution, or meatal bleeding suggestive of urethral injuries. A high-riding prostate on rectal examination may indicate posterior urethral disruption. A flank mass may signify trauma to the kidney or ureter, with hematoma or urine extravasation resulting. Examination of the urine is mandatory in any patient with abdominal, flank, or pelvic trauma. Gross or microscopic hematuria demands roentgenologic assessment of the urinary tract, beginning with intravenous pyelography (IVP) or contrast-enhanced computer tomography (CT). Radionuclide scanning or arteriography may be indicated if the contrast study reveals nonvisualization of the kidney, extravasation of contrast, or suspected vascular injury. Delayed films can help to visualize contrast extravasated along the course of the ureter or in the pelvis. In the setting of pelvic trauma or pelvic fracture, a retrograde urethrogram should be performed using aseptic technique, minimal pressure, and fluoroscopic guidance, if possible. This should be conducted before an attempt to pass a urethral catheter. If a catheter is already in place, the urethrogram can be done using a small feeding tube alongside the indwelling catheter. If the urethra is intact, a small, soft, well-lubricated catheter should be passed into the bladder for contrast studies. Conventional cystography should include a film with the bladder filled to capacity (or contracting if fluoroscopy is available), with oblique views, and a drainage film to look for extravasation.[13] CT cystography is being used more widely and is extremely sensitive to small bladder injuries as long as the bladder is adequately filled, either by retrograde instillation or during the IVP.[41]

Ureter

Injury to the ureter in adults is usually caused by knife or gunshot wounds. Ureteral injuries are less common in children but should be suspected after severe blunt trauma or penetrating injury. Fracture of the transverse process of a lumbar vertebra is a good indication of serious trauma that can also disrupt the adjacent kidney or ureter. The point of disruption in penetrating injuries can be at any level; however, injury involving blunt trauma is usually at the ureteropelvic junction.[61,68] Sometimes the injuries are bilateral.[6] The mechanism is a combination of exaggerated hyperextension of the spine with sudden acceleration or deceleration. The diagnostic finding by IVP or retrograde ureterogram is evidence of extravasation of contrast material at the site of injury. An associated renal contusion, however, may reduce contrast excretion and thereby mask the injury. Delayed films and careful inspection of the images are the keys to establishing the diagnosis. An enlarging flank mass in the absence of signs of retroperitoneal bleeding is an important clinical observation suggestive of urinary extravasation. CT imaging with enhancement is a very sensitive means of confirming a ureteral disruption.[42] Early diagnosis has been shown to improve the ultimate outcome.[51]

Treatment

Prompt repair is indicated once the diagnosis of a ureteral injury is established. A soft ureteral catheter should be passed endoscopically before exploring the flank to repair the ureter. An inlying catheter helps locate the ureter when there is hematoma, extravasated urine, or edema, thereby reducing the amount of dissection needed. This maneuver also aids placement of a soft Silastic stent through the distal ureter once the repair is completed.

A disrupted ureter is best repaired by excising the point of avulsion or penetration and preserving its adjacent blood vessels. Wide debridement of the injury may be necessary, particularly in high velocity missile injuries, which can devitalize tissue by the blast effect of the missile. The ureter is spatulated to increase the cross-sectional diameter of the anastomosis to prevent stricture. The ends are then joined using fine interrupted sutures of absorbable material.[12,87] A single- or double-J Silastic stent should fit loosely enough in the lumen of the ureter without causing pressure erosion of the ureteral wall. The stent is removed 2 to 3 weeks later using grasping forceps passed through a cystoscope.

The repair of an avulsion injury to the renal pelvis is simplified by mobilizing the kidney downward. This maneuver also lessens tension on the anastomosis if there has been loss of a short segment of ureter. A Malecot nephrostomy catheter to drain the kidney lends additional protection against postoperative extravasation. Watertight closure is desirable, but the anastomosis must be drained to prevent a retroperitoneal urinoma. Occasionally a renal pelvis is destroyed, so continuity between the kidney and ureter must be by anastomosis of the ureter to a lower pole calyx. It is important to prevent compression of the ureter by the renal cortex by excising scar or even a small wedge of parenchyma adjacent to the anastomosis.[24]

The lower ureter may be accidentally injured during any pelvic operation. Iatrogenic injuries during ureteral instrumentation are becoming more common with increased use of ureteroscopy. Acutely diagnosed ureteral injuries, usually ligation or division, may be repaired immediately or may be proximally diverted for delayed repair. Often the clinical setting dictates the timing of the repair, but one should aim to carry out any immediate intervention within 1 week while the tissues remain fresh and before fibrosis occurs; otherwise it is better to delay repair for several months until the tissues have softened. Most ureteroscopic injuries are manageable with stenting and patience. Percutaneous balloon dilatation of iatrogenic ureteral injuries has met with variable short-term success.[2]

Ischemic fibrosis or angulation of the ureter are two complications of reimplantation for vesicoureteral reflux that can be followed by extravasation of urine. The majority of injuries can be repaired by suitable reoperation,[29] which entails wide mobilization of the ureter to gain length, with reimplantation through a tunnel to prevent reflux. When there is a loss of length of the ureter other procedures may be necessary. One useful technique is "psoas hitch" in which the lateral aspect of the bladder is fixed to the ipsilateral psoas muscle lateral to the external iliac vessels.[65] This gains a little extra length and partially immobilizes the ureterovesical junction. The rolled bladder flap technique of Boari[5,8] is another method of overcoming shortness of the terminal ureter; however, we prefer to use another method in most cases, such as transureteroureterostomy or creating a ureter from a segment of intestine.

Transureteroureterostomy is an excellent technique for the management of the extremely short ureter or when the local operative field precludes safe reanastomosis because of sepsis, fibrosis, or hematoma.[33,79] The injured ureter is mobilized widely so that it can be brought retroperitoneally across to the normal contralateral ureter without tension. The contralateral ureter should never be mobilized toward the side of the short ureter. If the entire lower half of the ureter is absent, a transureteropyelostomy can be accomplished by joining the short ureter to the opposite renal pelvis. Mobilizing the kidney and fixing its lower pole medially can gain additional length for this maneuver. If the ureter is totally absent, a short segment of jejunum may be employed as the conduit from one renal pelvis to the other. Bowel can be used to substitute for an entire ureter.[14,30,36,66,80] An antireflux procedure is added except in adult patients with recurrent renal stones, for these patients free bladder drainage is a more important consideration than the absence of reflux. In the majority of instances a nonrefluxing union can be accomplished by making a very long submucosal tunnel diagonally across the trigone of the bladder. Autotransplantation of the kidney may be indicated in rare instances to provide adequate length to compensate for a short ureter.[36,37] The following cases will illustrate typical ureteral injuries and their management.

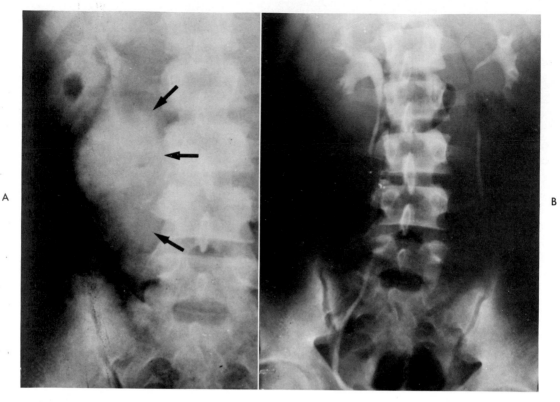

Fig. 18-1 Gunshot wound of right ureter in a 14-year-old boy. **A,** IVP shortly after admission showing extravasation of contrast in the right flank *(arrows)*. **B,** IVP 2 months after primary repair of disrupted ureter.

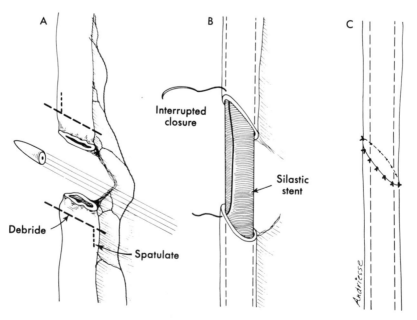

Fig. 18-2 Principles for repair of transected ureter. **A,** Debridement of site of injury and spatulation to increase diameter of anastomosis. **B,** Placement of interrupted absorbable sutures. Soft, loose fitting Silastic stent in ureter. **C,** Completed repair. Drain placed nearby.

CASE 1

A 14-year-old boy sustained a .25-caliber bullet wound to the right lower quadrant without a visible exit wound. IVP revealed marked extravasation from the right ureter (Fig. 18-1). Transabdominal exploration disclosed that the bullet had passed through the right mesocolon, divided the right ureter, and lodged in the paraspinal muscles. Repair consisted of debridement and primary reanastomosis over a stent (Fig. 18-2). The result was satisfactory.

CASE 2

A 4-year-old girl was struck in the right flank by an automobile and suffered an ecchymosis of the flank and a fracture of the fifth lumbar vertebra. IVP revealed extravasation of contrast material from the right kidney (Fig. 18-3). The kidney functioned well, but no contrast was seen in the ureter at anytime during the study.

An expanding right flank mass developed 24 hours after the injury, and a retrograde ureterogram with the child under anesthesia demonstrated gross extravasation of contrast material at the ureteropelvic junction. Exploration showed a large urine collection from the disrupted ureteropelvic junction. After debridement a primary spatulated anastomosis of the upper ureter to the renal pelvis was carried out over the ureteral stent placed during cystoscopy. Postoperatively the patient did well. The stent was removed 3 weeks later. Initially there was slight hydronephrosis, but IVP 1 year later showed normal findings.

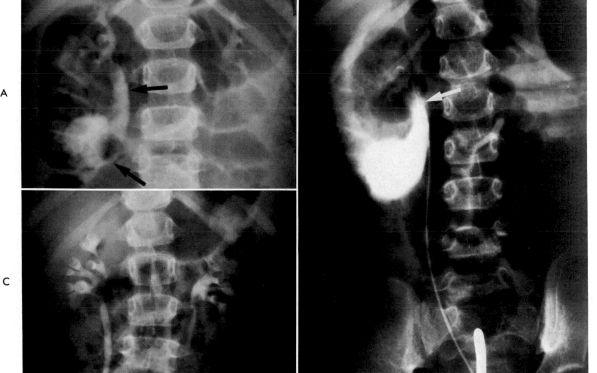

Fig. 18-3   Transection of ureteropelvic junction, right side in a 4-year-old girl after blunt trauma. **A,** IVP showing extravasation in right flank *(arrows),* good renal function, no visualization of right ureter. **B,** Retrograde pyelogram showing contrast extravasating at ureteropelvic junction *(arrow).* **C,** IVP 1 month after primary repair. Satisfactory result.

CASE 3

A 7½-year-old boy fell from a tree and was admitted to a local hospital with signs of intraabdominal hemorrhage and peritonitis. Injuries to the second part of the duodenum, bile duct, and pancreas were repaired. He did poorly, became anuric, and was treated with renal dialysis and hyperalimentation. Retrograde pyelography showed localized extravasation from the right kidney (Fig. 18-4). One flank was drained 1 month later, and within 2 weeks renal function improved enough to discontinue dialysis. IVP revealed some function on the right side but none on the left. Another laparotomy was performed to close a duodenal leak; at this time a nephrostomy tube was placed in the right kidney.

The boy was referred for reconstruction of his urinary tract 5½ months after the initial injury. BUN was 17 mg/dl and serum creatinine 1.7 mg/dl. Creatinine clearance was only 15 L/m²/24 hrs. Retrograde pyelography showed an atrophic left kidney and a separation of the ureter from the functioning upper pole of the right kidney. Further studies showed that the collecting system of the functioning upper pole communicated with a loop of small bowel. Aortogram showed that arterial branches to the lower pole of the right kidney and the main left renal artery were occluded. After 1 month of preoperative preparation, urinary reconstruction was performed through a thoracoabdominal incision (Fig. 18-5). The atrophic lower pole of the right kidney was mobilized and reanastomosed to the intrarenal collecting system of the upper pole and the kidney drained with a nephrostomy tube. A Whipple procedure was necessitated by recurrent bleeding from the duodenum.[49] The patient is well and has 40% of normal renal function. Great morbidity could have been prevented if primary repair had been accomplished at his first operation.

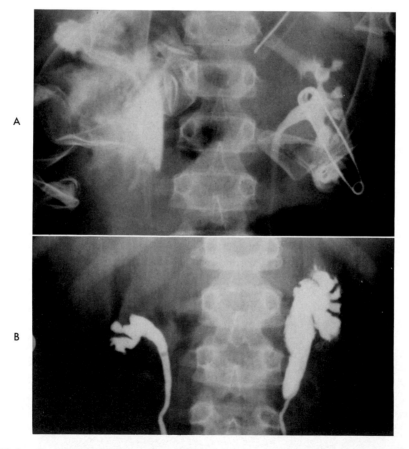

Fig. 18-4 Severe blunt trauma with avulsion of right renal pelvis from kidney and traumatic thrombosis of left renal artery. **A,** Retrograde pyelogram 1 month after injury. On right, extravasation of contrast. Intact collecting system, but kidney was anuric, that is, arterial thrombosis had occurred. **B,** Repeat study 5 months later when referred for reconstruction. On right, no continuity of renal pelvis with functional renal tissue. On left, atrophic kidney (contrast extravasated from overfilling during study).

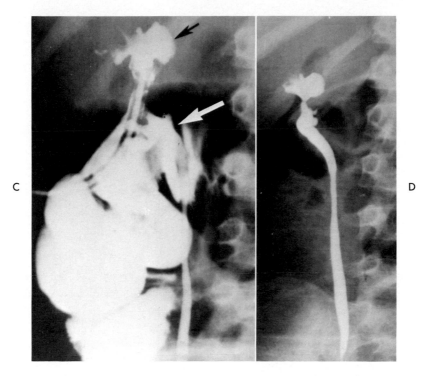

Fig. 18-4, cont'd   C, Simultaneous contrast injection of nephrostomy tube and retrograde catheter, showing wide separation of renal pelvis *(large arrow)* from upper pole *(small arrow),* the only remaining functional kidney tissue. **D,** Retrograde study 1 month after urologic reconstruction.

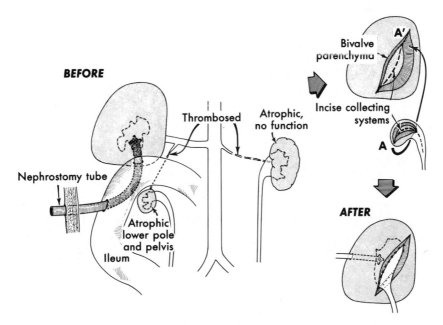

Fig. 18-5   Anatomy before and after reconstruction. The only remaining functional renal tissue, the right upper pole, had been drained via nephrostomy tube, which passed through a piece of ileum. The right renal pelvis and atrophic lower pole were mobilized and anastomosed to the intrarenal collecting system of the remaining right upper pole.

CASE 4

Bilateral uteral reimplantation for long-standing bilateral reflux with recurrent urinary tract infections in an 8-year-old girl was complicated by a urinary leak 1 week after operation (Fig. 18-6). IVP showed partial ureteral obstruction with extravasation at the ureterovesical anastomosis. The child had ischemic necrosis of the distal ureter at reoperation 5 weeks later. Transureteroureterostomy was performed. Subsequent roentgenograms showed a satisfactory result.

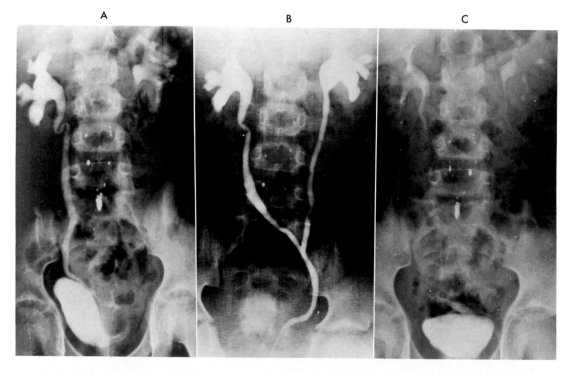

Fig. 18-6   Transureteroureterostomy in an 8-year-old girl after complication of ureteral reimplantation. **A,** IVP postoperatively with extravesical extravasation and partial obstruction, right side. There was a urinary fistula draining from the right lower quadrant drain site. Left side was normal. Leakage did not subside. Reexploration disclosed ischemic necrosis and complete dissolution of distal ureter, with considerable surrounding inflammatory reaction, making this unsuited for repeat reimplantation. The right ureter was mobilized, brought across the midline, and anastomosed to the left ureter. **B,** Retrograde pyelogram postoperatively. **C,** IVP 3 months later. Contrast medium overlying spine remains from previous myelogram.

Bladder

Simultaneous injury to the bladder occurs in about 20% of the children with pelvic fractures.[15,76] Approximately 80% of traumatic bladder injuries are associated with pelvic fractures. A full bladder usually ruptures at the dome, spilling urine directly into the peritoneal cavity. Peritoneal signs may not be immediate but will soon develop. Typically these patients have a serum urea nitrogen level elevated out of proportion to serum creatinine because of more rapid reabsorption of urea.[74,77] Extraperitoneal extravasation of urine, seen with about ½ of all bladder ruptures, produces more subtle signs. Its diagnosis may require IVP, retrograde cystography, or CT (Fig. 18-7). Falsely negative studies can result if there is inadequate bladder filling or failure to obtain oblique and drainage films.[10,13]

Catheter drainage can be used in small extraperitoneal bladder injuries, using urethral catheter or suprapubic drainage, well secured to the abdomen, for 7 to 10 days.[70] However, primary surgical repair of the ruptured bladder is the treatment of choice in cases of intraperitoneal bladder rupture or major extraperitoneal lacerations of the bladder, together with vesical and perivesical drainage. Drainage with a loose-fitting Silastic or Teflon-coated, nonreactive urethral catheter is usually sufficient unless continued bleeding necessitates a suprapubic tube. If in doubt, we do not hesitate to use dual drainage from above and below. Cystography to confirm complete healing of the bladder is performed before the drainage tubes are removed, usually 10 days after repair.

Massive pelvic trauma with avulsion of the bladder base and rectum precludes primary repair of pelvic structures. Fortunately these injuries are rare in children. They require diverting colostomy and some form of temporary urinary diversion, usually suprapubic cystostomy. Diverting urine flow by

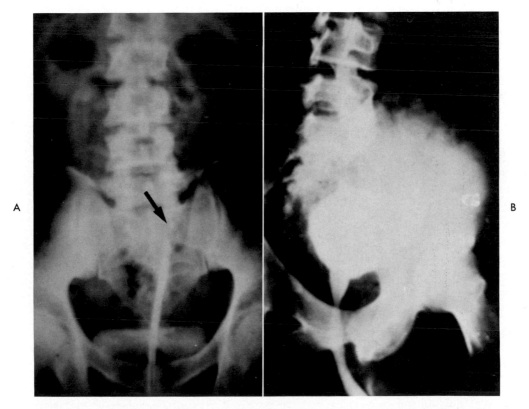

Fig. 18-7 Rupture of the bladder. **A,** Intraperitoneal rupture through dome of the bladder. Note straight catheter *(arrow)* passing through dome of bladder into peritoneal cavity. Bladder is filled with contrast from IVP. **B,** Perivesical extravasation of contrast during retrograde cystogram via the urethra.

skin ureterostomy can be followed by major complications (Figs. 18-8 and 18-9)[31] and should be avoided when possible. A massive wound involving bladder and both lower ureters would be best drained by temporary diversion into an isolated bowel segment brought to the skin for drainage.

Urethra

Injury to a child's urethra can be difficult to treat. Traumatic injury to the female urethra is rare,[53,89] except for iatrogenic injuries from operations on the bladder neck, excision of ectopic ureteroceles, or urethrotomy, each of which can cause stress incontinence or a urethrovaginal fistula.

Injury to the male urethra, however, is not so rare and is usually seen in boys with pelvic fracture and concomitant disruption of the urethra where it passes beneath the pubic arch. Management of this injury is controversial.[4,17,56,57,78] The membranous urethra (Fig. 18-10), located in the urogenital diaphragm between the two pubic rami, is subject to traumatic disruption when the pubic arch is fractured.[62,69] Urethral disruption can result also from a shearing of the prostatic urethra and bladder neck across the urogenital diaphragm and membranous urethra. The actual point of disruption may be closer to the bladder neck than seen with adults because of the smaller bulk of the immature prostate and the higher, more mobile child's bladder.

Urethral disruption should be suspected when a patient with a pelvic fracture is unable to void, particularly if there is blood at the urethral meatus. Furthermore, the bladder and prostate may be "high-riding" on rectal examination, and a butterfly perineal ecchymosis can be present. Approximately one quarter to one third of posterior urethral injuries are partial disruptions.[28] Careful initial management of these patients will prevent conversion of a partial tear to a complete injury. Retrograde urethrography should be performed under fluoroscopy using aseptic technique and minimal pressure. Partial injuries with urethral conti-

A   B   C

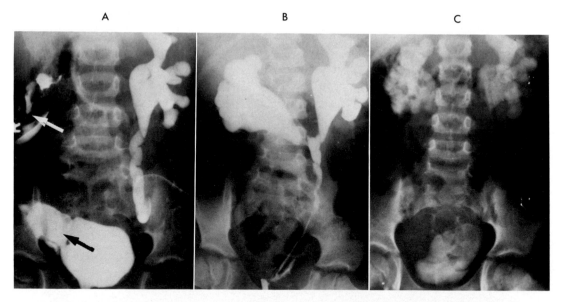

Fig. 18-8 Ischemic necrosis with loss in length of right ureter after cutaneous end ureterostomy *(white arrow)* and iatrogenic rupture of bladder *(black arrow)* during cystogram examination. This 3-year-old boy was referred for urinary reconstruction. Bilateral end cutaneous ureterostomy had been performed during early infancy with a loss in blood supply and sloughing of the right ureter. **A,** During preoperative assessment of the anatomy, shown in this film, filling of this long defunctionalized bladder with only moderate pressure resulted in extravasation. Subsequent elective reconstruction consisted of resecting the ureterostomy stomas, joining the short right ureter to the left side and the left ureter to the bladder. **B,** Retrograde study through ureteral stents shows the right-to-left transureteroureterostomy. **C,** Postoperative IVP showing adequate drainage of the upper urinary tracts. The patient has done well.

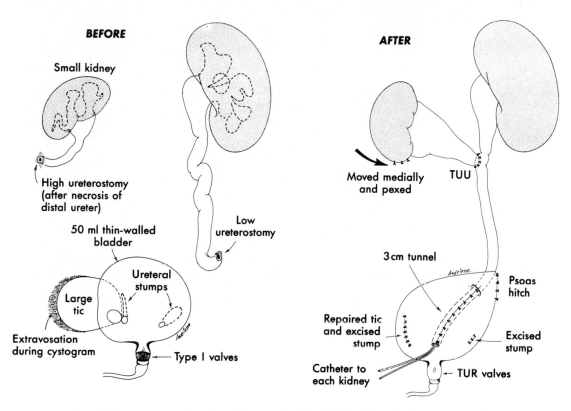

Fig. 18-9   Anatomy of patient illustrated in Fig. 18-8, before and after reconstruction.

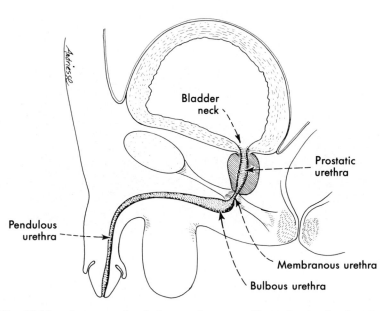

Fig. 18-10   Anatomy of male lower urinary tract illustrating levels of urethra.

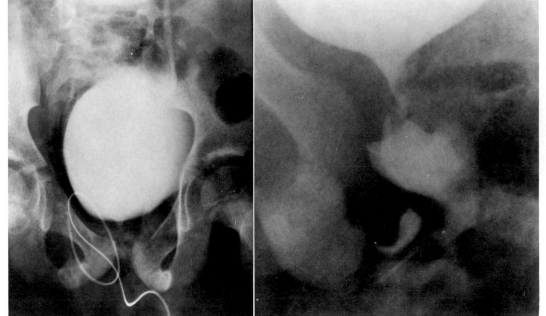

Fig. 18-11   **A,** Cystogram phase of IVP in a boy with a pelvic fracture, showing the urethral catheter passed outside the urinary tract through a posterior urethral disruption. **B,** Retrograde urethrogram in the same patient showing extravasation of contrast material around the disrupted posterior urethra.

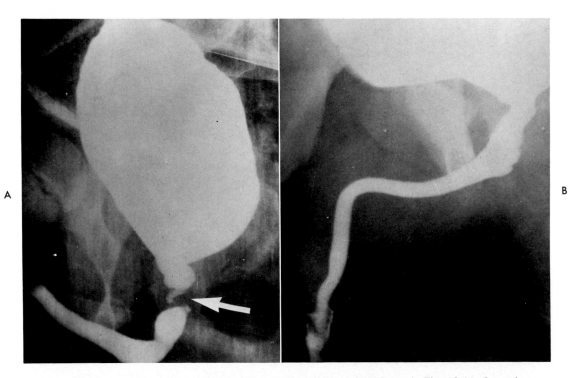

Fig. 18-12   **A,** Preoperative radiographic evaluation of the patient shown in Fig. 18-11, 6 months following injury. Combined voiding cystogram and retrograde urethrogram show the position and extent of the posterior urethral stricture *(white arrow)*. The stricture was repaired by mobilization of the distal urethra and primary anastomosis of the urethra. **B,** Postoperative urethrogram showing normal caliber urethra.

nuity will typically show localized extravasation. They may be treated with suprapubic cystostomy and follow-up urethrography to assess healing.

More often, however, disruption of the urethra is complete. Urethrography will demonstrate marked extravasation and discontinuity of the urethra (Figs. 18-11 to 18-13). Simple suprapubic bladder drainage is preferred, particularly if the child has other life-threatening injuries, followed by definitive repair several months later. Much controversy surrounds the issue of the appropriateness of early primary repair in this situation.[38,47,54] An increased risk of secondary impotence and recurrent stricture has been cited when repair is performed immediately at the time of injury.[58,85,86,88] If early repair is elected, it should be conducted only when the patient's general medical condition is stable. Pelvic clot that can be removed easily should be evacuated with the recognition of possible massive pelvic bleeding as a consequence. Adequate pelvic drainage is essential.

A third management option for complete urethral disruption is primary operative realignment of the urethra over a catheter.[23,54,63] Interlocking sounds manipulated through an open cystostomy regains continuity, and this is held in place with a Foley catheter. However, maintaining continuity of the injured urethra with downward traction on the bladder neck by a Foley catheter has several hazards. The balloon may either become deflated or cause pressure necrosis and contracture of the bladder neck and prostatic urethra. The latter complication of balloon treatment can result in incontinence because of interference with the bladder neck on which the patient will depend for continence, since the initial injury usually destroys the external sphincter.

Results of these different management schemes are often difficult to compare.[88] Immediate urethral repair or realignment is cited as having a stricture rate of 69% in contrast to 100% with cystostomy and delayed repair. The more useful comparison should be the persistent or recurrent stricture rate following definitive urethroplasty in the cases man-

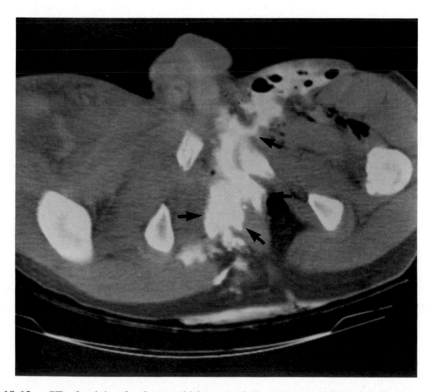

Fig. 18-13 CT of pelvis of a 9-year-old boy struck by an automobile and suffering a pelvic fracture and posterior urethral disruption. The scan shows contrast extravasation from the posterior urethra into the surrounding tissues *(arrows)*. CT images are also useful to image the orientation of the bony fragments for orthopedic reconstruction.

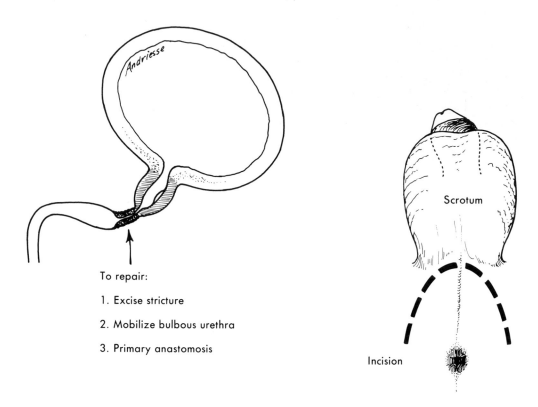

Andriesse

To repair:

1. Excise stricture

2. Mobilize bulbous urethra

3. Primary anastomosis

Scrotum

Incision

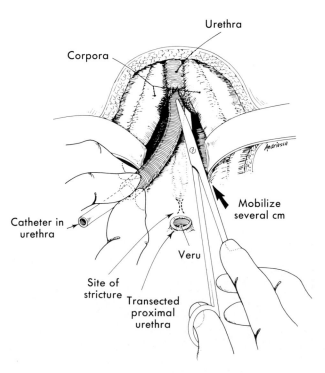

Urethra

Corpora

Mobilize
several cm

Catheter in
urethra

Veru

Site of
stricture

Transected
proximal
urethra

Andriesse

Fig. 18-14 Resection and primary anastomosis of stricture of membranous urethra. Spatulation of the proximal urethral stump is performed ventrally toward the veru montanum when adequate length is present distal to the veru, or dorsally when very close to the veru.

aged with delayed urethroplasty. Impotence is cited as occurring in 44% of patients undergoing immediate repair in contrast to 11.6% of those managed with delayed repair. Incontinence was more frequent following immediate repair, at 20% versus 1.7% for delayed management. The final conclusion seems to favor managing a complete posterior urethral disruption with initial suprapubic drainage and delayed definitive urethroplasty. Primary repair may be appropriate in unusual situations demanding exploration for associated conditions, including a very high-riding bladder, rectal laceration, bladder neck injury or continued bleeding.[88]

Technique of urethral repair

Immediate primary repair. The two ends of the urethra should be aligned over a soft, nonreactive catheter, fenestrated to permit drainage at all levels of the urethra. The ragged edges are debrided, spatulated, and the ends of the urethra approximated. Tension on the anastomosis can be prevented by using pull-out sutures through the prostate that are then tied over a bolster, such as a dental roll, on the perineum. We believe, however, that immediate repair is seldom the ideal choice of therapy for children.

Elective repair. Elective repair performed 4 to 6 months after injury should be preceded by simul-taneous contrast studies through the suprapubic tube and distal urethra to demonstrate the anatomic relationship of the prostatic and bulbous urethra (Fig. 18-12, *A*). Repair of the stricture can then be performed by several methods, shown in Figs. 18-14 to 18-18. The operative procedure should be determined in part by the length of the stricture. A short urethral stricture can be bridged by mobilizing the urethra and reanastomosing the ends. Long strictures require that the course of the urethra be changed (Fig. 18-15)[11,85] or that new tissue be brought into the site of injury as either a patch graft (Fig. 18-16)[22] or a tube graft (Fig. 18-17).[32,34,35] Staged definitive urethroplasty is used less frequently today than previously because of the excellent results achieved with single-stage graft repairs.

Endoscopic management of obliterated posterior urethral strictures has been reported.[20,48] However, we think such management of reaming out or dilating scar tissue will not be as apt to give a long lasting satisfactory passage, especially in a growing patient, as the other methods discussed earlier.

Traumatic disruption of the proximal urethra can lead to other serious complications as well, such as impotence and incontinence.[19,25,83,88] Assessment of erectile capability is recommended before reconstructive surgery is performed, especially in this

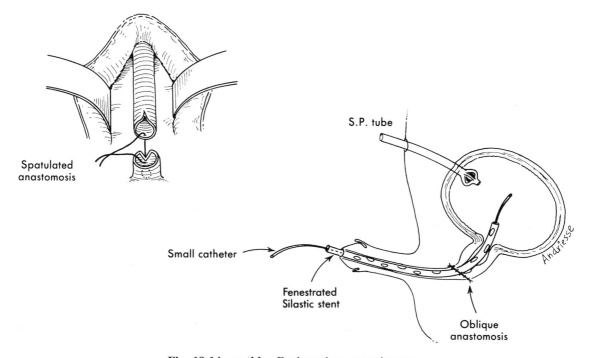

Spatulated anastomosis

S.P. tube

Small catheter

Fenestrated Silastic stent

Oblique anastomosis

Fig. 18-14, cont'd   For legend see opposite page.

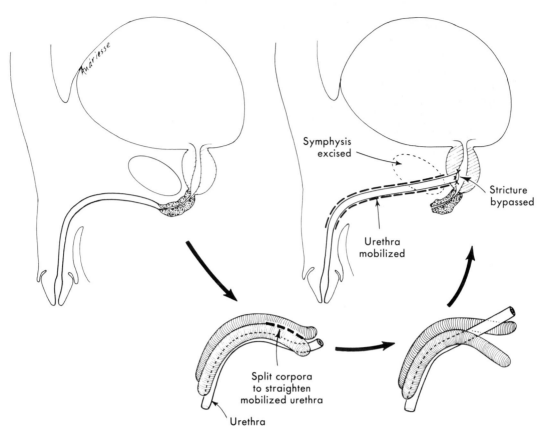

Fig. 18-15   Waterhouse repair using simultaneous approach from above and below. Bulbous urethra is mobilized; corpora are separated; center of pubis is resected; stricture is bypassed by anastomosis of bulbous urethra to anterior aspect of prostatic urethra, leaving stricture site intact.

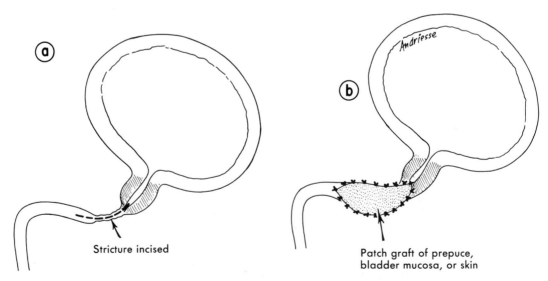

Fig. 18-16   Free patch graft technique. Prepuce, if available, makes the ideal free graft for this purpose. If prepuce is not available we use bladder mucosa. If neither of the above is possible, a free graft of non–hair bearing skin, $^{20}/_{1000}$ of an inch thick, can be used.

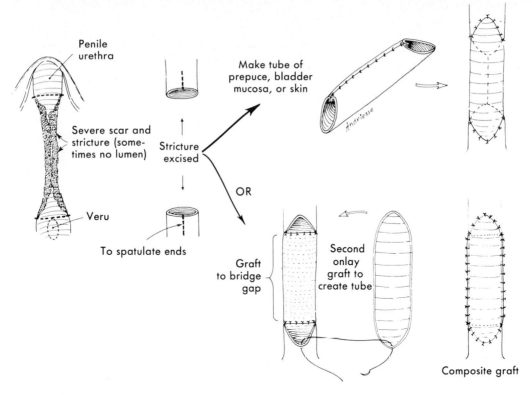

Fig. 18-17 Tube graft technique. A composite urethral tube may also be constructed when a single piece of graft tissue of adequate size is not available.

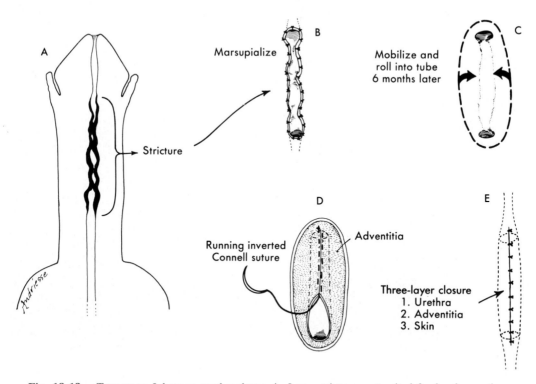

Fig. 18-18 Two-stage Johanson urethroplasty. **A,** Long stricture, not suited for local resection with anastomosis. **B,** Stricture marsupialized. **C, D, E,** At 6 months or more later that segment of urethra can be augmented by taking some skin from the penile shaft at the site of marsupialization and rolling it into a tube, with three-layer closure as illustrated.

day of rampant litigation. Portable nocturnal penile tumescence monitoring devices are available for this purpose.

Laceration or stricture of the distal urethra may follow straddle injury, hypospadias repair, or prolonged catheterization and instrumentation in the male.[21,43,60] The latter complication has become less common in recent years because of the availability of better equipment for cystoscopy of infants.

Anterior urethral strictures are treated by one of various methods including dilatation, injection of steroids and dilatation, endoscopic urethrotomy,[59] excision and reanastomosis, patch graft urethroplasty, or temporary marsupialization (Fig. 18-18).[39] The choice of treatment depends on the length and severity of the stricture.

The following cases illustrate some of the methods used for treatment of urethral strictures.

CASE 5 (Figs. 18-11 and 18-12)

An 8-year-old boy sustained a pelvic fracture when struck by a fire truck. Gentle passage of a small plastic catheter showed complete disruption of the urethra, with the catheter curled up outside of the urinary tract. Retrograde study showed the major disruption (Fig. 18-11, *B*). He was treated by suprapubic drainage. A later study showed noncontinuity of the prostatic and bulbous urethra (Fig. 18-12, *A*). Repair was performed by the technique shown in Fig. 18-14 and was successful.

CASE 6 (Fig. 18-19)

A 14-year-old boy developed a urethral stricture following resection of small urethral valves 7 years earlier. The patient's stream was satisfactory for a time but then became weak from a stricture in the bulbous urethra. The stricture persisted despite multiple dilatations. When he was referred, a satisfactory result was obtained with an onlay patch graft urethroplasty (Fig. 18-16) using a piece of penile skin.

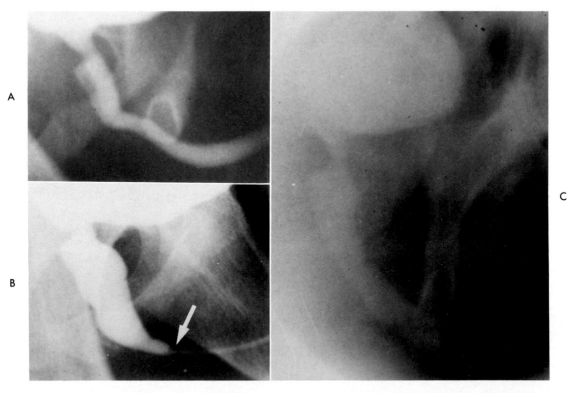

Fig. 18-19 Urethral stricture following endoscopic resection of valves. **A,** Voiding study at age 7 showing normal urethra; an endoscopic procedure was performed, resulting in stricture for which the patient was referred. **B,** Voiding study at age 14 with stricture of bulbous urethra *(arrow),* which was treated by onlay patch graft (Fig. 18-16). **C,** Voiding study 6 months postoperatively showing normal caliber of urethra.

CASE 7 (Fig. 18-20)

A 6-year-old boy was referred for urethral reconstruction. Severe posterior urethral valves had been noted at birth, and loop ureterostomies had been performed when he was 12 days old. His renal function was satisfactory, but he developed pyocystis and a urethral abscess. Endoscopic resection of the valves was conducted at 16 months of age, and the ureterostomies were closed 4 months later. He developed hydronephrosis and recurrent urinary tract infections. At 6 years of age he underwent bladder neck incision and perineal urethrostomy to improve drainage. He then developed day and night wetting through his perineal urethrostomy and continued to have infections.

When referred he had a bladder capacity of 130 cc and voided with high pressures. No reflux was demonstrated. There was a dense 2-cm urethral stricture distal to the perineal urethrostomy and a diverticulum next to it. The bladder neck was hypertrophied, and there was marked trabeculation. Repair of the urethra included resection of the stricture and diverticulum, as well as the perineal urethrostomy, and placing a composite graft from the prepuce (Fig. 18-17). When the stent was removed in 10 days he had a good stream and no residual urine. The suprapubic tube was removed. This patient may require more surgery, such as narrowing the bladder neck, which had been cut elsewhere, and augmenting the bladder if it remains small and noncompliant.

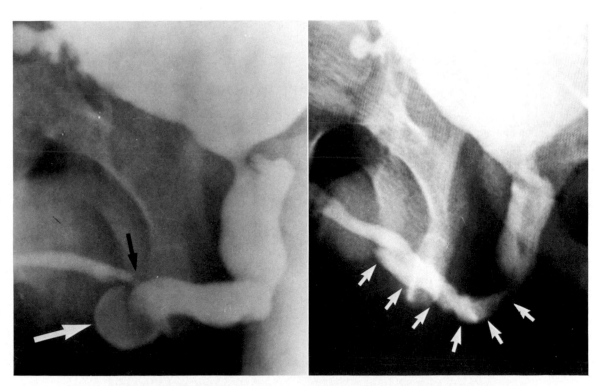

Fig. 18-20   Dense urethral stricture in a 6-year-old boy with previous posterior urethral valves referred for urethral reconstruction. The stricture was probably caused by the instrumentation, and a perineal urethrostomy was placed at the time of the bladder neck incision to treat high-pressure voiding. **A,** Preoperative urethrogram showing perineal urethrostomy and urethral diverticulum *(large white arrow)* and stricture distal to them *(small black arrow)*. Urethra was reconstructed using a tube graft after excision of stricture. Graft was a two-part composite as shown in Fig. 18-17. **B,** Postoperative urethrogram showing open urethra of normal caliber. Arrows indicate the extent of the graft.

CASE 8 (Fig. 18-21)

A 13-year-old boy with prune-belly syndrome had been managed by suprapubic drainage at 3 weeks of age for massive bilateral hydronephrosis and bilateral mega-ureter. The ureters were sequentially reimplanted at 5 and 6 years of age. When the boy was referred for "un-diversion" at age 13, the left kidney did not function, but the right kidney functioned well. There were multiple strictures of the penile urethra believed to be the result of previous instrumentation and catheterization. First stage Johanson urethroplasty was performed (Fig. 18-

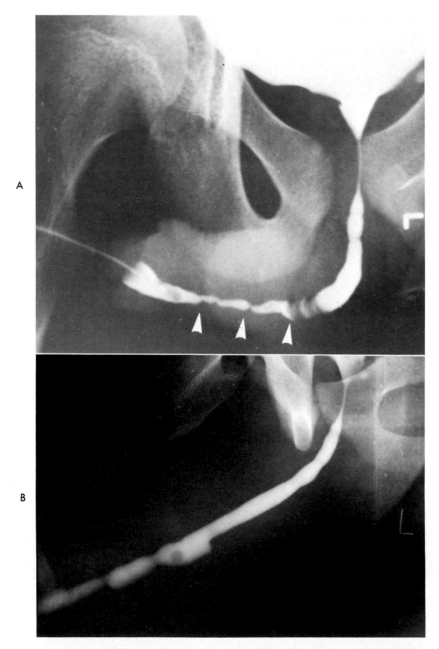

Fig. 18-21 Multiple strictures of penile urethra, possibly resulting from instrumentation, treated by marsupialization at time of extensive urinary tract reconstruction and by closure 1 year later (Fig. 18-18). **A,** Preoperative cystourethrogram showing extensive involvement of penile urethra *(arrows)*. **B,** Examination 1 year following closure of urethra.

18), together with transurethral resection of type I posterior urethral valves and upper tract reconstruction. Reconstruction included tapering and reimplanting the right ureter, right pyeloplasty, orchiopexy, cystostomy closure, left nephroureterectomy, and 50% cystectomy. Second stage urethroplasty was performed 1 year later. The patient has been well for the subsequent 14 years.

Penis

Penile trauma in infants and children in our experience most often follows circumcision[40] (Figs. 18-22 to 18-24). The complications observed include deskinning of the penile shaft, amputation of the glans, urethrocutaneous fistula, complete transection of the urethra, and even total coagulation necrosis of the entire penis by injudicious use of the electrocautery. Deskinning injuries of the shaft, usually a complication of a Gomco clamp

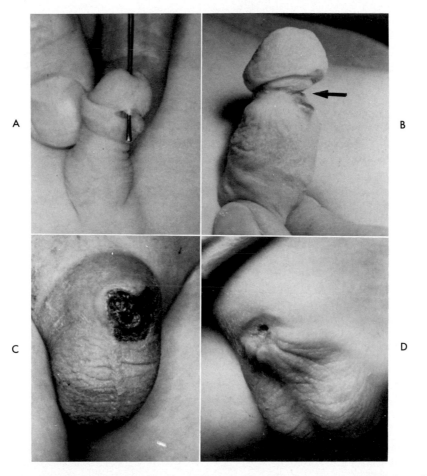

Fig. 18-22 Complications of circumcision. **A,** Urethral fistula at frenulum (note probe), probably the result of incisional trauma. **B,** Three-year-old boy with an almost transected glans from circumcision at birth; parents did not note the abnormality until the boy was 3 years of age. Urethra had been completely transected *(arrow)*. Repair included reanastomosing the ends of the urethra and repair of deep cleft surrounding the corpora. **C,** Neonate referred immediately after Gomco clamp circumcision in which all the skin of the shaft had been amputated. This is a fairly common complication caused by pulling too much skin up into the clamp and amputating it. Fortunately sometimes there is enough of the mucosal side of the prepuce to fold back to resurface the shaft (see Fig. 18-23), but some require a free skin graft. **D,** Six-month-old baby was referred after loss of the entire penis from cautery used during circumcision. Evidently both corpora had thrombosed and sloughed, so no phallus remained.

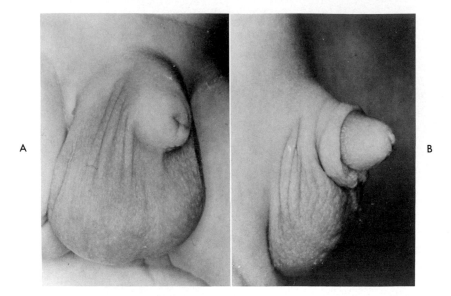

Fig. 18-23   Six-month-old baby after Gomco clamp circumcision similar to Figure 18-22, *C*. **A,** Stubby appearance of penis, the end of which appears to be missing, but in fact the glans and shaft were palpable beneath the small amount of remaining shaft skin. At operation the glans was liberated from beneath the cicatricial tissue at the tip of the penis, and there was enough of the mucosal surface of the prepuce to turn it back as skin for the shaft of the penis. **B,** Appearance at age 1.

circumcision, can often be repaired by resurfacing the denuded area with mucosa from the prepuce. More extensive injuries require a free skin graft. The variety of other penile and urethral injuries are best managed in accord with the principles of hypospadias surgery. In older males penile injury may occur from other causes, such as degloving by a piece of farm equipment or self-inflicted injury in the psychotic patient.

Strangulation injury with hair can be seen in the infant, with the hair acting as a tourniquet just proximal to the glans. This may be difficult to recognize in the face of severe edema, looking much like balanitis. Zipper injuries are not uncommon and may be managed in the emergency ward by cutting the zipper with a bone cutter.[71]

Scrotum

Injuries to the scrotum and scrotal contents require careful inspection of the testes, followed by appropriate debridement, repair, and drainage. Degloving injury with loss of scrotal tissues may require placing the testes into temporary subcutaneous pockets in the ipsilateral medial thigh until skin coverage is feasible.[50,55]

Testis

The infant or older child who has acute pain, swelling, and erythema of the scrotum may have had an injury, but this occurs most often from torsion of the testis.[7,52] In the newborn the twist usually involves the spermatic cord itself, whereas in older boys the testis twists within the tunica vaginalis.[75] In the latter there is the so-called "bell-clapper" deformity. The testis is attached loosely only at its upper pole, which predisposes to such a torsion (Fig. 18-25). The testis becomes swollen and exquisitely tender. A reactive hydrocele may develop after several hours. The testis is often higher in the scrotum than its unaffected mate, and the cremasteric reflex may be absent.[67] Differential diagnosis includes torsion of the appendix testis (Fig. 18-26), testicular neoplasm with acute hemorrhage, acute orchitis, and epididymitis.

Immediate exploration is indicated in cases of suspected torsion, since infarction of the testis is a frequent finding in children with a clinical history of longer than 6 to 8 hours. The ^{99m}Tc sodium pertechnetate scrotal scan has proven helpful in the differential diagnosis of orchitis and testicular torsion by demonstrating the presence or absence of

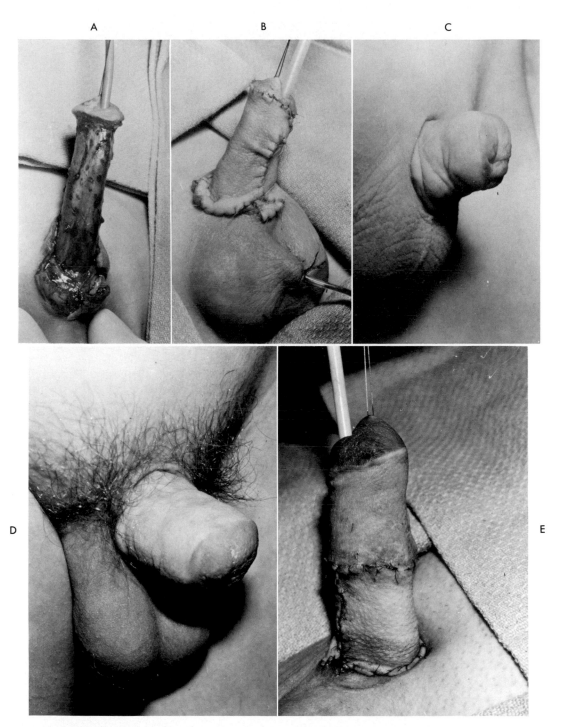

Fig. 18-24   Free skin graft to resurface penis. During ritual circumcision several years previously all the shaft skin and a part of the glans were amputated. **A,** Penis liberated from mons, where it had been buried. Length of the corpora is satisfactory, but there is no skin. **B,** A relatively thick ($^{18}/_{1000}$ inch) graft sewn in place. Note small suction catheter through scrotum to evacuate serum. **C,** Appearance 1 year later. **D,** Appearance of the same patient 12 years later, with inadequate penile skin to cover the postpubertal penis. A second free skin graft was placed proximally. **E,** Appearance after grafting.

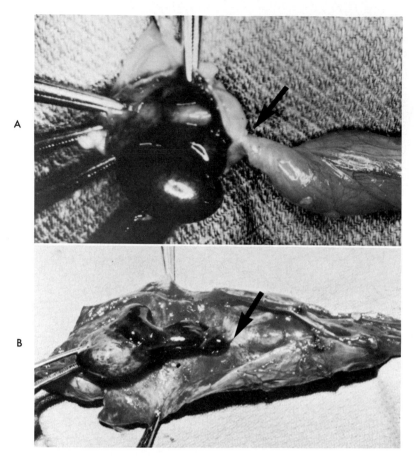

Fig. 18-25 Torsion of the testicle. **A,** Twisting of entire spermatic cord above the level of the tunica *(arrow)*. **B,** Intravaginal twisting with infarcted testis *(arrow)*.

blood flow.[9,82] However, if evaluation has been delayed increased blood flow from scrotal inflammation may be superimposed and mask the absence of testicular blood flow. The Doppler ultrasonic flowmeter has also been used to measure blood flow but is not as reliable as isotope scanning.[3,45] In general, the acute scrotum in the child should be explored, especially today when failure to diagnose torsion will invite malpractice litigation. Indeed it is our practice to recommend exploration whenever the diagnosis is not clearly epididymitis or torsion of the appendix testis, both of which can be treated nonoperatively. This practice will result in some negative explorations, which is better than losing a salvageable testis. The fact that the clinical history has been prolonged should not lessen the urgency for exploration, since partial torsion and venous obstruction may have a slower course toward irreversible testicular damage. Manual detorsion or

spermatic cord anesthetic block are rarely indicated because these maneuvers may only cloud the clinical picture.

A transcrotal approach is preferred, unless there is suspicion of a neoplasm. The torsion is reduced and orchiopexy performed to prevent recurrent torsion. Three permanent sutures placed into the septum and the testicular tunica albuginea provide adequate fixation.[44] The contralateral testis is also fixed to the septum at the same time. With a frankly nonviable testis, orchiectomy is performed. Incision of the tunica albuginea will show absence of fresh bleeding and dark necrotic seminiferous tubules. Doppler flow or fluorescein injection[72] may help make this determination. Experimental evidence has suggested that contralateral testicular damage may occur if the infarcted testis is left in place.[27,58] This has not been confirmed in humans. If viability is uncertain, orchiectomy is not indi-

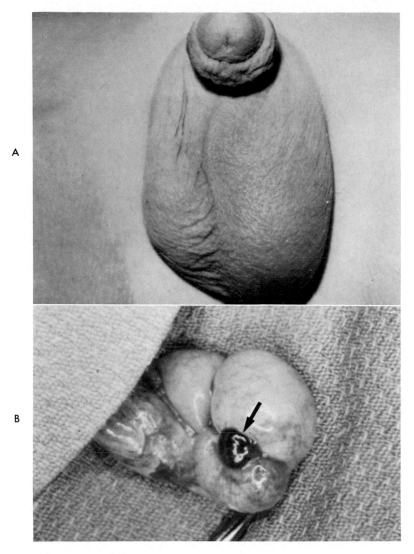

Fig. 18-26   Torsion of the appendix testis. **A,** Note considerable edema of left scrotum, which was tender and red. Exploration was carried out in this case because torsion of the testicle itself could not be excluded clinically, although this is often possible. **B,** Note gangrenous appendix testis *(arrow).*

cated, since endocrine elements may survive and surgical complications are uncommon. A testicular prosthesis may be inserted at the time of orchiectomy provided the scrotal incision does not directly overlie the prosthesis, which can cause it to extrude 8 to 10 days later. If inserting a prosthesis is contemplated, the incision should be made in the upper scrotum so that it will be remote from the prosthesis to be inserted through it and then down into the lower scrotum.

Children with torsion of the appendix testis have a normally positioned scrotal testis with maximal tenderness at the upper pole. The scrotum and spermatic cord usually become swollen and erythematous. Expectant treatment is indicated if the diagnosis is certain. The inflammatory process subsides a few days later as the appendix testis disappears. Some children will continue to experience enough discomfort to warrant surgical removal of a twisted appendix testis, especially if the tenderness is severe enough to make torsion of the testis itself a possibility.

Testicular rupture should be suspected in any patient with scrotal trauma and evidence of a hematocele.[16,81] Scrotal ultrasonography will demonstrate the hematocele and may show the actual capsular rupture.[1] Exploration, debridement of nonviable tissue, and repair of the capsule should be performed within 24 hours and usually will give a satisfactory result in terms of testicular appearance and function.[73]

Perineum

Penetrating Injuries

Impalement of the perineum may cause a penetrating injury to the rectum and damage the urethra, bladder, or vagina. The principles of treating a complex urethral injury with fecal contamination are similar to those of an isolated injury. Rectal penetration is best managed by diverting colostomy, debridement of the wound, and primary repair of the disrupted structures with thorough drainage and antibiotics. We have treated three children with this injury. One was impaled on a picket fence; the other jumped from a closet shelf and landed on a vacuum cleaner handle that passed through the rectosigmoid, small bowel, and mesentery and contused the pancreas. The third was run over by a garden tractor, opening rectum, vagina, and urethra. Primary repair was performed with successful outcome. The principles of treatment outlined proved effective in treating these cases.

Vulvar and vaginal lacerations may result from falls on a blunt object or from straddle-type injuries. Bleeding from a vaginal wall laceration requires careful endoscopy with sedation or general anesthesia, if necessary. The integrity of the vaginal wall is inspected to detect evidence of penetration into the bladder or rectum. The possibility of a coexistent bladder injury must be investigated by cystography or cystoscopy. Sterile instillation of dilute methylene blue into the bladder is a sensitive way of detecting small communications with the vagina.

Careful hemostasis of vaginal wounds is essential because of the risks of an expanding vulvar hematoma. The laceration is then repaired with fine absorbable sutures.

Rape

Rape is a special category of genitourinary trauma that should be mentioned to emphasize several points. Although the actual physical traumatic injury is not usually the paramount consideration, the psychologic and social implications of this crime can be great.[46,64] Because of medicolegal ramifications, accurate history, careful inspection, and the securing of appropriate specimens should be ensured. These include vaginal and perianal swabbings obtained with a moist cotton applicator; one smeared and air-dried on a glass slide and one placed in 0.5 ml of normal saline. These may confirm the presence of sperm, acid phosphatase, or both. Samples of pubic hair should be obtained to detect foreign hairs or sperm. Social and psychologic support of the patient are of great importance, as well as providing protection from possible venereal disease exposure and/or pregnancy. In addition to appropriate cultures, prophylactic treatment of gonorrhea infection, using amoxicillin and probenecid, is recommended within 48 hours. Testing for HIV infection can be offered; the legal applicability and ramifications of this vary with locality. Postmenarchial girls should receive a dose of synthetic estrogens within 72 hours of the assault or be given a course of diethylstilbestrol (DES), 25 mg twice daily for 5 days, to prevent pregnancy. Prompt referral of the victim to the appropriate sources of further counseling and support may well have the most important lasting benefit.

REFERENCES

1. Anderson KA et al: Ultrasonography for the diagnosis and staging of blunt scrotal trauma, J Urol 130:933, 1983.
2. Banner MP and Pollack HM: Dilatation of ureteral stenoses: techniques and experience in 44 patients, Amer J Roentgen 143:789, 1984.
3. Bickerstaff KI, Sethia K, and Murie JA: Doppler ultrasonography in the diagnosis of acute scrotal pain, Br J Surg 75:238, 1988.
4. Blandy J: Injuries of the urethra in the male, Injury 7:77, 1976.
5. Boari L, and Casati A: Communicazione all'academica delle contribute sperimental allo plastico dell'uretere, Scienze Med et Nat di Terrara Maggio (1894).
6. Boston VE and Smyth BT: Bilateral pelvi-ureteric avulsion following closed trauma, Br J Urol 47:149, 1975.
7. Bourne HH and Lee RE: Torsion of spermatic cord and testicular appendages, Urology 5:73, 1975.
8. Bowsher WG et al: A critical appraisal of the Boari flap, Br J Urol 54:682, 1982.
9. Brehmer B, Grunig F, and von Berger L: Radionuclide scrotal imaging: a useful diagnostic tool in patients with acute scrotal swelling? Scand J Urol Nephrol (Suppl) 104:119, 1987.
10. Brereton RJ, Philp N, and Buyukpamuku N: Rupture of the urinary bladder in children: the importance of the double lesion, Br J Urol 52:15, 1980.
11. Brock WA and Kaplan GW: Use of the transpubic approach for urethroplasty in children, J Urol 125:496, 1981.
12. Carlton CE Jr, Guthrie AG, and Scott R Jr: Surgical correction of ureteral injury, J Trauma 9:457, 1969.

13. Carroll PR, and McAninch JW: Major bladder trauma: the accuracy of cystography, J Urol 130:887, 1983.
14. Casale AJ et al: The use of bowel interposed between proximal and distal ureter in urinary tract reconstruction, J Urol 134:737, 1985.
15. Cass AS: Bladder trauma in the multiple-injured patient, J Urol 115:667, 1976.
16. Cass AS: Testicular trauma, J Urol 129:299, 1983.
17. Cass AS: Urethral injury in the multiple-injured patient, J Trauma 24:901, 1984.
18. Cass AS et al: Deaths from urologic injury due to external trauma, J Trauma 27:319, 1987.
19. Chambers HL and Balfour J: The incidence of impotence following pelvic fracture with associated urinary tract injury, J Urol 89:702, 1963.
20. Chiou RK et al: Endoscopic treatment of posterior urethral obliteration: long-term follow-up and comparison with transpubic urethroplasty, J Urol 140:508, 1988.
21. Churchill BM et al: Complications of posterior urethral valve surgery and their prevention, Urol Clin North Am 10:519, 1983.
22. Devine PC, Fallon B, and Devine DJ Jr: Free full-thickness skin graft urethroplasty, J Urol 116:444, 1976
23. DeWeerd JR: Immediate realignment of posterior urethral injury, Urol Clin North Am 4:75, 1977.
24. Duckett JW and Pfister RR: Ureterocalicostomy for renal salvage, J Urol 128:98, 1982.
25. Ellison M, Timberlake GA, and Kerstein MD: Impotence following pelvic fracture, J Trauma 28:695, 1988.
26. Feins NR: Multiple trauma, Pediatr Clin North Am 26:759, 1979.
27. Fisch H et al: Gonadal dysfunction after testicular torsion: luteinizing hormone and follicle-stimulating hormone response to gonadotropin-releasing hormone, J Urol 139:961, 1988.
28. Glassberg KI et al: Partial tears of prostatomembranous urethra in children, Urology 13:500, 1979.
29. Hendren WH: Reoperation for the failed ureteral reimplantation, J Urol 111:403, 1974.
30. Hendren WH: Urinary tract refunctionalization after prior diversion in children, Ann Surg 180:494, 1974.
31. Hendren WH: Complications of ureterostomy, J Urol 120:269, 1978.
32. Hendren WH, and Crooks KK: Tubed free skin graft for construction of male urethra, J Urol 123:858, 1980.
33. Hendren WH and Hensle TW: Transureteroureterostomy: experience with 75 cases, J Urol 123:826, 1980.
34. Hendren WH and Keating MA: Use of dermal graft and free urethral graft in penile reconstruction, J Urol 140:1265, 1988.
35. Hendren WH and Reda EF: Bladder mucosa graft for construction of male urethra, J Pediatr Surg 21:189, 1986.
36. Hensle TW, Burbige KA, and Levin RK: Management of the short ureter in urinary tract reconstruction, J Urol 137:707, 1987.
37. Hodges CV et al: Autotransplantation of the kidney, J Urol 110:20, 1973.
38. Jackson PH and Williams JL: Urethral injury: a retrospective study, Br J Urol 46:665, 1974.
39. Johanson B: Reconstruction of the male urethra in strictures, Acta Chir Scand Suppl 176:1, 1953.
40. Kaplan GW: Complications of circumcision, Urol Clin North Am 10:543, 1983.
41. Karp MP et al: The role of computed tomography in the evaluation of blunt abdominal trauma in children, J Pediatr Surg 16:316, 1981.
42. Kenney PJ, Panicek DM, and Witanowski LS: Computed tomography of ureteral disruption, J Comput Assist Tomogr 11:480, 1987.
43. Kiracofe HL, Pfister RR, and Peterson NE: Management of nonpenetrating distal urethral trauma, J Urol 114:57, 1975.
44. Kossow AS: Torsion following orchiopexy, NY State J Med 80:1136, 1980.
45. Levy BJ: The diagnosis of torsion of the testicle using the Doppler ultrasonic stethoscope, J Urol 113:63, 1975.
46. Livne PM and Gonzales ET Jr: Genitourinary trauma in children, Urol Clin North Am 12:53, 1985.
47. Malek RS, O'Dea MJ, and Kelalis PP: Management of ruptured posterior urethra in childhood, J Urol 117:105, 1977.
48. Marshall FF, Chang R, and Gearhart JP: Endoscopic reconstruction of traumatic membranous urethral transection, J Urol 138:306, 1987.
49. Marshall FF, Hendren WH, and Nason HO: Severe blunt trauma of upper urinary and intestinal tracts in a child, J Urol 118:315, 1977.
50. McDougal WS: Scrotal reconstruction using thigh pedicle flaps, J Urol 129:757, 1983.
51. McGinty DM and Mendez R: Traumatic ureteral injuries with delayed recognition, Urology 10:115, 1977.
52. Melekos MD, Asbach HW, and Markou SA: Etiology of acute scrotum in 100 boys with regard to age distribution, J Urol 139:1023, 1988.
53. Merchant WC III, Gibbons MD, and Gonzales ET Jr: Trauma to the bladder neck, trigone, and vagina in children, J Urol 131:747, 1984.
54. Meyers RP and DeWeerd JH: Incidence of stricture following primary realignment of the disrupted proximal urethra, J Urol 107:265, 1972.
55. Millard DR: Scrotal construction and reconstruction, Plast Reconstr Surg 38:10, 1966.
56. Mitchell JP: Injuries to the urethra, Br J Urol 40:649, 1968.
57. Morehouse DD and MacKinnon KJ: Management of prostatomembranous urethral disruption: 13-year experience, J Urol 123:173, 1980.
58. Nagler HM and DeVere White R: The effect of testicular torsion on the contralateral testis, J Urol 128:1343, 1982.
59. Noe HN: Endoscopic management of urethral strictures in children, J Urol 125:712, 1981.
60. Noe HN: Complications and management of childhood urethral stricture disease, Urol Clin North Am 10:531, 1983.
61. Palmer JK, Benson GS, and Corriere JN Jr: Diagnosis and initial management of urological injuries associated with 200 consecutive pelvic fractures, J Urol 130:712, 1983.
62. Palmer JM and Drago JR Jr: Ureteral avulsion from nonpenetrating trauma, J Urol 125:108, 1981.
63. Pierce JM Jr: Management of dismemberment of the prostaticmembranous urethra and ensuing stricture disease, J Urol 107:259, 1972.
64. Pokorny WJ et al: Perineal injuries in infants and children. In Brooks, BF, editor: The injured child, Austin, 1985, University of Texas Press.
65. Prout GR Jr, and Koontz WW Jr: Partial vesical immobilization: an important adjunct to ureteroneocystostomy, J Urol 103:147, 1970.

66. Prout GR Jr, Stuart WT, and Witus WS: Utilization of ileal segments to substitute for extensive ureteral loss, J Urol 90:541, 1963.

67. Rabinowitz R: The importance of the cremasteric reflex in acute scrotal swelling in children, J Urol 132:89, 1984.

68. Reda EF and Lebowitz RL: Traumatic ureteropelvic disruption in the child, Pediatr Radiol 16:164, 1986.

69. Reichard SA et al: Pelvic fractures in children—review of 120 patients with a look at general management, J Pediatr Surg 15:727, 1980.

70. Richardson JR Jr and Leadbetter GW Jr: Nonoperative treatment of the ruptured bladder, J Urol 114:213, 1975.

71. Saraf P and Rabinowitz R: Zipper injury of the foreskin, Am J Dis Child 136:557, 1982.

72. Schneider HC, Kendall AR, and Karafin L: Fluorescence of the testicle: an indication of viability of spermatic cord after torsion, Urology 5:133, 1975.

73. Schuster G: Traumatic rupture of the testicle and a review of the literature, J Urol 127:1194, 1982.

74. Shah PM et al: Elevated blood urea nitrogen: an aid to the diagnosis of intraperitoneal rupture of the bladder, J Urol 122:741, 1979.

75. Skoglund RW, McRoberts JW, and Ragde H: Torsion of the spermatic cord: review of the literature and an analysis of 70 new cases, J Urol 104:604, 1970.

76. Snyder HMcC and Caldamone AA: Genitourinary injuries. In Welch KJ et al, editors: Pediatric surgery, ed 4, Chicago, 1986, Year Book Medical Publishers.

77. Sullivan MJ, Lackner LH, and Banowsky LHW: Intraperitoneal extravasation of urine, JAMA 221:491, 1972.

78. Turner-Warwick R: Urethral strictures in relation to the sphincters, Br J Urol 40:677, 1968.

79. Udall DA et al: Transureteroureterostomy: experience in pediatric patients, Urology 2:401, 1973.

80. Ulm AH: Total placement of the ureter with small intestine: technique and results, J Urol 79:21, 1958.

81. Vaccaro JA et al: Traumatic hematocele: association with rupture of the testicle, J Urol 136:1217, 1986.

82. Valvo JR et al: Nuclear imaging in the pediatric acute scrotum, Amer J Dis Child 136:831, 1982.

83. VanArsdalen KN et al: Erectile failure following pelvic trauma: a review of pathophysiology, evaluation, and management, with particular reference to the penile rosthesis, J Trauma 24:579, 1984.

84. Waterhouse K: Injuries to the urinary tract in children. In Johnson JH and Scholtmeijer RJ, editors: Problems in pediatric urology, Excerpta Medica Monograph, 1973.

85. Waterhouse K: The surgical repair of membranous urethral strictures in children, J Urol 116:363, 1976.

86. Waterhouse K and Gross M: Trauma to the genitourinary tract: a 5-year experience with 251 cases, J Urol 101:241, 1969.

87. Weaver, RG: Basic surgical principles of ureteral repair, Surg Gynecol Obstet 110:594, 1960.

88. Webster GD, Mathes GL, and Selli C: Prostatomembranous urethral injuries: a review of the literature and a rational approach to their management, J Urol 130:898, 1983.

89. Williams DI: Rupture of the female urethra in childhood, Eur Urol 1:129, 1975.

19

Injury to the Immature Skeleton

John A. Ogden

Because injury to the developing skeleton and the subsequent reparative response differ from those of the mature skeleton, trauma involving a child usually requires different diagnostic and treatment approaches from those used with an adult with a comparable injury. Distinctions result from changing anatomy at both macroscopic and microscopic levels, physiology, mechanical response to fracture-producing forces, and rate of healing. These factors give rise to diverse types of skeletal injuries, diagnostic problems, treatment modalities, and long-term growth consequences. The primary determinant in considering the effect of trauma on the developing bones is the patient's skeletal rather than chronologic maturity.

Because of the varying anatomic, physiologic, and mechanical differences of immature bone, the biology of injury in children differs from that in adults in several important ways. Incomplete fractures—torus and greenstick types—are common in children. Also, the physis (growth plate) may be involved, creating the possibility of subsequent growth disturbance. Bone healing is quicker because of the periosteum's osteogenic potential. Normal processes of remodeling will correct some but not necessarily all loss of longitudinal alignment. Longitudinal overgrowth may correct length inequality resulting from fragment overriding. Fractures necessitate open reduction much less frequently than in adults.

The scope of this discussion is limited, since the chapter is part of a generalized textbook on care of the injured child. The reader interested in more detailed presentations concerning specific fractures should consult pediatric orthopedic trauma texts.[85,86,89,107]

ANATOMY AND PHYSIOLOGY

The tubular, or longitudinal, bones of the developing skeleton have several distinct anatomic areas (Fig. 19-1). The major portion of the ossified shaft is called the diaphysis. At birth this region is composed of fetal (woven) bone characteristically lacking haversian (osteon) systems. However, as periosteal-mediated appositional bone formation and remodeling enlarge the overall diameter of the shaft and the width of the diaphyseal cortices, mature bone with an osteonal pattern becomes dominant. The early bone is very vascular and more porous than the maturing bone of older children, adolescents, and adults. Subsequent growth leads to increased complexity of the haversian systems and elaboration of increasing amounts of extracellular matrix, causing a decrease in porosity and an increase in hardness. Compared with the adult periosteum, the periosteum in a child is thicker, more loosely attached to the underlying diaphysis, and capable of faster callus and membranous bone formation.[26]

At each end of the diaphysis the bony contour flares to form the metaphyses, which are characterized by decreased cortical bone and increased trabecular bone. The trabecular portion undergoes extensive remodeling as the primary spongiosa (a direct result of endochondral ossification) is transformed into more mature secondary spongiosa. The area of transformation of cartilage to bone is structurally weak. The metaphyseal cortex changes with time. Relative to the confluent diaphysis, the metaphyseal cortex is thinner and more porous. During the first years of life this cortex is filled with fenestrations connecting the marrow cavity with the subperiosteal space. The fenestrations are filled

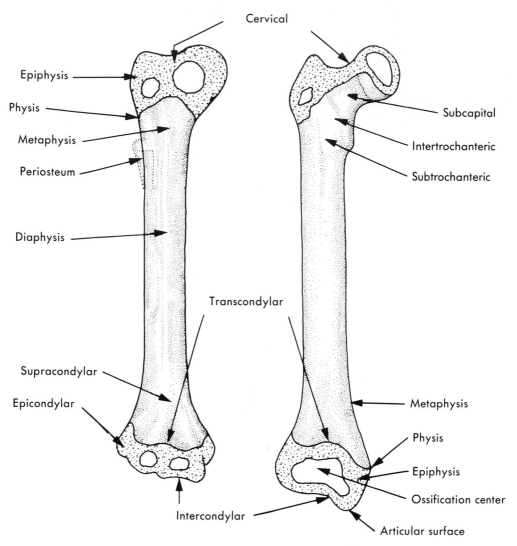

Fig. 19-1 Anatomic regions and terminology commonly applied to the description of fractures in children.

with fibrovascular tissue in continuity with endosteal tissue and the periosteum. As longitudinal growth continues, these fenestrations become less numerous, and the overall width of the metaphyseal cortex thickens.

At the end of each long bone is the epiphysis. With the exception of the distal femur, the epiphyses are completely cartilaginous at birth. At a characteristic time each chondroepiphysis develops a secondary ossification center that gradually enlarges, until the cartilage is completely replaced by bone at skeletal maturity. This process occurs by a variation of the endochondral ossification responsible for longitudinal bone growth.

Between the epiphysis and metaphysis is a dis-

coid structure, the physis (growth plate), which is responsible for endochondral ossification and longitudinal bone growth. The physis contains several cell zones that can be classified histologically or functionally. Juxtaposed to the epiphysis is the zone of resting cartilage. In the chondroepiphyseal stage this zone is indistinguishable from the adjacent hyaline cartilage; in the older child it is covered by the subchondral plate of the epiphyseal ossification center. Next to the zone of resting cartilage is the zone of proliferating cartilage, where both longitudinal and latitudinal cell division occurs. These first two histologic zones constitute the critical functional zone of cartilage formation, and they are necessary for continued longitudinal growth of the bone. Both zones depend heavily on a functioning vascular supply derived from the epiphyseal circulation.

A third epiphyseal zone contains the maturing or hypertrophic cells that form the columns characteristic of the physis and elaborate an extensive extracellular matrix among the cell columns. The final zone is that of cartilage transformation, where the extracellular matrix is calcified as a necessary prelude to capillary invasion and consequent formation of osteoid on the calcified cartilage framework (primary ossification). The periosteum, which is relatively loosely attached to the diaphyses and metaphyses, is densely attached to the periphery of the growth plate. Recent evidence suggests that the intrinsic contractility of the entire periosteum exerts some control over the physis' rate of growth.

Certain growth areas such as the tibial tuberosity have cellular modifications characteristic of a response to tensile rather than compressive forces.[91-93,99] The cell columns are replaced by fibrocartilage, which forms bone by membranous ossification rather than by endochondral ossification, although the two processes are completely integrated with regard to rates of growth. This type of functional modification of the physis appears to be associated with structures anatomically designated as apophyses. Although the "apophysis" is not directly involved in longitudinal growth, its contiguous relationship with the physis is such that damage to an apophysis could seriously impair the growth potential of the adjacent physis.

The physis has two primary sources of blood supply, the epiphyseal and metaphyseal circulatory systems. The epiphyseal circulatory pattern varies, changes with skeletal maturation, and is more susceptible to vascular compromise. In the small child the chondroepiphysis contains structures called cartilage canals that distribute to discrete areas of the germinal and proliferating zones of the physis, with minimal anastomosis between canalicular systems. As the epiphysis matures, arteries stem from the vascular network of the ossification center, penetrating the subchondral plate and supplying the aforementioned zones, still with a pattern of minimal anastomosis between vascular zones. This pattern of limited vessels with minimal collateralization gives rise to a risk of ischemia, especially in areas with highly selective vascular supply such as the proximal femur. If the blood supply is compromised, either temporarily or permanently, de-

creased or complete loss of function in the physis and consequent growth disturbance may result.

The metaphyseal circulation has a relatively unchanging pattern of sinusoidal loops throughout skeletal maturation. This system is also highly anastomotic. Fractures of the physis or metaphysis cause disruption of the metaphyseal circulation, but these vessels quickly recover to reestablish normal circulatory patterns. The transient loss of sinusoidal loop function causes widening of the physis, since the zone of hypertrophic cells cannot be invaded unless a functioning blood supply is present. However, once circulation is reestablished, this widened zone is rapidly invaded and restored to normal width. Disruption of the metaphyseal circulation, in sharp contrast to impairment of the epiphyseal circulation, rarely causes permanent growth disturbance.

BIOMECHANICS

Since immature bone undergoes continuous conversion of fetal bone to osteon bone, from less dense to more dense cortical bone, and constant remodeling in the metaphysis and diaphysis, the mechanics of skeletal failure vary with the changing biomechanical attributes of the bone and cartilage at any given time.[27] In addition to these changes in the hard tissue, the periosteum is also a significant factor contributing to a bone's overall capacity to respond to fracture-producing forces. The thick periosteum is less readily torn circumferentially, may prevent major displacement, and may be used as a "hinge" during closed reduction.

A common type of injury is the torus, or buckle, fracture (Fig. 19-2), which involves the metaphysis. Compact adult bone usually fails in tension. However, the more "porous" nature of immature metaphyseal bone allows failure in compression as well. The result is a compaction of the trabecular bone and a buckling of the cortical bone.[65] As previously discussed, the metaphyseal bone strengthens as the child grows, especially in weight-bearing bones. Torus fractures are relatively common in younger children; in older children epiphyseal changes are more common because metaphyseal changes render the junction of the physis and metaphysis the weakest area structurally.

A typical childhood injury is the greenstick, or incomplete, fracture (Fig. 19-2), which occurs because of changing microscopic anatomy. The less-dense bone of a young child can tolerate greater

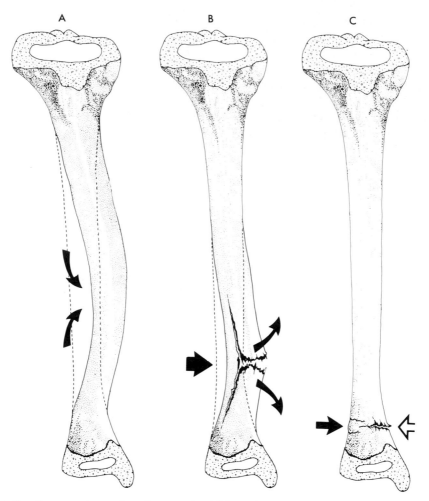

Fig. 19-2   Common incomplete fractures in children. **A,** Pure bowing or plastic deformation. **B,** Tensile greenstick fracture with plastic deformation (bowing) of the intact cortex. **C,** Compression greenstick fracture with buckling of intact cortex (torus injury).

degrees of elastic and plastic deformation before fracturing. Certain immature bones (for example, the radius and ulna) can be bent without failure (fracture), but if this deformation occurs in the plastic rather than the elastic phase of the deformation curve, permanent angular change may result.[11] In a greenstick fracture, failure occurs along the tension side of the bone. The fracture force becomes dissipated longitudinally along the neutral force line, whereas the compression side continues plastic deformation and may even buckle. At the maximal application of the fracture forces there may be considerable angular displacement. The elastic recoil of the soft tissues and unfractured bone usually improves the position. However, retained plastic deformation in the compressed bone may cause continued angular deformity and may necessitate completion of the fracture.

DIAGNOSIS

Although the cause of many injuries is readily evident, a definite history of the mechanism of fracture may be lacking, especially if the child was doing something wrong or in cases of child abuse. The injured extremity usually is painful, swollen, tender, and limited in function. However, the gross appearance may seem minimally deformed, since some types of fracture (greenstick, torus) are intrinsically stable.[61] A fracture may cause a febrile response, which may be the only sign in small infants or children with neuromuscular disorders, especially myelodysplasia.

Roentgenography is important in the diagnosis of childhood skeletal injuries. However, in contrast to evaluation of the adult skeleton, assessing the radiologic appearance of the immature skeleton presents several problems.[66] The epiphyses, which develop the secondary ossification centers in a reasonably predictable sequence, are variably radiolucent. Interpretation of roentgenograms must include consideration of the radiologically invisible contours, especially when evaluating injuries around joints, such as condylar, epicondylar, and supracondylar fractures of the distal humerus. To assist in interpretation of potential displacement of an ossification center, comparison views of the opposite, uninjured limb may be taken. Normal anatomic structures also may mimic fractures. The nutrient foramen may be long and oblique, resembling a spiral fracture. Children may develop thin, radiopaque lines parallel to the growth plate. These are called Harris's growth slowdown lines.[83]

Abnormal curvature in the bone sould be treated with suspicion, especially if the child has clinical signs of a fracture. As previously discussed, immature bone may undergo considerable deformation *without* fracture.[11,89] This is called bowing (Fig. 19-2). If a certain amount of plastic deformation is retained, the bone is susceptible to further injury.

TREATMENT

Most fractures involving the diaphyses should be treated by closed reduction and casting or by an appropriate period of skeletal traction followed by casting. However, certain fractures may benefit from open reduction and internal fixation. Among such injuries are intraarticular fractures, fractures of the femoral neck, certain types of epiphyseal and physeal injuries, and fracture of both bones of the forearm in an adolescent.

Nonunion is rare. However, the position of the fracture does affect the rapidity of healing and residual deformities. Distraction should be avoided, since it delays healing. Abnormal angulation may also delay healing because of the effect of muscle imbalance on callus maturation. The periosteum is very osteogenic in a child. In the age group of birth to 3 years, a femoral fracture develops a radiologically evident callus in 10 to 14 days, and stabilization may occur within 3 weeks. As the child gets older, callus formation and maturation take longer.

A torus fracture generally requires splinting. Manipulation generally does not affect the deformity. A greenstick fracture usually is best treated by applying a cast with three-point pressure. It may be necessary to complete the fracture if the deformity recurs, while casted, because of retained plastic deformation within the intact portion of the cortical bone.

Treatment of complete fractures may appear simple, but there are many possibilities for malunion. In adults, the deformity of a malunited fracture is permanent; in children, some deformities tend to correct with growth and remodeling, whereas others do not. Anyone treating childhood fractures should be aware of these conditions.

An angular deformity tends to correct, provided the plane of deformity conforms to the motion of the contiguous joint[77]; angulation not in the plane of joint motion is much less likely to correct. These principles apply primarily to "single action" joints such as the elbow, wrist, knee, and ankle. Furthermore, the closer the angular deformity is to the physis, the better the chance for spontaneous correction; the closer the deformity is to midshaft, the less chance for correction. An angular change of 20 degrees is the maximal that should be accepted during treatment.

When the fracture is complete, the fragment ends may be incompletely apposed or even side to side. Such positioning heals well with a large amount of callus that eventually will be remodeled. Every attempt should be made to keep the fragments aligned longitudinally when overriding is present. Shortening with side-to-side apposition can be accepted. Although figures of up to 2.5 cm have been given as acceptable, 1 cm is probably the best goal. This shortening is compensated by longitudinal overgrowth that undoubtedly results from two factors—the increased vascularity and the release of the normal periosteal control of longitudinal growth when this structure is completely disrupted. This phenomenon is most striking in the femur.

Rotational displacements must be corrected at the time of reduction. Residual rotational deformities do not correct spontaneously regardless of age or site of deformity. Such malunion may require corrective osteotomy.

COMPLICATIONS

Fractures in children are relatively free of serious complications. However, several major problems may occur. Injury around the physis may cause long-term growth disturbances. Open injuries may be complicated by osteomyelitis. Certain fractures about the elbow and knee may cause vascular compromise (Volkmann's ischemia/contracture). Joint injuries, especially of the elbow, may be complicated by myositis ossificans. Fat embolism and pulmonary embolism are rare. Refracture may occur,[4] but synostosis is infrequent.

FOLLOW-UP

Once a fracture heals in an adult, a static condition exists; but longitudinal growth in children presents the possibility of long-term problems, some of which may not become evident for many years. Children with fractures should be followed for at least 2 to 3 years, and if the fracture involves the growth plate, to skeletal maturation. This gives the physician the opportunity to assess growth disturbance early, when it may be correctable. A good example is the formation of an osseous bridge after a physeal fracture, a condition in which early resection may allow restoration of growth. The physician should also follow other potential problems. The child with a leg length inequality secondary to a femoral fracture may develop scoliosis.

OPEN INJURIES

Open fractures involving the immature skeleton tend to be deemphasized. Certainly they represent a small number of fractures in children, but they must be treated as carefully and aggressively as in the adult.[68,69] The mechanisms of injury, which usually involve violent trauma, are becoming more common through the use of go-carts, trail bikes, and riding lawn mowers.

The first step in treatment should be stabilization of the patient, since extensive injuries are not uncommon. The fracture may be splinted while appropriate diagnostic modalities are completed (for example, abdominal tap, liver-spleen scan). Once more serious injuries are ruled out or treated, attention may be directed to the open fracture. The objective is the eventual conversion of an open, dirty wound to a clean, closed wound. The patient should be taken to the operating room. Pretreatment wound cultures are essential, for these may give an early indication of an actual or potential infecting organism. The wound, including soft tissues and fracture ends, should be meticulously explored and debrided; this should be followed by profuse irrigation and, if available, pulsating lavage irrigation. In general, the wound should *not* be closed primarily, since there is usually some doubt as to the degree of peripheral tissue viability and contamination, especially by anaerobic organisms. Any wound that has been open for 8 to 12

hours, no matter how clean it might appear, must be left open. Similarly, all crush injuries should be left open. Although antibiotics are not a substitute for good surgical debridement, their prophylactic use is beneficial. A broad-spectrum antibiotic should be administered before and during surgery and for 48 to 72 hours after injury. Unless the wound was severely contaminated or is obviously infected, further use of the antibiotic is probably not necessary, unless cultures are positive. Secondary closure by granulation tissue or delayed primary closure becomes a matter of the surgeon's discretion. Use of external fixation allows appropriate management of the soft tissue injuries.

PATHOLOGIC FRACTURES

Although trauma is the major mode of injury to the developing skeleton, certain pathologic conditions may predispose a child to fracture with even minimal injury. In these cases the primary process renders the bone structurally weak and susceptible to fracture. Generalized abnormalities include osteogenesis imperfecta, osteopetrosis, vitamin deficiencies, endocrinopathies (including the use of exogenous steroids), neuromuscular abnormalities, and collagen disorders (especially juvenile rheumatoid arthritis).[36,89,105] More localized causes include osteomyelitis and benign and malignant tumors.[96] In fact, the usual initial sign of many skeletal tumors, whether benign or malignant, is pain consequent to fracture. Therapy must be directed at the primary cause, as well as the fracture.

PHYSICAL THERAPY

In sharp contrast to adult skeletal injury, immobilization, even for extended periods, rarely leads to long-term loss of joint motion or function. Early mobilization usually is not necessary and may even be contraindicated. Provided that the fracture is properly reduced, that the fragments have healed adequately, and that no soft tissue complications (fibrosis, myositis) have intervened, normal motion will return, and reasonably rapidly. Instinct usually guides the child as to functional limitations and restriction of activity. Active assisted exercise programs by a therapist or parent usually only cause continued protective muscle spasm and prolong functional return. However, in the poorly motivated child or in the child with a neuromuscular disorder, such as cerebral palsy or myelomeningocele, the active role of the therapist may be necessary. In the rare case when return of function is poor or does not occur because of fibrosis, heterotopic bone formation, or myositis ossificans, physical therapy may be beneficial, although surgical excision or release of the pathologic process may also be necessary.

EPIPHYSEAL AND PHYSEAL INJURIES
Types of Injury

Fractures involving the physis and epiphysis are unique to the developing skeleton. Neer and Horwitz[75] stated that at least 15% of fractures in children involved the epiphysis; 74% of 2500 cases involved the upper extremity, and 26% involved the lower extremity. The most commonly involved epiphysis was the distal radius (46%).

An adequate understanding of the diagnosis and treatment of these injuries is best acquired through systematic classification. Aitken[3] classified the injuries and relative prognosis. Salter and Harris[114] reviewed epiphyseal fractures and evolved a classification scheme comprising nine types of fractures based on radiologic appearance and prognosis. This system has been modified by Ogden.[81,82,88]

Type 1

In type 1 fractures the fracture line traverses the zone of cartilage transformation and may extend into areas of the primary spongiosa, especially where the physeal/metaphyseal contour is irregular.[112] This leads to complete separation of the epiphysis and separation of most of the physis from the metaphysis (Fig. 19-3). Since the zone of growth (that is, the germinal and proliferating zones) remains with the epiphysis, cell column formation and cell division continue. The metaphyseal disruption causes a delay in the vascular invasion of the hypertrophic cell columns and a relative "widening" of the physis. However, once the capillary circulation is reestablished, the widened hypertrophic region is quickly replaced and normal physeal thickness results. This type of fracture generally results from a shearing or avulsion force. It is most commonly seen in newborns and young infants, especially victims of child abuse, and in children with a pathologic predisposition such as myelomeningocele or the various types of rickets. The minimally disrupted periosteum prevents significant displacement in most cases. Treatment usually consists of closed reduction by gentle manip-

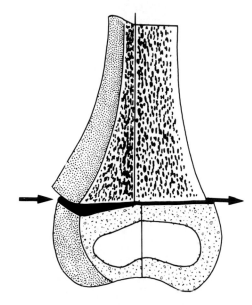

Fig. 19-3   Type 1 growth mechanism injury traversing the physis, with minimal displacement of the epiphysis.

ulation. Open reduction is necessary in unstable situations. Immobilization is continued for 3 to 4 weeks. The prognosis for normal future growth is excellent unless vascular compromise or compression damage to a localized area of the physis has occurred. Although those complications are rare, their occurrence should emphasize the need for adequate long-term follow-up.

Type 2

A type 2 fracture is the most common epiphyseal injury. As with type 1 fractures the mechanism is usually a shearing or avulsion force that propagates through the zone of cartilage transformation for an inconstant distance and then extends into the metaphysis, possibly through an area more structurally susceptible to continued propagation of the fracture-producing stresses. This produces a variably sized metaphyseal fragment that is still in continuity with the physis and is displaced along with the epiphysis (Fig. 19-4). If the epiphysis has no epiphyseal ossification center or only a small one, this metaphyseal fragment may be the only roentgenographic clue to the injury. The fragment was described by C. Thurstan Holland and retains his eponym.[43,47] The process of fracture healing is essentially the same as in type 1 injuries, except that bone-to-bone healing also occurs between the metaphyseal fragment and the remainder of the metaphysis. Treatment usually consists of closed re-

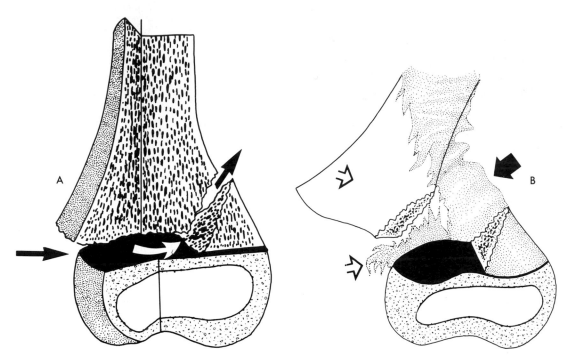

Fig. 19-4　**A,** Type 2 growth mechanism injury with a Thurstan-Holland metaphyseal fragment. **B,** Note how the periosteal sleeve remains intact on the "fragment side." This is an aid during reduction.

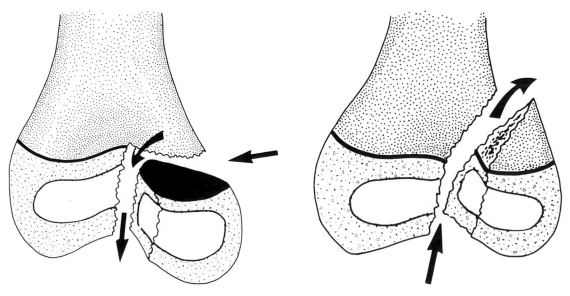

Fig. 19-5　Type 3 growth mechanism injury of the epiphysis. The physis and articular surfaces are both disrupted.

Fig. 19-6　Type 4 growth mechanism injury.

duction by gentle manipulation. The combination of the metaphyseal fragment and the intact periosteal hinge on the compression side affords some mechanical stability to the reduction (Fig. 19-4). As in type 1 fractures open reduction is indicated when closed reduction cannot be attained or maintained. Since the fracture line does not involve the germinal/proliferative zones, the prognosis for unimpaired growth is excellent. In rare cases small portions of the physis may be damaged and cause premature, localized closure of the growth plate, resulting in angular deformity.

Type 3

A type 3 fracture involves the epiphysis directly. It probably results from a combined compression/shearing force. The fracture line extends from the articular surface through the epiphysis and ossification center to the physis (Fig. 19-5). The fracture forces are then dissipated along the zone of cartilage transformation to the periphery. The fragment is frequently displaced, causing discontinuity of the articular surfaces. However, in some instances, especially with injuries to the distal femur, displacement may be minimal and stress roentgenography may be necessary to demonstrate the injury. When the fragment is displaced, closed reduction should be attempted first. However, open reduction usually is required to effect anatomic reduction of both the physeal and articular surfaces. This is especially important in the weight-bearing joints such as the knee and ankle, which commonly are affected by this type of injury. As previously described, the process of healing occurs along the physis/metaphysis separation and, additionally, by bone-to-bone healing within the split epiphyseal ossification center (if present). Articular defects heal by fibrocartilaginous ingrowth. The prognosis for future longitudinal growth is good. Long-term problems are more likely to be caused by intraarticular irregularity than by damage to the growth plate.

Type 4

Type 4 fractures involve portions of the epiphysis, metaphysis, and the intervening physis (Fig. 19-6). The most frequently involved area is the lateral condyle of the distal humerus. The combined fragment usually is displaced, causing disruption of normal physeal and articular relationships. If left anatomically inaccurate, displacement of either physis or joint surface or both could lead to significant long-term problems.

If displacement of the fragment is minimal, closed reduction initially may be attempted. However, it is imperative that roentgenograms be taken frequently to verify that subsequent displacement has not occurred as swelling subsides. Open reduction and internal fixation usually are necessary to restore anatomic continuity of both the joint surface and physis. Temporary, smooth Kirschner fixation pins may be used. Depending on the size of the fragments and ossification center, it may be possible to avoid crossing the physis with these pins. However, if the physis must be crossed, these thin, smooth wires should be removed within 4 to 6 weeks, and they should have no long-term effect on growth potential. If anatomic reduction is not accomplished, a bone bridge may develop between the epiphyseal ossification center and the metaphysis, resulting in an angular growth deformity. Concomitant joint incongruity could lead to joint stiffness and loss of normal motion mechanics. Because of these potential complications, the prognosis for normal growth is much more guarded in type 4 injuries than in the first three categories.

Type 5

A type 5 fracture is a rare injury resulting from a severe disruptive force, usually involving the knee or ankle (Fig. 19-7). The injury may be an isolated one affecting all or part of the physis, with the latter case being more likely. The injury also may accompany a type 1 or type 2 injury, involving the type 2 where the fracture begins to propagate into the metaphysis. Roentgenographic detection is virtually impossible at the time of acute injury. This type of injury was described by Salter and Harris as a crush injury.[114] However, more recent work suggests that microscopic disruption of the physeal periphery and ischemia are more likely causes.[88] Whatever the cause, all layers of the physis are involved, especially the zones of cartilage formation, leading to premature cessation of growth plate function. Vascular damage to the microscopic epiphyseal vessels may be the most important factor. If a large epiphyseal ossification center is present, a metaphyseal/epiphyseal osseous bridge may form. Since the seriousness of this injury often is not suspected, this fracture should be considered in any child with trauma to the knee or ankle joint that is accompanied by all the classic signs of fracture—pain, swelling, and limitation of motion. Treatment should consist of immobilization and non–weight bearing for 3 to 4 weeks. Adequate

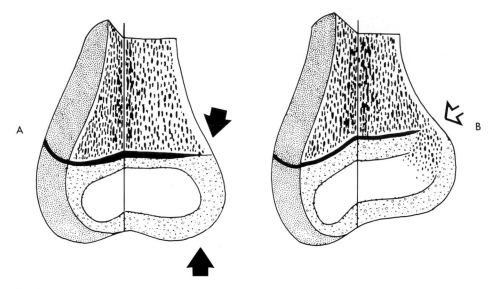

Fig. 19-7 **A,** Type 5 growth mechanism injury. Although originally conceived of as a physeal crushing, it is more likely that the "compressed" area sustains microscopic linear disruption between cell columns and ischemic damage. **B,** The end result is premature growth arrest and bridge formation.

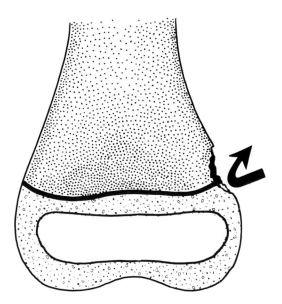

Fig. 19-8 Type 6 growth mechanism injury of the physeal periphery with damage to the zone of Ranvier.

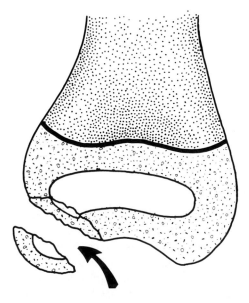

Fig. 19-9 Type 7 growth mechanism injury to create an osteochondral fragment. This fracture is completely within the epiphysis.

long-term follow-up is important because of the invariable complications of growth slowdown or arrest.

Type 6

A type 6 fracture is a shearing pattern of damage that particularly affects the physeal periphery (Fig. 19-8). Common mechanisms include catching the ankle in bicycle spokes, injuries caused by lawn mowers, and burns. This type of injury often leads to peripheral growth arrest and angular deformity.

Type 7

A type 7 fracture is an intraepiphyseal injury (Fig. 19-9; also see Fig. 19-27). It also represents a typical pattern of "ligament failure" in an adolescent. A small chondro-osseous fragment pulls away from the rest of the epiphysis, instead of damage occurring within the substance of the ligament. Tibial spine avulsion and Osgood-Schlatter's lesions are frequent type 7 injuries.

Type 8

A type 8 fracture is a temporary disruption of the metaphyseal circulation and the normal bone modeling/remodeling that occurs in this region (Fig. 19-10). This disruption includes a decreased rate of physeal replacement by primary spongiosa, effectively widening the physis and making it temporarily susceptible to epiphysiolysis.

Type 9

A type 9 fracture involves damage to the periosteum, the growth mechanism of the diaphysis (Fig. 19-11). If there is bone loss, along with periosteal loss, spontaneous repair of segmental defects is unlikely.[97] When debriding open fractures, the periosteal tube should be maintained as much as possible.

Apophyseal avulsions

Areas of growth that are primarily responsive to tensile stresses classically are called apophyses. These areas may be avulsed by violent muscular pull. This occurs frequently around the pelvis (for example, as with ischial tuberosity) but may also occur at the medial epicondyle and tibial tuberosity.[50,58,89] If the apophysis is minimally displaced, treatment should be relief of weight bearing or nonuse of the extremity, with cast, for 3 to 4 weeks. If displacement is significant, open reduction and internal fixation are indicated. It is often stated that

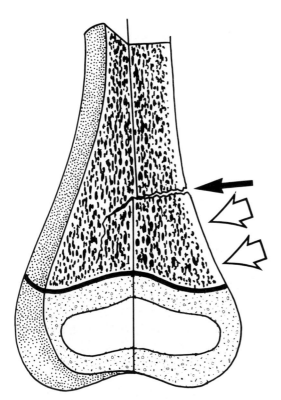

Fig. 19-10 Type 8 growth mechanism injury *(solid arrow)* leads to temporary vascular cutoff of the region between fracture and physis *(open arrows)*, disrupting osseous remodeling in the secondary spongiosa and preventing replacement of the hypertrophic/calcified physis by primary spongiosa.

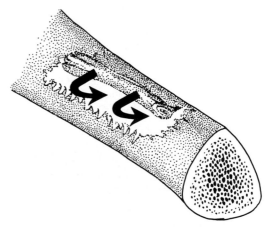

Fig. 19-11 Type 9 growth mechanism injury with torn periosteum rolling into a tube, which retains the capacity to make bone. Severe damage adversely affects the ability to repair a major osseous defect.

these avulsion injuries are not complicated by growth disturbances, but the physis and apophysis at the knee or elbow are fully integrated growth regions and can cause angular growth deformities by mechanically limiting growth in selected areas of the remainder of the physis. Apophyseal avulsions may also affect the spine.[64]

Diagnosis

An injury may be suspected clinically and easily confirmed roentgenographically, since most physeal fractures are associated with displacement. Diagnosis is more difficult if displacement is absent or minimal. However, stress roentgenography may confirm the injury. Even if radiographic evidence is lacking, clinical suspicion of the injury should guide treatment. This is especially important in a young child with minimal development of the epiphyseal ossification center, in whom roentgenographic interpretation is difficult. Comparison views may be helpful to demonstrate asymmetric relationships.

Fracture Healing

In general, much less time is required to effect fracture healing in epiphyseal fractures than in metaphyseal or diaphyseal fractures. Solid healing is obtained in 2 to 4 weeks. In the first three types of fractures, normal physeal cartilage growth and maturation processes continue, but the transformation of cartilage to bone is interrupted because of a temporary cessation of the metaphyseal circulation. This is analagous to the metaphyseal-vessel ischemia described by Trueta,[89] except that it is a transient phenomenon. This vasculature is quickly reestablished and, in conjunction with the normal processes of metaphyseal remodeling, leads to rapid reunification of bone and hypertrophied cartilage. Additional bone forms along the areas of intact periosteum. This is also a rapid process that contributes to overall stability.

In type 4 fractures healing is normal bone-to-bone callus formation in both the metaphysis and epiphyseal ossification center. The gap in the physis is bridged by fibrous or fibrocartilaginous tissue, which does not interfere with longitudinal growth. However, if reduction is not anatomic, this fibrous tissue may be replaced by callus and a transphyseal osseous bridge may form. In types 1 through 4 the process of healing usually is associated with vascular hyperemia and may cause a temporary or even permanent longitudinal overgrowth.

Treatment

The most important concept is *gentle* reduction. Forceful manipulation can disrupt areas of the physis and introduce additional injury into localized areas.[98] The reduction must be accomplished as soon as possible, since healing is rapid. In general, all types of epiphyseal fractures should be treated by closed reduction whenever possible. However, many type 3 injuries may require open reduction, and type 4 injuries almost always require open reduction. Transfixation of fragments with smooth Kirschner wires, which are removed 3 to 6 weeks later, should not affect continued physeal growth.

Growth Disturbance

About 85% of epiphyseal fractures are associated with normal long-term growth. In the remaining 15% partial or complete premature growth cessation (traumatic epiphysiodesis) may occur. Large areas of damage may preclude further longitudinal growth, whereas smaller areas may cause eccentric longitudinal growth and angular deformity.

The distal humerus and distal femur seem to be more prone to premature closure after major injury. Both involve joints with single-plane joint motion (flexion-extension). The fracture force is applied in an abduction or adduction manner, causing transmission of compression forces into the physis.

In the arm most growth occurs at the proximal humerus and distal radius and ulna, whereas in the leg most growth occurs in the distal femur and proximal tibia. Thus damage to these growth plates would have more effect than damage to the physes at the opposite ends of the respective bones.

Physeal damage in an 8 year old would be more serious than comparable damage in a 12 year old, because both longitudinal and angular growth deformities require a certain period of growth to become overtly manifest. Skeletal maturity rather than chronologic age is more important; a 10 year old may have a skeletal age quite different from his or her 10 years.

If the entire physis is destroyed, a progressive discrepancy in limb length results. If only a portion of the physis is damaged, both limb length discrepancy and angular deformity develop. If one of paired bones (radius/ulna, tibia/fibula) is affected, the length or angular inequality may affect the adjoining bone adversely.

If damage is complete, surgical epiphysiodesis of the contralateral growth plate can be considered. If the damage involves one of paired bones, surgical epiphysiodesis of the other bone may be performed to prevent relative overgrowth, or selective lengthening may be undertaken. Angular deformities present a greater problem. Small osseous bridges may be resected and the defect packed with fat or methyl methacrylate to prevent reformation of the bridge.[13,87] Larger bridging defects may not be resected as easily and may require completion of the epiphysiodesis and corrective osteotomy.[60,87]

Specific Epiphyseal Injuries
Clavicle

The medial end of the clavicle has a thin physis with dense ligamentous attachments to the sternum. This epiphysis is radiolucent until the eighteenth year, when a linear ossification center forms. Fusion of this growth plate is one of the last to occur, at about 22 to 25 years of age, rendering this area susceptible to injury long after physiologic fusion of the remainder of the physes. Separation through the physis may result in the metaphysis being displaced either anteriorly or posteriorly.[15,31] Pain, swelling, and a protuberant mass at the sternoclavicular joint after a fall on the shoulder suggest anterior displacement (Fig. 19-12). Posterior displacement, suggested by a concavity at the sternoclavicular joint, is of greater significance, since the bony fragment can enter the chest and damage the trachea, lungs, or mediastinum. Crepitation, although rare, strongly suggests a pulmonary laceration with dissection of air in the subcutaneous tissues. Computed tomography (CT) is useful in making the diagnosis of a posterior metaphyseal displacement, a diagnosis that may be difficult to make with standard roentgenograms. Anterior displacement usually can be treated by manual re-

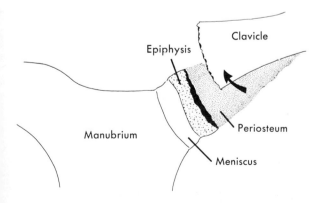

Fig. 19-12   Physeal fracture of the proximal clavicle, the childhood equivalent of sternoclavicular separation.

duction, with the periosteum and posterior sternoclavicular ligaments preventing overreduction into the chest. Closed reduction of a posterior displacement of the metaphysis is much more difficult and frequently unsuccessful. Open reduction is often indicated. If wire fixation is used, the ends of the wires must be bent at right angles to prevent migration into the thoracic cavity, and the wires should be removed in 4 to 6 weeks.

A thin epiphysis also is present distally. Trauma that usually produces an acromioclavicular separation in a young adult creates an epiphyseal injury in the younger patient (Fig. 19-13). The periosteal sleeve is intact and still attached to the coracoclavicular ligaments. Healing occurs within this sleeve, often leading to partial "duplication" of the distal clavicle.[84]

Proximal humerus

The proximal humeral physis becomes a conoid structure that resists direct shear displacement and usually results in a major metaphyseal fragment (type 2 injury) from the medial side of the metaphysis (Fig. 19-14). The lateral metaphyseal fragment is often displaced through a tear in the periosteum. This particular epiphysis seems most susceptible to injury in the adolescent.[3,29]

Radiologic diagnosis usually is easy. Treatment should be directed to both the patient's age and the degree of displacement. In young children a type 1 fracture usually is present. Major efforts at manipulation and reduction under general anesthesia are probably not justified because of the growth potential in this epiphysis. The proximal humeral growth plate contributes 80% of the longitudinal growth of the humerus and quickly corrects the deformity in the young child. The arm should be immobilized in a Velpeau-type dressing for 3 weeks until union begins. The arm can then be progressively immobilized.

In older children a type 2 fracture is more common. In cases of mild displacement, shoulder immobilization usually is all that is required, although reduction sometimes can be obtained by manipulation. When the proximal fragment is more severely angulated or displaced, closed reduction with the patient under general anesthesia is indicated. Because of the instability of the reduction, it may be necessary to maintain the arm in considerable abduction, forward flexion, and neutral rotation with a shoulder spica cast. Because complete anatomic reduction is not absolutely essential to acceptable shoulder function, open reduction is

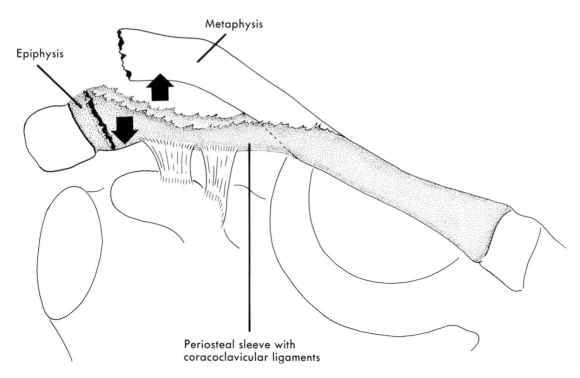

Fig. 19-13   Physeal fracture of the distal clavicle. Note the intact ligaments remain attached to the avulsed periosteal sleeve.

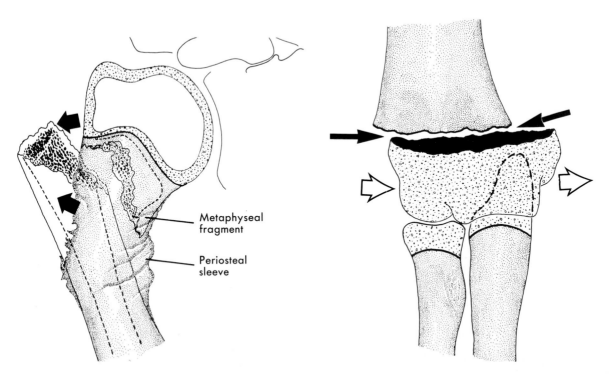

Fig. 19-14   Type 2 physeal fracture of the proximal humerus. The fracture displaces through a tear in the periosteal sleeve, which often makes anatomic reduction difficult, if not impossible.

Fig. 19-15   Type 1 physeal fracture of the distal humerus. This pattern is common in infancy, especially in cases of child abuse. Because of the lack of epiphyseal ossification, the injury is often misinterpreted radiographically as a dislocated elbow.

rarely indicated in the small child or even the adolescent. However, every effort should be made to correct angular malalignment. In rare instances damage to the growth plate may cause subsequent varus deformity of the proximal humeral epiphysis. This is usually a complication of injury in early infancy rather than in adolescence, since the concomitant metaphyseal fragment protects the physis from damage.

Distal humerus

Separation of the entire distal humeral epiphysis is rare (Fig. 19-15). It is much more common to encounter partial injury, with separation of the lateral condyle, medial condyle, and medial epicondyle (Fig. 19-16). These injuries are type 3 and type 4 epiphyseal separations and if not managed properly may have serious long-term growth consequences, resulting in major varus or valgus malalignment.

Lateral condylar injury usually is caused by a varus force with significant elbow subluxation or even dislocation.[23,48,54] The fragment, with the attached extensor mass, may be rotated 90 degrees to 180 degrees and displaced partially into the joint. Even if the fragment is not displaced initially, the pull of the extensor muscles may increase the deformity during immobilization. Because of muscle pull, the undisplaced fracture should be treated with the forearm in full supination to minimize the deforming force of the extensor mass. Since the fracture line crosses the physis and joint surface, accurate anatomic reduction is essential. If any displacement is present, open reduction and internal fixation, usually by Kirschner wires, is indicated. Either nonunion or malunion with premature growth arrest of the lateral portion of the growth plate may result in a progressive cubitus valgus deformity and a delayed ulnar nerve palsy.[38]

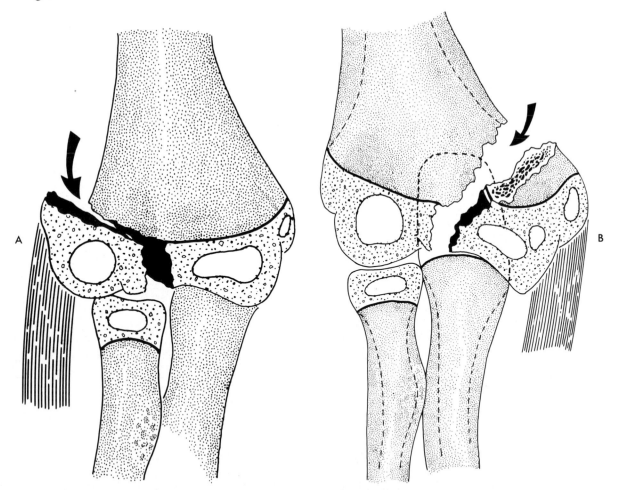

Fig. 19-16   A, Type 3 fracture of the lateral condyle. **B,** Type 4 fracture of the medial condyle.

On the opposite side of the distal humerus, the medial epicondyle rather than the condyle is the major area of injury.[10] However, an unossified medial condylar fracture may appear to be a medial epicondylar "injury."[35,44] The epicondylar fragment frequently is displaced and may even lodge in the joint, especially if it accompanies an elbow dislocation (Fig. 19-17). Ulnar nerve paresis may be a common acute complication of this injury, especially with displacement of the fragment. When the epicondyle is minimally displaced, joint immobilization at 90 degrees with the forearm in pronation usually is adequate. However, once displacement begins, open reduction and internal fixation must be considered. If the displacement is not accompanied by instability to valgus stress, treatment probably can consist of closed reduction and immobilization. When a major displacement of the fragment is accompanied by elbow instability, open reduction is definitely indicated. When undertaking such reduction, care must be taken to isolate the ulnar nerve and protect it during the surgical procedure. The fragment should be visualized, and if intact it should be reattached using Kirschner wires for stabilization. In the adolescent with fragmentation of the epicondyle, the bone may be excised and the flexor muscle mass reattached to the epicondylar region.

Proximal ulna

Injuries of the proximal ulna are comparable to adult fractures, except that the juxtaarticular portion of the physis is involved (Fig. 19-18). When displacement is minimal, treatment should consist of immobilization. Markedly displaced fragments of the olecranon, particularly those involving the distal tip with its epiphysis, should be treated with open reduction and tension band fixation.[42,76]

Proximal radius

Fractures involving the proximal radial epiphysis usually are type 2 fractures and are much less common than fractures involving the radial neck (metaphysis).[37] Depending on the mechanism of injury, the proximal radial epiphysis may be minimally, moderately, or severely displaced. In more severe instances the entire epiphysis may be displaced posteriorly or anteriorly into the joint.[122] Displacement is accompanied by an angular deformity and crush injury to the adjacent metaphysis. In treatment every effort should be made to reduce any angular deformity. This often can be accomplished by closed means, under adequate anesthesia, with direct pressure applied over the proximal radius. In those cases in which the proximal radial epiphysis has been displaced into the joint, open reduction and fixation is indicated. Injuries of the radial head always should be sought when a patient has a fracture of the shaft of the ulna (Monteggia injury), or when the elbow has been dislocated.

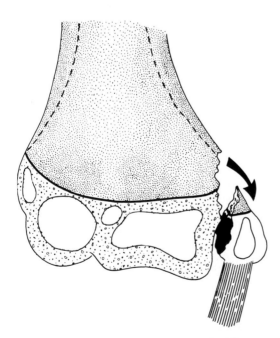

Fig. 19-17   Avulsion of the medial epicondyle.

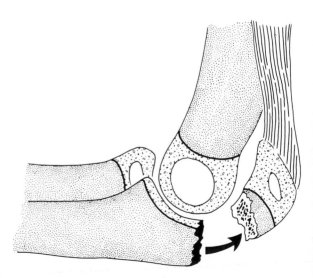

Fig. 19-18   Fracture of proximal ulnar epiphysis (olecranon, with displacement of the fragment by the triceps.

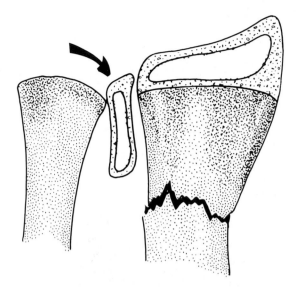

Fig. 19-19   Completely displaced type 1 physeal fracture of the distal ulna.

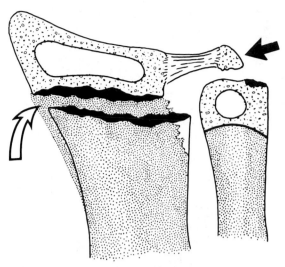

Fig. 19-20   Type 1 physeal fracture of the distal radius. A type 7 avulsion of the unossified ulnar styloid usually accompanies this fracture. This often will ossify separately from the rest of the ulnar epiphysis, creating a "radiologic nonunion."

Distal ulna

Injury to the distal ulna is uncommon but may accompany displacement of the distal radial epiphysis (Fig. 19-19). Closed reduction should be attempted. Open reduction may be necessary if the fragment is displaced into the interosseous region.

Distal radius

Displacement of the distal radial epiphysis is probably the most common epiphyseal injury encountered (Fig. 19-20), constituting approximately half of the cases in most large series.[12] It usually is caused by a fall on an outstretched hand with hyperextension, causing the epiphysis to be dorsally displaced. The most common injury is type 2, with the metaphyseal fragment being from the dorsal side of the metaphysis. This may be a solitary injury, or it may be accompanied by a greenstick injury of the ulna, separation of the distal ulnar epiphysis, or a separation through the ulnar styloid process. The injury usually is treated with a closed reduction and immobilization for 3 to 4 weeks. An adequate level of anesthesia should be used for the reduction to optimize the ability to reduce this type of fracture on the first attempt. Repeated attempts to reduce the injury may result in further damage to the growth plate. Since this is an area of major growth, angular deformities up to 20 degrees and 30 degrees and incomplete anatomic reduction usually correct over time, de-

pending on the patient's age. There is rarely any indication for open reduction of this fracture. Although diagnosis of a type 2 injury is easy, this area may be also affected by type 5 injuries, which are difficult to diagnose. A child with a history of a fall on a hyperextended hand with a painful, swollen wrist with no radiographic evidence of a type 1 or type 2 injury should be treated as potentially having a type 5 injury, with adequate immobilization for 3 to 4 weeks and follow-up over the next 2 to 3 years. The damage to the physis may be complete, with premature closure of the physis, or it may be localized to a small area.

Pelvis

A number of growth centers are present around the pelvis. Traction injuries commonly involve the iliac spines (Fig. 19-21). These injuries may occur when muscles are abruptly contracted, as in springing out of starting blocks, or may occur with more chronic, repetitive avulsion.[121] Disruption of the acetabulum is a fracture-dislocation of the hip and may lead to premature closure of the triradiate cartilage (Fig. 19-22).[17]

Proximal femur

The proximal femoral epiphysis and physis vary considerably in susceptibility to trauma, primarily

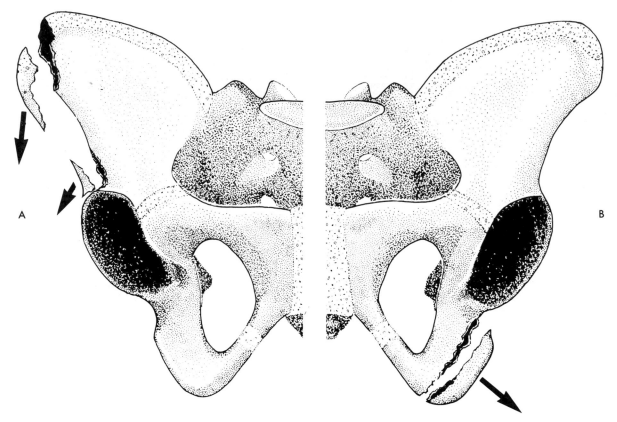

Fig. 19-21   **A,** Avulsion of the iliac superior or inferior spines (apophyses). **B,** Avulsion of ischial tuberosity.

because of changing anatomic structure during femoral neck development. Epiphyseal fractures involving the proximal femur are rare.[108] The entire proximal femoral epiphysis, which includes both the capital femoral and greater trochanteric regions, may be separated from the metaphysis by birth trauma (Fig. 19-23).[94] Examination and presentation mimic a child with unilateral hip dislocation, with one major exception—pain during range of motion examination. Separation of the capital femoral epiphysis may occur at any age, although it is most commonly a problem of adolescence, when the entity slipped capital femoral epiphysis is prevalent (Fig. 19-24). There is controversy over whether this represents a chronic gradual slip or a true fracture displacement. In many reported instances the history and presentation suggest an acute traumatic displacement of the capital femoral epiphysis. In these cases attempted reduction by gentle preoperative traction in bed (not forceful manipulation under general anesthesia) should be combined with transepiphyseal pin fixation. Dis-

ruption of the proximal femur in the midchildhood range is rare and often is associated with pathologic conditions such as rickets. In these situations manipulation, casting, and correction of the primary disease are necessary.

Distal femur

Fractures involving the distal femoral physis and epiphysis may cause major problems. This physis is the most active in longitudinal growth of the skeleton, contributing 70% of the femoral length and 40% of the overall leg length. Most of these injuries are type 2 (Fig. 19-25), and they may be further classified as abduction, hyperextension, or hyperflexion injuries.[117] It is imperative that major displacements be anatomically reduced.[21,110] In evaluating the possibility of this injury, stress views should be considered, since the injury may have been spontaneously reduced on cessation of the deforming force. Treatment should be directed at reduction, using a general anesthetic if necessary, and casting that is appropriate to the type of injury

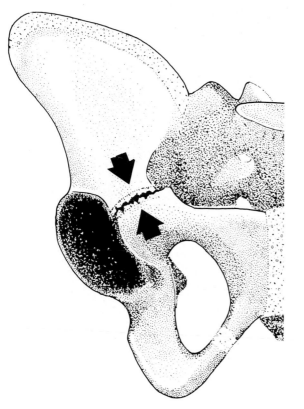

Fig. 19-22   Displaced fracture through the triradiate cartilage. This injury has a high risk of growth arrest.

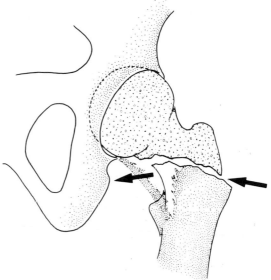

Fig. 19-23   Birth fracture of the entire proximal femoral epiphysis, a type 1 physeal injury involving both femoral head as well as greater trochanter.

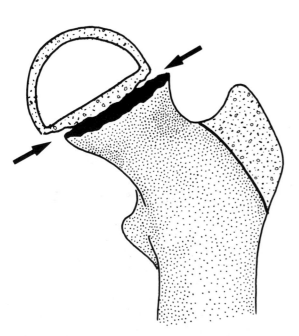

Fig. 19-24   Type 1 physeal injury in an adolescent creates slipped capital femoral epiphysis, either acutely or, more commonly, chronically.

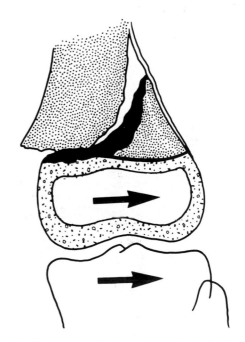

Fig. 19-25   Type 2 physeal fracture of the distal femur.

that occurs. The type of cast and position of the leg should be directed at preventing recurrent angular deformity. Type 3 and type 4 injuries require surgical intervention.

Proximal tibia

Injuries to the proximal tibia are rare (Fig. 19-26). Strain in the ligaments that might otherwise

cause separation of the epiphysis from the remainder of the bone is transmitted mainly into the metaphysis. Injuries, when they occur, should be followed closely, since this physis contributes 30% of the overall leg length. The injury usually results in posterior displacement of the shaft of the tibia

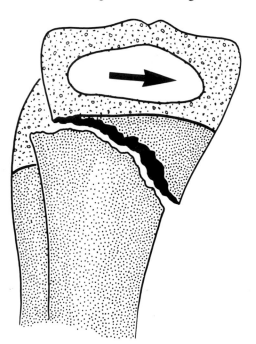

Fig. 19-26 Type 2 physeal fracture of the proximal tibia.

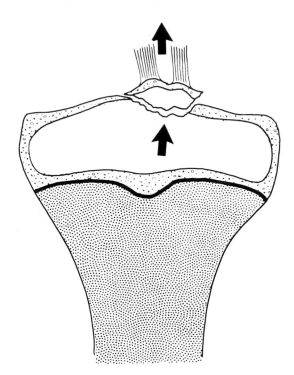

Fig. 19-27 Type 7 growth mechanism injury of the tibial spine.

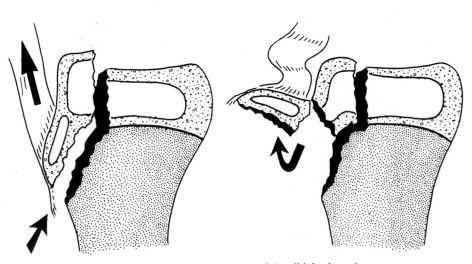

Fig. 19-28 Type 3 fractures of the tibial tuberosity.

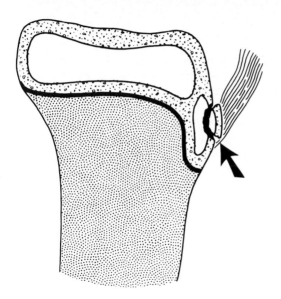

Fig. 19-29 Type 7 growth mechanism injury of the anterior tibial tuberosity. This is the Osgood-Schlatter lesion.

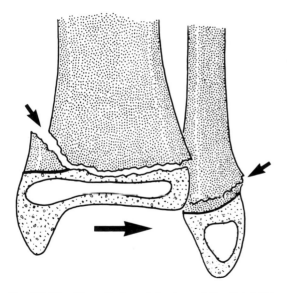

Fig. 19-30 Type 2 physeal fracture of the distal tibia combined with a metaphyseal fracture of the fibula.

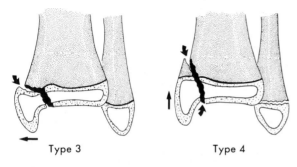

Type 3   Type 4

Fig. 19-31 Type 3 and 4 physeal fractures of the medial malleolus.

and may cause vascular and neural injury. Treatment initially should be closed reduction, although internal fixation may be necessary to stabilize the reduction. Exploration is indicated if the reduction does not improve the vascular status.

The tibial spines, especially the anterior one, may be avulsed along with the cruciate ligament (Fig. 19-27).[73] These represent ligament injury analogs in the child. If undisplaced, closed treatment is indicated. However, separation or delayed union of undisplaced fractures requires open reduction.

The tibial tuberosity presents unique problems (Fig. 19-28). The microscopic anatomy of the physeal region of the tibial tuberosity is specifically adapted to the tensile forces imparted by the pull of the quadriceps-patellar tendon mechanism. As such, direct avulsion of the tuberosity from the metaphysis is rare. If significant displacement occurs, open reduction and anatomic restoration is indicated.[46,100,104] Treatment should be directed toward soft tissue repair and metallic fixation.

The cause of Osgood-Schlatter's lesion has yet to be completely explained, but current anatomic and experimental studies suggest that the condition may represent an avulsion of portions of the patellar tendon and developing ossification center of the tibial tuberosity (Fig. 19-29), since this is a region that may more easily fail under tensile stress than the tuberosity physis itself.[85,93,99] Children with this injury generally respond to immobilization in a cylinder cast (for about 3 weeks) and a period of progressive rehabilitation of the quadriceps muscle.

Distal tibia

This region contributes approximately 20% of the overall length of the leg. Injuries may occur through a number of mechanisms: abduction, external rotation, adduction, plantar flexion, and axial compression (Fig. 19-30), resulting in a complex variety of fracture patterns.[25] Most of these injuries are type 2, with a variably sized metaphyseal fragment that may be quite large and spiral along the distal third of the tibial shaft. Less frequently, other types of injury may be present. The medial malleolus and a portion of the adjacent metaphysis may be separated as a type 3 or type 4 injury (Fig. 19-31). Comparably, the lateral portion of the distal epiphysis may be separated and may be displaced posteriorly or anteriorly as a type 3 injury (Fig. 19-32).[57] This may also be accompanied by a posterior or anterior metaphyseal fragment as a type 4 injury.

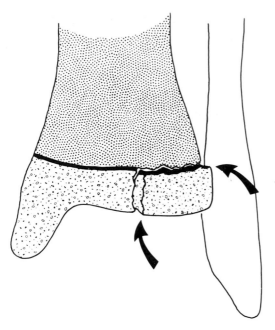

Fig. 19-32   Type 3 physeal fracture of the lateral side of the distal tibia. This is often referred to as the fracture of Tillaux.

The distal tibia is subjected to compression injuries more commonly than are the other epiphyses and physes. In any injury involving the distal tibial physis, possible compression injury must be considered, and the patient must be followed for an adequate period of time, since the effects of such injury may not be manifest for several years. Furthermore, injuries that appear to be primarily type 2 because of the twisting, compression mechanism that often causes the fracture, may also have areas of damage that would be more appropriately considered type 5.

Type 1 and type 2 injuries are treated with gentle closed manipulation under general anesthesia as early as possible after injury to minimize the effects of swelling that may compromise reduction efforts. Forceful manipulation to effect a reduction may cause compression injury to the physis and subsequent cessation or retardation of growth in portions of the physis. It is most important to try to correct varus and valgus angular deformities, although a valgus tilt of up to 15 degrees may be accepted. Angular deformity in the anteroposterior plane usually can be corrected by growth, since this is in the plane of motion of the joint. With type 3 and type 4 injuries the area should be opened and the damage repaired appropriately.[70]

In dealing with fractures involving the distal tibia, the orthopedist's most important role after initial treatment is to ensure adequate long-term follow-up. The physis may develop significant growth impairment, and it is imperative that such impairment be recognized as early as possible. If total growth arrest occurs, it may be necessary to epiphysiodese the distal fibula so that it will not overgrow and mechanically impair ankle function. When eccentric epiphysiodesis occurs, an osteotomy should be considered. An opening wedge osteotomy offers a better opportunity to regain some of the loss of leg length. If significant growth is still anticipated because of the child's age, epiphysiodesis of the remainder of the tibial physis and distal fibula also should be performed. Recognizing a limited epiphysiodesis early may allow removal of the osseous bridge.

Distal fibula

Injuries to the distal fibula may be isolated or may occur in conjunction with similar injuries to the distal tibia. Because the injury often causes minimal displacement of the epiphysis, diagnosis by routine radiologic methods is difficult. Stress views of the ankle sometimes can accentuate the injury. However, any injury with swelling and pain that localizes to the region of the distal fibular epiphysis and physis should be treated as a fracture. Often the only evidence is deposition of subperiosteal bone along the distal fibular metaphysis 2 to 3 weeks later.

Foot

Injuries involving the physis of the metatarsals and phalanges should be treated with closed reduction whenever possible. When closed reduction cannot be achieved, the types of fractures and specific treatment are analogous to treatment of similar injuries in the hand, and reference should be made to the section on injuries to the skeletal elements of the hand (see Chapter 21).

METAPHYSEAL AND DIAPHYSEAL (SHAFT) FRACTURES
Clavicle

Throughout the period of skeletal growth, fractures of the clavicle are the most frequent skeletal injuries.[19] The bone may be injured at birth because of shoulder compression or the use of forceps during delivery. Later the usual mechanism of injury

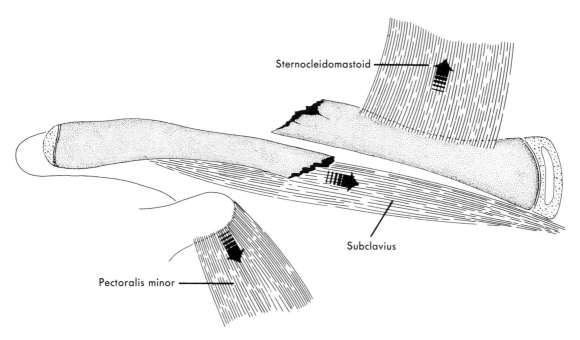

Sternocleidomastoid

Subclavius

Pectoralis minor

Fig. 19-33   Fracture of diaphysis of the clavicle. The various attached muscles become deforming forces.

is a fall, with the patient landing directly on the shoulder or outstretched arm.

The fracture involves the area between the middle and distal sections of the bone, at the distal curve; this area accounts for almost 90% of the fractures (Fig. 19-33). Younger children sustain a greenstick injury, whereas older children have a greater likelihood of complete and frequently comminuted fracture. In the younger group the fracture tends not to be displaced significantly. However, when the fracture is complete, the fragments are displaced. The attachment of the sternocleidomastoid muscle to the proximal fragment tends to pull it superiorly, whereas the pectoralis and subclavian muscles and the weight of the arm tend to pull the distal fragment inferiorly and cause some overriding of the fragments. Less frequently the distal third of the clavicle near the acromioclavicular joint is involved; such a fracture usually results from a direct blow to the shoulder. This fracture generally is transverse to the longitudinal axis of the clavicle and rarely is significantly displaced. The coracoclavicular ligaments in the child are quite strong and infrequently disrupted and thus contribute to the relative stability of the fracture.

The clinical diagnosis of clavicle fracture often is easy because of the pain and evident deformity.

However, fracture during infancy and early childhood may be accompanied by little pain or displacement and may become evident to the parents only after the exuberant callus characteristic of the fracture has formed. This prominent callus is disturbing to the parents, and it should be emphasized that it will disappear over 6 to 12 months as the bone remodels. Infants often are brought to the physician for failure to move the arm and shoulder, although the hand and forearm are functional. In such cases of pseudoparalysis, the roentgenogram demonstrates the cause.

Treatment can be accomplished by a sling in the small infant or a clavicle strap in the toddler. Since the fracture usually is incomplete (greenstick) and remodeling is relatively rapid in this age group, reduction is not necessary. The fracture usually heals sufficiently in 2 to 3 weeks to allow discontinuation of the immobilization. Treatment in older children should be dictated by the type of fracture. In general, greenstick fractures do not require reduction, whereas complete, overriding fractures require some reduction. Whereas the simple application of a clavicle strap may accomplish adequate alignment of fracture fragments immediately, the mild posterior displacement of the shoulders and adjustment of tension in the strap over 2 to 3 weeks may effect a gradual reduction. The parents can be instructed to adjust the tightness of the strap, but the physician should check it at intervals to ensure that undue pressure is not applied to the axillary regions, causing secondary neurovascular compromise. These children also should have the ipsilateral arm placed in a sling to minimize gravitational pull on the upper limb.

Humerus

In the proximal metaphysis/diaphysis region, two major types of injury are commonly encountered. Direct blows to the arm usually produce a transverse or comminuted fracture of the diaphysis or a torus (buckle) fracture of the proximal metaphysis (Fig. 19-34). This greenstick fracture is common. The fracture fragments are displaced contingent on the level of the fracture and associated muscle attachments that can act as deforming

forces. The major limiting muscle appears to be the deltoid. If the fracture occurs above the insertion of the deltoid, the pull tends to displace the distal fragment laterally and superiorly, whereas the proximal fragment is adducted and internally rotated by the combined effect of the pectoralis major, latissimus dorsi, and teres major muscles. In contrast, when the level of the fracture is below the insertion of the deltoid, this muscle, in combination with the rotator cuff musculature, pulls the proximal fragment into abduction and flexion, whereas the combined pull of the biceps and bra-

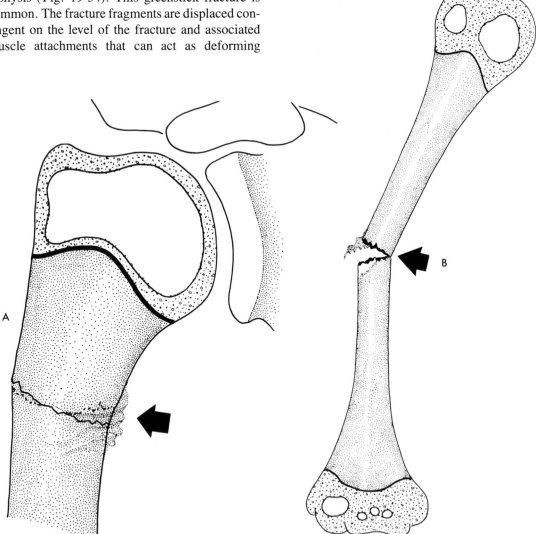

Fig. 19-34   **A,** Torus fracture of the proximal metaphysis of the humerus. **B,** Diaphyseal fracture of the humerus. The medial cortex *(arrow)* in young children may be intact (greenstick fracture).

chialis muscles pulls the distal fragment toward the shoulder, causing marked overriding.

Indirect trauma, such as a fall on an outstretched arm or a blow to the elbow, may transmit sufficient force into the humerus to create an oblique or greenstick fracture of the diaphysis or a torus fracture of the proximal metaphysis. These fractures are minimally displaced.

It is important to assess the possibility of associated neurovascular injury, particularly to the radial nerve, which has a close relationship to the humerus as it wraps around the musculospiral groove. Although paresthesias are relatively common, complete paralysis caused by severance of the nerve is uncommon in children, and nerve function almost always recovers with proper conservative management of the fracture.

Treatment should be dictated by the type of fracture and the presence of any associated injuries. When the fragments are markedly displaced, the initial step must be to attempt to reduce the fracture. This should include longitudinal traction to correct overriding and direct pressure over the deformed segments to bring them back into alignment. However, this approach may not be clinically stable and may result in recurrence of deformity. Overriding of approximately 1 to 1.5 cm usually is acceptable, although the patient's age must be considered. Length inequality is not as severe a problem as in the leg, but it may create a cosmetic problem. Of more importance is the correction of rotational and angular deformities and maintenance of normal longitudinal alignment (even if the overriding fragments are parallel). An angulation greater than 15 degrees to 20 degrees should not be accepted. If closed reduction can be accomplished, the child may be placed in a number of different immobilization devices. The child with a stable fracture may be placed in a sling and swathe or Velpeau stockinette shoulder device for 3 to 4 weeks and then started on an exercise program. The child with a potentially unstable fracture may be treated by a hanging cast or longitudinal plaster splints holding the elbow at 90 degrees. Roentgenograms should be taken after reduction to detect distraction of the fragments, which is not acceptable although much less likely to lead to nonunion than in an adult. The forearm should be left in neutral position. Unstable fractures and open fractures initially should be treated with skeletal traction. In the latter instance this allows observation and care of soft tissue injuries. When stable, one of the aforementioned devices may be used.

Supracondylar Humerus

Fractures involving the supracondylar region are some of the more common injuries in children (Fig. 19-35). They account for approximately 60% of elbow injuries in the 3- to 10-year-old range. Because of the anatomy of the region, acute neuro-

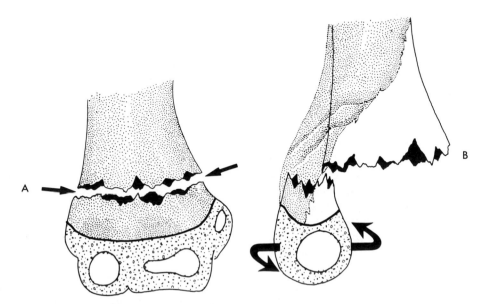

Fig. 19-35   **A,** Supracondylar fracture of the distal humerus. **B,** The distal fragment often rotates significantly.

vascular complications are a frequent accompaniment, and the problems of treatment in the first 2 to 3 weeks introduce a high probability of growth problems. The fracture line usually is at the epicondylar level and traverses both the coronoid and olecranon fossae. However, in many cases the fracture line may not be radiographically evident despite a clinical presentation that suggests skeletal injury. In such cases careful observation should be made for the "fat pad" sign on the lateral roentgenogram, since this may be the only definitive evidence of the fracture. This injury varies considerably with regard to the obliquity of the fracture line, the degree of comminution, the amount of rotational malalignment, and the direction of displacement of the distal fragment, although the distal fragment usually is displaced posteromedially. A significant number of supracondylar fractures are greenstick, with loss of the normal position of the condyles anterior to the longitudinal axis of the humerus and deviation into a varus position (plastic deformation). In evaluating any patient with a supracondylar injury, one of the most important aspects is an adequate assessment of the neurovascular status.[49] The brachial artery, in particular, is often damaged or placed in spasm by the displacement of the fragments.

Absolute anatomic reduction in the anteroposterior plane is not essential, as appositional overriding in this plane, being in the plane of normal joint motion, corrects with time through an active remodeling process.[5] However, two alignment problems must be corrected—malrotation and medial or lateral angulation. Rotational deformities do not correct spontaneously, but shoulder movements compensate reasonably well. However, this should not be used as an excuse not to correct malrotation as much as possible during reduction. Any lateral or medial tilting must be corrected, since it can easily lead to significant changes in the carrying angle of the elbow, which may require later corrective osteotomy.[28] When the fragments are moderately to severely displaced, reduction should be attempted with the child under general anesthesia; if successful, the child should be admitted for at least 12 to 24 hours of observation of the neurovascular status. If a stable reduction cannot be attained or if major neurovascular complications are present initially or after the reduction attempt, the child should be placed in skeletal traction, either overhead or side, with an olecranon pin or screw.[33] The pin should be inserted medial to lateral to pre-

vent damage to the ulnar nerve. Operative reduction may be accomplished acutely or several days later, when soft tissue swelling decreases.[20,39,40,106]

Circulatory injury is the most severe acute or chronic problem encountered in supracondylar fractures.[111] The arterial occlusion may occur through direct injury causing kinking or contusion (only rarely is the vessel lacerated, and this may be a subintimal tear), or through indirect compression as swelling in the fascial planes increases. The flexed position used during treatment may accentuate the occlusion. Several symptoms and signs help in diagnosing real or potential vascular problems. These signs are severe pain in the forearm or hand, numbness and coldness in the fingers, pallor and cyanosis of the fingers, inability to extend the fingers without great pain, and absence of the radial pulse. However, the absence of the radial pulse is not pathognomonic and may only indicate

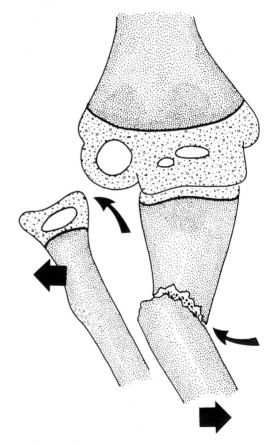

Fig. 19-36   Monteggia injury. This is a dislocation of the radial head accompanying a fracture of the ulna. Always look for this injury pattern when only the ulna appears injured on the radiograph.

vascular spasm. If the radial pulse is absent but the other signs also are absent and if capillary filling of the nailbeds is good, temporary occlusion is most likely. When major vascular compromise is detected, the first step is to reduce the fracture. If the vascular compromise appeared after reduction, less flexion should be used until the pulse is restored. When reduction fails to improve the status, open exploration is indicated. If untreated, vascular compromise can lead to Volkmann's ischemic contracture (as muscle infarction changes to muscle fibrosis and progressive flexion contracture), primarily of the flexor mass. Severe Volkmann's contracture may necessitate muscle excision or distal advancement.

Radius and Ulna

Fractures of the forearm bones are among the most common skeletal injuries in children; 75% of these fractures involve the distal third, 18% the middle third, and 7% the proximal third. It is not unusual for the fracture lines to involve different levels because of the differences in breaking strength of each bone at the same transverse level and because of the capacity of the interosseous membrane to transmit fracture forces. In many cases only one bone may be fractured. When such a diagnosis is made, great care must be taken to rule out a concomitant joint injury. Isolated fracture of the ulna may be accompanied by dislocation of the radiohumeral joint (Monteggia's injury) (Fig. 19-36), whereas isolated fracture of the radius may be accompanied by disruption of the distal radioulnar relationship (Galeazzi's injury).[6,16,74] Both bones may have a greenstick injury; however, it is not unusual to see one bone with a greenstick fracture and the other intact but with increasing bowing, or one bone with a greenstick fracture and the other completely fractured (Fig. 19-37). Again, this reflects differing mechanical responses of the two bones at any given transverse level.

Patterns of fracture differ with age and degree of skeletal maturation. A fall on the forearm, with the wrist dorsiflexed, probably will cause a torus or buckle fracture of the metaphysis in a 4 year old, a dorsally displaced radial fracture in a 7 year old, or a Salter epiphyseal displacement in a 9 year old.

Injuries to the proximal third usually are caused by direct blows on the elbow or upper forearm and frequently result in only one bone being fractured. When the proximal radial metaphysis is involved, significant angular deformity secondary to metaphyseal buckling may result and can severely impair normal radiohumeral and radioulnar interaction.[34,41] Gentle closed reduction with direct pres-

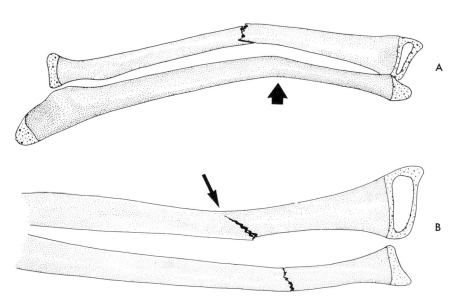

Fig. 19-37   **A,** Fracture of radius with bowing (plastic deformation) of the ulna. **B,** Fractures of radius and ulna. One is complete, whereas the other is greenstick *(arrow),* a relatively common combination.

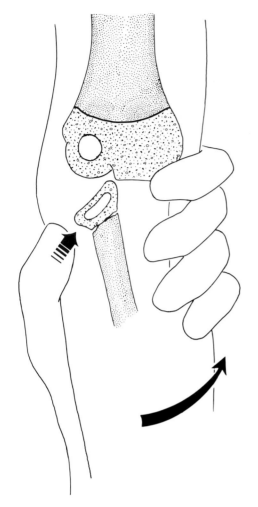

Fig. 19-38   Method of pushing the angulated metaphyseal fracture back into anatomic position.

sure over the radial head (Fig. 19-38) usually accomplishes reduction.[55,120] When the radial or ulnar fracture is a few centimeters distal to the elbow joint, the primary goal is correct alignment that avoids both rotational deformities of proximal and distal fragments and longitudinal malalignment causing narrowing of the interosseous space, the integrity of which is essential to restoration of supination and pronation.[22] Traditional teaching calls for immobilization in full supination. However, such a position may not always be necessary, and neutral may be just as stable and more conducive to healing with minimal rotational malalignment. Adequately spaced roentgenograms should be taken to follow any potential position changes while the area is casted.

Fractures of the middle third are among the most difficult to control. Injuries fall into two broad categories, undisplaced greenstick fractures and complete, displaced fractures. In the greenstick injury the bones are angulated, usually with the apex guided in the volar direction. If the bones are casted as is or after straightening, the likelihood of deformity recurrence is high (Fig. 19-39). An essential part of treatment may have to be gentle completion of the fracture by reversing the deformity. Usually the dorsal periosteum remains intact and aids in the stabilization. The arm should be placed in a long-arm cast in neutral or supination. When the fractures are complete and the fragments overriding, several problems must be corrected, including loss of length, rotational malalignment, and angular malalignment. Of the three, angular malalignment has the greatest potential for long-term functional impairment.[101] Some angulation toward the volar or dorsal surfaces can be accepted in the younger child. However, angulation of the

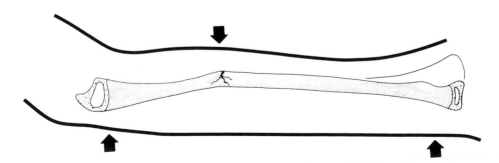

Fig. 19-39   Three-point pressure should be used to counter the plastic deformation of a greenstick injury.

fragments toward the interosseous space is unacceptable. Bayonet overriding is acceptable, providing both longitudinal and rotational deformities are corrected. If the fractures are not stable, repeat attempts at reduction can be made several days later, after swelling has subsided. If severe deformity is still present, two courses can be followed: The younger child can be placed in skeletal traction, and the older child, particularly the adolescent approaching skeletal maturity, can be treated by open reduction and plate fixation. However, such treatments should be reserved only for the most difficult cases, and every effort should be made to effect a closed reduction. When assessing reduction

attempts radiologically, comparison views of the opposite arm are essential. The forearm bones have gentle curves that can be deceiving, and these should be restored as much as possible.

The torus fracture of the distal third of the radius and of the ulna is one of the most common forearm fractures in children. The distal fragment usually is dorsally angulated, with the dorsal cortex buckled and the volar cortex reasonably intact. Manipulation usually is unnecessary, since angular deformity is not marked. A cast or splint should be applied for 3 weeks. True greenstick (not torus) fractures of the distal third must be reduced if more than 15 degrees to 20 degrees of angular deformity is present. This may involve complete reversal of the deformity during the manipulation. This fracture should be casted for 4 to 6 weeks.

The most difficult distal third fracture is the dorsally displaced radius and ulna (Fig. 19-40). Reduction requires good muscular relaxation and is

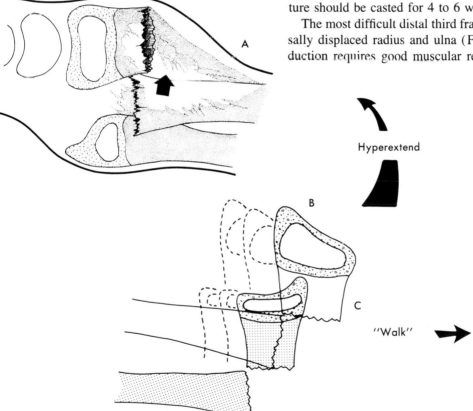

Fig. 19-40   A, Dorsally displaced fracture of distal radius. **B-D,** Method of reduction.

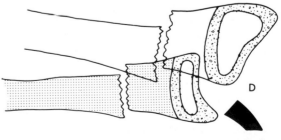

best accomplished under general anesthesia. The deformity is accentuated while traction is applied to the hand and direct pressure is applied to the distal fragment. The fragments are hooked together, and the hand is then brought down into palmar flexion. Although it is not necessary to completely restore anatomic position of the radial fragments, side-to-side aposition with maintenance of the complete dorsal displacement should be avoided. Keeping the hand in mild palmar flexion counterbalances the tendency of the distal fragment to angulate dorsally. However, if this causes any impingement of median nerve function, the flexion should be decreased. Neutral rotation is generally stable, although pronation may be more effective if only the radius is fractured.

Several factors aid in achieving the best outcome in forearm fractures. The cast should immobilize both the elbow and wrist initially, and it should be close fitting and adjusted as necessary to compensate for reduced swelling. Serial roentgenograms should be taken to detect any loss of position or reduction, as well as the accuracy of the initial reduction. The forearm should be immobilized in a position of rotation that maximizes stability and not necessarily in the classic textbook position. Greenstick fractures must be completed. The neurovascular status must be closely monitored. Volkmann's ischemia may occur in both bone forearm fractures and supracondylar fractures. Injury to the median nerve may occur in the dorsally displaced distal third fracture.

Femur

Other than acute separation of the capital femoral epiphysis, fractures involving the femoral neck are infrequent, accounting for approximately 20% of all femoral fractures in children.[56,59] Four basic types of femur fractures are recognized: type 1, transphyseal (acute slipped capital femoral epiphysis); type 2, transcervical (Fig. 19-41); type 3, cervicotrochanteric (base of the neck); and type 4, intertrochanteric. Type 2 and type 3 fractures are most common. A true femoral neck develops postnatally and gradually elongates as the child matures. Thus the chances of sustaining these fractures increases as skeletal maturity increases. It is important to realize that types 2 and 3, particularly, involve not only bone, which is easily evident on roentgenograms, but also hyaline and physeal cartilage, which is present along the superior and posterior femoral neck and which is essential to normal

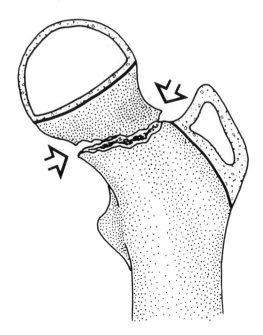

Fig. 19-41 Transcervical fracture of the femoral neck.

development of the femoral neck. This cartilage also is closely juxtaposed to the normal blood supply of the capital femoral epiphysis. The amount of epiphyseal cartilage along the femoral neck lessens with increasing skeletal maturation. In the first few years of life, when a significant amount of hyaline cartilage is present, type 2 and type 3 fractures are essentially analogous to type 4 physeal fractures and require the same sort of concise approach to reduction to minimize chances of subsequent growth deformities. In infants the proximal femur is one large mass of cartilage that is relatively resistant to injury. As such, fractures tend to go through the metaphyseal ("subtrochanteric") region. Such fractures, usually incurred during birth, mimic congenital hip dysplasia clinically and radiologically. However, irritability with movement of the hip should suggest trauma.

In contrast to the ease of fracture of the osteoporotic femur in the older patient, femoral neck injuries in children usually result from severe, direct trauma, and there is a high incidence of associated injury, especially to the thorax and abdomen.

The presence of a thick periosteum and cartilage along the femoral neck lessens the incidence of displacement. Many children do not have any external signs of deformity, compared with adults with a similar fracture, and roentgenography becomes essential to the diagnosis. However, because of the directional forces of various muscle groups, the structurally weak femoral neck that is initially minimally displaced gradually may be worsened to a significant varus deformity.

Categorical decisions regarding the best therapeutic approach should be discouraged. The orthopedist must consider the type of fracture; the plane or angle of the fracture line relative to joint reaction and muscle forces; the patient's age; the possibility of vascular damage, either from the original injury or the potential treatment method; and the disruption of the growth region along the femoral neck.

If the fracture is minimally or nondisplaced and stable to gentle manipulation, the patient may be placed in a hip spica. However, follow-up observation must be strict, since muscle spasm and even normal muscle forces may lead to a slowly progressive varus deformity. The child with any degree of displacement beyond minimal should be placed in traction, with the hip flexed to decrease intraarticular pressure caused by the intracapsular bleeding. Like fractures of the supracondylar humerus, these fractures often are best treated by open reduction and internal fixation, thus allowing reapproximation of neck cartilage and introducing an internal strut to minimize tensile stress along the superior femoral neck. Threaded pins can be used, but these should *not* cross the physis. If the level of the fracture dictates that the physis must be crossed, smooth pins should be used instead. Any varus deformity should be corrected by manipulation before pin placement.

Complications of these fractures are relatively common. Coxa vara should be prevented by appropriate observation and, when necessary, reduction and internal fixation.[52,109] Persistent varus deformity may predispose the femur to subsequent slipped capital femoral epiphysis. Delayed union, particularly if closed reduction and spica immobilization are employed, may occur because of the tendency to create the varus deformity. Normal muscular forces tend to place the femoral neck under tensile stress, delaying callus formation. Premature epiphysiodesis may also occur, especially if the fracture line is near the physis. Such closure may involve all or part of the physis. Because of the unique susceptibility of the blood supply of the femoral head, avascular necrosis may also supervene, although long after the initial injury. Finally, reactive hyperemia may cause femoral head and neck overgrowth, comparable to coxa magna of healing Legg-Calvé-Perthes disease.

Fractures of the femoral diaphysis and distal metaphysis are relatively common injuries in children, especially during the active summer months. They are usually a consequence of severe trauma (falls, automobile accidents) with the potential for multisystem involvement. With the exception of the first year of life, greenstick fractures are uncommon, since early weight-bearing stresses cause rapid remodeling and formation of harder osteon bone that tends to fracture completely. Approximately 70% of femoral fractures involve the middle third and 30% the distal third.

Two mechanisms and characteristic fractures are common. A direct blow, as by a car bumper, usually causes a transverse, displaced, and often comminuted fracture. A fall tends to cause an indirect torsional force that results in a spiral or oblique fracture, which has less tendency to override or to be displaced significantly (the periosteum usually is not as severely disrupted and creates some intrinsic stability). Displacement of the fragments is determined by the type of deforming force, the level of the fracture, and the muscles attached to the fragments. In general the distal femur and remainder of the leg are externally rotated. The quadriceps and hamstrings, which span the proximal and distal fragments, accentuate overriding of the fragments. If the fracture level is subtrochanteric, the proximal fragment tends to be flexed (iliopsoas), externally rotated (external rotator group), and abducted (glutei). The more distal the fracture level is, the more effective the adductor group becomes as an additional deforming force of the proximal fragment; when the fracture level is primarily above the adductor magnus insertions, the muscles accentuate overriding rather than adduction. In distal third fractures, the gastrocnemius may flex the knee. This can cause significant injury two ways. First, the proximal fragment tends to be anteriorly displaced into the intermedius and may cause muscle damage and scarring that eventually leads to decreased quadriceps excursion and may even require quadricepsplasty to improve function. Second, the posterior displacement of the distal fragment can lead to damage to the neurovascular bundle (femoral artery and sciatic nerve) and can cause vascular insufficiency syndromes (Volkmann's ischemia) even though the artery may not be completely severed.

The diagnosis of a femoral fracture usually is

made by observation, although an undisplaced fracture in a young child may not cause the characteristic deformity seen in most children. A presumptive diagnosis should be made before any diagnostic tests are undertaken, even roentgenographic studies. The child should be comfortably splinted in a Thomas splint as soon as possible. Any manipulation must be gentle to minimize triggering painful muscle spasms. An adequate assessment of the neurovascular status is mandatory. Once these steps are completed, the definitive diagnostic step, roentgenography, can be undertaken safely. Although rare, ipsilateral hip dislocation can occur, so roentgenograms must be taken of the entire femur. Since many of these fractures are associated with severe trauma, associated injuries should be sought. The thigh may easily accumulate significant amounts of blood. In general the child easily adapts to that degree of volume depletion, but if other injuries are present, such as a ruptured spleen, the child may quickly go into hypovolemic shock.

Treatment is dictated by a number of factors: the patient's age, associated injuries, local soft tissue damage, and the type of fracture.[18] As a rule, treatment should be directed to correction of length inequality, maintenance of normal femoral contours (the femur normally has an anterolateral bowing), and correction of rotation. The undisplaced fracture usually can be casted soon after injury. However, close observation is essential, since muscle spasm may cause sufficient displacement to require recasting.[30,51] Open reduction is not routinely applied for these fractures unless the patient is approaching skeletal maturity.[119]

Infants and children up to 2 years of age and not weighing more than 25 to 30 pounds may be treated by Bryant's traction. Skin traction is applied to both legs, with the knees in slight flexion and the malleoli well padded. The hips are flexed to 90 degrees, and the same amount of traction is applied to each leg. The total weight should be enough to just lift the buttocks and sacrum off the mattress. A chest restraint is helpful. The circulatory status must be closely and frequently observed, since various degrees of ischemia can supervene and create long-term problems. Any angular or rotational deformity should be corrected, as much as possible, by adjustment of traction.[120] Angulation in subtrochanteric fractures may require abduction of the traction; this should be done bilaterally, as in divarication for congenital hip disease. Traction adjustment every few days should be considered an integral part of the treatment; remodeling should not be relied on to correct the deformity. Stable callus usually forms rapidly in these small children, within 2 to 3 weeks, and allows early casting.

The treatment of older children and adolescents, unless a stable reduction can be attained by closed manipulation, should be one of several variations of traction: (1) skin traction in Russell's suspension, (2) skin traction with the leg extended on a Thomas splint placed at 30 degrees to 45 degrees, (3) skeletal traction with a Thomas splint and Pearson attachment, or (4) skeletal traction with 90-90 suspension. The choice should depend on the surgeon's experience, associated injuries, and the child's age. The older the child the more likely he or she will require skeletal traction. Pin placement for skeletal traction may be in either the proximal tibia or distal femur. In either case the pin should be at least 1 cm away from any physis. If a tibial pin is used, a short leg cast should also be applied to lessen the tendency for the pin to cut out anteriorly. Growth deformity caused by pin pressure has been reported; this is an unnecessary complication.[9] The pin's position and the degree of reduction should be checked after placement in trac-

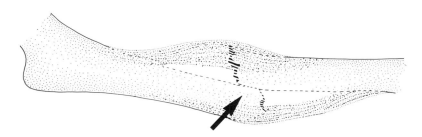

Fig. 19-42   Overriding does not prevent adequate healing and should be allowed in the 2- to 10-year range to counter the normal overgrowth response.

tion/suspension, and any adjustments undertaken. Frequent roentgenograms of the fracture allow further adjustment as indicated and show the progress of callus formation. When the fracture site is not tender and the femur can be moved comfortably as a unit, the child can be casted.

Complications of femoral shaft fractures can and should be avoided.[90] Rotation malalignment, because of the "universal" hip joint, can be more easily adapted to than a similar deformity in other bones. However, it may cause an asymmetric gait that is unacceptable to the parents and child. Adjustment of traction to correct rotational deformity is relatively easy and should be conducted on a daily basis if necessary. Angular deformities of 25 degrees or less probably will correct spontaneously, but the goal should be adjustment of traction to reproduce femoral bowing as much as possible. Persistent bowing accentuates length inequality and may cause later problems, such as slipped capital femoral epiphysis.[90] The major problem is inequality of leg length.[116,120] While 2 to 3 cm often is cited as an acceptable degree of overriding (Fig. 19-42), 1 cm is probably more realistic, and this only in the 2- to 10-year-old range. Children under 2 years of age and older than 10 years do not have the same propensity to reactive overgrowth and

may be left with a permanent deformity. Most length correction occurs during the first year after the fracture.[7,8] If a significant length inequality results, the child should be treated with an appropriate lift, observed for secondary deformity (scoliosis), and considered for well-leg epiphysiodesis at the appropriate time.

Knee

Fractures of the patella, when undisplaced, may be treated with an extension cast (Fig. 19-43). However, displacement requires open reduction. Thin pieces of bone, especially inferiorly, may indicate a sleeve fracture with avulsion of a large cartilaginous component. The bipartite patella may become symptomatic through a stress fracture.[95]

Tibia and Fibula

The patterns of fractures of the tibia and fibula are very much contingent on the child's age and the severity of the fracturing forces. The tibia undergoes major changes in its morphology, developing a thick cortex in the middle and distal thirds. This thick cortex becomes increasingly brittle and more susceptible to fracture, relative to the more resilient metaphyseal ends. However, the fibula does not form mature osteon bone and cortical

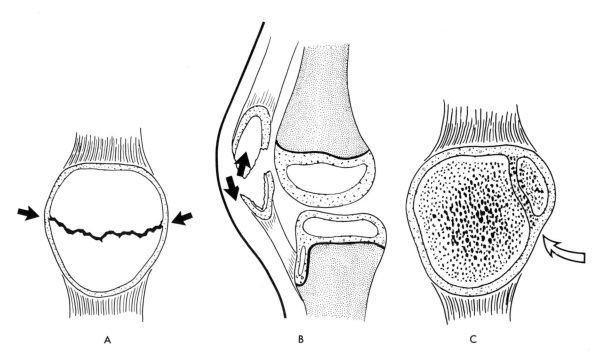

Fig. 19-43 **A,** Undisplaced patellar fracture. **B,** Displaced sleeve fracture of the patella. **C,** Bipartite patella.

thickening at the same rate and thereby maintains a resiliency that renders it less susceptible to fracture. In the child, approximately 30% of tibial fractures are associated with a fibular fracture. The high incidence of intact fibula, thick tibial periosteum, and interosseous membrane minimizes displacement of the tibial fragments, especially if the fracture line is oblique. Major displacement usually results from violent trauma (automobile accident). No matter what the patient's age, the most important concept to consider is that the tibia links two hinge joints with essentially parallel planes of movement. Varus, valgus, and rotational malalignment adversely affects the joint axis relationships and must be corrected.

In children up to 3 years of age, the usual injury is a spiral fracture of the tibial diaphysis, with an intact fibula. The mechanism is not always evident because of the child's inability to communicate. Such a communication difficulty also presents problems in localizing the injury. Manipulation of the foot may be more painful than palpation of the tibia, probably because of increased tension in muscles originating along the tibia. Fractures of the foot, especially in the young child, are uncommon, so the physician should always be suspicious of tibial injury in such circumstances. These fractures tend to be long, oblique disruptions with minimal displacement and overriding. The child should be treated with a long leg cast for 3 to 4 weeks.

From 3 to 6 years of age, coincident with a childhood growth spurt, the rapidly developing proximal tibia becomes more susceptible to injury. The fractures may result from direct violence, since this is a time of increased activity and exploration, or from torsional stresses. Fractures of the proximal tibial metaphysis are analogous to torsional fractures of the distal radius. Frequently the distal fragment has a valgus angulation, in association with an intact fibula (Fig. 19-44). This region seems to lack the complete remodeling potential of other metaphyses, and there is a tendency to maintain all or some of the valgus deformity, with the concomitant malalignment of the knee and ankle axes. An essential part of treatment must be the manipulative restoration of the normal longitudinal axis, followed by immobilization in a long leg cast. Manipulation may necessitate completing a greenstick fracture or even overcorrecting it, but if this is not done, the deformity may gradually recur, even in the cast. The child must not walk in the cast. This growth period is associated with the normal shift

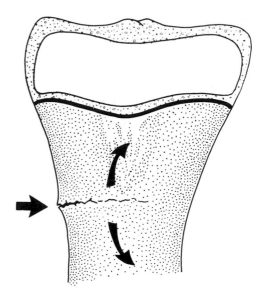

Fig. 19-44   Typical incomplete fracture of proximal tibial metaphysis. This fracture has a significant potential to overgrow medially, leading to *progressive* tibia valgum.

from varus to neutral or valgus posturing at the knee. Adequate long-term follow-up is mandatory because a significant potential complication is asymmetric overgrowth of the medial side of the physis, leading to genu valgum.[53,89] Bracing may prevent or correct the deformity. Severe malalignment may require corrective osteotomy, which should include fibular osteotomy.[113]

Older children, because of increasing thickness and hardness of the cortices of the middle and distal thirds of the tibia, are more prone to injury in this region. Because of increasing activity levels, these fractures have a greater tendency to be caused by violent trauma and to be compound. As the child grows, there is a greater likelihood of concomitant fibular fracture. Treatment should consist of closed manipulative reduction to correct both longitudinal and rotational deformity and any significant overriding. One centimeter of overriding should be the maximal accepted. The initial cast should be long leg, with a shift to a patellar–weight bearing cast after 3 to 4 weeks. These fractures usually heal in 6 to 8 weeks but may take longer in the adolescent approaching skeletal maturity. Long-term follow-up should assess both leg length equality and angular deformity at the fracture site and the metaphysis. A few cases have been described in which diaphyseal fractures, because of the direction of the deforming forces, caused concomitant damage to the proximal physis (type 5 injury), which may take many months to years to manifest.

Foot

Fractures of the tarsal and longitudinal bones of the feet are unusual in children. The tarsal bones, in particular, have a large cartilage component surrounding a central osseous portion. Undoubtedly this allows better resistance to forces that might otherwise produce a fracture in the mature skeleton. Most fractures result from direct, crushing injuries and are accompanied by significant soft tissue swelling. Because of this edema, it is wise to treat initially with elevation and a bulky compression dressing and to apply the appropriate cast only after swelling has subsided sufficiently. Although small portions of the tarsal and metatarsal bones may be fractures, great care must be taken to ascertain whether an apparent fracture is really one of a multitude of accessory bones.[63]

The talus most commonly is fractured through the neck, but significant displacement is rare.[102] Unlike with the comparable fracture in the adult, avascular necrosis rarely supervenes. Fractures of the calcaneus rarely involve the subtalar joint and usually are located between the subtalar joint and calcaneal apophysis, the region analogous to the metaphysis of a long bone.[71] Again, major displacement is uncommon. Metatarsal and phalangeal fractures are the most common foot injuries in children, and most can be treated by closed reduction. The eccentrically placed apophysis of the base of the fifth metatarsal should not be confused with a fracture line. The foot skeleton matures before the major long bones and thus may be subject to "adult" types of fractures in early adolescence.

DISLOCATIONS

Compared with adults, children infrequently sustain joint dislocations. Two factors seem to contribute to this difference of response. First, young children in general have more joint motion or capsular and ligamentous laxity. This hypermobility decreases as the child approaches skeletal maturity, making the growing child increasingly more susceptible to joint dislocations. In certain pathologic states, such as Down's syndrome and Ehlers-Danlos syndrome, the hyperlaxity is excessive, and joint subluxation and dislocation are relatively common. Second, the articular ligaments in a child

are strong and better able to withstand tensile stress than the adjacent physis. Thus instead of a joint dislocation or ligamentous tear, a child is more likely to sustain an epiphyseal fracture. Most ligaments and joint capsules insert into the epiphysis rather than into the metaphysis, which increases the likelihood of epiphyseal fracture. This is more evident in the knee, where the medial and lateral collateral ligaments insert into the distal femoral epiphysis and into the proximal tibial metaphysis. The proximal tibial epiphysis is comparatively free of ligamentous insertions. Injury to the distal femoral epiphysis is common, whereas injury to the proximal tibial epiphysis is rare. Generally, if a child has a swollen joint as a result of trauma, a fracture is more likely than a joint injury. When treating joint dislocations in children, early mobilization is not a factor because joint stiffness in children is rare, even after prolonged immobilization.

Upper Extremity

With the exception of the elbow, dislocations of the upper extremity are rare. As previously discussed, a dislocation of the sternoclavicular joint usually is an epiphyseal fracture. The acromioclavicular joint is strong, and a force that might cause conoid/trapezoid ligament rupture in an adult instead pulls the periosteum away with the ligaments. Subperiosteal new bone and remodeling rapidly occur, minimizing the likelihood of chronic acromioclavicular instability. Injuries that normally would produce a dislocated shoulder in a young adult instead usually are associated with a physeal fracture of the proximal humerus. Disruption of the distal radioulnar joint and wrist dislocations are rare.

In contrast to the aforementioned areas, elbow dislocations are more common in children than in adults and probably represent the most common dislocation of youth (Fig. 19-45). The radiohumeral joint may be dislocated in association with an ulnar fracture (Monteggia's injury).[6] Such a dislocation may occur without an ulnar fracture, although the ulna may be excessively bowed.[6,16,89] When only the radial head is dislocated, an osteochondral fragment may be knocked from the capitellum. This may effectively block reduction. Most commonly the elbow is subjected to a posterolateral dislocation (that is, the olecranon portion of the ulna is displaced posterolaterally), and the coronoid process may "lock" into the olecranon fossa of the distal humerus.

Dislocations often are accompanied by osseous

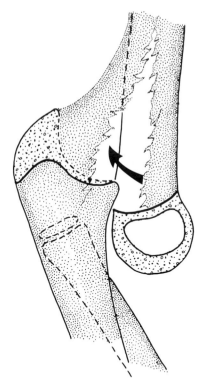

Fig. 19-45 Dislocated elbow with characteristic stripping of the posterior humeral periosteum.

injuries, especially osteochondral fragments, avulsion of the coronoid process, or fracture of the medial epicondyle. These osseous fragments may mechanically impede reduction. To reduce the dislocation, traction should be applied with the elbow extended but not hyperextended. Roentgenograms are essential after the reduction to evaluate small fractures and intraarticular fragments. Recurrent dislocation may affect the radiohumeral joint and is best treated by lateral capsular reinforcement.

The most common elbow injury in the young child up to 5 years of age is pulled elbow ("nursemaid's" elbow).[24,72] This results from excessive pull on an arm that is extended at the elbow and held in pronation. The child holds the forearm in pronation and resists supination. The annular ligament is loosely attached to the periosteum in this age group and may be avulsed enough to allow a portion of the radial head to subluxate into the tear or to allow a portion of the ligament to snap over the radial head (onto the articular surface).[115] Reduction is simple (Fig. 19-46). The physician places a thumb over the radial head and applies direct pressure while simultaneously rapidly supinating the forearm. Frequently a distinct click is felt, and the child immediately allows full supination and pronation. The arm should be immobilized in a sling for a few days until the child begins using the elbow spontaneously.

Dislocations of the hand, especially the interphalangeal joints, are common.[67] Diagnosis and treatment are discussed in Chapter 21.

Lower Extremity

As with the upper extremities, dislocations of the lower extremities are unusual in children. Dislocations of the joints of the foot (for example, Lisfranc's dislocation) usually result from severe, direct trauma. Ankle dislocations are rare, distal tibial epiphyseal separation being the usual injury

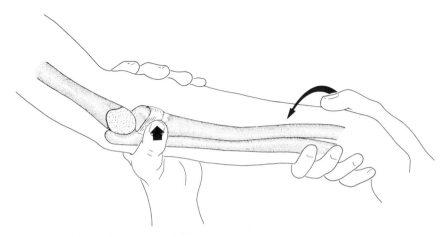

Fig. 19-46 Method of rapid supination with the thumb over the radial head to reduce the annular ligament to its normal position in a "nursemaid's elbow".

when the ankle is subjected to significant trauma. The most common joint disruptions in a child's lower extremities are subluxation and dislocation of the patella and dislocation of the hip.

Injuries to the hip joint are infrequent. Dislocation usually is posterior and, surprisingly, may result from seemingly minor trauma. Coincident damage to the acetabulum is less frequent than in adults, since the acetabular labrum is quite resilient, being composed of both hyaline and fibrocartilage. Closed reduction should be undertaken as soon as possible, since delay beyond 24 hours seems to predispose to avascular necrosis of the femoral head, especially in older children.[103] If possible the child should be kept non–weight bearing. Ischemia (avascular necrosis) is the most problematic complication.[45]

Dislocation of the knee is a problem primarily of adolescent athletes, and it may occur in any direction. The dislocation should be reduced promptly and any associated osseous or neurovascular injuries should be thoroughly evaluated. Damage to the popliteal artery is not uncommon and may require vascular reconstruction. The peroneal nerve is most commonly injured but is rarely disrupted, so immediate exploration is seldom indicated. Repair of ligaments should be reserved until the knee has been reduced and immobilized for several weeks. Many times stability is surprisingly good, and open repair is not necessary.

The normal laxity in the child may be a predisposing factor in subluxation or dislocation of the proximal fibula from the tibiofibular joint.[79] Closed reduction usually is successful in children.[78]

Dislocation of the patella is a complex problem. Acute dislocation laterally is a relatively common injury that is easily reduced; it must be immobilized for 3 to 4 weeks and followed by an aggressive quadriceps rebuilding program to minimize recurrent instability and potential redislocation. Care must be taken to evaluate possible osteochondral fragments. Recurrent subluxation of the patella is common, especially in young girls. It probably does not relate directly to acute trauma and is not discussed here.

ATHLETIC INJURIES IN THE CHILD

The times of maturation of the female and male skeletal systems coincide with periods of increased athletic activity, especially through the aegis of organized team sports.[2,80] The physician dealing with children participating in such sports must consider the variation in growth maturity and coordination of the musculoskeletal system, both during the preparticipation physical examination and in the treatment of specific injuries, particularly with regard to allowing the resumption of competition. It is essential that any abnormalities of skeletal development, whether localized or generalized, and any chronic disorders be evaluated on an individual basis that considers those activities that can be safely tolerated in view of the musculoskeletal problem(s). Certain types of injuries may effectively preclude participation in some sports but not others. As is discussed later in this section, "little league elbow" is essentially a disorder affecting a preadolescent pitcher. Simply putting the youngster in a fielding position or decreasing the amount of pitching may allow him or her to continue playing.[1,14,118]

Athletic trauma, whether incurred during organized or recreational sports, usually has a recognizable cause. The most important factors are the following:

1. *Conditioning*—The young athlete must learn the fundamentals of both a specific sport and generalized physical conditioning. Thus injury most commonly affects the novice participant in the early parts of the season. However, as the young athlete develops coordination, confidence, and experience, he or she lessens the risk of injury. It is recognized that ligament strength increases with conditioning. This is undoubtedly important in the older adolescent, but it may not be as crucial a factor in the younger child, since the physis and metaphysis, rather than the ligaments, appear to be the weakest areas.

2. *Endurance*—With continued physical conditioning and increased familiarity with the specific demands of the sport (learning to pace onself), the athlete becomes less susceptible to injury. Fatigue is an important predisposing factor.

3. *Antecedent injury*—Failure to diagnose and treat minor trauma can culminate in serious injury later. For example, repetitive, unprotected ankle "sprains" in a young gymnast can lead to a serious inversion injury with complete ligamentous disruption and the need for surgical reconstruction.

4. *Adherence to rules*—Many injuries are incurred during rule infractions, such as not wearing required protective equipment. It is the physician's responsibility to see that equipment rules in particular are strictly enforced.

Injuries to the musculoskeletal system involving the young athlete appear to be much less prevalent than in the older athlete, particularly when ligamentous injuries are considered. Larson[62] reported on a series of 4854 athletic injuries, of which 933 (19%) occurred in children under 15 years of age, even though that particular group represented the greatest number of participants in organized athletic programs. Selective examination of tackle football programs in this study showed the injury rate for the junior high school group was 11%, whereas the injury rate for the high school group was 33%. Similar differences were seen in other sports activities (basketball, baseball, track, gymnastics, wrestling, and cross-country); in these instances the junior high school students had an injury incidence of 2%, whereas the high school students had an injury incidence of 12%.

Most incidents of trauma in athletes involve localized soft tissue injury—contusion, abrasion, laceration, muscle, and tendon injury rather than skeletal injury. Certain sports seem to have prevalent injury patterns. Ice hockey, for example, is associated with a high incidence of cranial and facial trauma, a fact that underscores the need to wear protective headgear. Injuries to the low back are relatively common. These usually involve soft tissue inflammation and manifest as a loss of lumbar lordosis as a result of paravertebral muscular spasm. There appears to be an increase in discrete skeletal trauma to the low back in certain sports characterized by repetitive spinal stresses. Thus spondylolysis and spondylolisthesis are often seen in gymnasts and figure skaters.

One of the more common problems affecting the adolescent athlete has been called "epiphysitis" or "apophysitis."[62] These terms are used to describe inflammatory reactions involving the ligament or tendon insertions into an epiphysis primarily affected by tensile forces (for example, the ischial tuberosity, tibial tuberosity, and medial epicondyle of the distal humerus). The most publicized example is "little league elbow," a title that stems from the mechanism by which the inflammation is derived. Excessive duration of throwing or attempts to throw a curve ball with an immature elbow cause the elbow to be brought rapidly from acute flexion to forced extension with a supinated forearm. This causes excessive increase in muscular strain within the flexor-pronator muscle group and manifests as increased force at the medial epicondyle of the distal humerus. Similarly, compressive stresses can lead to damage of the proximal radial epiphysis or capitulum (osteochondrosis). Because of the hypervascularity associated with normal repair, these areas may be sites of excessive growth, causing either a cubitus valgus or cubitus varus deformity. Furthermore, when the capitulum is involved, there sometimes is fragmentation of the articular surface and creation of loose bodies within the joint. Limiting the amount of pitching to some degree probably would affect the incidence of these problems. A similar sort of problem occurs in young children who play intensive competitive tennis, in which the mechanism of the serve duplicates that of throwing a baseball. In the lower extremity the insertion of the Achilles tendon into the epiphysis of the os calcis sometimes can lead to apophysitis known as Sever's disease. This condition is best treated by rest and sometimes may benefit from the use of heel cups. The most frequent affected area in the lower limb is the tibial tuberosity, where the Osgood-Schlatter's lesion becomes manifest. Recent anatomic and experimental studies suggest that this lesion represents a chronic microavulsion of small portions of the patellar tendon from the tibial tuberosity as the ossification center is forming. This leads to formation of osseocartilaginous tissue and of a prominent deformity on the anterior tibia that may elevate the patellar tendon and patella enough to affect mechanical function along the patellofemoral axis. This condition also is best treated by rest and may require immobilization in a cylinder cast for 3 to 4 weeks. Around the pelvis the attachments of the rectus femoris to the anteroinferior iliac spine, the psoas to the lesser trochanter, and the hamstrings to the ischial tuberosity are areas of potential apophysitis and areas that can be completely avulsed because of excessive severe muscle contracture.

Epiphyseal fractures, although common in children, do not appear to be more frequent as athletic injuries. Although such fractures usually heal within 3 to 4 weeks, depending on the type, and are much stronger than healing fractures in the metaphysis or diaphysis during early phases of repair, return to athletic participation must be individualized with regard to the patient's overall ability, assessment of any damage to joint function (particularly when a type 3 or type 4 injury is involved), and appreciation of the sport's particular musculoskeletal demands. When the epiphyseal fracture involves a joint, it is recommended that the child abstain from contact sports for at least a year and that sports such as swimming, which allow joint exercise with lessened weight-bearing stresses, be emphasized.

Stress fractures are less common in children than in adults.[32] However, recognition and treatment follow similar parameters. Progressive conditioning in running sports is helpful in reducing the incidence of shin splints, a phenomenon becoming more common in young children and adolescents with the increasing emphasis on jogging.

REFERENCES

1. Adams J: Injuries to the throwing arm: a study of traumatic changes in the elbow joint of boy baseball players, Calif Med 102:127, 1965.
2. Adams J: Bone injuries in very young athletes, Clin Orthop 58:129, 1968.
3. Aitken A: Fractures of the proximal humeral epiphysis, Surg Clin North Am 43:1573, 1963.
4. Arunachalam V and Griffins J: Fracture recurrence in children, Injury 7:37, 1975.
5. Attenborough CG: Remodelling of the humerus after supracondylar fracture in childhood, J Bone Joint Surg 35B:386, 1953.
6. Bado J: The Monteggia lesion, Clin Orthop 50:71, 1967.
7. Barfod B and Christensen J: Fractures of the femoral shaft in children with special reference to subsequent overgrowth, Acta Chir Scand 116:235, 1959.
8. Bisgard J: Longitudinal overgrowth of long bones with special reference to fractures, Surg Gynecol Obstet 62:823, 1936.
9. Bjerkreim I and Benum P: Genu recurvatum: a late complication of tibial wire traction in fractures of the femur in children, Acta Orthop Scand 46:1012, 1975.
10. Bode W, Lefebvre A, and Rosman M: Fractures of the medial humeral epicondyle in children, Can J Surg 18:137, 1975.
11. Borden S: Traumatic bowing of the forearm in children, J Bone Joint Surg 56A:611, 1974.
12. Bragdon R: Fractures of the distal radial epiphysis, Clin Orthop 41:59, 1965.
13. Bright R: Operative correction of partial epiphyseal plate closure by osseous bridge resection and silicone-rubber implant, J Bone Joint Surg 56A:655, 1974.
14. Brogdon M: Little leaguer's elbows, Am J Roent 83:671, 1960.
15. Brooks A and Henning G: Injury to the proximal clavicular epiphysis, J Bone Joint Surg 54A:1347, 1972.
16. Bruce H, Harvey J, and Wilson J: Monteggia fractures, J Bone Joint Surg 56A:1563, 1974.
17. Bucholz RW, Ezaki M, and Ogden JA: Injury to the acetabular triradiate physeal cartilage, J Bone Joint Surg 64A:600, 1982.
18. Burton V and Fordyce A: Immobilization of femoral shaft fractures in children age 2-10 years, Injury 4:47, 1973.
19. Calandi C and Bartolozzi G: On 110 cases of fracture of the clavicle in the newborn, Riv Clin Pediatr 64:541, 1969.
20. Carcassone M, Bergoin M, and Hornung H: Results of operative treatment of severe supracondylar fractures of the elbow in children, J Pediatr Surg 7:676, 1972.
21. Cassenbaum W and Patterson A: Fractures of the distal femoral epiphysis, Clin Orthop 41:79, 1965.
22. Christensen J, Cho K, and Adams J: A study of the interosseous distance between the radius and ulna during rotation of the forearm, J Bone Joint Surg 46B:778, 1964.
23. Conner A and Smith M: Displaced fractures of the lateral humeral condyle in children, J Bone Joint Surg 52B:460, 1970.
24. Corrigan A: The pulled elbow, Med J Aust 2:187, 1965.
25. Crenshaw A: Injuries to the distal tibial epiphysis, Clin Orthop 41:98, 1965.
26. Crilly R: Longitudinal overgrowth of the chicken radius, J Anat 112:11, 1972.
27. Curry J and Butler G: The mechanical properties of bone tissue in children, J Bone Joint Surg 57A:810, 1975.
28. D'Ambrosia R: Supracondylar fractures of the humerus— prevention of cubitus varus, J Bone Joint Surg 54A:60, 1972.
29. Dameron T and Reibel D: Fractures involving the proximal humeral epiphyseal plate, J Bone Joint Surg 51A:289, 1969.
30. Dameron T and Thompson H: Femoral shaft fractures in children. Treatment by closed reduction and double spica cast immobilization, J Bone Joint Surg 41A:1201, 1959.
31. Denham R and Dingley A: Epiphyseal separation of the medial end of the clavicle, J Bone Joint Surg 49A:1179, 1967.
32. Devas M: Stress fractures in children, J Bone Joint Surg 45B:528, 1963.
33. Dodge H: Displaced supracondylar fractures of the humerus in children—treatment by Dunlop's traction, J Bone Joint Surg 54A:1408, 1972.
34. Dougall A: Severe fractures of the neck of the radius in children, JR Coll Surg Edinb 14:220, 1969.
35. Fahey J and O'Brien E: Fracture separation of the medial humeral condyle in a child confused with fracture of the medial epicondyle, J Bone Joint Surg 53A:1102, 1971.
36. Feil E, Bentley G, and Rizza C: Fracture management in patients with haemophilia, J Bone Joint Surg 56B:643, 1974.
37. Fielding J: Radio-ulnar crossed union following displacement of the proximal radial epiphysis, J Bone Joint Surg 46A:1277, 1964.
38. Flynn J and Richards J: Non-union of minimally displaced fractures of the lateral condyle of the humerus in children, J Bone Joint Surg 53A:1096, 1971.
39. Flynn J, Matthews J, and Benoit R: Blind pinning of displaced supracondylar fractures of the humerus in children, J Bone Joint Surg 56A:263, 1974.
40. Fowles J and Kassab M: Displaced supracondylar fractures of the elbow in children. A report on the fixation of extension and flexion fractures by two lateral percutaneous pins, J Bone Joint Surg 56B:490, 1974.
41. Gandhi R, Wilson P, and Mason Brown J: Spontaneous correction of deformity following fractures of the forearm in children, Br J Surg 50:5, 1962.
42. Grantham S and Kiernan H: Displaced olecranon fracture in children, J Trauma 15:197, 1975.
43. Grogan DP and Ogden JA: Thurstan-Holland fragment, J Bone Joint Surg 67A:980, 1985 (letter to the editor).

44. Grogan DP and Ogden JA: Differentiating lateral condylar from transepiphyseal fractures: pediatric elbow fractures need not be your nemesis, J Musculoskeletal Med 3:64, 1986.

45. Haliburton R, Brockenshire F, and Barber J: Avascular necrosis of the femoral capital epiphysis after traumatic dislocation of the hip in children, J Bone Joint Surg 43B:43, 1961.

46. Hand W, Hand C, and Dunn A: Avulsion fractures of the tibial tubercle, J Bone Joint Surg 53A:1579, 1971.

47. Holland CT: Radiographical note on injuries to the distal epiphyses of radius and ulna, Proc Roy Soc Med 22:695, 1929.

48. Holst-Nielson F and Ottsen P: Fractures of the lateral condyle of the humerus in children, Acta Orthop Scand 45:518, 1974.

49. Hordegen K: Neurologic complications of supracondylar humeral fractures in children, Arch Orthop Unfall 68:294, 1970.

50. Howard and Piha R: Fractures of the apophyses in adolescent athletes, JAMA 192:842, 1965.

51. Irani R, Nicholson J, and Chung S: Treatment of femoral fractures in children by immediate spica immobilization, J Bone Joint Surg 52A:1567, 1972.

52. Ireland D and Fisher R: Subtrochanteric fractures of the femur in children, Clin Orthop 110:157, 1975.

53. Jackson D and Cozen L: Genu valgum as a complication of proximal tibial metaphyseal fractures in children, J Bone Joint Surg 53A:1571, 1971.

54. Jakob R, Fowles J, and Rang M: Observations concerning fractures of the lateral humeral condyle in children, J Bone Joint Surg 57B:430, 1975.

55. Jones E and Esah M: Displaced fractures of the neck of the radius in children, J Bone Joint Surg 53B:429, 1971.

56. Kay S and Hall J: Fracture of the femoral neck in children and its complications, Clin Orthop 80:53, 1971.

57. Kleiger B and Mankin H: Fracture of the lateral portion of the distal tibial epiphysis, J Bone Joint Surg 46A:25, 1964.

58. Lagier R and Jarret G: Apophysiolysis of the anterior inferior iliac spine. A histological, clinical and radiological study, Acta Orthop Unfall 83:81, 1975.

59. Lam S: Fractures of the neck of the femur in children, J Bone Joint Surg 53A:1165, 1971.

60. Langenskiold A: An operation for partial closure of the epiphyseal plate in children and its experimental basis, J Bone Joint Surg 57B:325, 1975.

61. Larson B, Light TR, and Ogden JA: Nonunion and ischemic necrosis of the ossifying scaphoid, J Hand Surg 12A:122, 1987.

62. Larson R: Epiphyseal injuries in the adolescent athlete, Orthop Clin North Am 4:839, 1973.

63. Lawson JP et al: The painful accessory navicular, Skeletal Radiol 12:250, 1984.

64. Lawson JP et al: Physeal (end-plate) injuries of the cervical spine, J Pediatr Orthop 7:428, 1987.

65. Light TR, Ogden DA, and Ogden JA: The anatomy of metaphyseal torus fractures, Clin Orthop 188:103, 1984.

66. Light TR and Ogden JA: Metacarpal epiphyseal fractures, J Hand Surg 12A:460, 1987.

67. Light TR and Ogden JA: Complex dislocation of the index metacarpophalangeal joint in children, J Pediatr Orthop 8:300, 1988.

68. Lindseth R and DeRosa G: Fractures in children. General considerations and treatment of open fractures, Pediatr Clin North Am 22:465, 1975.

69. Love SM, Grogan DP, and Ogden JA: Lawn mower injuries in children, J Orthop Trauma 2:94, 1988.

70. Lynn M: The triplane distal epiphyseal fracture, Clin Orthop 86:187, 1972.

71. Matteri R and Frymoyer J: Fracture of the calcaneus in young children, J Bone Joint Surg 55A:1091, 1973.

72. McRae R and Freeman P: The lesion in pulled elbow, J Bone Joint Surg 47A:808, 1965.

73. Meyers M and McKeever F: Fracture of the intercondylar eminence, J Bone Joint Surg 41A:209, 1959.

74. Mikic Z: Galeazzi fracture-dislocations, J Bone Joint Surg 57A:1071, 1975.

75. Neer C and Horwitz B: Fracture of the proximal humeral epiphyseal plate, Clin Orthop 41:24, 1965.

76. Newell R: Olecranon fractures in children, Injury 7:33, 1975.

77. Nonnemann H: Grenzen der Spontankorrektur fehlgeleilter Frakturen bei Jugendlichen, Langenbecks Arch Chir 324:78, 1969.

78. Ogden JA: Dislocation of the proximal fibula, Radiology 105:547, 1972.

79. Ogden JA: Subluxation and dislocation of the proximal tibiofibular joint, J Bone Joint Surg 56A:145, 1974.

80. Ogden JA: The role of orthopaedic surgery in sports medicine, Yale J Biol Med 53:281, 1980.

81. Ogden JA: Injury to the growth mechanism of the immature skeleton, Skeletal Radiol 6:237, 1981.

82. Ogden JA: Skeletal growth mechanism injury patterns, J Pediatr Orthop 2:371, 1982.

83. Ogden JA: Growth slowdown and arrest lines, J Pediatr Orthop 4:409, 1984.

84. Ogden JA: Distal clavicular physeal injury, Clin Orthop 188:68, 1984.

85. Ogden JA: The uniqueness of growing bones. In Rockwood CA Jr, Wilkins KE, and King RE, editors: Fractures, vol 3: children, Philadelphia, 1984, JB Lippincott Co.

86. Ogden JA: Pocket guide to pediatric fractures, Baltimore, 1987, Williams and Wilkins, Inc.

87. Ogden JA: Current concepts review: the evaluation and treatment of partial physeal arrrest, J Bone Joint Surg 69A:1297, 1987.

88. Ogden JA: Skeletal growth mechanism injury patterns. In Uhthoff HK and Wiley JJ, editors: Behavior of the growth plate, New York, 1988, Raven Press.

89. Ogden JA: Skeletal injury in the child, ed 2, Philadelphia, WB Saunders Co (in press).

90. Ogden J, Gossling H, and Southwick W: Slipped capital femoral epiphysis following ipsilateral femoral fracture, Clin Orthop 110:167, 1975.

91. Ogden JA and Grogan DP: Prenatal skeletal development and growth of the musculoskeletal system. In Albright JA and Brand RA, editors: The scientific basis of orthopaedics, ed 2, New York, 1987, Appleton & Lange.

92. Ogden JA, Grogan DP, and Light TR: Postnatal skeletal development and growth of the musculoskeletal system. In Albright JA and Brand RA, editors: The scientific basis of orthopaedics, ed 2, New York, 1987, Appleton & Lange.

93. Ogden JA, Hempton R, and Southwick W: Development of the tibial tuberosity, Anat Rec 182:431, 1975.

94. Ogden JA et al: Proximal femoral epiphysiolysis in the neonate, J Pediatr Orthop 4:285, 1984.
95. Ogden JA, McCarthy SM, and Jokl P: The painful bipartite patella, J Pediatr Orthop 2:263, 1982.
96. Ogden JA and Ogden DA: Skeletal metastasis: the effect on the immature skeleton, Skeletal Radiol 9:73, 1982.
97. Ogden JA et al: Ectopic bone secondary to avulsion of periosteum, Skeletal Radiol 4:124, 1979.
98. Ogden JA and Southwick W: Adequate reduction of fractures and dislocations, Radiol Clin North Am 11:667, 1973.
99. Ogden JA and Southwick W: Osgood-Schlatter's disease and tibial tuberosity development, Clin Orthop 116:180,1976.
100. Ogden JA, Tross RB, and Murphy MJ: Fractures of the tibial tuberosity in adolescents, J Bone Joint Surg 62A:205, 1980.
101. Onne L and Sandblom P: Late results in fractures of the forearm in children, Acta Chir Scand 98:549, 1949.
102. Pathi K: Fracture neck of talus in children, J Indian Med Assoc 63:157, 1974.
103. Pennsylvania Orthopaedic Society: Traumatic dislocation of the hip in children, J Bone Joint Surg 50A:79, 1968
104. Polakoff DE, Bucholz RW, and Ogden JA: Tension band wiring of displaced tibial tuberosity fractures in adolescents, Clin Orthop 209:161, 1985.
105. Quilis A: Fractures in children with myelomeningocele, Acta Orthop Scand 45:883, 1974.
106. Ramsey R and Griz J: Immediate open reduction and internal fixation of severely displaced supracondylar fractures of the humerus in children, Clin Orthop 90:130, 1973.
107. Rang M: Children's fractures, ed 2, Philadelphia, 1983, J.B. Lippincott Co.
108. Ratliff A: Traumatic separation of the upper femoral epiphysis in young children, J Bone Joint Surg 50B:757, 1968.
109. Ratliff A: Fractures of the neck of the femur in children, Orthop Clin North Am 5:903, 1974.
110. Rogers L et al: "Clipping injury" fracture of the epiphysis in the adolescent football player: an occult lesion of the knee, Am J Roent 121:69, 1974.
111. Rowell P: Arterial occlusion in juvenile humeral supracondylar fractures, Injury 6:254, 1975.
112. Rudicel S et al: Shear fractures through the capital femoral physis of the skeletally immature rabbit, J Pediatr Orthop 5:27, 1985.
113. Salter R and Best T: The pathogenesis and prevention of valgus deformity following fractures of the proximal metaphyseal region of the tibia in children, J Bone Joint Surg 55A:1324, 1973.
114. Salter R and Harris W: Injuries involving the epiphyseal plate, J Bone Joint Surg 45A:587, 1963.
115. Salter R and Zaltz C: Anatomic investigations of the mechanism of injury and pathologic anatomy of "pulled elbow" in children, Clin Orthop 77:134, 1971.
116. Staheli L: Femoral and tibial growth following femoral shaft fractures in childhood, Clin Orthop 55:159, 1967.
117. Stephen D, Louis E, and Louis D: Traumatic separation of the distal femoral epiphyseal cartilage plate, J Bone Joint Surg 56A:1383, 1974.
118. Tullos H and Fain R: Little league shoulder: rotational stress fracture of the proximal epiphysis, J Sports Med 2:152, 1974.
119. Viljanto J, Linna M, and Kiviluoto H: Indications and results of operative treatment of femoral shaft fractures in children, Acta Chir Scand 141:366, 1975.
120. Viljanto J, Kiviluoto H, and Paananen M: Remodeling after femoral shaft fracture in children, Acta Chir Scand 141:360, 1975.
121. Winkler AR, Barnes JC, and Ogden JA: Break dance hip: chronic avulsion of the anterior superior iliac spine, Pediatr Radiol 17:501, 1987.
122. Wood S: Reversal of the radial head during reduction of fractures of the neck of the radius in children, J Bone Joint Surg 51B:707, 1969.

20

Sports Injuries

J. Kevin Lynch and Mark Galloway

More than 30 million children participate in organized extrascholastic athletic programs, and approximately 6 million take part in interscholastic athletic pursuits.[15] In the past 20 years the definition of "sport" has become more obscure, but the term "sports medicine" has become more popular.

The practice of sports medicine involves the treatment of microtrauma (overuse syndromes) and macrotrauma (acute anatomic disruptions), but it also offers a comparatively unique opportunity to prevent injury. It carries the responsibility of counseling in regard to the psychosocial impact of a child's athletic activity by becoming involved in nutritional advice; it is not concerned merely with returning the child to activity more rapidly than would otherwise be expected, although that seems to be the public's perception of sports medicine.

The role of the sports medicine practitioner should be to prevent long-term dysfunction, to encourage fitness, and to allow the young athlete to enjoy himself or herself while pursuing these goals.

Many excellent texts are available that deal with sports medicine in detail.[23,24] The goal of this chapter is to cover the more common problems that are dealt with in a sports medicine practice.

FITNESS

An important goal of sports medicine is to encourage fitness. In a complete sense, fitness requires three essential elements: psychologic well-being, nutritional awareness, and physical performance. There is an assumed risk in participating in sports. However, it is imperative to eliminate or diminish the risk of injuries that cause long-term disabilities or, when confronted with such injuries, to treat them optimally. The best way to achieve these goals is through fitness on the part of the patient and awareness on the part of the physician.

Psychologic Fitness

In a busy practice it often is difficult to be responsive to the psychologic implication of complaints. However, recognition of this aspect provides the only access to treatment and the avoidance of "burnout," which is not infrequent in young athletes. Although there may be many indications of a psychologic problem, the most commonly encountered signs at our center are: (1) the quiet child accompanied by an overly involved parent (for example, the "hockey mother"), (2) chronic inappropriate pain, and (3) the injury-prone child.

The latter two syndromes, particularly, are often a manifestation that the child no longer wants to participate in the sport, or that he or she is enjoying all the attention the problem is getting. Parents frequently say they have seen several doctors, but they complain that other doctors "have not been able to diagnose the cause of the pain"; "have not been able to provide the child with a brace to prevent chronic injury"; or "have not been able to return the child to activities as quickly as (the parents) would like." Although these complaints are always somewhat disheartening for the health professional interested in sports and in children, much can be accomplished through frank discussion. The child should realize that although it is important to do his or her best, it is not necessarily important to be the best. Parents and coaches also must understand this, and they must realize that they are mature adults dealing with an individual who frequently is both socially and psychologically fragile. Children are not small adults, and they frequently have difficulty dealing with the stress of participation; they certainly cannot deal with the additional stress of parental and coach pressure.

The psychologic benefits and potential impact of sports have been well documented, but the sports medicine practitioner must be aware of the possible implication of the syndromes just discussed so that he or she can offer the pediatric athlete optimal treatment.[1,18]

Nutritional Fitness

American children often are too fat and unfit. Recent studies have confirmed these findings,[20,21,30] which are of significant national concern. Being too fat and unfit not only affects a child's ability to pursue sports activities, but also has grave ramifications for the child's cardiovascular health as he or she becomes an adult. In the sports medicine setting, being overweight is one of the most difficult problems to deal with, but it also can be very rewarding to treat the patient.

Most overweight children have overweight parents, and in dealing with this problem it is almost impossible to isolate the child from the parents. In sports an unfortunate preselection appears to occur: The overweight child, at the very least, is simply assigned to take up room or, mistakenly, "big" frequently is related to "strong." Thus the overweight child is relegated to playing goaltender, catcher, or lineman or is assigned to throwing events in track and field. Consequently, these children are prone to injury from their peers or to self-inflicted injury caused by their body weight. Frequently such a child is the least conditioned child on the team.

Unfortunately, there often is no time for adequate nutritional counseling, and simply providing a patient with a diet usually is not enough. However, the pursuit of fitness as a family activity, involving both reasonable exercise and appropriate diet, can be effective although exceedingly difficult to accomplish.

As a guide to weight loss the following ideas are suggested:

1. Although either exercise or dieting will result in weight loss, the best program is a combination of the two. However, exercising is fun, and dieting is not. It should be pointed out that the amount of exercise required to produce effective weight loss very often is beyond the capability of the overweight patient and often leads to injury.
2. A slow weight loss of 3 to 4 pounds per week is probably the best plan. A relatively mild reduction in calories and a moderate increase in energy expenditure result in an effective weight loss without the patient feeling a sense of fatigue and without sacrificing lean body

mass. As a rule of thumb, approximately 1000 calories a day of appropriate food intake results in a 2-pound increase in lean body tissue per week. Eliminating approximately 1000 calories a day results in a weight loss of 2 pounds per week. This is also an important concept for young wrestlers trying to make or break weight.

An easy way to follow body weight is on the basis of triceps fat fold. The standards are readily available for this.[8]

Nutritional supplements are so widely advertised that young athletes often ask questions about their effectiveness; there is no scientific medical evidence to show that supplements have any benefit whatsoever. The exception to this is possibly iron supplementation. This subject has been controversial, and some believe that certainly there may be some indication for iron replacement in menstruating girls and women. Recent studies show fairly conclusively that in endurance athletes, both male and female, there is a definite risk for iron deficiency.[16,22] This condition is best determined by serum ferritin level, not by hemoglobin determination.

Water replacement is as necessary in young endurance athletes as it is in adults. There is no benefit to supplemented beverages as long as the child's diet is normal.

Inquiries about diet and supplementation often arise from a child's attempt to increase body size, change body image, increase the performance level, or hasten the healing process. In treating young athletes, the practitioner must be sensitive to these questions, particularly with the increasing availability of drugs, including steroids. The practitioner also must be alert to the possibility of eating disorders, which may originate with attempts to manipulate body weight.

Physical Fitness

Of all the elements of fitness, physical fitness is the most difficult to define. Obviously a fit swimmer is markedly different from a fit football player or tennis player.

Physical fitness means different things to different people, and being physically fit does not guarantee sports-specific performance, as noted by Mangi and Jokl.[13] These researchers' nine points for consideration in assessing fitness are given in the left box on p. 442.

Unquestionably, fitness in the broader sense (but

```
┌─────────────────────────────────────┐
│          PHYSICAL FITNESS            │
│                                      │
│       Aerobic capacity               │
│       Strength                       │
│       Endurance                      │
│       Agility                        │
│       Speed                          │
│       Muscle balance                 │
│       Flexibility                    │
│       Jumping ability                │
│       Body fat                       │
└─────────────────────────────────────┘
```

```
┌─────────────────────────────────────┐
│     RISK FACTORS FOR OVERUSE INJURIES│
│                                      │
│       Growth                         │
│       Muscle–tendon imbalance        │
│       Training error                 │
│       Cultural deconditioning        │
│       Deficient nutrition            │
│       Improper footwear              │
│       Hard playing surfaces          │
│       Malalignment syndrome          │
│       Coincidental disease           │
└─────────────────────────────────────┘
```

even in the more specific sense) is effective in reducing both the number and severity of injuries sustained in athletic performance. Unfortunately, in the pursuit of the competitive edge, young people are exposed to injury. Sports-specialty camps often are designed on a "survival of the fittest" basis. As noted by O'Neill and Micheli,[17] this type of regimen poses an additional risk factor in the production of overuse syndromes. Risk factors for overuse injuries appear in the box above, right.

Rather than having the young athlete concentrate on skills and strategy, an excessive amount of endurance work is done. It is impossible, even for a child, to become fit in a week. In attempting to achieve this, the child frequently is injured and at best is so fatigued that most of the skill training is wasted; at worst, the child develops a season-debilitating injury.

A good preparticipation training program should be designed with the particular sport in mind and should be conducted for at least 6 weeks before participation in the sport.

PREVENTION OF INJURY

Although the treatment of sports injuries has been glamorized and well publicized, the most important aspect of treatment is prevention. Millions of children participate in athletic pursuits, both organized and unorganized, and millions of injuries occur each year. In 1986 more than 600,000 junior varsity and varsity players were injured in football alone.[14] Of these injuries, 14,000 required surgery, and of that number almost 10,000 were knee operations. The socioeconomic impact of these figures must be obvious to the practitioner of pediatric sports medicine. Prevention therefore is as important as treatment.

Prevention involves three concepts: preparticipation screening, protective equipment, and fitness.

Preparticipation Screening

The efficacy of preparticipation physical examinations has been questioned in both children and adults. However, it is fairly clear that although the routine physical examination is probably not productive in prescreening, the sports-oriented specific physical examination is very productive.[9] One of the most valuable aspects of preparticipation examination is the opportunity to counsel both the child and the parents about general matters of fitness and injury prevention and occasionally to point out the inadvisability of pursuing a particular athletic activity, thereby avoiding the frustration of unrealistic ambitions and possible injury. Besides the medical evaluation, children should be instructed in warm-up techniques, stretching techniques, and strengthening techniques.

The issue of strengthening techniques has been controversial, but a statement by the American Academy of Pediatric Physicians helped clarify the issue by pointing out the difference between weight lifting and weight training.[31] Prepubescent children can gain significant strength with weight training,[25] and they can accomplish this without injury.[19]

The greatest number of athletic participants among children probably are in the age group of 8 to 14 years old. This is a time when children are undergoing their most rapid development, and they generally lack the speed, power, and coordination of older children. It is important to note that standard physical development charts indicate that in a given age group, it is not unusual for one child's body weight to be double another child's within two standard deviations. The Tanner scale also is useful, and generally a child at the lower end of this scale should not be competing with one at the upper end.

It is difficult to disqualify a child from participating for these types of reasons, but the physician often can point out potential problems and can suggest that the child pursue some other type of athletic activity or compete for another position on the team. Occasionally a physician must disqualify an athlete, and the guidelines recommended by the American Medical Association Committee on Medical Aspects of Sports[4] may be helpful on these occasions.

Protective Equipment

Injuries do not occur just during a game or during competition; they frequently occur during practice. Of all football injuries reported to the National High School Injury Registry in 1986, 62% occurred during practice.[14] Therefore appropriate protective equipment must be worn during practice as well as during the game. Appropriate clothing and shoes are just as important to runners as head and neck protection and padding are to hockey players and football players. Proper equipment certainly is not a guarantee against injury, but it has been shown to diminish the number and severity of injuries.

One controversial issue is the efficacy of prophylactic knee bracing. The question is not only whether prophylactic knee bracing works, but also whether use of a single upright brace preloads the knee, causing a higher incidence of injury. The preponderance of information available suggests that knee braces do not prevent knee injuries, and this is also the stand of the American Academy of Orthopedic Surgeons. Nevertheless, it must be recognized that two types of knee braces are used, prophylactic braces and functional braces. As the name suggests, prophylactic braces are worn by athletes who have not had knee injuries to prevent such injuries; the efficacy of these braces is controversial. Function braces are worn by athletes with knee dysfunction to eliminate or diminish the dysfunction. The efficacy of these braces also is questioned, but it generally is felt that they effectively diminish dysfunction, although they do not eliminate it.

Fitness

Fitness, which has already been discussed, is probably the most important aspect of prevention. Fitness is also an important consideration in re-

turning an athlete to competition. Most athletic injuries are minor but nonetheless require appropriate treatment and rehabilitation. Goldberg et al.[10] found that 23.5% of injuries were related to inadequate previous rehabilitation. The insistence on returning to participation, often before rehabilitation has been completed, is one of the day-to-day problems the sports medicine physician encounters. It is probably one of the reasons sports medicine has been popularized, but it also places a heavy responsibility on those who practice sports medicine.

TRAUMA

The type of trauma a sports medicine physician sees depends largely on the population to which the practitioner is exposed. Generally speaking, lower extremity injuries are more common than upper extremity injuries, and injuries reported in males increase with age from 8 to 18 years old, whereas injuries in females appear to remain stable over that period. The National High School Injury

Table 20-1   Comparative time loss injury rate

Location	Percentage of total	Projected number of injuries
Boys high school football		
Hip/thigh	17.9	114,002
Ankle/foot	16.6	105,849
Forearm/hand	14.6	92,665
Knee	14.6	92,665
Trunk	10.0	63,895
Shoulder/arm	9.7	61,375
Head/spine	9.0	56,927
Face/scalp	2.8	18,086
Other	4.8	30,835
Girls high school basketball		
Ankle/foot	29.7	37,532
Knee	17.3	21,877
Forearm/hand	14.0	818,666
Hip/thigh	12.4	15,655
Trunk	8.6	10,838
Other	7.5	9,433
Face/scalp	5.4	6,824
Head/spine	2.5	3,211
Shoulder/arm	1.9	2,408

From National Athletic Trainers Association: National High School Injury Registry, 1986.

Registry figures for girls basketball in 1987 and boys football in 1986 are listed in Table 20-1.

Generally, injuries fall into two broad categories, microtraumatic and macotraumatic. Microtraumatic injuries include the overuse syndromes such as tendinitis, bursitis, stress injuries involving bone or joints, and induced instabilities. Macrotraumatic injuries usually are acute anatomic disruptions either caused by contact or self-induced. Many of these injuries are dealt with elsewhere in this text and are mentioned here only as they relate to sports medicine.

CERVICAL AND LUMBAR SPINE INJURIES

Severe injuries to the cervical spine are among the most devastating an athlete can incur. Fortunately, most head and neck injuries in the immature athlete are minor and do not cause long-term disability. Major head and neck injuries are rare among children participating in organized sports, and especially uncommon in those under 11 years of age.[2] As a child reaches adolescence, gains in size and speed are accompanied by a higher incidence of cervical injury.[28] It must be emphasized that most sports-related neck injuries can be prevented by paying proper attention to physical conditioning, training, and use of protective equipment.

Brachial Plexus Injuries

Classification and treatment of neck trauma are based on the extent of injury. Stretch injuries of the brachial plexus (brachial plexus neuropraxias, burners, stingers) are the most common neck injuries encountered in sports.[27] They are the result of traction on the upper trunk of the brachial plexus from forceful lateral bending of the neck. Patients may complain of transient, burning pain radiating down the arm with associated weakness. The short duration of symptoms and full, painless range of motion of the neck differentiate this condition from more serious cervical spine injuries. Patients may return to competition if the motor and sensory deficits resolve swiftly and completely and if no neck tenderness can be elicited. Patients with prolonged neurologic deficits or recurrent episodes should be evaluated with roentgenograms of the cervical spine, electromyogram (EMG) studies, and serial neurologic examinations. Patients should not be allowed to return to activities until neurologic deficits are fully resolved. Neck strengthening exercises and neck rolls are useful in preventing recurrence.[27]

Cervical Sprains

Cervical sprains are stable injuries to the posterior ligaments and paraspinous musculature that result from hyperflexion of the cervical spine. Patients have neck pain that is nonradiating and unassociated with neurologic deficits. Roentgenograms in these patients may reveal loss of normal lordosis but no subluxation or fracture. These patients must be treated as if they have an unstable injury until it is proven otherwise. Roentgenographic evaluation is mandatory. Patients usually respond to a brief period of immobilization followed by range of motion and strengthening exercises.

Spinal Stenosis

Transient and permanent quadriplegia have been reported in patients with spinal stenosis following hyperflexion or extension injuries of the cervical spine.[29] Stenosis may be congenital or acquired, as with a herniated disc. Treatment of these patients should include initial immobilization and attention to the need for possible respiratory support. Patients should then be transported to a hospital for roentgenographic evaluation and serial neurologic examinations. Needless to say, after recovery patients should not participate in contact sports.

Fractures and Dislocations

Fractures and dislocations of the cervical spine are most commonly the result of forced flexion and rotation. Pain or neurologic deficit or both occur immediately, and initial treatment is the same as for spinal stenosis. Because of their increased ligamentous laxity, young children may have significant myelopathy secondary to cervical spine trauma without roentgenographic evidence of bony injury.[7] The history usually is remarkable for transient paresthesias at the time of injury, but the patient may have an intact neurologic examination. The natural history is that of steady progression to permanent neurologic deficit.

Patients who have chronic complaints about or actual injuries to the cervical spine should be evaluated for congenital anomalies, even in the absence of persistent findings. Such evaluations are accomplished by CT or magnetic resonance imaging (MRI) studies (Figs. 20-1 and 20-2).

In the lumbar spine, most problems relate to overuse microtraumatic injuries secondarily related to hyperlordosis. Although these injuries are not common in a general sports population, they may be seen frequently if a sports practitioner is dealing with a large group of gymnasts. Hyperlordosis is also encountered in swimmers. Besides causing mechanical low back pain, upper lordotic posturing has been incriminated in stress fractures of the pars interarticularis. Scheuermann's disease also can account for low back pain in a child. For the most part these conditions can be treated by reducing activity, taking nonsteroidal antiinflammatory drugs, pursuing selective physiotherapeutic programs, using a modified Boston brace, and following a graduated return to activity.

The other conditions seen in the lumbar spine are spondylolysis and spondylolisthesis. These conditions also can be treated conservatively with appropriate exercise and bracing. A child with spondylolisthesis with a grade I or grade II slip should not be involved in contact sports, even with a brace.

UPPER EXTREMITY INJURIES

Although skeletal injuries to the upper extremity are not infrequent, the most common upper ex-tremity problems seen by the sports medicine practitioner are those related to overuse, and these are seen primarily in the throwing athlete. Most injuries involve soft tissue around the shoulder. In contrast to an adult, the young throwing athlete rarely exhibits degenerative disorders or tears of the rotator cuff.

To understand the cause and biomechanics of these injuries, one must understand the biomechanics of pitching a baseball (see the box on p. 446).

The following syndromes appear to occur in the throwing athlete:

1. *Anterior shoulder pain* can be caused by stretching of the anterior rotator cuff in the late part of stage 2, the cocking phase. However, during true acceleration rotator cuff activity actually is minimal, and anterior shoulder pain probably is caused by straining of the pectoralis major.
2. *Posterior shoulder pain* is a deceleration injury probably caused by strain of the posterior portion of the supraspinatus. This sort of dysfunction causes imbalance and leads to subacromial impingement.
3. *Subacromial impingement* is caused by overpull of the deltoid and forward subluxation of the shoulder.

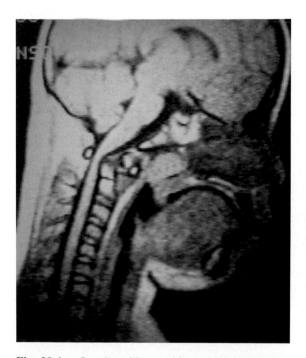

Fig. 20-1   Os odontoideum with cord impingement.

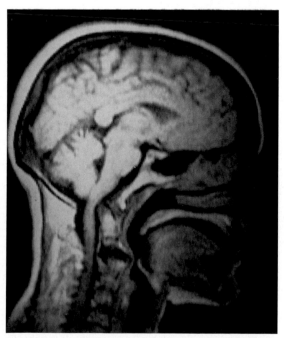

Fig. 20-2   Klippel-Feil syndrome with cord impingement.

FIVE STAGES OF PITCHING

Stage 1   Windup

Stage 2   Early cocking: The shoulder at this stage is approaching full adduction and marked external rotation, and the forward foot is approaching the ground.

Stage 3   The shoulder has reached maximal external rotation, the forward foot is well planted on the ground, and the trunk has begun forward motion.

Stage 4   Acceleration phase: This stage starts with internal rotation of the humerus and ends with initial release of the ball.

Stage 5   This stage constitutes the follow-through or deceleration phase.

Diagnosis is easier when the pain is associated with specific phases of throwing and occurs specifically anteriorly or posteriorly in the shoulder. However, this is not always the case, and diagnosis sometimes is difficult because the findings on examination are subtle. Pain at night or at rest often indicates an early rotator cuff tear. On physical examination, localized tenderness may indicate biceps tendinitis posterior and anterior rotator cuff involvement or subacromial bursitis. The grimace and apprehension test may be positive in both impingement and subtle subluxations, whereas the relocation test (that is, the grimace and apprehension test conducted with posterior force placed on the shoulder) will relieve the pseudoimpingement of subluxation but not change true impingement.

Additional tests such as isokinetic testing may help locate muscle deficiencies, and occasionally CT arthrography and MRI may be helpful. Generally, plain roentgenograms are not particularly helpful, but in a chronic situation bony changes may be observed in the glenoid both posteriorly and anteriorly.

Jobe and Kzitene[12] described the following four categories of shoulder dysfunction:

Group 1   Patients with pure impingement

Group 2   Patients with pseudoinstability, that is, instability caused by impingement and secondary muscle dysfunction

Group 3   Patients with pure instability and no impingement

Group 4   Patients with instability caused by hyperelasticity; differentiated from group 2 patients by other findings of hyperelasticity

In addition to anterior instability, posterior instability is not as uncommon as was once thought. The practitioner must be aware of the multidirectional instability and physiologic instability not infrequently seen in children.

Most instabilities and impingements can be treated conservatively. Since most of these injuries result from repetitive microtrauma, the initial step is cessation of throwing. Using ice and nonsteroidal antiinflammatory drugs also can be beneficial. A graduated program of internal-external rotator cuff strengthening and strengthening of the pectoralis major and biceps muscles are important. Flexibility is important for impingement and for unopposed muscles in instabilities, but it is important to avoid flexibility exercises that encourage instability. A strengthening sequence usually involves the internal and external rotators and the supraspinatus with progression to the scapula rotators (trapezius, serratus anterior, and latissimus dorsi).

If conservative treatment fails, surgical intervention is occasionally required, but surgery should be recommended cautiously for the throwing athlete. Regardless of the patient's wishes, tolerance of instability should not be accepted or recommended, and occasionally the physician may have to recommend that the patient's activity level be reduced to avoid instability.

Other causes of shoulder dysfunction in the young athlete include the following:

1. *"Little league" shoulder*   Persistent, proximal humeral pain associated with repetitive throwing can result in epiphyseal fractures. Proximal humeral growth alterations have been reported by Cahill.[3] The child should cease throwing until this diagnosis has been ruled out.

2. *Osteolysis of the distal clavicle*   This condition may occur through trauma, but it is seen more frequently in older children who participate in weight lifting; it is particularly associated with bench pressing. The condition usually responds to a reduction of activity, although surgery is occasionally necessary.

3. *Biceps tendinitis*   As an isolated condition, this is probably unusual and likely relates to subacromial impingement.

Sports Injuries   **447**

With regard to the elbow, most problems in this area involve epiphyseal disorders, which are described in Chapter 19.

LOWER EXTREMITY INJURIES

Lower extremity injuries are more common in the pediatric athlete than upper extremity injuries. Microtraumatic, or overuse, injuries are the most common type of injury, and the knee requires more physician visits than any other part of the lower extremity.

In general, injuries are categorized as (1) strains (injury to a muscle or a muscle-tendon unit), (2) sprains (injury to ligaments), and (3) fractures (breakage involving bones or joints).

Sprains or ligament injuries frequently are categorized according to anatomic area, but in general they may be classified as the following:

Grade I   Ligamentous disruption without instability
Grade II   Ligamentous disruption with mild instability
Grade III Ligamentous disruption associated with significant instability

Injuries of the lower extremity in the immature athlete encompass a wide variety of pathologic conditions. Children are subject to the same symptoms commonly encountered in adults, but in addition a child's growth plate predisposes him or her to unique patterns of injury. As was discussed elsewhere, the physis is the weakest link in the bone ligament complex. Consequently, children more commonly suffer a fracture through the physis than major ligamentous disruption. However, major dislocations are rare in the pediatric patient.

Classification and treatment of pediatric fractures are discussed elsewhere.

Knee Injuries

The knee comprises both the patellofemoral and tibiofemoral joints, and although they are anatomically related, functionally they are quite different. Review of the knee injuries seen at our center reveals that the most common complaint involved the patellofemoral joint (Fig. 20-3).

Patellofemoral joint

Most of the injuries to the patellofemoral joint are overuse injuries. The anatomy of the patellofemoral joint comprises the quadriceps muscle, the patella, and the patellar tendon. Dysfunction usually relates to the relationship of these components to the trochlear groove of the femur. Most overuse syndromes of the patellofemoral joint involve various degrees of malalignment. Therefore many factors contribute to patellofemoral pain, and an understanding of this concept is a prerequisite to the

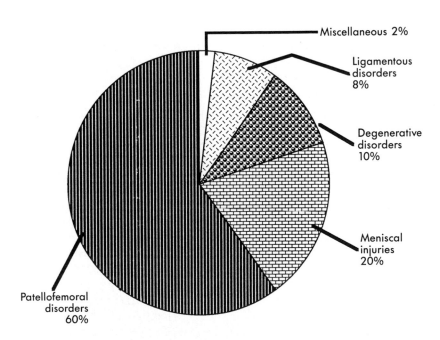

Fig. 20-3   Patellofemoral disorders.

CAUSES OF PATELLOFEMORAL PAIN

Suprapatellar causes

Vastus medialis obliquis hypoplasia
Vastus lateralis hyperplasia
Internal femoral torsion (anteversion)
Retinacular tightness

Infrapatellar causes

Genu valgum
External tibial torsion
Pronation
Lateral placement of tibial tubercle

Patellofemoral causes

Hypoplastic femoral trochlea
Abnormal patellar configuration

---

therapeutic advice. A simple way to assess the patellofemoral joint so that these contributing factors are not overlooked is to establish a regional anatomic inventory delineating potential contributions to the function of the patellofemoral joint. Such an outline is given in the box above.

Quadriceps hypoplasia, particularly vastus medialis obliquis hypoplasia, is not infrequent after an injury to the knee that involves swelling. Quadriceps atrophy occurs as a result of a knee effusion, and although functional return may seem apparent, very often there is residual dysfunction of the medial aspect of the quadriceps, leaving the patellofemoral joint unbalanced and subject to overuse. Some children developmentally have poor definition of the vastus medialis obliquis and occasionally demonstrate an abnormally high insertion of this portion of the muscle.

Internal femoral torsion, or anteversion, is a frequently encountered abnormality in the pediatric age group. This condition presents a problem because the femoral groove that provides the patellofemoral joint with geometric stability is internally rotated relative to the position of the patella; in a dynamic environment, this can lead to excessive pressure in the lateral facet of the patella, subluxation, dislocation, or all three.

Some children exhibit vastus lateralis hyperplasia, which also leads to imbalance and lateralization of the patella in reference to the femur. Retinacular tightness tends to hold the patella in a lateral position or tilted laterally, causing excessive

pressure over the lateral facet and resulting in pain, feelings of instability, or both.

Genu valgum, or knockknee deformity, effectively causes lateralization of the patella, as do lateral placement of the tibial tubercle and external tibial torsion, since they affect the insertion of the patellar tendon and can lead to lateral instability of the patellofemoral joint. Abnormalities of the femoral trochlea, particular trochlear hypoplasia, result in a lack of inherent stability; a similar condition can be produced by abnormal configuration of the patella itself. Pronation of the foot frequently is associated with these syndromes, and tight hamstrings also may contribute to the problem. Mild genu recurvatum can have a markedly adverse affect on patellofemoral function.

Roentgenographic assessment of the patellofemoral joint can be helpful. Lateral views frequently reveal the presence of patella alta, and appropriate patellofemoral views should be ordered if the knee dysfunction is presumed to be caused by the patellofemoral joint.

Many of the structural problems encountered in patellofemoral pain syndromes are difficult to deal with, since problems such as femoral anteversion and genu valgum or trochlear dysplasia are difficult to treat. However, depending on the number of components contributing to the patient's problem and the degree to which each component is contributing, a patellofemoral program can be established for young athletic people that frequently reduces or eliminates their complaints, presuming that they are otherwise fit.[5]

The following program often is effective:

1. *Quadriceps development* is important. Simple straight-leg raises can increase quadriceps strength. Occasionally, in full extension, particularly in a child with patella alta, the patella is in fact tilted and partially subluxed, and in this case straight-leg raises probably are not the best way to exercise. Instead, the knee can be bent to approximately 15 degrees and leg raises done in this position with the patella contained within the trochlea. Short-arc quadriceps exercises also have been recommended, but the short arc occasionally is also a painful arc and in that case should be avoided. Leg press–type activity or the use of a rowing machine with progression to cycling frequently is effective.
2. All these patients must do *hamstring stretches*. Tight hamstrings increase the work

of the quadriceps and seem to accentuate patellofemoral problems. In addition, instructions in iliotibial band stretching and retinacular stretching are helpful.

3. *Pronation* may be associated with these problems even though not symptomatic in itself. It can be treated with orthotic devices, which seem to be helpful in diminishing the patellofemoral pain.

More extensive programs also can be designed for the patellofemoral joint, and certainly working with a physical therapist or trainer can be helpful if a simple home program is not effective.

Chondromalacia is a term often used to describe the general problem of patellofemoral pain. Chondromalacia is a pathologic diagnosis, not a clinical one, and probably should not be used to describe anterior knee pain syndromes.[6] Chondromalacia actually is not frequent in young people, and not all patellofemoral crepitus is caused by chondromalacia. If the practitioner presumes a diagnosis of chondromalacia, the question that must be answered is why that condition has occurred and what are the contributing causes. This will lead to a well thought out therapeutic approach.

Besides exercise, nonsteroidal antinflammatory drugs and regular periodic use of ice are helpful in easing symptoms. Surgery occasionally is required to relieve anterior knee pain, but this should be reserved for the persistently symptomatic child in whom aggressive conservative treatment has failed, including a reduction in the child's activity level. Procedures such as lateral release and patellar shaving are not panaceas and are not effective in the overweight, poorly conditioned child.

Anterior knee pain in the pediatric patient occasionally is caused by a suprapatellar plica. This also can be treated conservatively, but if conservative treatment fails, it does respond to surgical excision. However, plicae are a common finding in the knee; not all of them are pathologic, and they should not routinely be incriminated as the cause of pain. In our experience the association of plicae with patellofemoral instability is fairly high and in fact may be part of the instability of the pathologic condition. In this case surgical excision without dealing with the underlying problems does not relieve the symptoms.

A note of caution: Knee pain can be caused by disorders of the hip such as slipped capital femoral

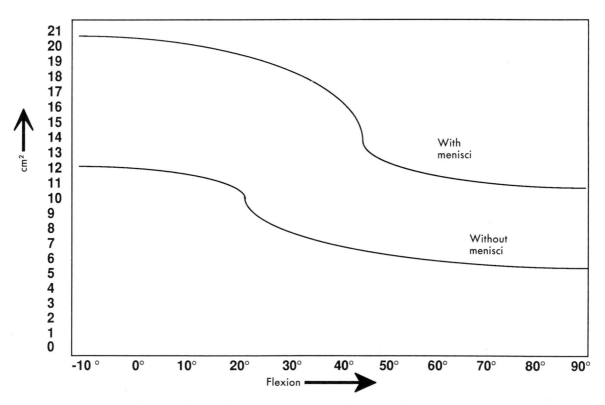

Fig. 20-4   Loadbearing function of the meniscus.

epiphysis or Legg-Calvé-Perthes disease. Persistent knee pain should always call for clinical and roentgenographic evaluation of the hip.

Tibiofemoral joint

Major knee joint trauma was once thought to be rare in younger children, but it is being seen more frequently, possibly because more children are participating in contact sports and possibly related to the higher level of participation.

The structures most commonly injured in the tibiofemoral joint are the menisci, collateral ligaments, and anterior cruciate ligament. The ligaments of the knee provide stability; the menisci provide load bearing. The physician should not try to treat ligamentous injuries optimally while treating meniscal injuries less than optimally.

Meniscal injuries. The sports medicine practitioner must consider the function of the meniscus rather than what type of tear it has. The meniscus assists in load bearing, and its contribution in this regard is substantial (Fig. 20-4). Consequently, surgical or traumatic deprivation of meniscal tissue results in long-term dysfunction of the knee. The long-term consequences of substantial meniscectomy in the pediatric patient are universally significant, with demonstrable degenerative changes at an early age.[11,26]

The meniscus usually is damaged through injury, although congenital discoid menisci can become symptomatic. The onset usually is sudden with pain over the joint line followed by swelling. Occasionally the knee may lock at the time of injury, or the initial symptoms may resolve, only to be followed by chronic, intermittent pain, locking, or a feeling of slipping as the child returns to activity. The physical signs may vary, but the most consistent finding probably is joint line tenderness. Occasionally a McMurray test (induction of pain or catching with rotational testing) may also be positive. Roentgenograms usually are normal and not particularly helpful in making the diagnosis. The most accurate and specific way of diagnosing meniscal injury in children is magnetic resonance imaging. It is accurate, painless, and noninvasive (Figs. 20-5 to 20-7).

Meniscal tears in children occasionally can be treated by immobilization with the expectation of healing. However, if the meniscal tear does not heal, it should be treated by repair and not excision, since the long-term consequences of substantial meniscal excision are significant. Repair is partic-

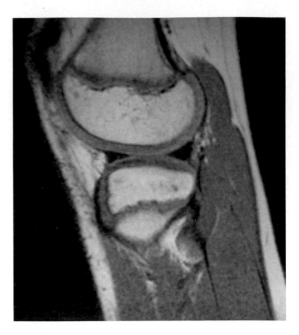

Fig. 20-5   Magnetic resonance image of normal knee.

ularly recommended for patients 15 years old or younger, since the success rate is high.

Collateral ligaments. The most common ligamentous injury in the pediatric age group is a tear of the medial collateral ligament. This injury usually is incurred by a twisting injury or contact and manifests with pain over the medial collateral ligament, varying degrees of swelling, and varying degrees of instability on examination. However, the vascular supply to the medial collateral ligament is abundant, and if the injury is an isolated one, it can be treated conservatively by immobilization followed by functional bracing, adequate rehabilitation, and return to activity.

Torn anterior cruciate ligament. A torn anterior cruciate ligament can be a devastating injury. Although it happens infrequently in the younger pediatric age group, it is not unheard of and is being seen more often. The injury is quite common in the older pediatric and high school age groups. It frequently is associated with meniscal tears, and the mechanism of injury is similar to that of other knee injuries in that it frequently results from a twisting injury or a twisting mechanism precipitated by contact. In basketball, volleyball, and skiing, it is frequently self-inflicted. The patient often tells of hearing or sensing a "pop" and notices swelling within 12 hours. This history, along with

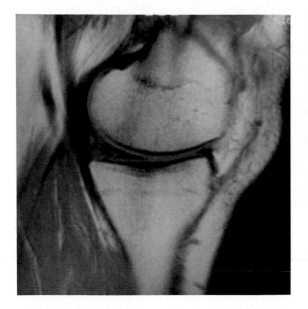

Fig. 20-6   Magnetic resonance image of torn medial meniscus.

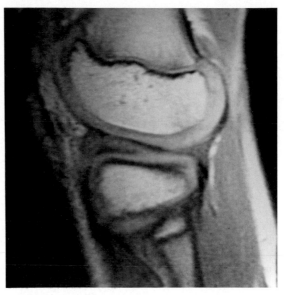

Fig. 20-7   Magnetic resonance image of discoid lateral meniscus.

instability at the time of examination and the presence of a hemarthrosis, frequently indicates an anterior cruciate ligament tear. Besides revealing evidence of a torn meniscus or associated collateral ligament injuries, physical examination frequently reveals a positive Lachman sign. MRI is invaluable in establishing not only the diagnosis of anterior cruciate ligament tear but also the presence or absence of associated meniscal tears.

Compared with the medial collateral ligament, the anterior cruciate ligament has a fragile blood supply and does not heal well.

Anterior cruciate ligament tears are fairly frequent injuries in the older pediatric patient, and some controversy surrounds the best way to approach these problems. We have found that if the following two points are emphasized, the correct treatment becomes easier to choose:

1. Knee dysfunction manifests itself in three ways: pain, swelling, and instability. Although pain and swelling are not desirable, they may cause physiologic deprivation and frequently are tolerated by the patient. However, instability should not be tolerated. Accepting instability and persisting in the activity that produces it leads to inevitable compromise of knee function.

2. It is essential to discuss in detail with the patient the anticipated activity demands on the knee. Some patients are perfectly willing to reduce their activity level to control stability and to avoid more aggressive treatment.

The therapeutic protocols for an isolated anterior cruciate ligament tear involve conservative treatment or surgical treatment. Conservative treatment calls for an exercise program involving concentration on hamstring strength. Normally, quadriceps strength is greater than hamstring strength, and the exercise program should attempt to create a more equal ratio between the two. Cycling is a simple way of accomplishing this, along with hamstring curls, but more aggressive conservative exercise programs are available. Exercise alone sometimes can control instability, but if it does not, other conservative measures should be added. Functional bracing using a derotational brace also helps in returning the athlete to activity. For the patient who is being treated conservatively and who is returning to contact sports or sports involving twisting, turning, or jumping, functional bracing probably is an appropriate suggestion.

The conservative treatment protocol can return a large percentage of people to activity, but it does not work in all cases. One problem is that there are very few predicators that would indicate who is going to be a successful candidate for conservative treatment as opposed to who will need surgery. Unfortunately, the failure of conservative treatment also is associated with additional injury to the knee, but then not all surgical remedies are successful in treating these injuries.

Surgical intervention is directed at reconstruction of the anterior cruciate ligament and repair of associated meniscal and ligamentous tears. This probably is the best solution for patients who do not want to reduce their activity level. Meniscal repairs can be done without repairing the anterior cruciate ligament, but this puts the meniscal repair at risk if the patient returns to high levels of athletic activity. Although the success rate with meniscal repair is fairly high, not all patients return to their original level of activity. Bracing may be helpful on returning to activity, but the effectiveness of bracing and the degree to which it might help are unclear.

ANKLE INJURIES

Ankle injuries are the second most frequently encountered injury at our center. Most of these are ankle sprains with varying degress of ligamentous disruption, usually incurred by inversion of the plantar-flexed ankle. The lateral collateral complex (that is, the anterior talofibular and calcaneofibular ligaments) is mostly involved. The medial ligamentous ligaments or deltoid complex occasionally is injured, but since it is a stronger structure, this is seen less frequently.

Ligamentous injuries of the ankle may be classified as follows:

First degree	Fibers are stretched or torn but not to the extent that instability results.
Second degree	The ligament is partly ruptured with some detectable clinical instability.
Third degree	Complete disruption has occurred with significant detectable instability.

Most injuries fall into the grade I or grade II categories. Examination reveals varying degrees of tenderness around the fibula, particularly anteriorly. Because of associated swelling, clinical instability sometimes is difficult to establish, but ecchymosis below the fibula on the lateral part of the foot and ankle often is associated with grade III injuries. A history of chronic instability often is associated with clinically detectable instability. However, a history of chronic recurrent sprains without associated instability in conjunction with

limited subtalor motion suggests a tarsal coalition. Roentgenograms should always be obtained, particularly with the immature patient; if it involves a significant cartilaginous component, small chip fractures may be more pertinent than otherwise would be the case. Roentgenograms also reveal mortis widening, and stress roentgenograms are useful in determining stability.

Grade I and grade II injuries usually are treated by relative immobilization, ice, and non–weight bearing until the immediate symptoms have subsided. Thereafter functional immobilization with protection of the injured ankle is advised with progressive weight bearing. This is followed by a progressive increase in weight bearing, rehabilitative exercises, and a return to activity. Frequently a medial lateral orthosis is worn on return to activity for additional protection.

Treatment of grade III injuries is somewhat controversial, although the results of conservative treatment have been good. The rehabilitative aspects of grade III injuries are continued for a significant period of time before a patient returns to change-of-direction sports, such as tennis, basketball, or volleyball. In addition to range of motion and strengthening exercises, agility training is essential for a good final outcome. Prolonged symptoms or inability to return to high levels of activity may suggest an unrecognized subchondral fracture and possibly osteochondritis dissecans of the talus, which has been associated with ankle sprains.

Shin Splints

The symptom of leg pain in young atheletes can be somewhat confusing. Four clinical conditions account for leg pain in atheletes: shin splints, medial tibial stress syndrome, compartment syndrome, and stress fracture.

Shin splints are somewhat unusual in young children, probably because their body weight is not sufficient to induce this sort of stress. However, shin splints do occur in older children, not only because of increased body weight and activity levels but also in association with growth spurts. The growing child tends to become relatively "tight," since muscle length occurs by adaption, whereas bone length occurs because of growth. The elastic components of soft tissue lengthen with relative ease, but the fibrous tissue component, or collagen, does not and fails. The normal physical properties of fibrous tissue take a surprisingly long time to return to normal and are readily reinjured if the patient returns to activity prematurely and does not complete rehabilitation.

Several clinical conditions frequently are associated with shin splints, including weak or imbalanced musculature, tight heel cords, pronated foot, and tibiavara. Physical factors common to other overuse syndromes also are often associated with shin splints, such as poor running shoes, inappropriate running surfaces, and an inappropriate increase in mileage or speed.

Clinically, pain usually is found over the anterolateral or posteromedial portion of the leg. Roentgenograms usually are normal, since the term "shin splints" should be applied only to inflammatory conditions of the musculotendinous unit, and the bone scan also is usually within normal limits. Shin splints are treated by reduction in activity, ice, and nonsteroidal antiinflammatory drugs. Exercise is permitted to maintain conditioning, but it should not be excessive. Therapeutic stretching and compensatory exercises are performed after the symptoms subside. Once the patient is made aware of conditions that might have led to the shin splints, he or she may slowly return to activity on a graduated basis.

Medial Tibial Stress Syndrome

Medial tibial stress syndrome usually is seen in runners, but it also is seen with repetitive, highbolistic activity. The symptoms frequently are similar to those of posteromedial shin splints. Roentgenograms are often normal, but they may exhibit periosteal reaction in the painful area. A bone scan also can differentiate this syndrome from true shin splints. The bone scan can be positive, and it presents a picture different from a stress fracture in that a diffuse pattern is seen rather than a localized one, as is the case with stress fractures. Occasional elevation of the compartment pressure also differentiates this syndrome from posteromedial shin splints. However, the compartment pressure is never elevated to the level that might be expected in true compartment syndrome. The treatment for medial tibial stress syndrome is similar to that for shin splints, but the patient's return to activity sometimes can be delayed.

Compartment Syndrome

Compartment syndrome can be acute or chronic, and the most common syndrome is the chronic form. This is particularly seen in runners but can be seen in other athletes as well. Muscles of the anterior compartment can undergo a 10% increase in girth, resulting in muscle and nerve ischemia. This increase in pressure appears to relate to the speed of movement and frequently is bilateral. The patient complains of weakness, aching, and pain over the involved compartment and also may complain of paresthesias over the dorsum of the foot.

Compartment syndrome can be confused with shin splints or stress fractures, but it can be distinguished by intracompartmental pressures. In the normal individual, resting pressure in the anterior compartment usually is 0 to 5 mm of mercury. With activity the pressure rises above 50 mm but rapidly returns to normal. Usually the pressure is back to the preexercise level within 5 minutes. In people with chronic compartment syndromes, the resting pressure usually is greater than 15 mm of mercury, rises higher than 75 mm, and does not return to normal within 5 minutes. Acute compartment syndrome also can occur, but it usually is associated with trauma. The treatment for these syndromes is fasciotomy of the involved compartment.

Stress Fracture

Although stress fractures may occur in many places, the area most commonly affected is the tibia. Stress fractures also are common in the metatarsals and the fibula. Pain usually is constant and becomes worse with activity. Physical examination usually reveals point tenderness over the involved area. Roentgenograms can be normal for several weeks or may never show prominent signs. The bone scan is the most sensitive method for early diagnosis, and it usually is positive within 48 to 72 hours after injury. A word of caution: The practitioner must bear in mind that bone tumors seen in children frequently appear to be associated with a history of inconsequential trauma. Physical and roentgenographic findings can be similar in the early history of bone tumors and can be confused with stress fractures. Stress fractures usually respond to reduction of applied stress. Occasionally, immobilization is required, and healing frequently can be prolonged.

Tendinitis

Tendinitis is one of the many overuse syndromes involving the lower extremity. The term often is used somewhat loosely, but it is important to differentiate peritendinitis, tendinitis, and tendinosis, particularly with regard to the Achilles tendon and the patellar tendon. Essential differences are manifest in the extent of inflammation and usually can be determined on the basis of symptom duration and response to conservative measures. Peritendinitis implies an inflammation of the tendon sheath, whereas tendinitis is an inflammation of the tendon proper (Figs. 20-8 and 20-9). Both of these conditions are reversible and usually respond to rest or antiinflammatory drugs and ice. This regimen usually is followed by stretching exercises, rehabilitative strengthening exercises, and correction of any train faults that might be detected. Other physiotherapeutic programs may also be beneficial, but injection into the area is discouraged. Tendinosis is a more chronic form of a disease and implies mucinous degeneration and calcification within the substance of the tendon. This is an important distinction because tendinosis usually is recalcitrant to conservative measures. Because of the subcutaneous position of both the Achilles and patellar tendons, ultrasound often is useful in detecting cystic degeneration and calcification within the tendon. When involvement in the tendon is this extensive, surgery usually is indicated, with debridement of the degenerative cysts. Epiphyseal and apophyseal overuse syndromes are discussed in Chapter 19.

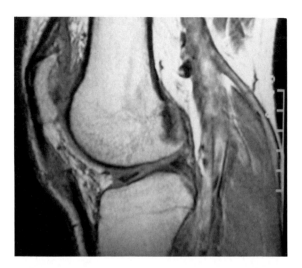

Fig. 20-8   Traumatic tendonitis of patellar tendon.

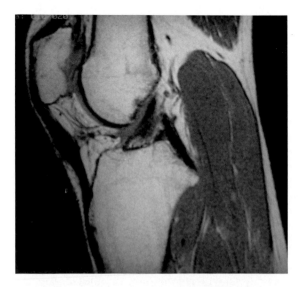

Fig. 20-9   Healed tendonitis of patellar tendon.

REFERENCES

1. Brown RS: Exercise and mental health in the pediatric population, Clin Sports Med 1:515, 1982.
2. Bruce DA, Shut L, and Sutton LN: Brain and cervical spine injuries occurring during organized sports activities in children and adolescents, Clin Sports Med 1:495, 1982.
3. Cahill BR: Little league shoulder, J Sports Med 2:115, 1970.
4. Craig TT, editor: Comments in sports medicine, Chicago, 1973, The American Medical Association.
5. DeHaven KE, Daldon WA, and Mayer PJ: Chondromalacia of the patella in athletes: clinical presentation and conservative management, Am J Sports Med 7:5, 1979.
6. Ficat RP and Hungerford DS: Disorders of the patellofemoral joint, Baltimore, 1977, Williams & Wilkins.
7. Fielding JW and Hesinger RN: Fractures of the spine. In Rockwood CA, editor: Fractures in children, Philadelphia, 1984, JB Lippincott Co.
8. Frisancho A: Triceps skinfold and upper arm muscle size norms for assessment of nutritional status. J Clin Nutr 27:1052, 1974.
9. Goldberg B et al: Preparticipation on sports assessment—an objective evaluation. Pediatrics 66:736, 1980.
10. Goldberg B et al: Children's sports injuries: are they avoidable? Physician and Sports Medicine 7:93, 1979.
11. Huckell JR: Is meniscectomy a benign procedure? Can J Surg 8:254, 1965.
12. Jobe FW and Kzitene RS: Shoulder pain in the overhand or throwing athlete, Orth Rev 18:963, 1989.
13. Mangi R, Jokl P, and Dayton W: Sports fitness and training, New York, 1987, Pantheon Books, Inc.
14. National Athletic Trainers Association, National High School Injury Registry, 1986.
15. National Federation of State High School Associations: Sports participation survey indicates overall increase, Nat Fed Press, vol 2, October 1981.
16. Nickerson NL: Decreased iron stores in high school female runners, Am J Dis Child 139:1115, 1985.
17. O'Neill DB and Micheli LJ: Recognizing and preventing overuse injuries in young athletes, J Musculoskeletal Med 6:21, 1989.
18. Pillemer F and Micheli L: Psychological considerations in youth sports, Clin Sports Med 7:679, 1988.
19. Raines CB et al: Weight training in prepubescent males: is it safe? Am J Sports Med 15:43, 1987.

20. Ross JG and Gilbert GG: The national children and youth fitness study: a summary of findings, JOPERD 56:45, 1985.

21. Ross JH and Pate RR: The national children and youth fitness study II: a summary of findings, JOPERD 58:51, 1987.

22. Rowland TW, Black SA, and Kelleher JF: Iron deficiency in adolescent endurance athletes, J Adolesc Health Care 8:322, 1987.

23. Schneider RC and Kennedy JC: Sports injuries: mechanisms, treatment, and prevention, Baltimore, 1985, Williams & Wilkins.

24. Scott WN, Nisonson B, and Nicholas JA: Principles of sports medicine, Baltimore, 1984, Williams & Wilkins.

25. Siewald BS and Michele AJ: Strength training for children, J Pediatr Orthop 6:143, 1986.

26. Taper EN and Hoover NW: Late results after meniscectomy, J Bone Joint Surg 51A:517, 1969.

27. Torg JS: Management guidelines for athletic injuries to the cervical spine, Clin Sports Med 6:53, 1987.

28. Torg JS et al: The national football head and neck injury registry: report and conclusions, 1978, JAMA 241:1477, 1979.

29. Torg JS et al: Neuropraxia of the cervical spinal cord with transient quadriplegia, J Bone Joint Surg 68A:1354, 1987.

30. Updyke WF: Physical fitness program, Chrysler Fund AAU.

31. Weight training and weight lifting, information for pediatricians policy statement, Amer Acad Pediatr Sports Med 35:7, 1982.

21

The Injured Hand

Frederick Finseth

Hand injuries are common in children. In the rough and tumble child's world the little hand explores, fights, strikes the ground first in a fall, and clumsily gets into doors, machines, and places the experienced adult hand avoids. The little hand is a complex precision tool, so anatomically intricate that a small cut or injury can seriously diminish function. The initial care of pediatric hand injuries is of primary importance, since the surgical care at the time of injury is the predominant factor influencing an optimal functional result. Commissions and omissions in this initial care can irrevocably compromise the functional result. Accordingly, a sound knowledge of the principles and capabilities of hand surgery is essential for undertaking the proper care of hand injuries.

The ultimate impact of the surgical result on the individual is immense. One should not underestimate hand use in the overall functioning of the individual. Good hand function has a profound effect on future occupational choice, education, and socioeconomic potential. Psychologic consequences of hand deformity and decreased function can also be significant.

Children's hands are notable for their repair potential—flexor tendon repairs and grafts do better, nerves recover function better and faster, joints do not get stiff so easily, and they recover motion more readily[41,62,76] when deformed or limited in motion or function. These little hands possess a clever adaptability and versatility. All this works to the advantage of the surgeon, influencing the approach to the surgery of repair and reconstruction. However, the principles for hand surgery are the same as for the adult. In this chapter these common surgical principles and the special requirements and circumstances of surgery for pediatric hand trauma will be emphasized.

EXAMINATION

Examination of the hand is the first step in formulating a rational treatment plan.[33,58,72,77] It is essential to determine the nature and extend of the injury and which structures are involved. Errors in diagnosis can compromise the opportunity for an optimal result. A proper and careful examination of the hand in children is at best difficult. The high emotion and pain associated with the injury diminish the possibility for willful cooperation or verbal communication with which one usually can approach the adult. Therefore a high index of suspicion for injury to any and all structures in the traumatic field is critically important. It is better to explore with the child under anesthesia in an operating room than to miss a significant injury. For instance, in young children with a volar wrist laceration, the median and ulnar nerves, as well as all flexor tendons, should be checked carefully for possible injury.

The history is clearly an important part in evaluating the injury and planning the repair. The mechanism of injury gives useful information about the severity of the injury and what may be involved. It is important in determining the type of wound, which in turn greatly influences the surgical approach. For instance, crush and avulsion injuries, such as a wringer injury, involve more soft tissue injury, skin devitalization, and reactive edema than does a tidy incising injury. The timing and method of surgical repair are very difficult, as will be discussed later. A fall on the outstretched hand may imply a carpal fracture or dislocation. Forceful abduction of the thumb, as occurs in a ski pole injury, suggests possible injury to the thumb metacarpophalangeal joint ulnar collateral ligament. Many other examples would simply confirm that history is a significant component in diagnosis and, accordingly, in developing a rational treatment plan.

Most information about the injured child's hand is gathered by observation alone, rather than by efforts to test for sensation or for specific motions. The posture of the hand provides a wealth of information. The extended finger from loss of flexor tone signals the possibility of flexor tendon injury. Wrist drop implies a radial nerve problem. Marked localized swelling on a closed injury suggests a possible fracture. Angulatory or rotating deformity of the digits may indicate a fracture, a ligamentous injury, or a tendon injury, as in a mallet finger or boutonnière deformity. Analysis of spontaneous movement yields information on the integrity of musculotendinous units, the status of their innervation, the condition of joints, and so forth. As pain limits motion, these data are necessarily incomplete.

For the older child, with whom some level of informed cooperation can be achieved to test for specific functions, a useful survey can be accomplished to assess for injury to major structures

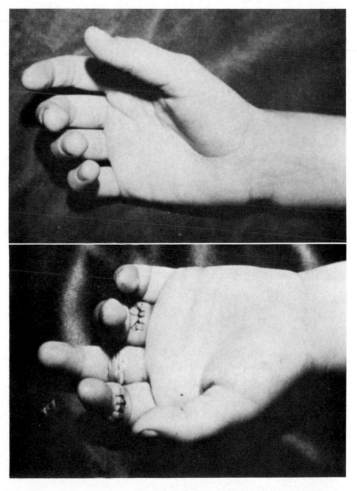

Fig. 21-1   The normal hand. Observation alone yields a wealth of information in examination of the hand. The posture of the fingers is a result of the static forces of the musculotendinous units that attach to the digit. Note the ulnar increments of increasing flexion. Severence of the flexor tendons to a digit results in a loss of flexor tone, and the posture of the finger is in greater extension relative to the other fingers. Flexor digitorum profundus is specifically tested for by noting flexion of the distal joint while the middle phalanx is stabilized. Flexor digitorum sublimis is specifically tested for by holding all other digits in full extension and examining for active flexion at the proximal interphalangeal joint. This maneuver blocks the action of flexor digitorum profundus to the finger being examined. Flexor pollicis longus is examined by noting interphalangeal joint flexion while stabilizing the proximal phalanx of the thumb.

within the hand and forearm. Each tendon, nerve, bone, and joint should be assessed for potential injury. A good knowledge of the functional anatomy of the hand is essential to examine and assess the injured hand (Fig. 21-1).[4,23,51]

Flexor digitorum sublimis is examined for by holding the other digits in complete extension, thus blocking the common action of flexor digitorum profundus and observing proximal interphalangeal joint flexion. Flexor digitorum profundus is tested for by stabilizing the middle phalanx and observing for distal interphalangeal joint flexion. Flexor pollicis longus is checked by stabilizing the thumb proximal phalanx and examining interphalangeal joint flexion. The extrinsic digital extensors— extensor digitorum communis, extensor indicis

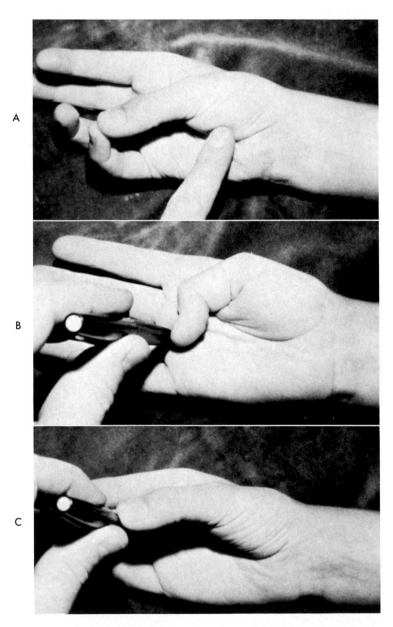

Fig. 21-2   **A,** Median nerve motor function is examined by observing and palpating the activity of the thenar muscles. **B** and **C,** Median nerve motor function is further assessed by noting true pronation of the thumb, which can be observed by noting the rotation of the plane of the thumb nail while abducting the thumb.

proprius, and extensor digiti quinti—are observed by noting full extension at the metacarpophalangeal joint. An extension lag here heralds injury to the extrinsic extensor to that digit. Note that intertendinous connections can mimic partial extension but not full extension at the metacarpophalangeal joint. Moreover, the index and little fingers have double extensor tendons; injury to only one often will not result in an observable extension deficit.

Injuries to the digital extensor mechanism are tested for by observing the posture of the digits.[62] Distal injuries result in a mallet finger, with loss of active extension of the distal interphalangeal joint, and resultant flexion deformity. Injuries to the central slip of the digital extensor apparatus at the proximal interphalangeal joint result in a boutonnière or button hole deformity, with loss of extension of the proximal interphalangeal joint, producing a flexion deformity of the proximal interphalangeal joint and secondary hyperextension of the distal interphalangeal joint.

Instabilities of joint ligamentous injuries are assessed generally by radial and ulnar lateral stress.

Fractures are indicated by bony instability, deformity, and sites of marked pain and swelling. Careful x-ray film review is clearly essential to assess for fractures.

Median nerve motor function is tested by observing for true abduction and pronation of the thumb (Fig. 21-2). Awareness that thumb flexion is not true opposition is important in accurately examining median motor function. Ulnar nerve motor function is noted by the palpable activity of the first dorsal interosseus muscle and of the hypothenar muscles during pinch and by the ability to abduct and adduct the digits with the hand held flat. The ulnar palsied hand shows clawing of the ring and little fingers—hyperextension of the metacarpophalangeal joints and flexion of the interphalangeal joints—due to the loss of intrinsic muscle function (Fig. 21-3). Additionally, the pinch is weak with loss of adductor pollicis and first dorsal interosseus. The compensatory deformity involves thumb interphalangeal joint flexion (Froment's sign) and thumb metacarpal adduction (Fig. 21-4).

A reliable nerve examination in an apprehensive

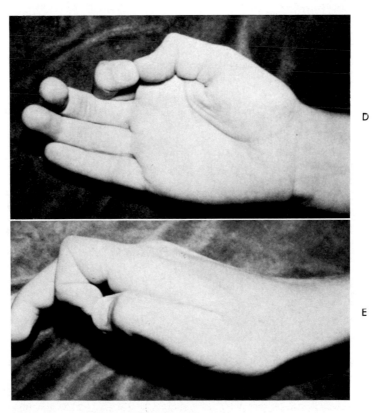

Fig. 21-2, cont'd   D and **E,** Median nerve palsy is manifested by an adducted position of the thumb with loss of true opposition and pronation of the thumb.

child is either questionable or impossible. The hand will not necessarily be held in a position to demonstrate the claw deformity of the ulnar deficient hand. The trick motions of the thumb using flexor pollicis brevis or crossover innervation from the ulnar nerve to the median motor distribution can stimulate median nerve motor function.

Integrity of nerve sensibility can be objectively evaluated in the absence of valid cooperation by noting the presence or absence of sudomotor ac-

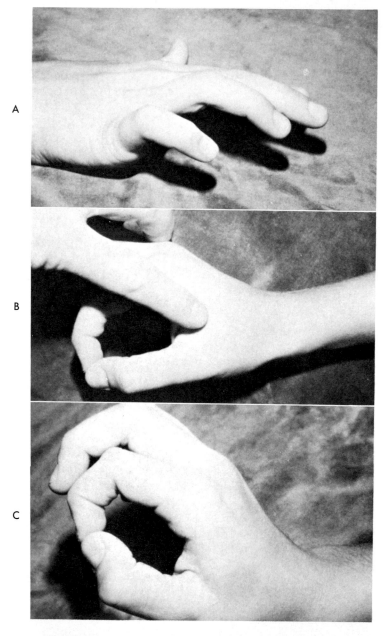

Fig. 21-3   **A,** Ulnar nerve palsy results in the loss of 14 intrinsic muscles of the hand, which profoundly disturbs its dynamic balance. This manifests as a claw deformity of the little and ring fingers with hyperextension of the metacarpophalangeal joint and flexion of the interphalangeal joints. This is the intrinsic minus position of the digits. **B,** The first dorsal interosseus can be observed and palpated for in testing for ulnar motor function. **C,** Ulnar nerve palsy results in sharp flexion at the interphalangeal joint of the thumb during pinch (Froment's sign).

tivity, reflecting sympathetic nervous activity. The tactile adherence test of Harrison is useful in assessing sudomotor activity (Fig. 21-5).[26]

When cooperation is possible, test for soft touch and pain sensibility. Touching with a cotton-covered wood tip and gently pricking with a pin about the autonomous cutaneous area of a nerve in older children will provide a basic estimate of sensation. Two-point discrimination is a more refined assessment of sensibility. Check for partial nerve injuries where only one portion of a nerve's territory is affected or where an area is hypesthetic and not anesthetic.

The vascular supply is evaluated by capillary blanching and refill of the skin and of the nail beds and by the character of radial and ulnar arterial pulses. Pallor, pain, paralysis, and pulselessness indicate an acute vascular problem requiring immediate attention to a compression syndrome with loss of circulation.

The adequacy of skin cover should be carefully determined. Astute observation of skin loss, vascularity, and crush of avulsion is essential to formulate an adequate and rational treatment plan. Finally, x-ray studies complete the examination and provide further objective data on suspected fractures or foreign bodies.

A careful record of all components of the hand examination should be prepared when the injured hand is first seen. Aside from the legal requirements, it proves that a thorough examination indeed was performed (Figs. 21-6 and 21-7). It assists in organizing and clarifying the nature and extent of the injury, and it provides the necessary

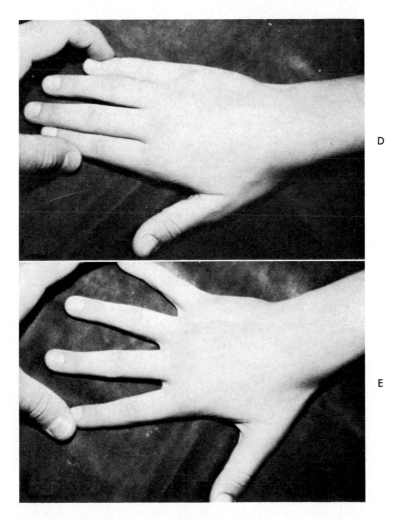

Fig. 21-3, cont'd **D** and **E,** Abduction and adduction of the fingers against resistence checks for the dorsal and the volar interossei muscles, respectively.

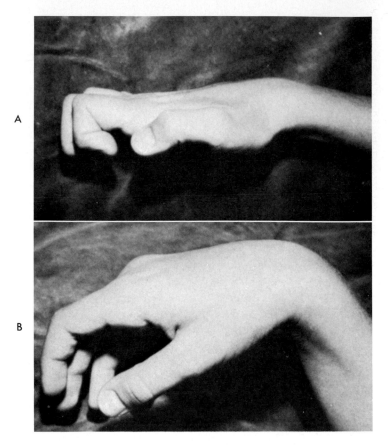

Fig. 21-4 **A,** Combined median and ulnar nerve palsy results in clawing of all the digits and adduction collapse of the thumb due to paralysis of all intrinsic muscles of the hand. **B,** Radial nerve palsy shows the wrist drop with inability to extend the wrist, the metacarpophalangeal joints, and the thumb. An injury at or below the elbow can result in loss of digital and thumb extensors only with preservation of the radial wrist extensors, since their innervation is above the elbow.

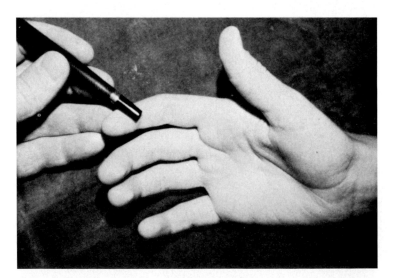

Fig. 21-5 The tactile adherence test, as described by Harrison, examines for the presence of sudomotor activity—sweat gland function mediated by sympathetic fibers in the peripheral nerve. This is particularly useful in peripheral nerve examination in children when reliable testing of sensation is difficult or impossible. Innervated skin possesses a characteristic tactile adherence of a smooth object. Denervated skin is dry, slick, and smooth with loss of tactile adherence.

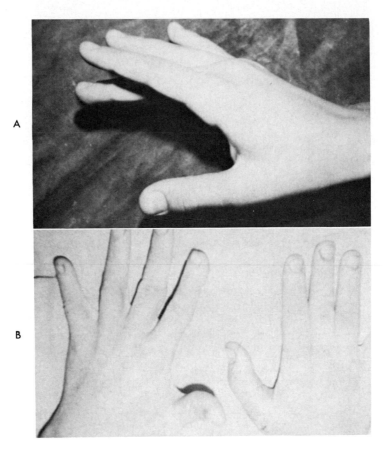

Fig. 21-6   A, An extensor lag at the metacarpophalangeal joint implicates laceration of the extrinsic extensor tendon to that finger. **B,** Inability to extend the thumb implicates injury to the extensor pollicis longus and/or extensor pollicis brevis.

information for review if there is a complication or a postoperative problem questioning the circumstances of the original injury.

The basic principles in evaluating hand injuries in children are to suspect injury to any structure in the traumatic field, to realize the inherent limitations of examination, to observe and to analyze carefully, and then, when necessary or in doubt, to conduct an exploration with the child under anesthesia in the operating room, and to be prepared to carry out the necessary repair. The operating surgeon should proceed to the operating room with as complete a set of examination data as is possible, culled from observation and analysis of spontaneous motion, and, for older children, assisted by specifc tests and motions. There is then full knowledge of what is injured and what might be injured, as well as a careful plan of repair and reconstruction.

SURGICAL PRIORITIES AND OBJECTIVES

The primary objective in surgery of the injured hand is to restore function. This involves experience, flexibility in choice of a range of procedures, and skill in the planning and conduct of the reparative surgery. The principal responsibility of the surgeon is to provide fundamental wound care,[33,62,72,77] which includes the following:

1. Wound cleansing and debridement of foreign material and devitalized tissue. This is the most important step in preventing infection and in providing the circumstances for expeditious wound healing.

2. Stabilization of the skeleton. This is usually accomplished by Kirschner wires or interosseous screws or plates judiciously placed to immobilize fractures and to prevent skel-

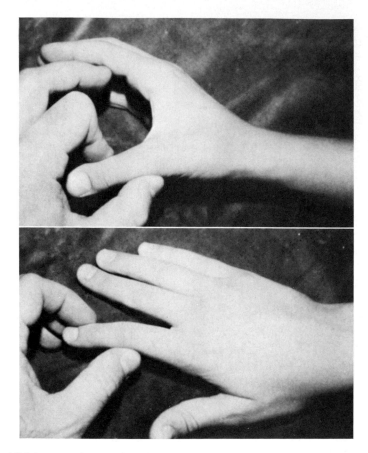

Fig. 21-7   All joints must be examined for instability to assess for ligamentous injury and fracture dislocations.

etal instability from increasing and compounding the soft tissue damage.

3. Provision of skin cover. This is the major obligation of the surgeon along with adequate wound debridement, with skin coverage taking priority over repair of deep injured structures.

4. Repair of tendons and nerves. This assumes a lesser priority than debridement and skin coverage.

5. Proper dressing and splinting of the hand for immobiliziation of both the soft tissues and the skeletal framework. In young children requiring plaster immobilization, the plaster needs to extend to the axilla, with the elbow at 90 degrees of flexion to secure the hand adequately. In older children, the customary forearm splint of cylinder cast is adequate as in adults. A proper hand dressing and splint are important parts of the technical surgery performed.

WOUND ANALYSIS AND SURGICAL IMPLICATIONS

Depending on the agent, the mechanism, the environment of injury, and the time since injury, hand wounds fall into two basic clinical categories.[62] One major type of wound is the tidy or simple wound. This is an incising clean wound with minimal contamination by foreign material and is seen within 6 hours of injury. In these wounds, the degree of bacterial contamination, as assessed by quantitative bacteriologic tests,[35] is predictably low; therefore they are suitable for primary closure and repair of deep structures such as nerves and tendons.

The other basic type of hand wound is the untidy or complicated wound. These wounds involve the crushing, avulsion, or blasting injuries in which the extent of injury often is not immediately apparent and in which devitalization of skin is considerable. There is also major contamination and lodgment of foreign material such that there is a

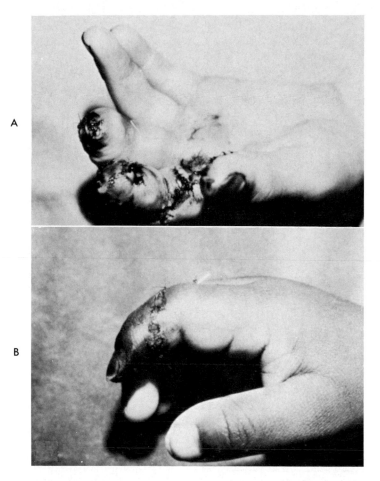

Fig. 21-8   A, Crush injuries can result in severe soft tissue damage. This crush injury with partial amputations of index and long fingers was primarily closed. Five days following injury, considerable skin loss, necrosis, and infection had developed, requiring more proximal amputation levels. This crush injury would have been well managed by delayed primary wound management. **B,** This crush injury associated with phalangeal fractures was considered viable at the time of immediate wound care. Some 8 days following injury, dry gangrene of the crushed digit was evident. This sort of injury must carry a high index of suspicion of considerable soft tissue injury.

high risk of bacterial contamination.[35] Accordingly, these wounds require extensive debridement of foreign material, devitalized, or damaged tissue, and skin in which there are excessive bacteria (greater than 10^5 bacteria per gram tissue).[35] They are therefore not suitable for primary closure or primary repair of deep structures.

Primary closure carries high risk of infection and of further tissue loss and damage. The dangers of immediate wound closure in the untidy or complicated wound involve possible coverage of necrotic tissue, the enclosure of contaminants, the lack of egress for serous fluid or blood collection, tension in the closure, and the formation of a dead space,

all factors that contribute to the development of wound infection (Fig. 21-8).

The correct surgical approach is to perform adequate surgical debridement and skeletal stabilization and to leave the wound open. Delayed primary management of wound closure and skin coverage are generally performed 5 days after the injury. However, under certain circumstances the wound can be left open for longer periods, provided there has been adequate debridement and skeletal stabilization. Delayed primary wound management provides for optimal control of the wound and allows for adequate second-stage debridement. Severed tendons and nerves are repaired secondarily

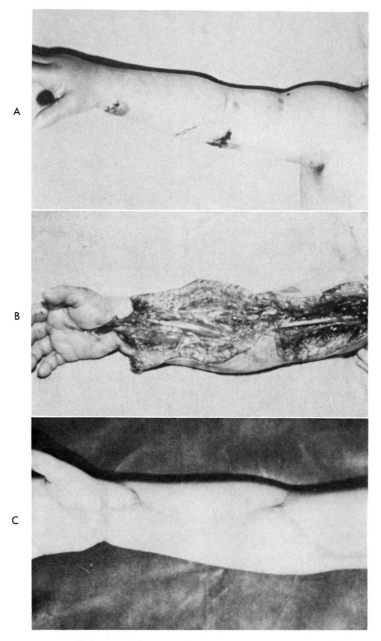

Fig. 21-9   A, Compression syndromes of the upper extremity with resulting compromise of the circulation require prompt decompression. Compression syndromes can develop from several causes, such as crush injuries, humeral fractures, circumferential burn injuries, severe infections, and intraarterial injections of adverse compounds. This completely ischemic extremity with no evidence of any circulation was related to a transfusion infiltrated through the axillary vein into the axilla. **B,** Restoration of the circulation required decompression of the extremity from the axilla to the hand including complete fasciotomies and release of the carpal tunnel. Amniotic membrane was applied as a biologic dressing to the open wound. Delayed closure of the wound was possible 10 days following decompression. **C,** With prompt restoration of the circulation by decompression, no late functional or anatomic loss has occurred. The extremity has normal circulation, normal nerve function, and normal musculotendinous units.

after the wound has been controlled and has healed.

It should be remembered that the indeterminate wound or the intially untidy wound, in some cases, can be converted by adequate surgical debridement and wound cleansing to a clean and tidy wound with a bacterial contamination of less than 10^5 organisms per gram of tissue, so primary repair of injured structures and wound closure is feasible.

Crushing injuries of the hand and forearm are a special problem in the group of untidy injuries. The extent of soft tissue damage is difficult to appreciate initially. Second-stage debridement is often useful as a preliminary to delayed primary closure.

Reactive edema and swelling from crush injury is marked and, when involving the forearm, produces a compression syndrome with the expansion of skeletal muscle within a closed fascial compartment, thus compromising the vascular supply. In the hand this can involve the dorsal interossei muscles. Recognition of a compression syndrome is extremely important, and surgical decompression by fasciotomy is essential to restore the circulation. In the forearm, decompression involves incision of the skin and fascia over the flexor compartment from the wrist to the elbow and should be combined with carpal tunnel release at the same time (Fig. 21-9). For crush injuries of the hand, decompression of the doral interossei should be considered.[8,28]

Wringer injuries of the hand and forearm involve a crushing injury and avulsion of the skin from its blood supply resulting from the tremendous shearing forces.[16,24,28] The amount of skin loss due to the shearing avulsion is often much more than originally suspected, and a second delayed debridement in 5 to 7 days is important. The injury requires close observations for circulatory compromise, which would mandate immediate decompression.

WOUND CLOSURE AND SKIN COVERAGE

Whether wound closure is being performed as a primary or as delayed primary management, the provision of adequate skin coverage to the hand is a high surgical priority. Primary repair or secondary reconstruction can be undertaken only when there is adequate surface coverage. The principle is to provide the simplest possible coverage—coverage that is adequate for deep structures and for preservation of function. For injuries involving skin loss, free skin grafting is the simplest method

for wound coverage and closure. It requires a suitable vascular bed for the graft to take. When there is exposure of bone, joint, tendon, nerve, or an avascular bed, free skin grafting is not suitable, and flap coverage, either local or distant, is indicated.

Split-thickness free skin grafts can be taken with either a dermatome or a free hand knife. The upper inner arm and the upper thigh and buttock are suitable donor sites. Stents are generally not required for skin grafts on the hand because there is no difficulty in having the graft conform to the recipient bed, which is generally firm. A molding, conforming, mildly compressive hand dressing with plaster immobilization is the key to dressing and immobilizing grafts on the hand during the healing process. Unless there are reasons for an early dressing change, the hand dressing is left intact for 7 days. Mobilization is then permitted, and the grafts generally require only a protective dressing at that point.

Full-thickness grafts, which can be taken from the wrist, elbow, or groin creases, are rarely indicated in the acutely injured hand. They generally are reserved for secondary reconstruction procedures in which free skin grafting is required on the volar surface of the digits or the palm, where the thickness, durability, and minimal contracture of the graft are important considerations.

Under some circumstances, a skin graft is inadequate for the functional purpose of the surface area requiring coverage. A variety of local flaps are available that provide better reconstruction. The fingertip is notable for having special requirements, which include durable padding, sensibility, and preservation of length. Volar advancement flaps, cross-finger flaps, triangular V-Y advancement flaps, and thenar flaps all have been used to advantage on the fingertip.[1,41,62,63] Dorsal transposition flaps are used for pliable coverage in the first web space for thumb adduction contracture releases. Various single and multiple Z-plasties are used throughout the hand for different contracture deformities.[49] Local sensory flaps are available about the hand for redistributing sensation to critical areas.[29] The principal sensory flap is the neurovascular island pedicle, which is transferred from a digit to the thumb, where sensation is critical to hand function.[43] The major limitation of local flaps on the hand is their maximal possible size, which does not make them suitable for large defects.

When hand wounds requiring flap coverage are

of such a size that local flaps are not feasible, then distant flap coverage is necessary. Major skin loss with exposure of bone, tendon, joint, nerve, or a region requiring future deep reconstruction are conditions requiring flap coverage to the wound (Fig. 21-10).[4,62,78] The application of the flap can be immediate, delayed for 5 days following debridement and skeletal stabilization, or secondary following temporary closure of the wound with a graft.

A major source for the provision of distant flap coverage to the hand is the groin flap, described by McGregor and Jackson in 1972.[50] It is an au-tonomous vascular cutaneous territory, based on the superficial circumflex iliac artery and vein, an axial pattern flap of prodigious length compared with the older abdominal pedicle flap. The versatility of the groin flap accrues from the considerable length that can be achieved following adaptation to large and complex wound defects. The flap is robust and reliable. Its carrying limb is long and can be tubed, leaving no raw surface area. The donor site often can be primarily closed, again leaving no raw surface area that would otherwise require skin grafting. Because of the groin flap's

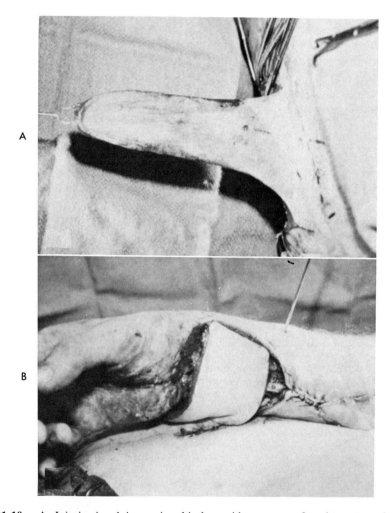

Fig. 21-10   **A,** Injuries involving major skin loss with exposure of tendon, nerve, bone, or joint where a free skin graft is inadequate coverate, skin flap surfacing is necessary for optimal functional results. The groin flap is an extremely useful flap for hand injuries. Its remarkably long length commends it for the repair of complex, extensive defects, and for the ease of immobilization, and for its facility to tube proximally, eliminating any raw surface area and any need for skin grafting. **B,** This groin flap was used to surface a volar forearm tissue loss resulting from an electrical injury where there was exposure of both tendon and nerve following debridement.

length, immobilization is simple; this is a great advantage in children requiring flap coverage to the hand. Moreover, the amount of subcutaneous fat is less in the groin skin than in skin on the abdomen.

The groin flap has a further and distinctive capability in the repair of complex hand injuries when bone in addition to flap coverage is required for reconstruction. With a groin flap, iliac crest bone can be imported simultaneously with flap coverage in the anticipation of ultimate reconstruction in complex injuries.[21] For instance, a tube flap complete with bone can be obtained immediately at the time of injury for primary thumb reconstruction after thumb amputation.

When the groin flap is not available or not feasible for distant flap coverage to the hand, there are a number of other possible flaps. These include the abdominal pedicle flap, the submammary flap, and the cross-arm flap. Each is patterned after a template of the wound defect and applied. The donor defects of these flaps require grafting, and the carrying limb of the flap has a raw surface. Since the length of the carrying limb is necessarily short, the problems of immobilization to prevent tension, kinking, and distortion are considerable.

Free flap transfer with immediate microsurgical revascularization should be considered for children with hand injuries that require flap coverage, be-

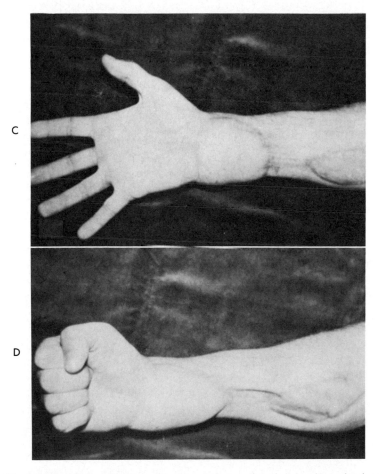

Fig. 21-10, cont'd   C and **D,** Proper tendon and nerve function can be maintained when there is adequate surfacing by a skin flap. Three months after the application of the flap, this patient underwent tenolysis and neurolysis. Six months after the original injury, full extension and full flexion were obtained, along with full ulnar nerve recovery, median motor nerve recovery, and the recovery of sensation to thumb and long finger. Further nerve work is planned for the residual sensory deficits. Carefully planned multistaged procedures are called for from the beginning in such complex injuries. The varied capabilities and principles of the reconstructive surgeon are brought into demand in such cases.

cause of its rapid reconstruction, the absence of prolonged immobilization, and the possibilities of early mobilization. The free transfer of composite flap tissue through restoration of the circulation by microvascular anastomoses was conceived by Krizek et al.[37] in 1965 and clinically demonstrated in 1973.[13] Numerous reports of successful free flap transfer have since been published.[25,57] It seems that this method may be of singular advantage in children, who cannot tolerate prolonged immobilization of a hand to a skin flap on the abdomen or groin. A free flap transfer is the most expeditious reconstruction. It permits early motion and movement of the joints of the hand. It diminishes prolonged immobilization and hospitalization. Selection of patients, timing of surgery, as well as the skill of the surgeon in microvascular surgery are all vitally important to the success of this surgery.

AMPUTATIONS

In general, all amputated parts should be saved for evaluation by the treating hand surgeon. The tissues should be wrapped in a saline-moistened sponge, placed in an impervious plastic bag, and then covered in an ice solution, avoiding direct contact of the tissues with the ice.

Depending on the level and mechanism of injury, the age and condition of the patient, and the caliber and quality of the digital vessels, microvascular replantation may be elected. In some cases, especially in infants and young children, amputated tips may be applied as nonrevascularized replants or composite grafts with reasonable hopes of success. In many cases, the tips may be defatted for application as skin grafts.

FINGERTIP INJURIES

The fingertip is the most commonly injured portion of the hand, especially in children. Special functional requirements for a satisfactory surgical reconstruction of the fingertip are tip sensibility, a pain-free scar, durable surfacing, and preservation of length (Fig. 21-11). There are multiple ways of managing a nonreplantable amputated finger, and the selection principally depends on the level of amputation and the angulation of the amputation.[51,63]

In distal soft tissue fingertip amputations, when incised with a knife or glass and seen within the first 2 hours of injury, direct replacement of the amputated part can be considered in young children, as revascularization of small distal amputated portions can occur. Alternatively, for the sharply incised clean injury, the distal amputated soft tissue part can be defatted and the portion used as a full-thickness skin graft, provided there is a suitable wound bed.

Small distal fingertip skin losses are best managed in children by conservative dressing and secondary wound healing and contracture. Excellent results are obtained from allowing the secondary healing and contracture to occur, since it results in good padding, good sensation, and generally a pain-free tip.

Larger areas of fingertip skin loss are well managed by split-thickness skin grafting. However, the use of a full-thickness free graft from a plantar toe surface could be considered for application to the fingertips, since this area carries a high density of sensory end organs, which is considered to improve the ultimate quality of sensibility.

Finger amputations through the middle of the distal phalanx require local flap arrangements for satisfactory closure, preservation of length, and provision of an adequate surface over the bone. The volar, triangular, subcutaneous-based V-Y advancement flap provides an excellent solution for the transverse amputation through the middle portion of the distal phalanx.[1] It meets all the necessary criteria.

For the more proximal injury, either transverse, proximal to the distal interphalangeal joint, or oblique removing the majority of the volar pulp tissue of the fingertip, other local flaps are more useful. The cross-finger flap is a versatile flap, when preservation of digital length is important and when there has been considerable loss of volar fingertip pulp skin.[12,70] It is a reliable procedure, transferring dorsal digital skin to the injured fingertip. Adequate mobilization of the flap most often requires release of Cleland's ligament. Flap division is generally at 17 to 21 days. Late sensory reinnervation is observed to a variable degree. For a similar type of proximal fingertip injury, a thenar flap is available when preservation of length is critical.[22,51] This procedure has been criticized because it involves complications of interphalangeal joint stiffness and painful donor site scars on the thenar eminence. However, children are not prone to stiffness following this immobilization, nor do they necessarily develop dysesthetic scars. Accordingly, it is a procedure that can be considered

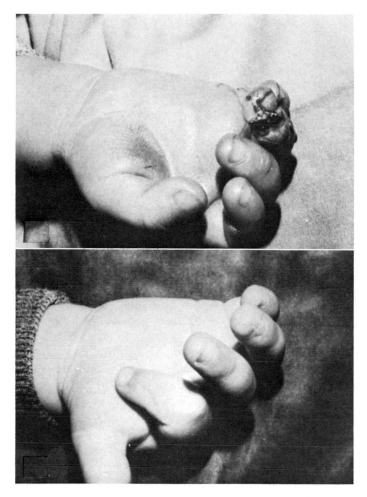

Fig. 21-11   Fingertip injuries are common in children. With attention to the principles of wound management, healing can be sound and infection prevented.

in children. The volar advancement flap, so useful in thumbtip injuries, is a possible alternative in these more proximal fingertip amputations. This provides the surface and sensibility but carries the potential liability of a flexion deformity of the proximal interphalangeal joint.

Proximal digital amputations should be considered for replantation in children, since the anticipated functional recovery can be satisfactory.[56] This requires an experienced team in microvascular work. Potential indications for replantation include an amputated thumb, amputated index finger, or multiple digital amputations. Avulsion and crush injuries are unsuitable for replantations. If a microvascular team is not available, the chances for successful replantation are small, and alternate methods of management must be considered.

For children, a fingertip injury is not trivial, and following one of these reparative procedures, adequate immobilization for soft tissue healing is essential.

RECONSTRUCTIVE MICROSURGERY

The development of reliable microsurgical technique and methods has been a major advance in the management of hand trauma.* Since the late 1960s and early 1970s, replantation of amputated parts of the hand and upper extremity has become a reliable reconstructive procedure, widely used by surgeons with training and experience in microsurgery and the management of such complex hand

*References 10, 11, 45, 55, 65, 74.

trauma. With the establishment of effective micro-surgical techniques, instrumentation, and the development of anatomic knowledge regarding blood supply, the free transfer of vascularized tissue for reconstruction has become a reality. Proper skin debridement, skeletal stabilization, and vascularized flap coverage of the adequately debrided wound need to be followed to achieve a successful microsurgical revascularization result.

There are many donor resources available for free transfer, depending on the reconstructive requirements. Toe-to-hand transfer can be carried out for thumb and digit reconstruction. Free functional muscle transfer of the gracilis, serratus anterior, or the latissimus dorsi muscle can be carried out for loss of the flexor muscle in the forearm. Skin flap coverage can be provided from a groin flap, a scapular flap, a lateral arm flap, or by use of a free muscle transfer combined with skin graft coverage to establish flap coverage. Free vascularized joint transfer from the foot to the hand is also possible, and free vascularized live bone transfer can be carried out from within the fibula or the ilium for reconstruction of segmental bone loss. This approach eliminates the 3-week period of attachment of the hand or extremity to a pedicle flap, a situation very difficult to maintain in a very young patient. Immediate transfer without attachment provides complete vascularization and wound closure, which is of particular advantage to the pediatric patient.

Microsurgical revascularization may be indicated when injury causes partial amputation with vascular injury and ischemia. Restoration of the circulation can salvage injured components of the hand and improve the circulation, thereby augmenting healing time.

Replantation of the completely amputated part of the hand is indicated for thumb amputation, for multiple digit amputation, and for amputation through the metacarpal level, the wrist, and the forearm. Contemporary microsurgical technique and capability are such that the smaller sized blood vessel in the pediatric patient does not preclude microsurgery for replantation or reconstruction.

FLEXOR TENDON INJURIES

The key to the management of pediatric flexor tendon injuries is to maintain a high index of suspicion in volar lacerations to the hand or forearm, which conceivably could result in flexor tendon injuries. In young children, examination is difficult if not impossible, and exploration in the operating room with the child under anesthesia and under proper conditions is often required to determine whether there has been a flexor tendon injury. A proper exploration is required if the best results of nerve and tendon injuries in this age group are to be obtained.

In children, the nature of the wound permitting, several flexor tendons should be primarily repaired within 6 to 8 hours of injury, at whatever level (Fig. 21-12.)[34,62,75] With meticulous surgery, children do exceptionally well with consistently good to excellent results from primary repair of flexor tendons. The problems attending the adult injury do not apply directly to children. However, the principles of wound management as discussed previously must be attended to, and not all flexor tendon injuries will be possible to be primarily repaired because of wound complications.

At the wrist level, all injured structures should be primarily repaired when possible. These include the nerves and the tendons. Each digit has two flexor tendons, and it is thought that optimal digital function and better digital balance result from restoring normal anatomy and providing each digit with both flexor tendons. However, there is controversy over this point. At a minimal the profundus tendons require repair, and the index sublimis tendon can be considered as well for primary repair.

When multiple structures are repaired at the wrist level or any structure is repaired in the proximal or midpalm level, a carpal tunnel release should be performed. The carpal tunnel is a noncompromising closed space carrying nine tendons and one nerve. The expected edema from the injury and wound healing when multiple structures are involved or any involvement in the carpal tunnel region means that there is a predictable compression, and adverse results can be anticipated if the volar carpal ligament is not released. When the repair is at or just proximal to the beginning of the flexor digital sheath, the proximal portion of the sheath can be incised to minimize the fibrosis of the repair from being contiguous with the flexor sheath.

Flexor tendon injuries within the digital flexor sheath, which extends from the distal palmar crease to just distal to the proximal interphalangeal joint crease, should be primarily repaired, the wound circumstances permitting.[34] If possible, both flexor tendons should be repaired to restore a more normal anatomy and to obtain an ultimate better digital balance and power. A window of flexor sheath is excised over the site of repair to minimize the fibrosis between the repair and the adjacent flexor sheath. The vinculae are the thin dorsal structures that restrain the proximal retraction of the tendons when severed. It should be observed that the vinculae carry an important blood supply to the flexor tendons; when intact they should not be injured in the dissection, but should be preserved. Should a proximal end of a tendon be difficult to retrieve, a separate plamar incision can be made to assist, from whence the tendon can be found and led out to the digital wound. The digital injury incision is usually extended both proximally and distally, depending on the location and orientation of the

wound. For a transverse wound, it is often convenient to convert this to a T-shape with a midaxial extension proximally and distally. For oblique incisions, extension involving the Bruner type of incision is useful. This is a volar "zigzag" incision.

The isolated profundus injury should be primarily repaired when the level involves the proximal half of the middle phalanx. For a level involving the distal portion of the distal phalanx, profundus advancement with reinsertion into the distal phalanx is performed.

For wounds seen late after injury, for example 12 to 18 hours, and for wounds in which there is a significant degree of contamination or more extensive soft tissue damage from crushing, primary repair of the flexor tendons and nerves should not

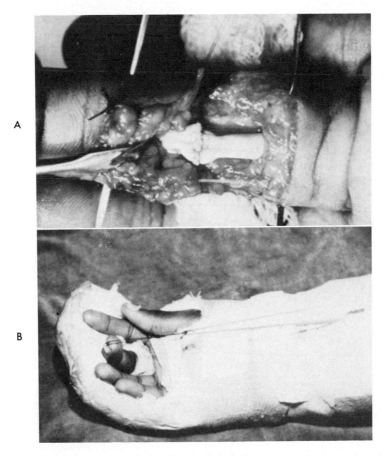

Fig. 21-12 **A,** Flexor tendon injuries in the digital fiberosseous flexor tendon sheath can be primarily repaired in children if the wound is tidy and incising without tissue loss, compound injury, gross contamination, or an excess period of time since injury. In this knife cut injury, primary repair of flexor digitorum profundus was performed using transfixion needles to relieve tension at the junction during tendon repair and excision of a window in the flexor tendon sheath. **B,** When the child is old enough to cooperate, as was the case with this 11 year old, controlled early motion is employed.

Continued.

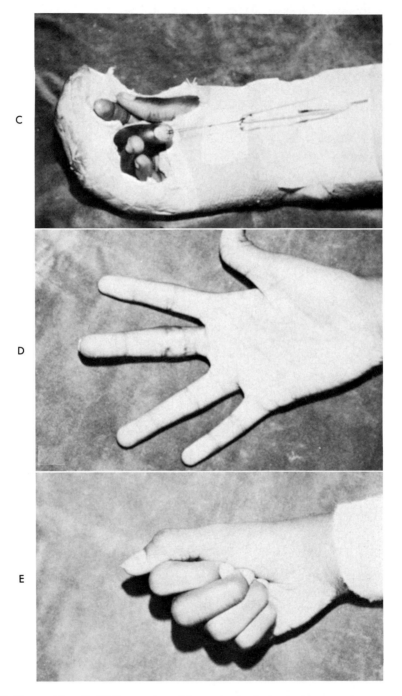

Fig. 21-12, cont'd **C,** Gliding motion of the tendon is obtained without tension across the tendon junction. The hand is splinted for 3½ weeks before active motion and therapy is commenced. **D** and **E,** One month out of the plaster cast, the patient has an excellent result with a full range of motion.

be undertaken. A delayed primary repair should be considered for these circumstances. Initially, the wound is thoroughly debrided, cleansed, and closed. Antibiotics are given for 2 to 3 days. About 5 to 7 days after the initial treatment, the healing of the wound can be evaluated and assessed. If there is infection, evidence of inadequate debridement, greater soft tissue injury then initially appreciated, or marked soft tissue reaction, the secondary flexor tendon repair would be indicated following sound healing of the hand wound. However, in the presence of wound healing with absence of infection and minimal wound reaction, a delayed

primary repair can be proceeded with. With the planned delay, one has ensured proper wound circumstances, yet at a time before fibrosis and retraction have proceeded where a primary suture repair of tendon or nerve cannot be performed.

There are several good techniques for end-to-end suture of severed tendons.[4,34,51] Through an incision allowing adequate exposure, the severed tendon ends are transfixed proximally and distally through soft tissue with straight needles. This relieves tension and permits careful suturing of the tendon ends. In younger children, the repair is with 5-0 monofilament nylon, and in older children, 4-0

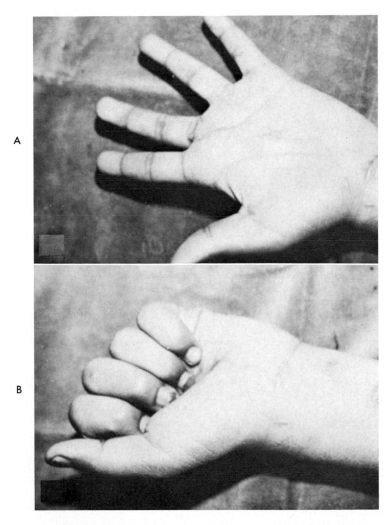

Fig. 21-13 **A,** When primary flexor tendon repair has not been done, then secondary flexor tendon grafting is required. In this case, for reasons of extensive fibrosis throughout the flexor mechanism, a preliminary Silastic rod was placed on a first stage to flexor tendon grafting. A flexor tendon sheath forms about the rod. Subsequently, a flexor tendon graft replaces the rod in the new sheath. **B,** Full extension and full flexion were achieved from this two-stage flexor tendon grafting procedure.

monofilament nylon. A single criss-cross suture is used in such a way that the knot is placed between the severed tendon ends. Then a running 6-0 or 7-0 synthetic braided suture material is continuously run around the margin of the tendon repair for precision in coaptation of the tendon ends. The tendon is handled only on its cut surface, is exposed for a minimal amount of time, and is kept moist at all times, thus minimizing injury along its gliding surface, which would encourage fibrosis and compromise quality of results.

Secondary flexor tendon grafting is required when both flexor tendons have been injured and primary repair not performed (Fig. 21-13).[19,60,71] Thorough healing and fully mobile joints are essential. The digit and palm are then fully exposed through appropriate incisions. The flexor tendon sheath is cleared with preservation of three pulleys and removal of remaining flexor tendon segments. A free flexor tendon graft of palmaris longus or plantaris tendon is inserted, using either flexor digitorum profundus or flexor digitorum sublimis as a motor, passing through the pulleys and inserting on the distal phalanx. Palmaris longus is preferable as the tendon graft; the plantaris tendon serves as the back-up choice. The distal insertion is done first using a pull-out wire taken through the distal phalanx over a button on the nail. The proximal tendon junction is done last using a Pulvertaft weaver (the interweaving of two tendons for a mechanically secure tendon junction), which permits easy adjustment of the tension and length of the graft to be used. The hand is immobilized for 3½ weeks, following which a graded, progressive rehabilitative program is undertaken. In very young children, this is not really possible, and the continuous daily hand motions at play become excellent physiotherapy. A removable protective night splint is used for the first 2 weeks after mobilization.

In secondary flexor tendon reconstruction where there is diffuse and prolific scarring with destruction of the flexor tendon bed and obliteration of pulleys, a two-stage reconstruction is required.[27] A Silastic rod is placed in the flexor tendon bed with or without pulley reconstruction to form a new flexor tendon sheath. Flexor tendon grafting is then performed through this new sheath.

The pediatric hand is notorious for its difficulty in proper immobilization. Great care and attention must be taken to the dressing of the hand and the plaster immobilization. For flexor tendon injuries, the digits are held in flexion in the posture they assume with 30 degrees of wrist flexion. Children under 10 years of age require a plaster cylinder cast extending to the axilla (Fig. 21-14). A stockinette is then applied to the entire extremity, wrapped across the opposite axilla and about the neck to secure the upper extremity against the torso. It should be applied so that the tips of all digits can be visualized. For the older child in whom understanding and cooperation are realistic, the adult

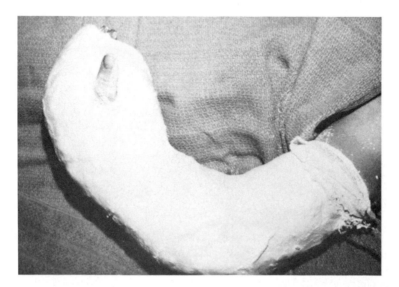

Fig. 21-14   In younger children, adequate hand immobilization for flexor tendon injuries as well as for other injuries requires cylinder plaster involving the entire extremity to the axilla.

form of dressing is applied, consisting of a short arm cylinder cast with a dorsal hood to block extension. These are personal preferences. Many other techniques of dressing and immobilization are used and are effective.

In this latter method for the older child, controlled early motion is instituted on the third postoperative day, following primary repair of flexor tendons.[34] This has been demonstrated to be an important component in postoperative care for primary repair of flexor tendons in the digital flexor sheath in the adult. It permits gliding motion of the tendon during the healing process. An exercise device is built into the short arm cast as follows. An elastic band is connected to a suture applied to the nail at the time of surgery. The band is then attached to a cleat built into the plaster cast on the volar forearm. This exercise arrangement provides a dynamic flexor restoring force to the digit. Active extension is permitted up to the dorsal plaster extension block, and elastic then provides the restoring flexion force, thus reducing any forces across the tendon repair, yet maintaining the gliding function. Plaster immobilization for all circumstances is 3½ weeks.

EXTENSOR TENDON INJURIES

Extensor tendon injuries of the hand are fundamentally divided into two different groups, depending on their level of injury. The first are injuries to the extensor tendons in the dorsal areas of the hand and wrist, proximal to the metacarpophalangeal joint level. These injuries are principally manifested by an extensor lag at the metacarpophalangeal extension of the middle and little fingers, despite interruption of extensor digitorum communis to those fingers.[68] This can confuse the diagnosis.

The other major category involves injury to the digital extensor apparatus distal to the metacarpophalangeal joint level. These can result in mallet finger or boutonnière deformities (Fig. 21-15).

The repair of extrinsic extensor tendons to the hand is equally important as the repair of flexor tendons to the hand.[17] Given satisfactory wound conditions as discussed above, primary repair is indicated and produces good functional results in children. With avulsion injuries and major tissue loss to the dorsum of the hand, however, flap coverage is required as a first stage.

In all tendon work, the tendons are kept moist and are not handled with forceps on their gliding surface. For extensor tendons, a criss-cross suture is used for repair, leaving the knot between the ends of the severed tendons. The extensor apparatus near the metacarpophalangeal joint level and the digital extensor mechanism are broad, flat structures for which horizontal mattress sutures are used. A tendon suture of 5-0 nylon in younger children and 4-0 in older children is used.

Approximately 4 to 6 weeks of immobilization are important for the satisfactory repair of these tendons. An extensor tendon repair needs to be protected for a longer period because of the greater force of the flexor tendon across the finger joints. The position of immobilization is critical; this should involve the wrist in 45 degrees of extension, the metacarpophalangeal joint in 30 degrees of flexion, and the interphalangeal joints in 20 degrees to 30 degrees of flexion. The metacarpophalangeal joints do not have to be placed in full extension to relieve tension at the site of extensor tendon repair. This is principally controlled by wrist extension. If the metacarpophalangeal joints are incorrectly held in full extension or hyperextension for this period, inevitable limitation of flexion results. This can be a serious disability, involving a long period of rehabilitation and, in certain cases, further surgery.

Extensor tendon injuries of the thumb are relatively common. Lacerations of extensor pollicis brevis and extensor pollicis longus, with wound conditions permitting, are best treated with primary repair, followed by 4 to 6 weeks of immobilization of the wrist and all thumb joints in extension, for example, a thumb spica dressing.

Digital extensor mechanism injuries are special problems, can easily go unrecognized, and require precise reconstruction for adequate results. The dorsal surfaces of both the proximal interphalangeal joint and distal phalangeal joint are exposed and therefore are frequent locations of laceration. Injury to either site should provoke suspicion about injury to the digital extensor mechanism. Laceration of the central portion of the digital extensor mechanism overlying the proximal interphalangeal joint results in a boutonnière deformity with flexion of the proximal interphalangeal joint and hyperextension of the distal interphalangeal joint.[18,44,67] This requires direct surgical repair. The earlier the surgical management, the better the possibilities for a good result. For the immediately recognized injury, a direct primary repair of the extensor mech-

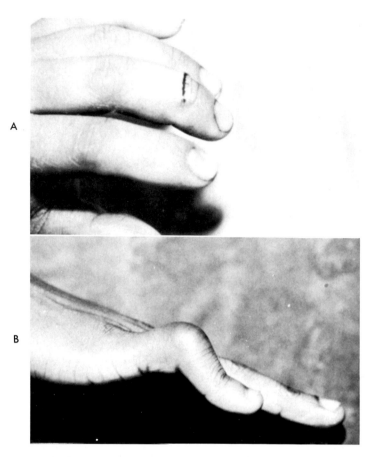

Fig. 21-15 **A,** Injuries to the digital extensor mechanism at the distal interphalangeal joint result in mallet finger deformity. When closed, these can be treated conservatively by 6 weeks of splinting. However, in some cases a k-wire is needed for adequate internal splinting. In open injuries, the tendon injury is directly repaired, and a k-wire is placed across the distal interphalangeal joint. **B,** Injury to the central slip of the digital extensor mechanism over the proximal interphalangeal joint results in a boutonnière deformity. Whether open or closed, direct surgical repair is necessary. A k-wire is placed across the joint for adequate immobilization for 4 weeks.

anism with horizontal mattress sutures of 4-0 or 5-0 nylon is required, and a k-wire is placed across the proximal interphalangeal joint with the joint in full extension. This k-wire is required for satisfactory immobilization. In general, the k-wire is removed after a 4-week period, following which active flexion exercises are permitted. The best time for correction of an injury to the digital extensor mechanism at the proximal interphalangeal joint level is immediately. Often, however, the injury is not immediately recognized, and it appears as a boutonnière deformity some 4 to 6 weeks after injury, perhaps from an incomplete extensor mechanism laceration, which proceeds to completion in time. When the injury is seen late, a direct surgical

repair is needed, with advancement and suturing of the central extensor mechanism, dorsal reefing of the lateral bands, and k-wire immobilization of the proximal interphalangeal joint.

The mallet finger deformity results from injury to the conjoined extensor tendon at the distal interphalangeal joint. The distal joint then assumes a flexion deformity with loss of active extension. In general, the treatment requires 6 weeks of immobilization with the distal interphalangeal joint in extension.[4,48,51,62] As this is impossible to maintain in younger children, internal fixation with a Kirschner wire is often necessary. When there is a fracture—dislocation of the dorsal base of the distal phalanx—a second k-wire is useful in anchoring the fractured fragment, diminishing the proximal pull on it by the intact extensor tendon. Conservative external splinting for the closed injury, as applicable to adults, is useful only in the older child. For the open injury, direct suture of the severed tendon is necessary with k-wire immobilization.

The key to boutonnière and mallet finger deformities from digital extensor mechanism injuries is to recognize them initially and to repair then accordingly. Their late deformity and late repair involve problems and uncertain results that are best prevented.

NERVE INJURIES

Peripheral nerve injuries are difficult to diagnose in children, particularly in younger children, in whom a reliable sensory examination and evaluation of motor function is not possible. A high index of suspicion must be kept in mind for any laceration or injury, since it may involve a peripheral nerve, depending on the location. Often exploration with the child under anesthesia in the operating room is required to determine the presence or absence of a nerve injury. This approach is particularly useful for the partial nerve injury when the emergency room evaluation by examination can be so deceptive.

For the clean, tidy wound, primary repair of the injured nerve is performed (Fig. 21-16). Secondary repair of the injured nerve is indicated for the complicated wound that is either initially untidy or contaminated or requires soft tissue coverage and sound healing before repair of the injured deep structure (Fig. 21-17).[62] Because of their exceptional healing and regenerative properties, children do consistently better than adults in terms of recovery of nerve function following repair, either primarily or secondarily.[47,62,64]

Regarding the technique of nerve repair, operative magnification is widely considered to be essential for precision in the coaptation of nerve ends, as it permits appreciation of the intraneural topography to achieve optimal alignment of nerve fascicles.[32,66] For direct end-to-end suture, four epineural sutures are placed, spaced 90 degrees from each other using 6-0 synthetic suture material. Proper alignment and rotation can be achieved by noting the location of the longitudinally disposed blood vessels and by observing the pattern and shape of the fascicular bundles. With operative magnification through either an operating microscope or four-power loupes, specific fascicular alignment and coaptation is obtained by interrupted 10-0 nylon perineural sutures to the major fascicular bundles. Usually from five to eight are used. The epineural sutures provide a structural integrity to the repair, and the perineural sutures provide precision in fascicular coaptation. One is balancing off precision in fascicular coaptation against factors that increase fibroplasia at the repair site—the amount of suture material left intraneurally, surgical trauma, and total operative time with nerve exposure. This method is one used personally and represents a middle position between the classical epineural suture method and the multifascicular repair with resection of epineureum, a large number of fascicular sutures, and a long operative time. The technical objectives are to achieve optimal precision in coaptation with a minimal of surgical trauma, suture material at the repair site, tension across the nerve junction, and operative time.

If the extent of injury to the nerve is indeterminant or over a considerable length, or if the wound is crushing, avulsed, contaminated, or lacks coverage, then primary repair should not be undertaken, and secondary repair is mandated. Epineural sutures, however, are placed to maintain the length of the nerve under these circumstances to limit the amount of retraction during wound healing before the secondary repair.

For the secondary repair of the injured peripheral nerve, the suture technique is the same. All fibrosis and injured nerve are debrided by transverse sections with a razor blade back to normal nerve proximally and distally. Operative magnification is of great use in this determination. One looks for pliable, protruding fascicles free from the characteristic inelastic fibrosis to indicate that normal nerve has been reached. In either the primary or secondary repair, immobilization is for 3 weeks, following which a removable protective splint is provided for a further 2 weeks.

In the complicated peripheral nerve injury in which there has been loss of considerable nerve tissue, reoperative surgery for neuroma formation at the site of a former repair, or complications such as wound infection attending the original injury, a large gap may exist between the proximal and distal ends of the nerve at the time of secondary repair. End-to-end suture then necessarily involves a certain amount of tension, and the coincident wide mobilization of the nerve deprives a portion of the blood supply to the nerve. Millesi[52,53] introduced interfascicular nerve grafting in an effort to improve results under these complicated circumstances. Free grafts of sections of the sural nerve are placed under operative magnification between corresponding fasciculi or groups of fasciculi to bridge the gap in the nerve, thus relieving tension and making wide mobilization unnecessary (Fig. 21-18). The adjacent epineureum is resected, and the fascicular graft coaptations are staggered in an effort to minimize fibrosis at the site of repair, which can compromise the number of axons traversing the repair sites. A key point is the relief of tension on the repaired nerve. Millesi's long-term follow-up on a larger series reported excellent results, better than the large series reported by Seddon and by Sakellarides using the standard method of direct end-to-end suture for all circumstances, as cited by Millesi.[53] Millesi states that any gap over 2 cm measured with the wrist in neutral and all joints in extension should be grafted.[52] There is no consensus on this, however, and the relevant studies are pending. Interfascicular nerve grafting should be considered for the complicated nerve

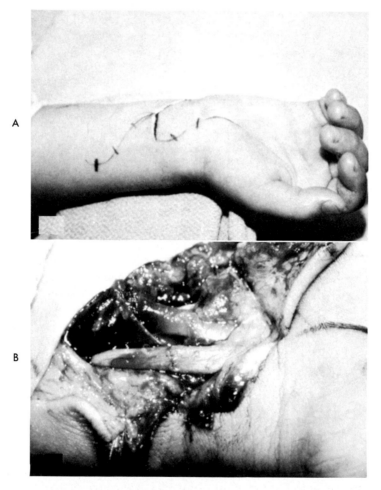

Fig. 21-16   A, A distal volar forearm glass laceration resulted in median nerve injury with loss of thumb opposition and anesthesia in the median nerve distribution. **B,** Primary nerve repair was performed using several interrupted epineural sutures combined with six perineural 10-0 nylon sutures applied to major fascicular bundles to assist in the precision of coaptation of the nerve ends. The two flexor tendon lacerations at this level were simultaneously primarily repaired. The immobilization period was 3½ weeks. Excellent motor and sensory function were recovered after this injury, including full motor recovery and sensibility for pain, soft touch, two-point discrimination of 8 mm, and functional tactile gnosis as assessed 9 months after injury.

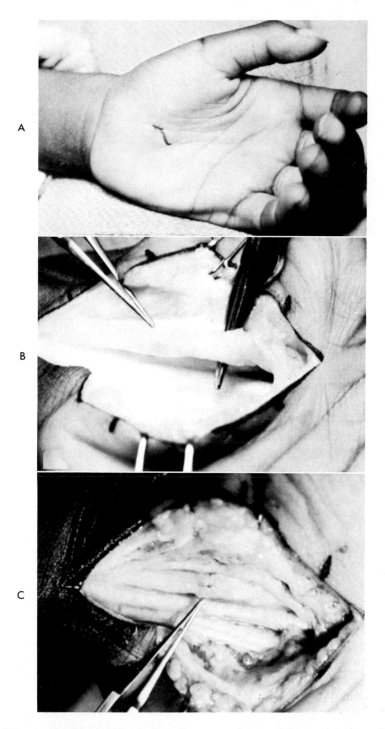

Fig. 21-17 **A,** Small lacerations in the palm can result in partial nerve injuries, which must be examined for carefully. This young patient complained of anesthesia in the index finger and the adjacent side of long finger 4 weeks following a glass injury to the palm. **B,** Exploration demonstrated a neuroma to a portion of the dividing median nerve in the proximal palm. **C,** Resection and nerve suture under operative magnification was performed. Eight months following injury, this patient had good recovery of sensation including two-point discrimination and tactile gnosis.

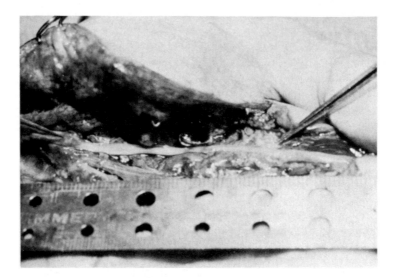

Fig. 21-18   This patient sustained a blast injury to the palm of the hand with a partial median nerve injury consisting of blast loss of the common digital nerve to the radial side of the index finger. Subsequent nerve grafting was performed under operative magnification using the sural nerve as a donor and grafting the common digital nerve to radial side of index finger for a gap of 5 cm. The graft seen here is sutured in place with the nerve junctions of the graft indicated by forceps proximally and distally. Recovery of sensation was excellent with restoration of pain and soft touch sensibility, along with 6 mm two-point discrimination and appreciation of tactile gnosis.

injury when there is a large gap between the proximal and distal ends of the injured nerve and when direct end-to-end suture involves significant tension.[20]

Digital nerve injuries, wound circumstances permitting, are best managed by primary suture repair.[64] Operative magnification is required, and between two to four interrupted 10-0 nylon sutures are used with careful attention to precise coaptation of the severed nerve end.

FRACTURES AND JOINT INJURIES

The principles of management of fractures and dislocations in the pediatric hand are basically the same as for the adult.[4,5,23,51,69] Children have the remarkable capacity for rapid healing and remodeling of a fracture site to accommodate for lack of perfect reduction. In children, particular attention must be given to the epiphysis, since epiphyseal injuries can result in subsequent growth deformity. Surgery itself can injure an epiphysis, resulting in a growth disturbance.

The objectives of management of a fracture are: (1) to provide an acceptable reduction, (2) to secure adequate fixation during skeletal healing, and (3) to obtain a functional hand with full joint mo-

bility. Reductions are either open or closed. Most fractures can be managed with closed reduction, with the provision of external plaster for stabilization. Open reduction is indicated only if the reduction can be substantially improved and maintained by the direct visualization and manipulation of the fractured segments. Unstable fractures at times require open reduction and the provision of internal fixation to stabilize the reduction. Stable fractures usually can be maintained in reduction by external plaster.

Fractures involving the articular surfaces of the joints are of particular concern, since slight imprecision in the anatomic reduction can have long-term adverse consequences on the joint. Accordingly, open reduction is often indicated to provide precise anatomic reduction and maintenance with k-wire internal fixation. Fractures involving joint surfaces with unstable dislocations require open reduction and k-wire fixation.

Phalangeal fractures are common in children. Tuft fractures of the distal phalanx require no special treatment other than managing the usually associated soft tissue injury, dressing, and externally splinting the finger. Fractures involving the articular surface of the distal or proximal interphalangeal joint require a precise anatomic reduction and maintenance, usually with k-wire fixation if the fracture involves more than 25% of the surface. Shaft fractures, either spiral or transverse, of the middle or proximal phalanges can be managed by closed reduction when stable, with attention given to precise correction of angulatory and rotatory deformity. In older children, a short arm cast or a volar plaster wrist extension splint with an incorporated aluminum extension splint to the digit is adequate for immobilization. In smaller children, a complete careful hand dressing with plaster extending to the axilla with the elbow in a 90-degree angle is required for hand fracture immobilization, as for other sorts of injuries. However, when reduction cannot be maintained by such external measures, then either a percutaneous k-wire fixation or open reduction and k-wire fixation is required.[40]

Metacarpal fractures are most often managed by closed reduction and molded plaster extending from the forearm to the proximal interphalangeal joint level. It is important to maintain flexion at the metacarpophalangeal joint to prevent stiffness in extension from developing. A degree of dorsal angulation of the metacarpal can be accepted, since functional limitations do not result, and the long-term remodeling is excellent. Careful attention to digital rotation in both full extension and flexion should be made to ensure proper rotation in the reduction position.

Carpal fractures and dislocations are managed as in the adult. Fractures are often not initially apparent on x-ray films, especially in pediatric hands. An index of suspicion should be exercised, and the wrist and forearm should be immobilized for 3 weeks for follow-up x-ray studies if the nature of the injury and the findings on examination imply the possibility of a fracture.

Full joint mobility is an objective of successful fracture management. This implies early joint motion. In general, joint motion is allowed after 3 weeks of immobilization. By then, there is usually sufficient healing to maintain skeletal stabilization, even though radiologically bone healing is not complete. Early motion is essential to obtain joint mobility and to minimize stiffness. Certain unstable fractures, however, require longer periods of immobilization to obtain greater stability before motion is allowed. Protective splints are useful during heavy activity and at night during the period of early mobilization of joints.

Three injuries are of special concern, since they

may require open surgical repair. These are thumb and index metacarpophalangeal joint dislocations and Bennett's fracture.[9,30] With complete disruption of the ulnar collateral ligament of the thumb metacarpophalangeal joint, there is gross instability and at times volar subluxation of the proximal phalanx on the metacarpal head. The anatomy is such that the collateral ligament is displaced, and the adductor pollicic insertion interposes and prevents apposition of the torn collateral ligament on closed reduction. Accordingly, the ulnar collateral ligament fails to heal. The joint itself can become painful, weak, and osteoarthritic. When there is gross instability with complete disruption of the ulnar collateral ligament of the thumb metacarpophalangeal joint, direct surgical repair is indicated to reconstruct the ulnar collateral ligament and to restore the normal anatomic relationship. Thumb spica plaster immobilization is required for 3 weeks. For the chronic established instability from a former injury, a free tendon graft is used to reconstruct the ulnar collateral ligament.

Surgery is usually necessary for index metacarpophalangeal joint dislocation when there is dorsal dislocation of the proximal phalanx on the metacarpal head.[2,30] The metacarpal head is trapped between the flexor tendons, the lumbrical, and the transverse metacarpal ligament, and dorsally the volar plate is attached to the base of the proximal phalanx. This is a situation that prevents manipulative reduction, necessitating operative reduction.

Bennett's fracture is an articular fracture-dislocation of the trapeziometacarpal joint of the thumb. The volar lip of the bone of the first metacarpal is fractured off, and the thumb metacarpal subluxates in a radial and dorsal direction, with adduction collapse of the metacarpal. The strong torque at the fracture site exerted by the combined action of the adductor pollicis and abductor pollicis longus obviates against stability and makes adequate fixation by plaster immobilization most difficult. Either open reduction and k-wire fixation or closed reduction with percutaneous k-wire fixation is necessary to hold the fracture adequately during healing. Inadequate reduction of this articular fracture produces a disturbance in the complex functional anatomy of this joint and can result in a painful traumatic osteoarthritis requiring either arthroplasty or arthrodesis. Nonunion or displaced union of the fracture with radiodorsal capsular weakness associated with thumb metacarpal adduction collapse seen early—before destructive joint complications develop—can be treated by operative reduction and ligamentous reconstruction of the trapeziometacarpal joint by partial tendinous slips from flexor carpi radialis, abductor pollicis longus, or extensor carpi radialis longus, reinforcing the attentuated radiodorsal capsule.

THUMB INJURIES AND THUMB RECONSTRUCTION

Since the thumb represents perhaps 50% of the total function of the hand, thumb injuries and their surgical reconstruction are of major importance in rehabilitating the injured hand and in providing it with optimal function. Injuries to the thumbtip involving skin loss are handled much like the other fingertips. Small areas of skin loss can be allowed to heal secondarily with good final results. Larger areas require skin grafting.

Loss of the distal volar pulp in the thumb can be well managed by a volar advancement flap, since this preserves length and sensibility to the working surface of the thumb (Fig. 21-19).[59]

Thumb sensation is a critically important factor and is a feature preserved by a volar advancement flap. Only limited advancement can be obtained, however; for larger areas of volar skin loss to the thumb, a volar advancement is inadequate, and flap tissue must be provided for coverage. The preferred reconstruction of major volar skin loss to the thumb is a neurovascular island pedicle flap taken from the ulnar surface of the long or ring finger.[43,73] Its major asset, aside from being a local flap, is that it imports intact sensibility from one region of the hand to the critical volar pulp surface or working area of the thumb. In adults, late diminution and alteration of the quality of sensation has been reported.[54] Some of the best results from this procedure have been in younger people.

For amputations at the metacarpophalangeal joint level or more proximal, there are basically three methods of thumb reconstruction. One is the osteoplastic thumb reconstruction involving a tube flap with bone graft, which is subsequently followed by neurovascular island pedicle for sensory reconstruction. This can be expedited by using a groin tube flap composite with iliac bone in a single procedure.[21] Another major method of thumb reconstruction is index pollicization.[6,42.] With proper technique and care for the extrinsic muscle balance, excellent results from pollicization can be achieved. A final method of total thumb reconstruc-

tion that is possible is a toe-to-thumb transfer with immediate restoration of the circulation by microvascular anastomoses combined with direct digital nerve repair.

INFECTION

Infections of the hand are a serious problem and unless aggressively treated can result in major disability. The principles of treatment of infections of the hand include immobilization, elevation, antibiotics, and adequate surgical drainage of suppurative collections.[4,23,51,62] In children, except for the most simple and spontaneously draining subcutaneous abscesses, adequate surgical incision and drainage require general anesthesia and operating room conditions (Fig. 21-20). This also applies to felons, suppurative tenosynovitis, volar space abscesses, and large subcutaneous abscesses. Cellulitis and lymphangitis are treated by immobilization, elevation, antibiotics, and frequent observation with attention to the possible evolution of a suppurative collection, which would require drainage.

Immobilization and elevation are essential in all infections. In children, immobilization can be difficult, as has been emphasized, and requires meticulous attention to application of a dressing with plaster extending to the axilla with the elbow at a 90-degree angle (Fig. 21-21). The whole hand is immobilized, and each of the fingertips and the thumbtip are left slightly protruding for observation of vascularity. Stockinette is then applied to the upper extremity, where it is split 2:1 at the axilla and carried around to the opposite axilla and back around over the neck. The tail of the stockinette coming off the hand is then wrapped around the neck and back upon the forearm portion of the dressing, thus holding the upper extremity against the anterior chest and providing satisfactory immobilization. With the child lying in bed, this provides elevation, since the hand is above the heart level.

A felon is an abscess of the fingertip pulp space (Fig. 21-22). Due to the multiple compartments formed by the vertical fibrous septae compromising the fingertip pulp space, adequate surgical drainage is not as simple as might first be supposed. In children, general anesthesia is required with a tourniquet for an asanguinous field. When the suppuration is clearing pointing and is about to drain spontaneously, the drainage incision is directly

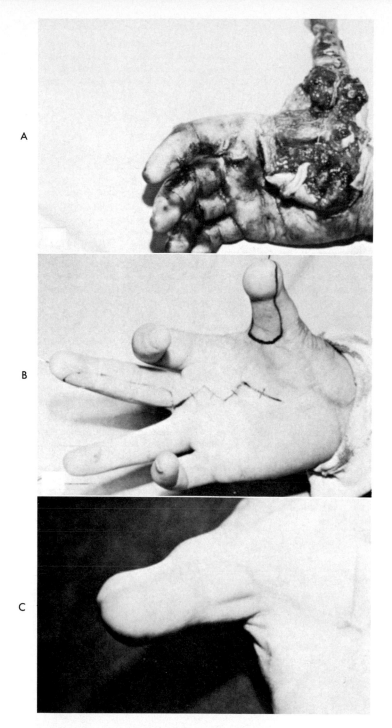

Fig. 21-19   **A,** An exploding chemistry set produced this injury. Both thumb digital nerves were avulsed from the median nerve proximally in the distal forearm. Viable thumb components were reconstructed. However, the thumb was insensate and without the possibility of nerve repair. **B,** Thumb sensation is critically important to overall hand function. When it is irreparably lost, a neurovascular island pedicle flap from either the ulnar border of the long or ring fingers is a useful reconstructive method to restore sensation to the thumb. A skin island is raised on its neurovascular bundle based in the proximal palm and transferred to the thumb. It is preferrable to make it large enough to encompass the whole working surface of the thumb during grasp and pinch. **C,** The same neurovascular island pedicle flap for sensory thumb reconstruction, healed. Two years after surgery, the sensation is essentially normal with normal two-point discrimination and tactile gnosis. In complex hand injuries, a total reconstructive effort must begin from the time of the original injury and the primary surgery.

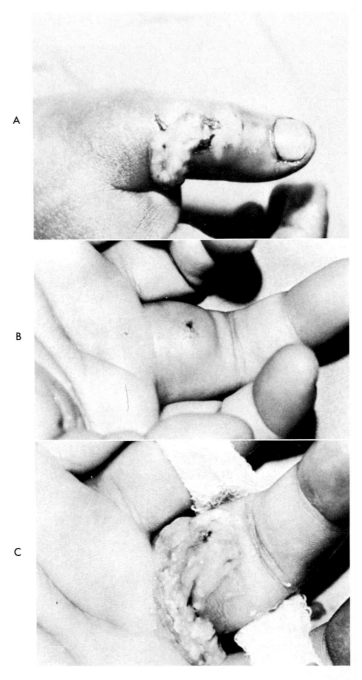

Fig. 21-20   **A,** Abscesses of the hand require adequate incision and drainage. In children, adequate anesthesia often implies general anesthesia. This subcutaneous abscess extended from the thumb to the dorsum of the hand and involved the first web space dorsally. **B** and **C,** Subcutaneous abscess formation of the digit requires distinction from suppurative tenosynovitis. This is a localized abscess formation associated with a foreign body that did not transgress the flexor sheath.

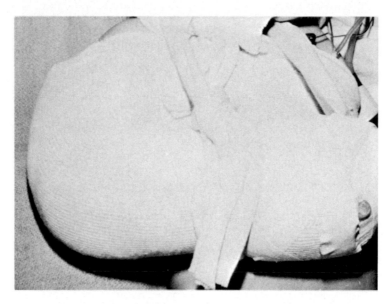

Fig. 21-21   A pediatric hand dressing for adequate soft tissue immobilization requires an entire upper extremity dressing. As in this case of syndactyly repair in which full-thickness grafts required immobilization for healing, the entire extremity is dressed and in plaster from the hand to the axilla with the elbow at a 90-degree angle. A stockinette is applied over the dressing, split 2:1 at the axilla, and carried around the opposite axilla and in varied manners about the neck and thence down over the forearm for suspending and securing the extremity against the torso in a comfortable and safe manner.

over that area (Fig. 21-23), even though it is on the volar surface of the pulp.[31] When the suppuration is diffuse and not clearly pointing, then a dorsal lateral hockey stick incision is made with the distal end just under the margin of the nail. A rubber drain and a wet dressing are applied, and the upper extremity and digit properly immobilized. The wet dressing aids in diminishing crusting and wound closure, which impede continuous drainage. Thereafter daily dressing changes are undertaken until the sepsis is controlled and the finger healed.

Paronychia can be more simply managed. With adequate sedation of the child, the cuticular margin can be elevated for drainage. A gauze wick or rubber drain is readily inserted to maintain the drainage. A metacarpal digital block is useful for this procedure in the absence of cellulitis. When there is subungual extension and collection, resection of the base of the nail is required for adequate drainage. In older children, a metacarpal block can be adequate, but in young children general anesthesia is required.

Palmar and thenar space abscesses are manifested by evidence of marked localized sepsis in-

cluding swelling, redness, pain, and fluctuance. When there is diffuse cellulitis and the issue of closed space suppuration is uncertain, a course of systemic antibiotics is necessary both to control the cellulitis and to permit observation for localization and the possible formation of a purulent collection. Adequate surgical drainage requires general anesthesia in the operating room and is done through appropriate palmar incisions.

Suppurative tenosynovitis of the flexor tendon sheath is manifested by marked uniform swelling and redness of the entire digit, a posturing of the digit with flexion at each joint with exquisite pain on either extension or flexion of the digit. Incision and drainage through a midaxial incision is essential. Flexor tenosynovitis must be distinguished from a cellulitis or a subcutaneous abscess of the digit. This is not always simple; use of antibiotics and repeated observations under conservative management are required to make the decision. It is useful in uncertain circumstances to puncture the digit with a needle to clarify whether a subcutaneous abscess is present. If there is a suppurative tenosynovitis, then opening of the flexor sheath and drainage are mandatory. However, if there is cel-

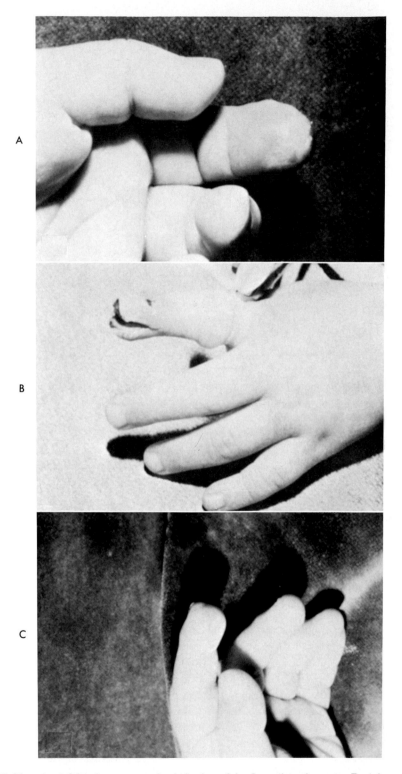

Fig. 21-22   **A,** A felon is a suppurative infection of the fingertip pulp space. **B,** Adequate incision and drainage are necessary, with the patient under adequate anesthesia, which in children usually involves general anesthesia. Due to the skin necrosis along the dorsal margins, the soft tissues of the fingertip simply fell away from the distal phalanx. In general, a hockey stock incision placed dorsally and next to the nail margin is adequate for drainage. Postoperatively, the incision is kept open with a temporary drain, and appropriate antibiotics are used. **C,** The same fingertip healed.

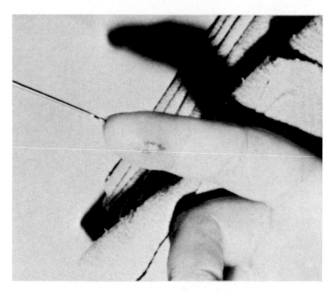

Fig. 21-23   When a suppurative infection of the fingertip pulp space has a distinct focal point, incision and drainage are directly into that area, as in this case, in which there was a foreign body associated with the felon.

lulitis or a subcutaneous abscess, masquerading as a tenosynovitis, then it would be extremely hazardous to open the flexor sheath, thereby introducing sepsis into that complex anatomic region.

ACUTELY BURNED HAND

Burns of the hand often attend a larger burn injury and understandably are of secondary importance to the initial lifesaving resuscitative efforts. However, given that the patient is going to survive the thermal injury, the individual's ultimate rehabilitation and integration into a productive role in society will depend to a considerable degree on the functional results with the hands. A child's future is very much influenced by the loss of hand function. Accordingly, proper emphasis must be placed on management of the thermal injury to the hand.

In general, the earlier a burn wound of the hand is debrided and cleared of all nonviable tissue and the wound closed with skin grafts, the better will be the ultimate functional result.[3,36,46] The longer an open burn wound with necrotic tissue is left untreated the greater the development of edema, infection, and fibrosis, which leads inevitably to joint stiffness, contracture deformity, and loss of hand function. Early wound closure, by contrast, permits early motion and early recovery of function with minimal stiffness and contracture deformity.

When the patient with a burned hand is seen in the emergency room, the immediate care consists of cleansing the burn wound, applying an appropriate antibacterial agent (silver sulfadiazine at our institution) to the burn wound surface, dressing and splinting the hand, and placing the hand and extremity in elevation. The hand should be splinted so that the wrist is in extension, the metacarpophalangeal joints are in flexion, and the interphalangeal joints are in extension.

For first-degree and superficial second-degree or superficial dermal burns to the hand, spontaneous healing can be expected in less than 2 weeks. The dressing is changed daily, and the hand is put through motion exercises to maintain joint mobility. For deep second-degree or deep dermal burns, full healing of the burn wound may not occur in 14 days. Spontaneous healing could occur after that time from the scattered islands of epithelialization, but the ultimate functional result is often not acceptable with unstable epithelium, hypertrophic scar formation, and a deficiency of skin on the dorsum of the hand. Accordingly, if after a 2-week period there is unsatisfactory spontaneous healing of the burn wound, then either tangential or complete excision with immediate skin grafting is undertaken to obtain an acceptable result.[38]

For burn wounds of the hand that are clearly third-degree or full-thickness, primary excision and skin grafting are performed, provided the patient's overall general condition and response to resuscitation are satisfactory and stable. In general, this is performed 3 to 5 days following the burn injury. With tourniquet control of bleeding, the burn eschar is excised. Care is taken to preserve the dorsal veins if they have not been coagulated by the thermal injury. If there is difficulty in securing hemostasis after the tourniquet is released, then delayed grafting is performed 24 hours later.

Kirschner wires are used at times to maintain skeletal position and stabilize the hand during the healing period.[3] In particular, it is useful to place crossed k-wires between the first and second metacarpal bones to maintain thumb abduction. This is noteworthy, as thumb adduction contracture is a relatively frequent deformity after excision and grafting of the burned hand.[3,46] When there is thermal injury to the digital extensor apparatus or the interphalangeal joints, then a Kirschner wire is placed across both interphalangeal joints to maintain the position in extension. This is not performed when early mobilization can be anticipated directly on healing of the skin graft.

Circumferential burns are a special problem, since a compression syndrome can develop that could compromise the circulation. Decompression can be either surgical, with direct escharotomy to restore the circulation, or enzymatic (Travase).* Close immediate attention to the circulation needs to be paid in such circumferential burns.

With rapid debridement and closure of the burn wound to the hand, edema, fibrosis, and infection are diminished, joint stiffness is minimized, and potential loss of function is alleviated.

CONCLUSION

In this chapter the broad spectrum of surgery of the hand as it specifically applies to children has been reviewed. The principles that any surgeon can apply in providing basic surgical care to an injured hand have been emphasized. Analysis of the wound and the recognition of significant injury are fundamental. The next major responsibility of the surgeon is to provide proper wound care through debridement and adequate skin cover in wound closure. Complex injuries, repair of deep structures, and secondary reconstruction are problems often best left to those experienced in surgery of the

hand. Disaster can attend misguided attempts at repair and reconstruction and make a good result impossible.

Results of careful, thoughtful, and precise surgery can be gratifying in these young patients, since healing can be rapid and recovery of function quick. The young patient can then return to family, society, and a long future with the best possible tools—functional hands.

REFERENCES

1. Atasoy E et al: Reconstruction of the amputated fingertip with a triangular volar flap, J Bone Joint Surg 52A:921, 1970.
2. Becton JL et al: A simplified technique for treating the complex dislocation of the index metacarpophalangeal joint, J Bone Joint Surg 57A:698, 1975.
3. Boswick JA: The management of fresh burns of the hand and deformities resulting from burn injuries, Clin Plast Surg 1:621, 1974.
4. Boyes JH: Bunnell's surgery of the hand, ed 4, Philadelphia, 1964, JB Lippincott Co.
5. Brown PW: The management of phalangeal and metacarpal fractures, Surg Clin North Am 56:1393, 1973.
6. Buck-Gramcko D: Pollicization of the index finger, J Bone Joint Surg 53A:1605, 1971.
7. Burkhalter WE: Thoughts on delayed closure of hand wounds. In Cramer LM and Chase RA, editors: Symposium on the Hand, vol 3, Educational Foundation of The American Society of Plastic and Reconstructive Surgeons, St Louis, 1971, The CV Mosby Co.
8. Burkhalter WE et al: Experiences with delayed primary closure of war wounds of the hand in Vietnam, J Bone Joint Surg 50A:945, 1968.
9. Campbell CS: Gamekeeper's thumb, J Bone Joint Surg 37B:148, 1955.
10. Chen Z, Yang D, and Chang D: Microsurgery, Berlin, 1982, Shanghai Scientific and Technical Publishers, Springer-Verlag.
11. Cormock GC and Lamberty BGH: The arterial anatomy of skin flaps, Edinburgh, 1986, Churchill Livingstone, Inc.
12. Curtis RM: Cross-finger pedicle flap in hand surgery, Ann Surg 145:650, 1957.
13. Daniel RK and Taylor GI: Distant transfer of an island flap by microvascular anastomoses, Plast Reconstr Surg 52:111, 1973.
14. Eaton RG: Joint injuries of the hand, Springfield, Ill, 1971, Charles C Thomas.
15. Eaton RG and Littler JW: Joint injuries and their sequelae, Clin Plast Surg 3:85, 1976.
16. Edgerton MT and Golden GT: Wringer (crush) injuries of the upper extremity. In Littler JW, Cramer LM, and Smith JW, editors: Symposium on reconstructive hand surgery, Educational Foundation of The American Society of Plastic and Reconstructive Surgeons, St Louis, 1974, The CV Mosby Co.
17. Elliott RA: Injuries to the extensor mechanism of the hand, Ortho Clin North Am 1:335, 1970.
18. Elliott RA: Boutonnière deformity. In Cramer LM and Chase RA, editors: Symposium on the hand, vol 3, Edu-

---

*Travase brand of sutilains, Flint Laboratories, Division of Travenol Laboratories, Morton Grove, Illinois.

cational Foundation of the American Society of Plastic and Reconstructive Surgeons, St Louis, 1971, The CV Mosby Co.

19. Entin MA: Flexor tendon repair and grafting in children, Amer J Surg 109:287, 1965.
20. Finseth F, Constable JD, and Cannon B: Interfascicular nerve grafting, Plast Reconstr Surg 56:492, 1975.
21. Finseth F, May J, and Smith RJ: Composite groin flap with iliac bone flap for primary reconstruction, J Bone Joint Surg 58A:130, 1976.
22. Flatt AE: The thenar flap, J Bone Joint Surg 39B:80, 1957.
23. Flatt AE: The care of minor hand injuries, ed 3, St Louis, 1972, The CV Mosby Co.
24. Golden GT, Fisher JC, and Edgerton MT: "Wringer arm" reevaluated: a survey of current surgical management of upper extremity compression injuries, Ann Surg 177:362, 1973.
25. Harii K, Ohmori K, and Ohmori S: Successful clinical transfer of 10 free flaps by microvascular anastomoses, Plast Reconstr Surg 53:259, 1974.
26. Harrison SH: The tactile adherence test estimating loss of sensation after nerve injury, Hand 6:148, 1974.
27. Hunter JM and Salisbury RE: Use of gliding artificial implants to produce tendon sheaths: techniques and results in children, Plast Reconstr Surg 45:564, 1970.
28. Jabaley ME and Peterson HD: Early treatment of war wounds of the hand and forearm in Vietnam, Ann Surg 177:167, 1973.
29. Joshi BB: Sensory flaps for the degloved mutilated hand, Hand 6:247, 1974.
30. Kaplan EB: Dorsal dislocation of the metacarpophalangeal joint of the index finger, J Bone Joint Surg 47A:522, 1957.
31. Kilgore ES et al: Treatment of felons, Amer J Surg 130:194, 1975.
32. Kleinert HE and Griffin JM: Technique of nerve anastomosis, Orthop Clin North Am 4:907, 1973.
33. Kleinert HE and Lister GD: Selecting the operation and the patient. In Littler JW, Cramer LM, and Smith JW, editors: Symposium on reconstructive hand surgery, Educational Foundation of The American Society of Plastic and Reconstructive Surgeons, St Louis, 1974, The CV Mosby Co.
34. Kleinert HE et al: Primary repair of flexor tendons, Orthop Clin North Am 4:865, 1973.
35. Krizek TJ and Robson MC: Biology of surgical infection, Surg Clin North Am 55:1261, 1975.
36. Krizek TJ, Robson MC, and Wray RC: Care of the burned patient. In Ballinger WF et al, editors: The management of trauma, 1973, WB Saunders Co.
37. Krizek TJ et al: Experimental transplantation of composite grafts by microsurgical vascular anatomoses, Plast Reconstr Surg 36:538, 1965.
38. Krizek TJ et al: Delayed primary excision and skin grafting of the burned hand, Plast Reconstr Surg 51:524, 1973.
39. Krizek TJ et al: Emergency nonsurgical escharotomy in the burned extremity, Orthop Rev 4:53, 1975.
40. Leonard MH and Dubravcik P: Management of fractured fingers in the child, Clin Orthop 73:160, 1970.
41. Lindsay WK: Hand injuries in children, Clin Plast Surg 3:65, 1976.
42. Littler JW: The neurovascular pedical method of digital transposition for reconstruction of the thumb, Plast Reconstr Surg 12:303, 1953.
43. Littler JW: Neurovascular pedicle transfer of tissue in reconstructive surgery of the hand, J Bone Joint Surg 19A:1285, 1967.
44. Littler JW and Eaton RG: Redistribution of forces in the correction of the boutonnière deformity, J Bone Joint Surg 49A:1267, 1967.
45. Maaktelow RT: Microvascular reconstruction, Berlin, 1986, Springer-Verlag.
46. McCormack RM: Problems in the treatment of burnt hands, Clin Plast Surg 3:83, 1976.
47. McEwan LE: Median and ulnar nerve injuries, Aust NZ J Surg 32:89, 1962.
48. McFarlane RM: Treatment of extensor tendon injuries of the hand, Can J Surg 16:1, 1973.
49. McGregor IA: The z-plasty in hand surgery, J Bone Joint Surg 49B:448, 1967.
50. McGregor IA and Jackson IT: The groin flap, Br J Plast Surg 25:3, 1972.
51. Milford L: The hand. In Crenshaw AH, editor: Campbell's Operative Orthopaedics, ed 7, St Louis, The CV Mosby Co.
52. Millesi H, Meissl G, and Berger A: The interfascicular nerve grafting of the median and ulnar nerves, J Bone Joint Surg 54A:727, 1972.
53. Millesi H, Meissl G, and Berger A: Further experience with interfascicular grafting of the median, ulnar and radial nerves, J Bone Joint Surg 58A:209, 1976.
54. Murray JF, Ord JVR, and Gavelin GE: The neurovascular island pedical flap, J Bone Joint Surg 49A:1285, 1967.
55. O'Brien BMcC: Microvascular reconstructive surgery, Edinburgh, 1977, Churchill Livingstone, Inc.
56. O'Brien BMcC: Replantation surgery, Clin Plast Surg 1:405, 1974.
57. O'Brien BMcC et al: Free flap transfers with microvascular anastomoses, Br J Plast Surg 27:220, 1974.
58. Patterson TJS: Hand injuries. In Stack HG, editor: The proceedings of the Second Hand Club, London, 1975, British Society for Surgery of the Hand.
59. Posner MA and Smith RJ: The advancement pedical flap for thumb injuries, J Bone Joint Surg 53A:1618, 1971.
60. Pulvertaft RG: Treatment of tendon injuries. In Stack GH, editor: The proceedings of the Second Hand Club, London, 1975, British Society for Surgery of the Hand.
61. Rang MD: Children's fractures, Philadelphia, 1974, JB Lippincott Co.
62. Rank BK, Wakefield AR, and Hueston JT: Surgery of repair as applied to hand injuries, Baltimore, 1968, Williams & Wilkins.
63. Sandzen SC: Management of the acute fingertip injury in the child, Hand 6:190, 1974.
64. Seddon HJ: Surgical disorders of the peripheral nerves, Edinburgh, 1972, Churchill Livingstone, Inc.
65. Serafin D and Buncke HJ: Microsurgical composite tissue transplantation, St Louis, 1979, The CV Mosby Co.
66. Smith JW: Microsurgery of peripheral nerves, Plast Reconstr Surg 33:317, 1964.
67. Smith RJ: Boutonnière deformity of the fingers, Bull Hosp Joint Dis 27:27, 1966.
68. Smith RJ: Balance and kinetics of the fingers under normal and pathological conditions, Clin Orthop 104:92, 1974.
69. Swanson AB: Fractures involving the digits of the hand, Orthop Clin North Am 1:261, 1970.

70. Thompson HG and Sorokilit WT: The cross-finger flap in children, Plast Reconstr Surg 39:482, 1967.

71. Tubiana R: Incisions and technique in tendon grafting, Am J Surg 109:339, 1965.

72. Tubiana R: Planning of surgical treatment, Hand 7:223, 1975.

73. Tubiana R and DuParc J: Restoration of sensibility in the hand by neurovascular skin island transfer, J Bone Surg 43B:474, 1961.

74. Urbaniak JR: Microsurgery for major limb reconstruction, St Louis, 1987, The CV Mosby Co.

75. Verdan CE: Primary and secondary repair of flexor and extensor tendon injuries. In Flynn JE, editor: Hand surgery, Baltimore, 1966, Williams & Wilkins.

76. Wakefield AR: Hand injuries in children, J Bone Joint Surg 46A:1226, 1964.

77. Weeks PM: A basic approach to the injured hand. In Littler JW, Cramer LM, and Smith JW, editors: Symposium on reconstructive hand surgery, Educational Foundation of The American Society of Plastic and Reconstructive Surgeons, St Louis, 1974, The CV Mosby Co.

78. Woolhouse FM: Resurfacing problems in the hand, Clin Plast Surg 3:13, 1976.

22

Insect and Spider Bites

Dennis J. Hoelzer

Millions of persons are bitten by insects each year. Usually these injuries can be managed conservatively and will not result in serious sequelae. It is estimated that eight of every 1000 people are allergic to insect bites and that four of these individuals are severely sensitive.[3,10] Approximately 25,000 people per year suffer hypersensitivity reactions. From 40 to 50 people die each year as the result of insect stings or bites.[3,5,10,12] These deaths are attributed almost exclusively to anaphylactic reactions and not to the direct effect of insect venom.

ANAPHYLAXIS

Table 22-1 summarizes the characteristics of an anaphylactic reaction. Mild symptoms of pruritus, erythema, urticaria, and angioedema should be treated with epinephrine injected subcutaneously or intramuscularly (Table 22-2), followed by oral diphenhydramine or hydroxyzine (Table 22-3).[4] If necessary, additional doses of epinephrine may be repeated every 15 to 20 minutes in either the same or smaller doses. If the patient improves without progression of anaphylaxis, an injection of long-acting epinephrine should be given and oral antihistamines continued for 24 hours.[4]

Patients with severe bronchospasm, laryngeal edema, cardiovascular collapse, and shock require intravenous epinephrine (Table 22-2).[4] A continuous infusion of epinephrine should be titered, with appropriate monitoring. Supplemental oxygen and intravenous volume expansion (saline solution or colloid) should be considered. Airway patency must be maintained, and endotracheal intubation or emergency tracheostomy may be required. Patients with persistent and more severe systemic anaphylaxis may require intravenous corticosteroid therapy followed by daily oral steroids. H_2-receptor

blockers are recommended to supplement epinephrine and steroid therapy (Table 22-3).[4]

All patients with anaphylaxis should be observed for several hours until symptoms resolve and the progression of anaphylaxis ceases. Severe systemic anaphylaxis necessitates hospitalization.

The emergency room treatment of individuals sensitive to insect bites should include patient education about desensitization programs; the availability of emergency kits; the risk of serum sickness, which can occur from 1 to 2 weeks after a systemic reaction; and the advisability of wearing Medic Alert identification.*

---

*Medic Alert Foundation, Turlock, CA 95381 (1-800-344-3226).

Table 22-1 Characteristics of anaphylactic reactions

Effects	Characteristics
Local	Pain and swelling at injury site
Systemic	Pruritus, urticaria, flushing of the skin, dyspnea, weakness, anxiety, nausea, abdominal cramps, loss of consciousness
Respiratory	Dyspnea, rhinitis, sneezing, cough, bronchospasm, wheezing, angioedema, respiratory arrest
Gastrointestinal	Abdominal cramps, diarrhea, sudden involuntary defecation, nausea, vomiting
Cardiovascular	Vasodilation with hypotension, cardiac arrhythmias, syncope, circulatory collapse
Late	Urinary incontinence, uterine contractions, serum sickness

Table 22-2 Primary treatment of anaphylaxis—epinephrine

Route/type of epinephrine	Dosage
Subcutaneous or intramuscular	
1. Aqueous epinephrine (1:1000)	0.01 mg (0.01 ml)/kg
	May be repeated every 15-20 minutes
2. Long-acting epinephrine (in thioglycolic acid)	0.005 mg/kg as a single dose
Intravenous	
1. Initial infusion	100 μg given at a rate of 10-20 μg/min
1:100,000 dilution of epinephrine (Mix 0.1 ml of 1:1000 aqueous epinephrine with 10 ml of saline solution. Resulting concentration of epinephrine is 10 μg/ml.)	Infuse over 5-10 minutes
2. Continuous infusion	Infuse at a rate of 0.1 μg/kg/min (maximum, 1.5 μg/kg/min)
1:200,000 dilution of epinephrine (Mix 0.5 mg [0.5 ml] of 1:1000 aqueous epinephrine in 100 ml of 5% D/W. Resulting concentration of epinephrine is 5 μg/ml.)	Increase infusion as needed to maintain blood pressure

Table 22-3 Treatment of anaphylaxis—secondary drugs

Drug/route	Dosage
Diphenhydramine (Benadryl)	
Oral	5 mg/kg/day in 4-6 divided doses (maximum, 300 mg daily)
Intramuscular or intravenous	5 mg/kg/day in 4-6 divided doses (maximum, 300 mg daily)
Hydroxyzine/oral	10-25 mg 3-4 times daily
Corticosteroids	
Hydrocortisone/intravenous	100-200 mg every 4-6 hours
Methylprednisolone/intravenous	20-40 mg every 4-6 hours
Prednisone/oral	Daily decreasing doses: 30, 25, 20, 15, 10, 5 mg
Cimetidine/intravenous	25-40 mg/kg/day in 6 divided doses

INSECT BITES AND STINGS

Insects that bite may be divided functionally into two groups: the *stinging arthropods,* which inject their venom by a stinger located posteriorly (bees, wasps, hornets, yellow jackets, ants, scorpions), and the *biting and piercing arthropods,* which inject their venom with an apparatus located anteriorly or associated with their mouth parts (tarantula, centipede, kissing bug, black widow and brown recluse spiders).

Stinging Arthropods

Yellow jackets, wasps, hornets, and honeybees

The major offenders of the order of stinging arthropods are the yellow jacket, wasp, hornet, and honeybee.[3] Only the female members can inflict injury because the stinging apparatus is a modification of their ovipositor. The honeybee is unable to remove her stinger after introduction; as the bee exits, a portion of her abdomen and venom sac remains with the victim, resulting in the bee's subsequent death. The stinger of the yellow jacket, wasp, and hornet usually is contaminated with bacteria, whereas that of the honeybee is seldom colonized. The venom of these insects contains histamine, serotonin, acetylcholine, and dopamine, as well as other chemicals.

The yellow jacket bite is the most likely to produce anaphylaxis, but cross-sensitivity exists among these insects, and one insect's bite may

---

MANAGEMENT OF PATIENTS WITH STINGS FROM BEES, WASPS, HORNETS, AND YELLOW JACKETS

Local reactions

Scrape stinger out of injury site.

Wash site with soap and water.

For itching: administer diphenhydramine (Benadryl), 5 mg/kg/24 hr orally in 4 divided doses.

For pain: use topical application of cold compresses, calamine lotion, steroid cream or lotion, aerosol spray of benzocaine, aerosol spray of diphenhydramine (Benadryl); acetaminophen, aspirin.

Systemic reactions

See Tables 22-2 and 22-3.

---

trigger an allergic reaction to that of any of the others. The extent of the patient's reaction depends on several factors: the amount of venom injected, the site and number of bites, and the individual's age, size, and degree of sensitivity. Multiple stings (10 or more) may produce toxic reactions, including vomiting, dizziness, muscle spasm, and convulsions. Patients who have severe reactions should be warned that they may develop serum sickness (morbilliform rash, urticaria, arthralgias, fever) 10 to 14 days after their injury. Treatment is presented in the box above.

Fire ants

Two species of fire ants, *Solenopsis richteri* and *Solenopsis invicta,* were introduced into the United States in the 1920s.[6] These ants now can be found in 13 southern states, extending from the East Coast to Texas, Oklahoma, and Arkansas.[11] Fire ants are small (2 to 5 mm in length) and reddish brown to black in color. They are highly mobile, easily provoked, aggressive creatures that live in colonies and build mounds.

The attack of the fire ant is a two-part process. Initially the ant attaches to the victim's skin with its mandible. After fixation the ant inserts its lancet-shaped abdominal stinger and releases its venom. By using its head as a pivot, the ant can rotate its body and produce multiple stings in one area.

The venom of the fire ant contains low-molecular-weight proteins that are believed to cause the allergic reactions associated with fire ant envenomation. The venom also contains dialkylpiperidines, which have a direct toxic effect on mast cell membranes. Subsequent histamine release accounts for the edema, pruritus, erythema, pain, and burning that result from a bite.

Within seconds after envenomation, a wheal-flare reaction occurs. Depending on the amount of venom injected and the victim's sensitivity, this skin reaction may vary from 1 to 2 mm to 10 cm in size. Several hours later, a superficial vesicle containing clear fluid and surrounding edema develop. Within 8 to 10 hours, the fluid within the vesicle becomes cloudy. Systemic allergic reactions may occur, but the most common complications of fire ant envenomation are secondary infection and cellulitis.

Treatment is symptomatic and consists of cleaning the skin with soap and water, applying ice compresses, and monitoring for secondary infection. A small percentage of children will develop a local skin response greater than 10 cm and may require hospitalization.

Biting and Piercing Arthropods
Spider bites

Almost all the 100,000 species of spiders are venomous and can bite. Fortunately, most spiders do not have chelicerae (jaws) strong enough to penetrate human skin. Of the 50 to 60 species of spiders that have been documented to cause human injury, only the tarantula, brown recluse spider, and widow spiders are of major clinical significance in the United States.[22]

Spiders are universally feared and maligned. This unfounded fear has resulted in many claims of spider bites that, when carefully reviewed, have revealed other insects to be the perpetrators.[16] For appropriate therapy to be initiated, every effort should be made to identify the offending spider.

Running, golden orb weaver, wolf, green lynx, black jumping, broad-faced sock, and parson spiders. These spiders have been documented to bite humans. Their bites are painful and are associated with edema, erythema, induration, vesicle formation, and pruritus. Often a pustulelike lesion followed by a small ulceration of the skin will develop at the site of the bite. Skin necrosis is rare but has been reported following the bites of running, golden orb weaver, and wolf spiders.[1,2]

Treatment is largely symptomatic and consists of immobilization, elevation of the involved extremity, tetanus prophylaxis, analgesics, antihistamines, and oral antibiotics for secondary infection.

Tarantulas. The largest of all spiders belongs to the family Theraphosidae, the typical megalomorphs Americans mistakenly refer to as tarantulas.[7] Thirty to 40 species live within the United States, predominantly in the Southwest, but they may be found west of the Mississippi River, extending to California, Oregon, Utah, and southwestern Idaho.

Tarantulas have an unearned sinister reputation. They are quite restrictive in habit, staying close to their burrows and hunting only at night within yards of their dens, and attack only when vigorously provoked or roughly handled. Tarantulas can become quite large, spanning 15 to 18 cm. They produce a venom composed mostly of hyaluronidase and a protein toxic to cockroaches.[20]

The bite of the North American tarantula may vary from being almost painless to a deep, throbbing pain lasting for an hour. Treatment is symptomatic and consists of immobilization and elevation of the injured part, tetanus prophylaxis, and analgesics.

Many of the species possess urticaria-producing hairs on the dorsal surface of the abdomen that the spider can "flick" toward an aggressor. Contact with these hairs may produce pruritus and wheals that can last several weeks. Treatment with topical corticosteroids and oral antihistamines is usually effective, but patients with severe symptoms may require administration of oral corticosteroids for 1 to 2 weeks.[22]

Black, brown, and red widow spiders. Five species of widow spiders, *Latrodectus,* are found in the United States, and all are capable of inducing significant neurotoxic symptoms in humans. The southern black widow, *L. mactans,* is found from the South extending to southern New England. The northern black widow, *L. variolus,* has been identified from the East Coast west to eastern Texas. The habitat of the western black widow, *L. hesperus,* ranges from the Midwest to the Southwest. The red widow, *L. bishopi,* is found throughout Florida, but the brown widow, *L. geometricus,* has been identified only in southern Florida.[22]

Widow spiders are web weavers that spin strong webs varying in size from the space of a small burrow to a meter or more in diameter. The webs are placed in or close to the ground in protected places, such as vacant rodent burrows, under stones and logs, and in littered areas. Widow spiders stay close to their webs and normally live up to 2 years.[18]

Adult female widow spiders are large, sometimes measuring more than 12 mm in length. They are most often jet black in color and characteristically have a red hourglass marking on the underside of their large, globe-shaped abdominal section (Fig. 22-1). The males are much smaller and retain the bright colors of their immature stages. Widow spiders were so named because it was believed that the females devoured their mates after copulation. Most often, however, the male escapes by weaving a web around the stuporous female after copulation.[17]

The various species of *Latrodectus* have similar poisons and cause similar neurotoxic reactions in humans. The venom of the widow spider is an oily, yellow mixture of proteins, lipids, and carbohydrates.[7] The venom is composed of at least six active components, with molecular weights ranging from 5000 to 130,000 daltons.[21] These components cause a neuromuscular transmission block with the initial release of acetylcholine and catecholamine from synaptic terminals, followed by exhaustion. The depletion of neurotransmitter at

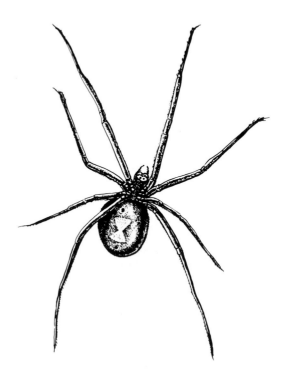

Fig. 22-1 Black widow spider *(Latrodectus mactans),* ventral view. Note the hourglass-shaped marking on the abdomen.

motor endings is believed to cause these patients' neuromuscular symptoms as well as the tachycardia and hypertension seen after envenomation. Envenomation in various animal models results in necrosis of epithelial tissue as well as of the blood vessels of the liver, kidneys, spleen, lungs, pericardium, lymph nodes, thymus, adrenal glands, and neural tissues. Experimentally, a seasonal variation in the spiders' toxicity has been demonstrated, with the highest toxicity noted in the autumn and the lowest in the spring.[8]

The bite of the female widow spider can be followed by severe systemic symptoms and signs but rarely death. Usually the bite is experienced as little more than a sharp pinprick, but it may be painless.[22] Slight erythema and edema soon surround the entrance site of the spider's fangs, which leave two tiny red marks on the victim's skin. Within 10 minutes to an hour after the bite, dull cramping to severe pain and numbness can spread from the injury site to involve the entire torso. Abdominal pain suggestive of a surgical abdomen can become excruciating and is especially common after a bite on the lower extremity. Chest pain mimicking a myocardial infarction has been reported after a bite to the upper extremity.

The pain characteristically peaks after 2 to 3 hours but may last for several days. Multiple symptoms and signs may result from the envenomation, including extreme anxiety, headaches, dizziness, weakness, fever, diaphoresis, salivation, nausea, vomiting, speech disturbances, chest tightness, backache, respiratory distress, priapism, urinary retention, tremors, hyperactive deep tendon reflexes, muscle fasciculations, peripheral paresthesias, and burning of the plantar surfaces.[22] Flexor muscle spasm may cause the victim to assume the fetal positon.

In healthy individuals these symptoms usually resolve without treatment in 2 to 3 days, but they may last for an entire week. Death is more likely in young children, the elderly, and those individuals with severe hypertension and cardiac dysfunction. Complications include renal failure (anuria, proteinuria), convulsions, shock, cardiac and respiratory failure, cerebral hemorrhage, and bacterial infection at the injury site.

Initial treatment should include washing the injury site with soap and water and applying an ice pack to reduce local pain. Patients younger than 16 years of age should be hospitalized and, after appropriate horse serum sensitivity testing, should

receive one ampule (2.5 ml) of intravenous Lyovac antivenin in 10 to 20 ml of saline solution. One ampule of antivenin is generally sufficient, providing relief of symptoms within 1 to 2 hours.[19,22] A second dose of antivenin may be administered if necessary. Because of the small volume of antivenin necessary for treatment, the patient rarely experiences serum sickness.

Pain relief may be accomplished with acetylsalicylic acid, acetaminophen, or intravenous morphine sulfate (0.05 to 0.2 mg/kg/dose). Patients with muscle spasms respond to intravenous calcium gluconate (0.1 ml/kg of a 10% solution), and the dose may be repeated every 4 to 6 hours as needed. Methocarbamol and diazepam are also useful.[22]

The box below outlines treatment for black, brown, and red widow spider bites.

Brown recluse spiders. Of the 10 species of *Loxosceles* found in the United States, six have been reported to bite humans and cause necrotic wounds.[7,20] These spiders can be found throughout the entire United States, including Hawaii, thanks to central heating and the moving van. The largest concentration of brown spiders is found in the South because of the warm, moderate winters.

MANAGEMENT OF PATIENTS WITH BLACK, BROWN, AND RED WIDOW SPIDER BITES

Wash wound with soap and water.
Apply ice pack.
Administer antivenin (Lyovac): 2.5 ml intravenously in 10-20 ml of saline solution (after negative skin test for horse serum sensitivity).
Administer analgesics:
  Mild pain: acetylsalicylic acid or acetaminophen
  Severe pain: intravenous morphine sulfate (0.05-0.2 mg/kg/dose)
Treat muscle spasm:
  Calcium gluconate: 0.1 ml/kg (10% solution) intravenously slowly; may be repeated every 4-6 hours as needed (check for bradycardia)
  Methocarbamol (Robaxin): 15 mg/kg/dose intravenously slowly; may be given every 4-6 hours as needed
  Diazepam (Valium): 0.1-0.3 mg/kg/dose intravenously slowly; may be given every 4 hours as needed
Hospitalize if patient is younger than 16 years of age.

The brown recluse spider, *Loxosceles reclusa,* has the widest geographic distribution and can be found from South Carolina west to Texas and from Indiana south to Alabama. It is seen most frequently in Missouri, Arkansas, eastern Kansas, and Tennessee. *L. unicolor* and *L. arizonica* are found in the Southwest, Arizona, New Mexico, Nevada, Texas, Utah, and southern California. *L. rufescens* is seen along the southeastern and Texas Gulf coasts. *L. devia* can be found in southern Texas, and *L. laeta,* a South American brown spider, is now an inhabitant of Los Angeles.[22]

The brown spiders are shy, nocturnal hunters who avoid light and disturbances, if possible. They have only three sets of eyes and are dull yellow to light brown or gray on the cephalothorax and olive-tan on the abdomen. They range in size from 10 to 15 mm in length and 4 to 6 mm in width, with a leg span greater than 25 mm. On the dorsal surface of the cephalothorax is a dark-brown violin-shaped marking, thus the name "fiddle-back spider" or "violin spider" (Fig. 22-2). Unfortunately, this characteristic marking is very faint in some species and does not appear at all on *L. unicolor.*[22]

The brown spider's natural habitat is outdoors, beneath rocks, logs, and boards and in holes and caves. Central heating has enticed the spider to live in homes, warehouses, and other buildings, where they establish residences in dark, dry, undisturbed

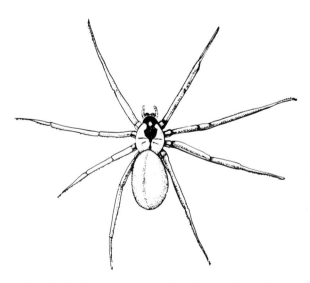

Fig. 22-2   Brown recluse spider *(Loxosceles reclusa),* dorsal view. Note the violin-shaped marking on the cephalothorax.

areas such as attics, closets, garages, and packing crates.

Loxosceles venom is potentially lethal and more potent than that of a rattlesnake.[22] The venom of the brown recluse, *L. reclusa,* has been studied extensively. It is a clear, viscous fluid that contains several enzymes, including alkaline phosphatase, 5′-ribonucleotide phosphohydrolase, hyaluronidase, esterase, and protease.[23] It has been shown that a phospholipase D (sphingomyelinase D) component is the toxic factor responsible for both the cutaneous and the systemic reactions seen with this spider's bite.[9,13]

Early histologic examination of the brown recluse spider bite is characterized by dermoepidermal separation, full-thickness dermal edema, thrombosis of small arterioles, moderate to extensive inflammatory infiltration with neutrophils and eosinophils, and severe extravasation of red blood cells. Polymorphonuclear leukocyte accumulation is seen within 24 to 72 hours and precedes necrosis of the epidermis and dermis with ulceration.[1] The healing process is accomplished by granulation and fibrocollagenous tissue beneath and surrounding the bite eschar.

The brown recluse spider is quite shy and bites only when forced into contact with skin, such as when a person puts on clothing in which the spider is residing. Clinical manifestations of the brown recluse bite depend on the amount of venom injected and the person's age and health. The site of the bite also influences severity. Fatty areas, such as the proximal thigh and buttocks, show more cutaneous reaction and damage. Systemic manifestations occur more often when the injury is to an area of thin skin and little subcutaneous tissue.[22]

The initial bite of the brown recluse spider may be painless or may be felt as a minor sting. During the first 8 to 10 hours after the bite, the person usually experiences only local pain, stinging, and pruritus, but it may take up to 24 hours for these symptoms to develop. Within a few hours to several days, a characteristic hemorrhagic, blue-gray macular halo lesion develops around the puncture site from local hemolysis and arterial spasm. This may progress to become a gangrenous eschar with surrounding erythema, edema, and purpura resembling a "target." The peripheral edema may spread to involve an entire extremity or a large portion of the torso, with lymphangitis and regional lymphadenopathy. Within 4 to 7 days, the central portion becomes necrotic and sloughs, resulting in a deep, sharp, defined ulceration (Fig. 22-3). This area, which can be very large, may take weeks to months to heal and may require skin grafting.

As the size of the necrotic lesion expands, systemic signs become more prevalent and severe. Malaise, restlessness, jaundice, generalized urticaria, arthralgia, myalgia, headache, convulsions, hemolysis, disseminated intravascular coagulation, high fevers, vomiting, diarrhea, hemoglobinuria, hematuria, anuria, delirium, shock, and coma have been reported. In general, these systemic complications will occur within 72 hours of the bite or not at all.

The diagnosis of a brown recluse spider bite can be made by identification of the spider and the presence of a characteristic wound. If the spider cannot be identified or if the bite is atypical, a passive hemagglutination inhibition test is available. This assay detects small quantities of venom expressed from the site of the bite up to 24 hours after the injury. An in vitro lymphocyte transformation test may be used to diagnose earlier bites. Patients with skin necrosis greater than 1 cm should be tested for free serum hemoglobin and thrombocytopenia because they are at risk for systemic complications.[22] Severe loxoscelism occurs more

often in children, with deaths attributed to massive intravascular hemolysis. Systemic manifestations require prompt attention and hospitalization.

Renal function should be monitored closely if hemolysis is detected, with serial measurements of serum and urine hemoglobin levels. Coagulopathies, as demonstrated by thrombocytopenia, fibrinogenemia, and prolongation of the clotting time, should be treated with early hydration, appropriate blood products, and systemic steroids during the acute phase. Broad-spectrum intravenous antibiotics should be given to patients with secondary infections. Leukocytosis may be greater than $30,000/mm^3$ during the acute phase of the illness, and proteinuria can persist for as long as a year.

The treatment of brown recluse spider bites is controversial.[14,15] Intralesional and oral steroids, high-dose hydroxyzine hydrochloride, early surgical excision of the bite site, and dapsone have been advocated. At present, most investigators do not recommend early excision of the bite site. Dispersion of the venom in the dermis is known to be rapid, and the bite site may not correspond to subsequent areas of skin necrosis; therefore excision is not believed to be beneficial.

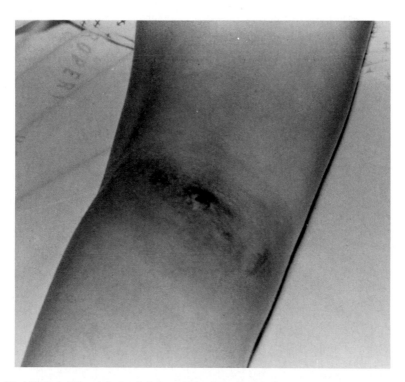

Fig. 22-3 "Target lesion" 4 days following painless brown recluse spider bite.

Dapsone (50 to 100 mg orally for 14 days), an inhibitor of polymorphonuclear leukocytes, has been shown to reduce the need for surgical excision and reconstruction in two limited studies.[14,15] If dapsone is used, however, caution is indicated because it can produce a dose-dependent hemolytic anemia despite normal levels of glucose-6-phosphate dehydrogenase.

If the patient does not develop signs or symptoms of a severe bite (bullae formation, cyanosis, hyperesthesia) within 8 hours after the injury, it is unlikely that extensive therapy will be required. Appropriate care for these patients includes ice packs for local pain relief, pain medication, wound care with sterile dressings, splinting of the involved extremity, rest, tetanus prophylaxis, and daily observation for 3 to 4 days, followed by weekly visits until wound healing is complete.

Necrotic ulcers should be kept clean with antiseptic scrubs and may benefit from topical antibiotic ointments to prevent secondary infections. Smaller ulcers can be allowed to granulate, but excision should be considered for large ulcers. Reconstructive surgery, skin grafts or flaps, should be delayed for at least 2 months because early intervention usually fails.

Children with large lesions (necrotic centers of 2 cm or more) or systemic manifestations should be hospitalized and screened for the presence of hemolysis and coagulopathies. Most authorities recommend systemic intravenous steroids (prednisone, 1 mg/kg) continued for 4 to 5 days, especially if renal and coagulation problems emerge.[2] If significant hemolysis occurs, renal function should be maintained with adequate hydration and periodic assessment of serum and urine hemoglobin levels. Patients with coagulopathies, thrombocytopenia, fibrinogenemia, and prolongation of the clotting time should be followed closely with appropriate use of blood products. Those with secondary infections require systemic broad-spectrum antibiotic treatment.

REFERENCES

1. Alexander JO: Spider bites. In Arthropods and human skin, New York, 1984, Springer-Verlag, Inc.
2. Anderson PC: Necrotizing spider bites, Am Fam Physician 26:198, 1982.
3. Barnard JH: Studies of 400 Hymenoptera sting deaths in the United States, J Allergy Clin Immunol 52:259, 1973.
4. Committee on Infectious Disease: Treatment of anaphylactic reactions. In Peter G et al, editors: 1986 Red Book, ed 20, Elk Grove Village, Ill, 1986, American Academy of Pediatrics.
5. Ennik F: Deaths from bites and stings of venomous animals, West J Med 133:463, 1980.
6. Ginsburg CM: Fire ant envenomation in children, Pediatrics 73:689, 1984.
7. Hunt GR: Bites and stings of uncommon arthropods. 1. Spiders, Postgrad Med 70:91, 1981.
8. Keegan HL, Hedeen RA, and Whittemore FW Jr: Seasonal variation in venom of black widow spiders, Am J Trop Med Hyg 9:477, 1960.
9. Kurpiewski G et al: Platelet aggregation and sphingomyelinase D activity of a purified toxin from the venom of *Loxosceles reclusa,* Biochim Biophys Acta 678:467, 1981.
10. Light WC and Reisman RE: Stinging insect allergy: changing concepts, Postgrad Med 59:153, 1976.
11. Parrino J, Kandawalla NM, and Lockey RF: Treatment of local skin response to imported fire ant sting, South Med J 74:1361, 1981.
12. Parrish HM: Deaths from bites and stings of venomous animals and insects in the United States, Arch Intern Med 104:198, 1959.
13. Rees RS et al: Interaction of brown recluse spider venom on cell membranes: the inciting mechanism? J Invest Dermatol 83:270, 1984.
14. Rees RS et al: Brown recluse spider bites: a comparison of early surgical excision versus dapsone and delayed surgical excision, Ann Surg 202:659, 1985.
15. Rees RS et al: The diagnosis and treatment of brown recluse spider bites, Ann Emerg Med 16:945, 1987.
16. Russell FE and Gertsch WJ: Toxicon 21:337, 1983 (letter to the editor).
17. Russell FE: Jaws that bite, things that sting, Emerg Med 10:25, 1978.
18. Russell FE: Venomous animal injuries, Curr Probl Pediatr 3:1, 1973.
19. Russell FE: Muscle relaxants in black widow spider *(Latrodectus mactans)* poisoning, Am J Med Sci 243:159, 1962.
20. Schanbacher FL et al: Composition and properties of tarantula *Dugesiella hentzi* (Girard) venom, Toxicon 11:21, 1973.
21. Spider bites, Lancet 2:133, 1980 (editorial).
22. Wong RC, Hughes SE, and Voorhees JJ: Spider bites, Arch Dermatol 123:98, 1987.
23. Wright RP et al: Hyaluronidase and esterase activities of the venom of the poisonous brown recluse spider, Arch Biochem Biophys 159:415, 1973.

23

Early Management of Burns

James A. O'Neill, Jr.

Accidental injuries cause more deaths in childhood than all the other causes combined. Although vehicular injuries rank first in terms of mortality, burn injuries are second in children up to 4 years old and third behind drowning and vehicular injuries in children over that age.[1] Presumably, most of these deaths are preventable. At present, more than 1500 children die from burns every year, and three times that many have permanent disabling injuries.

Boys sustain twice as many burn injuries as girls. Approximately 90% of injuries occur in the child's own home. In children under age 3 years, hot liquid scalds are responsible for most minor and major burns. Minor burns usually occur when children pull a pot of boiling liquid over themselves, whereas major injuries more frequently result from bathtub immersions. In infants who have sustained bathtub scald injuries, full-thickness burns frequently result. In children over age 3 years, flame burns occur more often than scalds, and both boys and girls suffer equally. Flammable fabrics, space heaters, matches, outdoor fires, and house fires are the most common etiologic factors involved. Flame burn injuries are usually full thickness and constitute most major fatal burns.

PATHOPHYSIOLOGY OF BURNS IN CHILDHOOD

Although many commonalities exist in the principles of burns management for children and adults, patients under 2 years present major differences.

Young subjects have almost three times the body surface area/body weight ratio than adults.[13] Since surface area is proportional to metabolic rate, related considerations, such as caloric expenditure, water turnover, protein utilization, susceptibility to infection, and other metabolic factors, are quite different. The metabolic differences between children and adults slowly diminish as the child grows older and are approximately equal by puberty. However, significant variations in the rate of evaporative water loss make approaches to fluid therapy quantitatively different. The same is true for the magnitude of stress response reflected in glucose metabolism.

Infants have thinner layers of skin and insulating subcutaneous tissue than adults, which means that they lose more heat and water and lose these faster than adults. In infants under 6 months, the mechanism of temperature regulation is at least partially based on nonshivering thermogenesis, which further accelerates metabolic rate because of an increased rate of oxygen consumption and production of excess lactate.

Although cardiopulmonary function is generally normal and efficient in children, since their metabolic rate is relatively greater than that in adults, reserve may be limited, so these functions may fail rapidly if not sufficiently supported. Furthermore, the evaluation of the cardiovascular status of an infant who is being resuscitated with fluids following burn injury may be difficult, since mottling of the skin and peripheral vasoconstriction occur so often in this age group.

By the time an infant is 1 year of age, renal function is normally comparable to that found in the adult. On the other hand, in infants under 6 months, osmolar concentrating capacity is limited, and free water clearance by the kidney is less efficient as time and water loading progress. For this reason, these infants are prone to water retention, which may be reflected not only as peripheral edema but also as pulmonary impairment. This is

501

somewhat counterbalanced by increased evaporative water loss, but use of diuretics may be necessary for this age group.

INITIAL EVALUATION

Although occasionally children who sustain minor burns are taken to physicians' offices, those with larger burns are usually taken to emergency rooms in community hospitals. At this level, thorough initial evaluation is important because it helps determine appropriate emergency treatment and decision making with regard to hospitalization, referral to a burn center, or outpatient care. A rapid history should be obtained first to determine the details of the mechanism and timing of the injury. This will help in evaluation of the burn's severity, since scald injuries are usually partial thickness and flame burns full thickness. The circumstances also are important to elicit because burns sustained in a closed space may indicate possible inhalation injury. If an explosion has occurred, there may be associated internal injuries that might not be anticipated otherwise. Also, one must find out about the child's past history of congenital or acquired disease, immunization status, drug allergy, and medication history.

The details about the circumstances and mechanism of injury and the physical examination permit one to decide whether to hospitalize the child and whether intravenous fluids are required. Additional factors in this history taking include the home situation and whether the possibility of child abuse exists. Minor and major burns are frequently a manifestation of child abuse.[18] With minor burns and many bathtub immersion injuries, if the pattern of burn distribution cannot be explained by the history offered, a thorough evaluation for child abuse is necessary to prevent subsequent lethal injury.

To determine the extent of injury, *depth* is best estimated by knowing the cause of the burn and seeing its appearance, and surface area is best estimated by using either the rule of nines in children over 10 years or the Lund and Browder chart in younger children (Figs. 23-1 and 23-2).[13] The latter method of estimating surface area is based on infants and young children having a relatively greater surface area for the head and a somewhat lesser surface area for the lower extremities. A full-thickness burn is considered to be twice as lethal and metabolically significant as a partial-thickness burn.

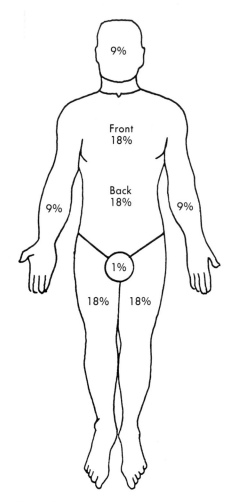

Fig. 23-1 The rule of nines is a practical guide to rapid estimation of surface area involvement in burn-injured individuals older than 10 years of age. A more accurate method is described in Fig. 23-2. (From O'Neill JA: Early management of burns. In Touloukian RJ: Pediatric trauma, ed 1, New York, 1978, J Wiley & Sons.)

Hospitalization is indicated for any child who is suspected to have an inhalation injury. Patients who have partial-thickness burns of less than 10% or full-thickness burns of less than 2% of body surface may be treated as outpatients. In infants under age 6 months, however, even injuries of this magnitude may be physiologically significant, and thus hospitalization should be considered. Patients with partial-thickness injuries of 10% to 20% of body surface area or full-thickness burns of 3% to 10% of body surface area can usually be cared for in community hospitals equipped to treat burn patients. Patients with larger burn injuries or those with inhalation injuries, however, should probably be referred to a specialized burn center.

Area	Age				
	Infant	1-4	5-9	10-14	Adult
Head	19	17	13	11	7
½ Thigh	5½	6½	8	8½	9½
½ Leg	5	5	5½	6	7

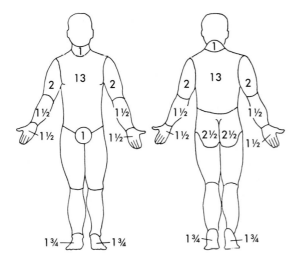

Fig. 23-2   This diagram is a modification of the Lund and Browder chart. It takes the differences in surface area distribution in the various age groups into account. Note that the main differences relate to the head and the lower extremities. (From O'Neill JA: Early management of burns. In Touloukian RJ: Pediatric trauma, ed 1, New York, 1978, J Wiley & Sons.)

When evaluating the depth of burn from physical characteristics, one should know that a first-degree burn resembles sunburn and is characterized by redness. Second-degree burns may be either superficial or deep; superficial second-degree burns are red and wet with blister formation. Patients with deep second-degree and full-thickness burns or with third-degree burns tend to have diminished or absent sensation in the injured area, which may be dry with a pale or brown surface and sometimes with visible coagulated blood vessels. The periphery of a full-thickness burn is usually partial thickness.

EARLY TREATMENT
Minor Burns

Patients with minor burn injuries are those who can be treated as outpatients, as previously defined. Most do not require intravenous fluids for their care, although supplemental oral intake may be desirable. The principles of care relate primarily to patient comfort, wound management for the promotion of expeditious healing, and prevention of infection and other forms of morbidity.

Most minor burns are caused by scalds with hot liquids or flash burns related to outdoor fires. If the child is seen a short time following injury, minor burns may be either immersed in cold water or have ice packs or towels soaked in ice water applied.[7] This is only meant as a temporary first-aid maneuver to reduce pain and edema, but the injury may be worsened if topical hypothermia is applied excessively.

Basically, two methods of wound care are available. For most patients the most practical method is topical application of 1% silver sulfadiazine cream applied twice daily with twice daily baths. If the child tends to rub the topical agent off too quickly, a single thickness of roller gauze may be applied, but excessive thickness should be avoided or the antibacterial agent will be inactivated. For minor burns it is best to leave blisters intact because then patients are more comfortable and healing progresses more rapidly. Under most circumstances, minor partial-thickness burns treated in this fashion will heal within 7 to 10 days, occasionally longer if portions of the injury are deep.

An alternative, more traditional method of care for minor burns is with nonadherent, occlusive dressings. We have found that with this treatment, dressings are best changed daily if superficial infection is to be avoided. This makes this method more expensive than open therapy with a topical antibacterial cream, but it is preferable for burns of certain body areas, such as the hands or feet. Office follow-up is best performed once or twice a week, depending on the parents' ability to manage the child. Topical therapy is usually sufficient to manage potential infection, and systemic antibiotics are only indicated when secondary infection occurs or if another systemic illness is present.

Pain control is ordinarily managed quite well with oral codeine or meperidine.

Patients with small third-degree burns may be treated through the phase of eschar separation and formation of a good bed of granulation tissue on an outpatient basis. Then they may be admitted for definitive skin grafting.

Major Burns
Airway and breathing

As with all trauma, the ABCs constitute the primary principles of care for patients with burn injuries. The most common cause of death in the first few hours following burn injury in a child is respiratory problems.[8] The most frequent inhalation injury in a child is related to upper airway edema, so the threshold for either naso- or endotracheal intubation in a child, particularly the infant, should be lower than in the adult. A history of being burned in an enclosed space or physical findings of singed nasal hairs; burns of the lips, tongue, or palate; or wheezes heard in the chest strongly suggest a significant inhalation injury. In the lung and distal tracheobronchial tree, toxic inhalation may produce progressive hypercarbia and hypoxemia, which are best treated by endotracheal intubation and controlled ventilation. If respiratory acidosis and hypoxemia are not addressed early enough, lethal cardiac arrhythmias or permanent central nervous system damage may occur.

The manifestations of injury related to inhalation of toxic substances are severe bronchospasm and progressive pulmonary edema, but these findings and roentgenographic confirmation may not be evident immediately and may take up to 36 hours to be demonstrable. Frequently, monitoring of blood gases may provide early information on these problems before x-ray studies show typical findings of inhalation injury. Another form of toxic inhalation injury is carbon monoxide poisoning, which results in severe hypoxemia.[2] Although we and others use hyperbaric oxygen therapy to treat hypoxemic patients, it is unclear whether this provides any additional benefit over careful ventilatory management.

When endotracheal intubation is difficult, when ventilation is anticipated for longer than 7 days, or when tracheobronchial toilet is expected to be difficult, tracheostomy is recommended. At times, therapeutic bronchoscopy may be useful in the management of patients with severe inhalation injuries who develop copious, tenacious secretions that cannot be evacuated by conventional suctioning methods. This may help to prevent atelectasis. Patients with carbon monoxide blood levels in excess of 30% are at great risk and must be treated aggressively.[21]

Gastric decompression

Children who sustain significant burn injuries usually have an associated gastric and intestinal ileus, which is best treated by nasogastric suction. In addition, children respond to burn injury with tachypnea to provide adequate oxygenation, which may accentuate the likelihood of gastric dilation.

This is a particularly important consideration for patients who are to be transported from one facility to another, since lethal vomiting may occur if gastric decompression is not performed. Within 48 hours, even in patients with severe injuries, this normally is no longer a concern, and the tube then may be used for the provision of milk and other nutrient feedings.

Fluid therapy

A large-bore, secure intravenous catheter should be placed either percutaneously or by means of a cutdown, preferably in an unburned extremity. Since the burn wound is expected to be colonized by bacteria, strict aseptic technique and use of sterile dressings must be followed to avoid the serious infectious complications with intravenous catheters that occur so often in burn patients with colonized wounds.[19] Although in patients with severe burn injury, central venous pressure or Swan-Ganz catheter monitoring may be desirable, it is best not to place such catheters in the superior vena cava as the initial intravenous access. The same is true of percutaneous placement of subclavicular subclavian catheters, particularly in infants, who have a high incidence of pneumothorax and other complications. Simultaneous with placement of the intravenous catheter, blood should be drawn for complete blood count, electrolytes, carboxyhemoglobin level, and arterial blood gases, if necessary. A Foley catheter should be passed to monitor hourly urine output, but such balloon catheters should be avoided in infant and preschool-age males because of the potential for stricture formation at the membranous urethra. In these patients a small, straight catheter or feeding tube may be less traumatic to the urethra, and it may be stabilized in place easily with adhesive tape or occasionally a suture. One must remember that once peripheral edema has become evident following intravenous fluid replacement, percutaneous cannulation of peripheral veins may be impossible, and thus careful immobilization and fixation are vital.

Many methods of estimating fluid requirements are available for burn-injured children, and although they differ in some respects, all such methods estimate higher fluid requirements for children than adults. This is probably because of the greater extent of evaporative water loss in children. It is well known that all children with extensive burn injuries require large amounts of intravenous fluid replacement, but the extent of such replacement varies greatly and differs in almost every patient. Regardless of the formula used, all must be modified to fit individual needs based on the patient's response to therapy, since no two burn injuries are exactly alike in terms of their extent or depth and associated factors such as inhalation injury. Common approaches to fluid resuscitation in the burned child have been reported by various authors. All formulas use Ringer's lactate as the primary resuscitation fluid. The Brooke group (Graves et al.[11]) recommends supplying maintenance volume and initiating burn resuscitation at 3 ml/kg/% burn. Baxter[5] recommends 4 ml/kg/% burn according to the Parkland regimen. Merrell et al.[14] found that somewhat more than this was required for their patients.

In a recent study the author noted a linear relationship between the amount of surface area burned and the amount of fluid required for satisfactory resuscitation.[17] Although patients with burns over 25% to 35% of body surface had fluid needs of approximately 3 ml/kg/% burn, as described by Graves et al.,[11] those with larger injuries were more effectively treated by the Parkland regimen (see box below). This would appear to be related to the greater magnitude of metabolic rate and insensible water loss associated with a larger surface area in children as compared with older subjects.

Although we and others have found that inhalation injury in children increases the fluid requirements for resuscitation following burn injury,

Navar, Saffle, and Warden[16] actually quantitated the amount of additional fluid needed in patients with inhalation injuries to be approximately 1 to 1.5 ml/kg/% burn. Although our study using linear regression analysis indicated an increase in fluid requirements related to the amount of surface area burned, Merrell et al.[14] found the strongest predictor to be age rather than increase in burn size with younger children requiring greater amounts of fluid, again on the basis of increased surface area compared with older subjects. We have emphasized more aggressive fluid replacement in children with inhalation or very deep, extensive full-thickness burns, since in our experience they have required additional amounts of fluid replacement in a nonlinear fashion. However, none of our patients has developed evidence of even mild pulmonary edema, although we have used diuretics routinely to accelerate the rate of water excretion. This would parallel the experience of Navar, Saffle, and Warden.[16]

Colloid in the form of 5% albumin is generally beneficial when administered after capillary leak has abated during the second 24 hours following the injury.[10] No general agreement exists as to whether earlier administration is possibly beneficial or not, but we have not encountered any particular disadvantage by withholding it for the first 24 hours after the burn. The new Brooke and Parkland formulas appear to be the most practical and economic approach to fluid resuscitation in the burned child, reserving colloid for the second postburn day. Regardless of the method used to estimate fluid requirements, however, preservation of normal organ function and restoration of normal physiology must be the goal of resuscitation.

The rate of fluid administration with Ringer's lactate alone during the first 24 hours following injury may be estimated at approximately one-half the requirement given during the first 6 to 8 hours and the remaining half over the next 16 hours. This is based on a chronology of fluid leak, with capillary permeability at its greatest during the first 12 hours after injury. Also, between 18 and 36 hours (usually about 24), capillary integrity is restored and Starling's law of the capillary is once again functional. Similarly, the basis for all fluid resuscitation therapy is water and sodium.

The aim of fluid resuscitation is to provide adequate amounts of fluid to prevent shock but not so much as to result in pulmonary edema. The objective is to maintain vital organ function

---

ESTIMATION OF PATIENT'S FLUID NEEDS DURING FIRST 48 HOURS FOLLOWING BURN INJURY

First 24 hours:
  Ringer's lactate—3 ml/kg/% burn (25%-35% burn); 4 ml/kg/% burn (more than 35% burn)
Second 24 hours:
  D$_5$ 0.5 N saline—½ to ¾ first day's needs
  5% albumin—as indicated
Guidelines for rate of fluid administration:
  Hourly urine volume
  Vital signs
  Clear sensorium
  Peripheral circulation
  Hematocrit, electrolytes, pH
  Central venous pressure

through adequate support of cardiac output and replacement of plasma volume without producing excessive edema. Edema in excessive amounts is known to have deleterious effects, particularly locally in the burn wound and in the lung. We have noted that accumulation of excessive edema within the burn wound of a child has the potential to transform an initial partial-thickness injury to a full-thickness one.

The most accepted and effective method of judging the adequacy of fluid resuscitation is measurement of hourly urine output. This is best done with an indwelling urinary catheter, as mentioned earlier. The acceptable range of urine output is considered to be 0.5 to 1.5 ml/kg/hour, but the most useful guideline is 1.0 ml/kg/hour. On the other hand, reliance on the level of urine output alone is insufficient in any patient and particularly in the child. Our studies indicate that patients with apparently adequate urine flow may have significant measurable decreases in renal plasma flow and glomerular filtration rate.[20] The latter parameters would appear to be restored to normal only after improvements in cardiac output. Consequently, some measure of estimating the adequacy of cardiac output is considered essential in addition to measurement of hourly urine flow. Since cardiac output cannot be measured easily in children, clinical estimations are useful. In addition to normal vital signs, adequate cardiac output is indicated by good quality of peripheral skin circulation, normal sensorium, and absence of metabolic acidosis. In infants with serious burn injuries, significant metabolic acidosis seen during the first 4 hours after injury may require the administration of sodium bicarbonate before a favorable response to fluid resuscitation is noted. The same is true for prevention of extreme hypothermia.

Since great increases in peripheral resistance are noted in the burned patient, central venous pressure monitoring is not as helpful as in patients with hemorrhage. Serial measurements may be useful, however, and Swan-Ganz catheter monitoring may be helpful as well in extreme cases. Use of a Swan-Ganz catheter may be particularly beneficial in those children with severe inhalation injuries as a guide to continuing fluid replacement. If cardiac output is measured using a Swan-Ganz catheter, findings may exceed the "normal" cardiac index of 2.5 to 3.5 liters/min/m². Within 24 hours following injury, most children with large burns appear to require higher levels of cardiac output, some-times as much as three times the normal resting values.

As mentioned, after the first 24 hours, water and sodium requirements diminish as capillary integrity is restored (again, best judged by appropriate monitoring), and fluid therapy is probably best provided in the form of D_5 0.5 N saline, with added potassium based on measurement of serum electrolytes. Also, after the first 24 hours, supplemental 5% albumin may be indicated, particularly in patients with large full-thickness burns. Evidence of hemoconcentration will help to determine whether or not colloid administration might be beneficial. As an estimate, the fluid requirements during the second postburn 24 hours are generally 50% to 75% of the first 24 hours' total fluid requirement.

After 48 hours following injury, fluid losses and sodium requirements change greatly because at this time the losses are primarily related to evaporation of water from the skin surface, and because the hormonal response to injury promotes water loss and sodium retention.[15] For this reason, hypernatremia and hyperosmolality are common electrolyte disturbances in patients with extensive burns who have had inadequate replacement of evaporative water loss beginning on the third postburn day. We have found the requirement for fluid therapy at this interval to be whatever is required for maintenance plus 1 to 2 ml/kg/% burn/24 hours (see box below). This formula for estimating the requirement for evaporative water loss is based on precise measurements of evaporative water loss we performed in a group of burned children. It has been determined that evaporative losses are approxi-

---

FLUID REQUIREMENTS 48 HOURS AFTER BURN INJURY—EVAPORATIVE WATER LOSS PHASE

Daily maintenance: D_5 0.2 N saline; according to individual needs
Evaporative loss: D_5 0.2 N saline; 1-2 ml/kg/% burn
Potassium: as indicated
Blood: as indicated
Guidelines for fluid needs after 48 hours:
    Body weight measured daily
    Serum sodium, potassium, osmolality; blood urea nitrogen
    Daily urine volume

mately 85% free water, and this may be effectively replaced with D_5 0.2 N saline with added potassium, again based on serum electrolytes and osmolality. Most patients who have had burns in excess of 35% of body surface will have gained weight that is 15% to 20% in excess of their basal weight. Also, diuresis usually takes approximately 5 to 7 days unless accelerated by administration of diuretics. Daily determinations of body weight and serum electrolytes are the best guides to fluid replacement during this time. This type of monitoring is required whether the child is receiving intravenous fluids, oral fluids, or a combination until a significant portion of the burn has either reepithelialized or been skin grafted.

Another occasional consideration in fluid therapy concerns the child who has a particularly extensive, deep thermal burn associated with hemoglobinurea or myoglobinurea. This is usually a possibility during the first few hours following the burn, and if tubular necrosis is to be avoided, administration of mannitol and additional fluids should be considered until the pigment has cleared.

One should remember that oral fluid requirements are generally slightly greater than intravenous requirements when replacing evaporative water losses, since the gastrointestinal tract is not as efficient a route for fluid supplementation as the vascular system.

Blood replacement

Thermal injury to the skin results in immediate destruction of red cells circulating through that capillary bed, as well as in partial damage and a diminished life span in some of the remaining red blood cells; thus plasma loss is the predominant consideration during the first 48 hours following injury. However, polycythemia is generally evident in such patients early, and blood replacement is contraindicated. On the other hand, after the first several days and particularly after the first week following injury, anemia may become evident and administration of packed red blood cells may be required. We generally try to maintain the hematocrit level in the range of 35% to 40%, particularly in infants. Patients with large burn injuries tend to have poor red cell production capability. As they undergo debridements and skin grafting, repeated transfusions are usually required to maintain adequate oxygen-carrying capacity in these severely ill, hypermetabolic children.

Pain control

Narcotic analgesia should be withheld initially until the child is hemodynamically stable and burn shock is no longer a concern. After that, intravenous morphine or meperidine can then be given in graduated small doses as indicated for pain control. When the child is taking oral fluids, oral meperidine or codeine may be administered, particularly before dressing changes or debridement sessions. In addition, administration of diazepam in appropriate doses may be helpful. In patients who have an itching problem, diphenhydramine may be helpful.

Early wound care

The principles of skin grafting are addressed in Chapter 24. Initially the wound should be cleansed with water at body temperature without soap unless the wound is severely contaminated; in this case soap should be used and thoroughly rinsed away because otherwise it may produce toxicity. Blisters should be left intact, except perhaps in very large burn injuries, where bacterial colonization may occur if undebrided tissue is left in place. Extremities that have sustained circumferential burns should be elevated to minimize edema.

If the burns are full thickness, the necessity for escharotomy must be considered during the first 24 to 48 hours when fluid resuscitation is in progress. With massive fluid therapy, not only burned but unburned tissue becomes edematous. Because of this, circumferential full-thickness burns of the trunk may cause respiratory impairment, or those of the extremities may result in vascularly compromised hands or feet. Evaluation of pulses using a Doppler is an extremely helpful guide to determine the need for escharotomy. If respiratory compromise is anticipated or if an indication of diminishing flow to the hands or feet exists, escharotomy is recommended, as described by Pruitt, Dowling, and Moncrief.[22] This involves only incision of eschar on the lateral and medial aspects of the extremity or thorax throughout the burn area. Fasciotomy is not required unless associated fractures or other injuries are present. Escharotomy may be performed at the bedside with minimal pain when the incisions are made through full-thickness burns. Escharotomy is usually sufficient to relieve pressure to the point where blood flow is adequate. Application of topical antibacterial therapy to the escharotomized site normally is sufficient to prevent infection.

In the past, children with burn injuries were treated with topical antibacterial therapy and daily debridement in a hydrotherapy tank until partial-thickness burns reepithelialized or full-thickness burn eschar could be removed and skin grafting performed after approximately 3 weeks. In recent years, early aggressive burn wound excision has been performed to accelerate the rate of wound coverage with beneficial effects.[23] This is addressed in detail in Chapter 24.

Infection control

Although topical antibacterial therapy, usually with 1% silver sulfadiazine, is the mainstay of infection control for the patient with a burn wound, at times *systemic* antibacterial therapy is advised. However, this is based on careful monitoring of the patient. Prophylactic systemic antibiotics are not indicated in burned patients. In the past, prophylactic penicillin was administered for the first 3 to 5 days following burn injury to prevent invasive streptococcal infection, but topical antibacterial therapy has changed this approach. On occasion, children are admitted with upper respiratory infections, and under these circumstances, prophylactic antibiotics may be given. In addition, children treated with topical therapy occasionally develop superimposed streptococcal or staphylococcal cellulitis, and these patients also may benefit from systemic antibiotics, but not on a prophylactic basis. Numerous studies have now indicated that prophylactic penicillin therapy during the first postburn week is not beneficial and may even promote the development of resistant organisms.[9] We have administered prophylactic antibiotics to patients undergoing aggressive debridement or skin grafting, since evidence indicates that prophylactic antibiotics are beneficial under these circumstances in preventing sepsis and early graft loss.

Fundamental to the use of any antimicrobial agent is the performance of frequent bacteriologic cultures not only of the burn wound, but also of blood, urine, intravenous catheters, pulmonary secretions, and other possible sources of infection. Appropriate sensitivities will indicate the type of antibiotic needed and how long it will be required. This is particularly important in patients with large burn injuries who are prone to develop infections with opportunistic organisms not ordinarily encountered in surgical populations.

The patient with a burn injury may be considered the same as any other patient with a traumatic injury to the skin in terms of tetanus immunization. Since antibody response normally is adequate in patients who have previously been immunized against tetanus within the prior 7 to 10 years, and since sensitivity to tetanus toxoid is occurring more frequently now than before, patients who have received tetanus toxoid over the previous 5 years need not receive it. If patients have not previously been completely immunized, tetanus immune globulin should be administered as well as tetanus toxoid.

The true value of gamma globulin has not been proved, but known changes in burn-injured patients appear to support its use, particularly in children with large burns. Arturson et al.[3] and Bjornson[6] have demonstrated that all classes of globulins in burn patients are usually depressed for the first month following the injury, so administration of gamma globulin may be helpful. Also, Alexander et al.[2] have demonstrated that administration of fresh frozen plasma may be helpful in terms of replacing other immune substances such as opsonins in patients with very large burn injuries, particularly those who have demonstrated sepsis. However, continuing good nutrition appears to be the most helpful way to maintain adequate levels of the various immunoglobulins and other immune substances.

Nutrition

In recent years, much information about the various metabolic consequences of severe thermal injury have been reported.[4,12] In the past, physicians routinely noted that young patients with burns in excess of 40% of body surface would often lose as much as 20% of their basal weight. It was demonstrated that patients such as these had great increases in vaporizational heat and water loss accompanying a severe hypermetabolic state. Aulick and Wilmore[4] and others have described hormonal changes that appear to be related to continuing catabolism and negative nitrogen balance. Also, severe malnutrition has been known for many years to be associated with poor wound healing and diminished graft acceptance and more recently with diminished immunologic function and a higher incidence of sepsis. Conversely, patients with good nutrition have been shown to have a lesser incidence of sepsis and a lower mortality.

As mentioned, the burned patient has increased need for water because of losses caused by evaporation from the wound surface. Increased caloric and nitrogen intake are also required to satisfy the tremendously increased needs of these hypermetabolic patients.[12] If at all possible, the gastrointestinal route should be used because of the potentially increased incidence of sepsis related to intravenous catheters required for hypercaloric intravenous nutrition. Although intravenous nutrition may be required temporarily because of bouts of ileus or diarrhea, the patient's own gastrointestinal tract is still the best route for providing maximal amounts of calories and protein.

If patients are unable to take adequate meals and dietary supplements, tube feedings may be required. The smallest tube possible should be used to avoid esophagitis from gastroesophageal reflux, and the patient should be placed in a slightly elevated position to minimize this problem further. Tube feedings are particularly helpful in the management of the infant and very young child with a large burn. These same patients tend to have high rates of evaporative water loss, so one must remember that tube feedings should have no more than one half to two thirds of a calorie per milliliter of feeding if hyperosmolality is to be avoided. At times, only night feedings are required in addition to regular meals and diet supplements during the day. If possible, one should try to achieve an intake of 100 calories/kg/24 hours and approximately 3 g/kg/24 hours of protein equivalent. When tube feedings result in temporary diarrhea, various elemental and semielemental diets are now available that may be helpful. Ongoing ingenuity may be required in this area of nutritional support to achieve the desired result of minimal weight loss. This has proved to be one of the prime keys to survival, particularly in patients who are undergoing early and repeated wound debridements and excision.

Rehabilitation

Rehabilitation should start the moment the patient is admitted to the hospital with daily visits from the physical therapist. Injured extremities should be appropriately splinted and elevated and, as early as possible, active and passive motion exercises instituted. Early rehabilitative treatment may prevent a disability from burn injury that cannot be treated later. Although early physical therapy is only one part of the long-term continuum of rehabilitation considerations, it is among the most important in terms of providing a satisfactory long-term result for a child who has many years of life ahead.

REFERENCES

1. Accident facts, Chicago, 1982, National Safety Council.
2. Alexander JW et al: A sequential, prospective analysis of immunologic abnormalities and infection following severe thermal injury, Ann Surg 188:809, 1978.
3. Arturson G et al: Changes in immunoglobulin levels in severely burned patients, Lancet 1:546, 1969.
4. Aulick LH and Wilmore DW: Hypermetabolism in trauma. In Girardier L and Stock M, editors: Mammalian thermogenesis, New York, 1983, Chapman and Hall.
5. Baxter CR: Fluid resuscitation, burn percentage, and physiologic age, J Trauma 19:864, 1979.
6. Bjornson AB: Effects of burn injury on humoral components of host resistance. In Pruitt BA, editor: Proceedings of the International Burn Research Conference, San Antonio, 1984, US Army Institute of Surgical Research.
7. Boykin JV et al: Cold-water treatment of scald injury and inhibition of histamine mediated burn edema, J Surg Res 31:111, 1981.
8. Charnock EL and Meehan JJ: Postburn respiratory injuries in children, Pediatr Clin North Am 271:661, 1980.
9. Durtschi MB et al: A prospective study of prophylactic penicillin in acutely burned hospitalized patients, J Trauma 22:11, 1982.
10. Goodwin CW et al: Randomized trial of efficacy of crystalloid and colloid resuscitation on hemodynamic response and lung water following thermal injury, Ann Surg 196:520, 1983.
11. Graves TA et al: Fluid therapy in the burned child, J Trauma 28:1656, 1988.
12. Kagan RJ et al: The effect of burn wound size on ureagenesis and nitrogen balance, Ann Surg 195:70, 1982.
13. Lund CC and Browder NC: The estimation of areas of burns, Surg Gynecol Obstet 79:352, 1944.
14. Merrell SW et al: Fluid resuscitation in thermally injured children, Am J Surg 152:664, 1986.
15. Moncrief JA and Mason AD: Evaporative water loss in the burned patient, J Trauma 4:180, 1964.
16. Navar PD, Saffle JR, and Warden GD: Effect of inhalation injury on fluid resuscitation requirements after thermal injury, Am J Surg 150:716, 1985.
17. O'Neill JA: Fluid resuscitation in the burned child—a reappraisal, J Pediatr Surg 17:604, 1982.
18. O'Neill JA: Child abuse. In Welch KJ et al: Pediatric surgery, Chicago, 1986, Year Book Medical Publishers, Inc.
19. O'Neill JA, Pruitt BA, and Moncrief JA: Suppurative thrombophlebitis, a lethal complication of intravenous therapy, J Trauma 8:256, 1968.
20. O'Neill JA, Pruitt BA, and Moncrief JA: Studies of renal function during the early postburn period. In Matter P: Research in burns, Bern, 1971, Hans Huber Publishers.
21. Parish RA: Smoke inhalation and carbon monoxide poisoning in children, Pediatr Emerg Care 2:186, 1986.
22. Pruitt BA, Dowling JA, and Moncrief JA: Escharotomy in early burn care, Arch Surg 96:502, 1968.
23. Rutan TC et al: Metabolic rate alterations in early excision and grafting versus conservative treatment, J Trauma 26:140, 1986.

The Burn Wound: Coverage and Rehabilitation

Donald H. Parks

The mortality rate in hospitalized burned children has decreased rather dramatically in recent years, largely because of the advent of burn centers and the burn team approach, aggressive nutritional support, the development of effective topical antimicrobial drugs, and early surgical excision of the burn wound, among other factors. An enhanced interest recently in maximizing the quality of life following burn injury by emphasizing physical and psychosocial rehabilitation has been particularly encouraging. Methods of burn wound care and early surgical excision, along with principles of physical rehabilitation, are emphasized in this chapter.

CARE OF THE BURN WOUND
Pathophysiology

Thermal injury to skin results in loss of the mechanical barrier it provides, compromising total body temperature regulation, protection of the internal milieu, and many systemic events. The severity of skin injury depends on the agent, the intensity and duration of the heat exposure, and the specific cellular sensitivity in the injured tissue.[34,35] Jackson[14] has described the thermal burn wound pathologically as consisting of a central zone of coagulation necrosis or avascular debris surrounded by an ischemic zone, the zone of stasis, and a peripheral zone of hyperemia (Fig. 24-1). Further vascular implications have been elucidated by Massiha and Monafo,[22] who noted vascular stasis initially on the venous side of the microcirculation and progressive thrombosis into the proximal capillary bed and ultimately to the arterial side of the microcirculation, with resultant ischemia. Such ischemia results in progression of irreversible tissue damage during the first 24 hours. Robson and Heggers[35] have corroborated this, implicating an arachidonic acid metabolite, thromboxane, in pro-

gressive dermal ischemia. Whatever the mechanisms and therapeutic implications, however, it is critically important to note that the burn wound is an avascular or ischemic wound and thus serves as an excellent culture medium for microbes, particularly pathogenic bacteria of the skin and environment. In addition, the delivery of systemically administered antibiotics to bacteria in the wound is inhibited.

Host defense mechanisms

Local nonspecific and specific host defense mechanisms are severely compromised by the presence of thermally injured tissue.[25] The phagocytic system of resistance is compromised through impairment of chemotactic activity normally induced by wound inflammation and the stimulus of invading microorganisms, as well as by decreased phagocytic activity and bacteriocidal ability of the phagocytes.[38] Furthermore, the immune system is dramatically altered by the burn wound, resulting in a state of generalized immunosuppression. The factors and mechanisms responsible for immunosuppression induced by the burn wound have not been thoroughly elucidated. Substances released from the wound itself, produced by cells in response to the wound, and released by or stimulated by bacteria in the wound have been implicated.

Infection remains the major cause of death among hospitalized burn patients. Loss of the mechanical skin barrier, the presence of an avascular and ischemic wound, and the severely immunocompromised state of the burn victim contribute to a high susceptibility to infection. It is thus critical that early wound coverage be expedited.

Isolation Techniques and Hydrotherapy

Control of the patient's environment is critical in decreasing the risk of infection, both from the external environment and from nosocomial

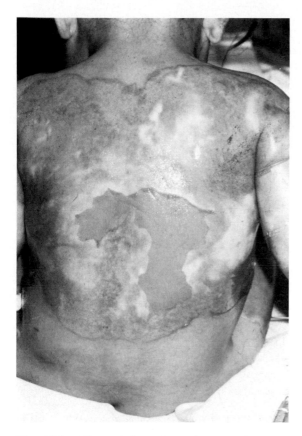

Fig. 24-1 Thermal flame burn demonstrating deep second-degree injury and gross characteristics of zones of necrosis, stasis, and hyperemia marginally.

sources. Initial evaluation of the burned child is performed in a warm environment, with personnel directed to use protective disposable paper gowns, caps, masks, and sterile gloves. Clean linen and waterproof drapes are used. Only when obvious gross contamination has occurred are admission cultures obtained in our center. On the burn unit, hydrotherapy is often used on admission if the patient is stable and generally once or twice daily when indicated later. Chlorhexidine gluconate (Hibiclens) is used preferentially for wound cleansing and during hydrotherapy. This product is relatively nontoxic, broad spectrum, and well tolerated and leaves a residual on the wound. Dakin's solution (dilute sodium hypochlorite) is also used as a compress when heavy contamination or colonization is identified, but it is not routinely used on open wounds because it may be toxic to human cells.[18]

Strict isolation is invoked when patients have

burns on greater than 60% of total body surface area and are particularly susceptible to infection, such as diabetic patients or those taking immunosuppressive drugs. Strict reverse isolation may be invoked when patients have multiresistant organisms or heavy colonization or invasion of the wound.

Generally the open unit concept of care is practiced, allowing children a much better psychologic environment and access to activities on the unit and with other children.

Strict principles of handwashing by all personnel at the burn unit or center and by visitors between patients are mandated. Gowns, gloves, caps, and masks are used during dressing changes. In-service education is frequently provided and emphasizes infection control principles. Sinks, showers, and all hydrotherapy and respiratory therapy devices often harbor large numbers of gram-negative bacteria because of their moist environment and must be monitored and cleaned frequently according to established policies.

Topical Antimicrobials

Topical antimicrobials have evolved as a standard of care for burn patients since the middle 1960s and have had a profound effect on the survival of patients with burns over 40% to 60% of total body surface area. Such agents are applied as early as practical to control surface flora and reduce the risk of subsequent colonization. Early effective topical therapy may reduce progressive dermal ischemia in the zone of stasis by controlling bacterial proliferation.[49] The ideal therapeutic agent should maintain broad-spectrum antiseptic activity, prevent or retard the development of resistant microbial strains, and permeate eschar without loss of activity. An ideal agent should not be absorbed systemically and should be nontoxic both locally and systemically if absorbed. It should not interfere adversely with wound healing or water and heat losses. Such agents should be applied easily, soothing to the patient, and be cost effective not only in its price but also in its application.

Among the more widely used topical agents are 1% silver sulfadiazine, 10% mafenide acetate cream (Sulfamylon), and 0.5% aqueous silver nitrate solution. The characteristics of these agents are summarized in Table 24-1.[24]

Silver sulfadiazine is currently the topical antimicrobial of choice in most burn centers and approaches the ideal agent.[8] The major disadvantages

Table 24-1 Advantages and disadvantages of widely used topical agents for burns

Agent	Advantages	Disadvantages
Silver sulfadiazine	Wide spectrum of activity Painless and easy to apply Nontoxic	Fair eschar penetration Transient leukopenia
Mafenide acetate (Sulfamylon)	Broad spectrum of activity Good eschar penetration Ease of application	Pain on application Sensitivity rash Metabolic acidosis (carbonic anhydrase inhibition) Inhibits epithelialization
0.5% Silver nitrate soaks	Broad spectrum of activity No resistant organisms Painless	Severe biochemical changes (hyponatremia, hypokalemia) Messy and time consuming Discoloration of wound Poor eschar penetration

From Moncrief JA: Topical antibacterial therapy of the burn wound. In Moncrief JA: Clinics in plastic surgery, 1974, Philadelphia, WB Saunders Co.

include lack of eschar penetration, the emergence of resistant organisms (particularly Enterobacteriaceae),[2] transient leukopenia,[17,46] and cutaneous sensitivity. Another agent often used is 10% mafenide acetate (Sulfamylon), often alternated with silver sulfadiazine because it readily penetrates eschar.[29] Its major disadvantages are pain on application and metabolic acidosis caused by carbonic anhydrase activity of the absorbed drug. Also, frequent application of mafenide is necessary. Silver nitrate, 0.5% aqueous, is occasionally used in children; leaching of minerals and absorption with hyponatremia are major disadvantages.[23] In addition, silver nitrate may be impractical because it tends to discolor the wound, possibly obscuring the diagnosis of wound complications, and is very messy, staining the environment.

Rarely, other agents are used in specific circumstances or centers. Undoubtedly in the future, agents possessing more of the ideal characteristics will be developed.

Dressings

A modification combining the exposure technique described by Wallace[45] with the concept of bulky occlusive dressings has evolved and appears to have many advantages. This wound therapy consists of the application of a layer of the appropriate antimicrobial cream to the wound followed by a layer of interrupted lengths of fine-mesh gauze retained by elasticized netting (Fig. 24-2). Fine-mesh gauze is easily removed once or twice a day as appropriate, provides a light dressing that facili-

tates joint mobility and thus early rehabilitation, and keeps an antimicrobial cream against the wound surface. Medicated fine-mesh gauze and elasticized netting are convenient, effective, and acceptable to the staff and patients.

Monitoring the Burn Wound

Daily inspection by experienced physicians and well-trained personnel, including nursing staff and burn technicians who receive frequent in-service training that emphasizes wound appearance and characteristics, provides the most accurate approach to wound monitoring.

Suspicious wound changes are immediately reported to the attending physicians; if indicated, surface swab cultures are obtained. If local or both local and systemic evidence of sepsis exists, two 5 mm punch biopsies are obtained from the suspicious area(s), and quantitative microbiologic and histologic bacteriologic examinations are obtained (Fig. 24-3). The presence of bacteria in quantities greater than 10^5 per gram of tissue, with histologic evidence of invasion into viable subjacent tissue, indicates burn wound sepsis. Parenteral antibiotics and possibly surgical debridement may be instituted.[41,42] Other supportive measures are simultaneously instituted.

In summary, control of burn wound flora through careful aseptic technique in handling the patients, use of hydrotherapy, administration of antiseptic solutions, appropriate use of topical antimicrobial agents, and early wound coverage have contributed to decreased morbidity and mortality in burn pa-

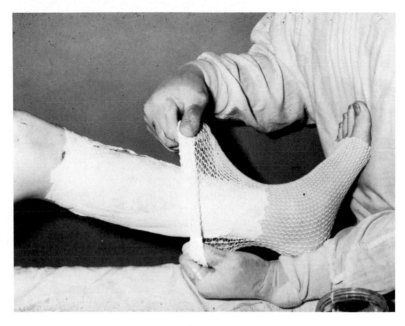

Fig. 24-2   Typical burn wound dressing consisting of topical antimicrobial agent (silver sulfadiazine), single layer of fine-mesh gauze, and elasticized netting.

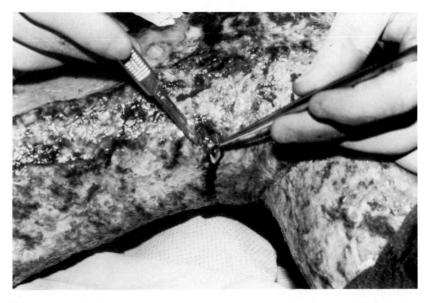

Fig. 24-3   Method of obtaining full-thickness burn wound biopsy by scalpel incision. Two specimens side by side are obtained and submitted for quantitative and qualitative microbiologic studies.

tients. Daily wound examination and a judicious use of quantitative microbiologic studies and pathologic examination may identify potentially lethal wound infections before the patient becomes irreversibly compromised. Burn care facilities should have an organized therapeutic plan in approaching the patient that is directed to rapid conversion of the fresh, open burn wound to a healed wound.

EARLY SURGICAL EXCISION

Successful burn wound management in children demands conversion of the open wound to a closed wound as rapidly as possible.

The concept of early removal of the burn eschar and immediate wound closure with permanent or temporary biologic cover recently has gained widespread acceptance. The concept waxed and waned in popularity in the early twentieth century, and little improvement in mortality was reported. More recently, however, advances in anesthetic technique, the availability of blood for transfusion, and a further understanding of the burn injury's pathophysiology with the development of specialized burn facilities have provided support for instituting early aggressive eschar removal and physiologic wound closure. Evidence accumulating in both laboratory and clinical settings suggests that early eschar removal is effective in decreasing morbidity and improving mortality.[1,44] Several methods of obtaining accelerated eschar removal and wound closure are practiced.

Augmented Spontaneous Separation

Spontaneous separation of the burn eschar occurs gradually from 3 to 6 weeks following injury. This separation occurs through the secretion of proteolytic enzymes from bacteria and leukocytes or through the effects of migrating epidermis dissolving denatured protein beneath the eschar.[47] This process may be augmented by careful tearing of eschar from the underlying viable bed with scissors or by superficially excising the eschar daily during hydrotherapy. This approach is carried out in conjunction with hydrotherapy and topical antimicrobial treatment, requires analgesia, and ideally results in the gradual development of a granulation bed 4 to 6 weeks following the burn.

The major disadvantage of allowing spontaneous separation is an association with high morbidity and mortality related to the prolonged presence of dead tissue, with attendant severe metabolic and nutritional deterioration of the patient with the ever-present threat of burn wound sepsis. This technique is tedious and time consuming for hospital personnel and generally is rarely indicated today.

Enzymatic Debridement

The use of enzymatic debriding agents to obtain early debridement is part of the therapeutic regimen in some centers.[28,37] An enzymatic extract of *Bacillus subtilis* incorporated into a hydrophobic ointment base (Travase) has gained acceptance. This enzyme splits polypeptide chains of necrotic tissue into water-soluble amino acids without affecting viable tissue.

Travase may be applied every 6 to 12 hours directly to the eschar. A topical agent such as silver sulfadiazine on fine-mesh gauze is applied directly over the enzyme to activate it. Some physicians alternate Travase with an antimicrobial dressing every 6 to 12 hours. Treatment generally starts on the second to fifth postburn day, and the enzymes should be applied to burned areas no larger than 15% to 20% of the body surface area. In most cases, debridement should be complete in only a few days, and thus final debridement and grafting can be carried out earlier.

Travase has been used effectively as a chemical escharotomy agent in deeply burned limbs. We have used enzyme debridement in elderly high-risk patients to avoid multiple general anesthetics.

The major complications of enzymatic debridement include increased fluid losses and increased incidence of sepsis.[13] Other adverse effects include pain and local bleeding. Appropriate use over small burned areas has made Travase a valuable agent in our burn treatment armamentarium.

Surgical Management
Preparation

Early surgical debridement of the burn wound has proved to be extremely important in improving mortality and morbidity of burn patients. Except when major respiratory injuries or other rare acute complications occur, burn patients are generally physiologically most able to withstand a surgical procedure early in their hospital course as opposed to later, when nutritional, septic, and other factors intervene. During the initial hours of evaluation, an experienced team of anesthesiologists, operating room staff, and support personnel must develop a coordinated, efficient plan and work together to provide the best overall surgical care.

The patient must be hemodynamically sound and in optimal acid-base and fluid and electrolyte balance. Adequate blood, whether designated donor or pooled packed red blood cells, must be available in the operating room at surgery.

Preoperative parenteral antibiotics are not used routinely in our center. However, when resuscitation has been compromised, the wound is already invaded with organisms before surgical excision, or potential infections exist, particularly beta-streptococcal, such as in children with preexisting upper respiratory illness, then parenteral antibiotics may be administered preoperatively. Patients with compromising systemic disease such as diabetes should also be treated perioperatively with parenteral antibiotics.

Anesthesia

Inhalation anesthesia may be used, but appropriate preoperative assessment, premedication technique, and intraoperative monitoring must be available. With children, tact is especially necessary, and the anesthesiologist must gain their confidence. An effective anesthesia management plan should be developed preoperatively for each patient, taking into account specific circumstances. An effective protocol has been described by Larson.[20] Depolarizing muscle relaxants specifically must be avoided because related severe hyperkalemia and cardiac arrest have been described.[36] Also, patients require several-fold elevated doses of nondepolarizing muscle relaxants, and thus it is critical that anesthesiologists familiar with all aspects of burn anesthesia be available.

Ketamine is an extremely valuable agent as well and has been used very successfully, particularly in burn anesthesia in children.

Tangential excision

Tangential excision was first described by Janzekovic[16] in 1969, and the technique further elucidated by Jackson in 1969[14] and Jackson and Stone[15] in 1972 in classic papers. This surgical approach to the burn wound is diagnostic as well as therapeutic for deep dermal burns. (See the following box for classification of early excision procedures.)

Tangential excision implies the removal of thin slices of eschar until profuse pinpoint bleeding from the white, moist, viable deep dermal surface is observed, followed by immediate grafting with thin sheets of autograft. The procedure is ideally

---

CLASSIFICATION OF PROCEDURES USED IN EARLY EXCISION[26]

1. Tangential excision
2. Tangential debridement
3. Excision to fascia
   a. Small, local third-degree burns
   b. Burn wound sepsis
   c. Massive burns

---

performed between the second and fifth postburn day. However, later excisions may be successful (Figs. 24-4 to 24-7).

We recommend a maximal excision of 15% of the total body surface area. Excision begins on the most distal portion of an involved extremity. We now advocate the use of a tourniquet for the control of bleeding, which has been a significant deterrent to tangential excision in the past. As excision is carried proximally in a definite predetermined excisional pattern, green sterile hospital towels are firmly wrapped with Ace wraps, and the tourniquet is deflated and removed. It is more difficult to obtain hemostasis on the trunk, but adequate control of bleeding may be accomplished with the aid of electrocautery and pressure, again with towels while skin grafts are being harvested. Mesh grafts are used in most body areas, except for the hands and face as well as other functional or aesthetic areas. In any event, we rarely expand the skin but rather apply it with the meshes closed. We strongly believe that this allows for drainage of hematoma, which can be devastating to the take of fresh autografts. Delayed autografting following tangential excision is rarely indicated but may be warranted when persistent, relatively uncontrolled bleeding is encountered. In these circumstances, grafts may be harvested and applied 24 hours later with good results.

Postoperatively, we retain the autografts with Nterface, Kerlix, and elastic wraps on the extremities or Nterface and elasticized netting on the face and trunk.

The advantages of tangential excision in the treatment of partial-thickness burns include early eradication of necrotic tissue and therefore decreased morbidity, shortened hospital stay, and decreased hypertrophic scar formation.

Complications are minimal, but blood loss has been a reported problem that can be controlled as

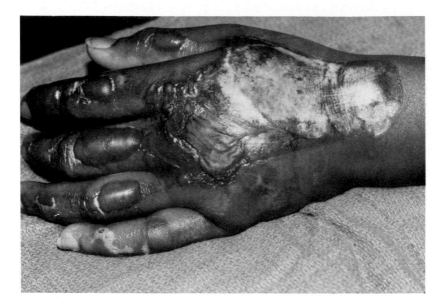

Fig. 24-4   Deep second-degree hot-press burn to dorsum left hand.

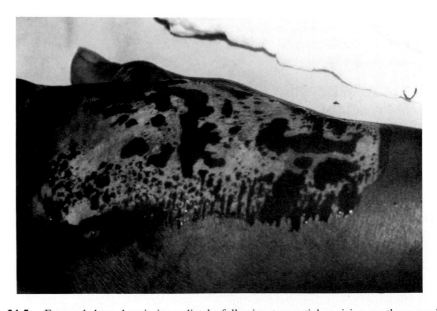

Fig. 24-5   Exposed deep dermis immediately following tangential excision on the second day after the burn. This wound is now ready for grafting.

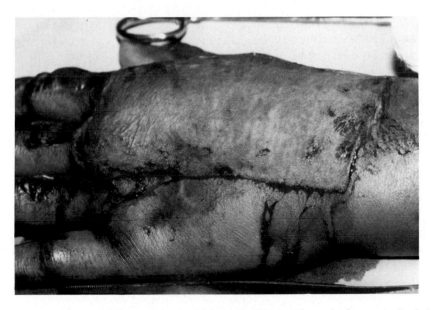

Fig. 24-6   Sheet autograft from patient's thigh applied to freshly excised wound. Graft is approximately 8/1000 inches thick and retained with occasional chromic catgut stitches.

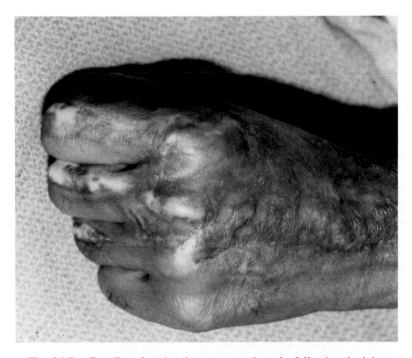

Fig. 24-7   Excellent functional recovery at 6 weeks following the injury.

indicated. Occasionally, small inclusion cysts and overgrafting of skin occur but are of relatively minor importance.

The donor sites are routinely managed by the use of scarlet-red gauze, applied to a donor site where hemostasis has been ensured by pressure.[7]

Tangential debridement

Tangential debridement is indicated in third-degree burns and implies excision of necrotic burn tissue in an effort to reduce the mass of burn eschar. It is used primarily when the wound may be several days old and has become soft and necrotic or when obviously deep, full-thickness eschar exists. In many cases, fat or fascia may ultimately be exposed by the debridement.

The technique is similar to tangential excision, but the accuracy of depth of excision is not as critical as it is with tangential excision. If a relatively clean, viable base can be reached in the subcutaneous fat and appropriate donor sites are available, grafting with autograft is the procedure of choice. Some concern exists regarding successful take of autograft on a bed of fat; in our experience this has been well founded. In this situation, the application of porcine xenograft or other biologic dressing, or alternatively, an antimicrobial-impregnated mesh dressing directed toward the ultimate development of granulation tissue as a graft bed,

have proved to be acceptable alternatives. The choice of wound coverage must be determined at surgery (Figs. 24-8 to 24-10).

Tangential debridement is basically a method of reducing the mass of necrotic tissue that provides an ideal environment for the proliferation of microorganisms, allowing for the development of early granulation tissue and thus for successful skin grafting. Overall, tangential debridement is our most frequently used method of debriding and grafting in adult patients with larger burns.

Burn wound excision

Excision of the burn wound to fascia is performed primarily in three circumstances:
1. Rapid reduction of wound size in massive burns
2. Excision of fat in which invasive burn wound sepsis is present
3. Deep third-degree burns

Reduction of burn wound size in massive burns. The mortality in children with burns over 60% of the total body surface area and greater has remained high despite the advent of topical antimicrobial therapy and improved adjunctive measures.[44] Several methods have been advocated recently for the early excision of the burn wound in these children and have led to significantly improved mortality figures.

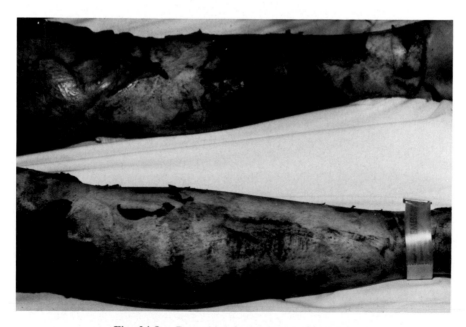

Fig. 24-8   Deep third-degree burns of both legs.

Herndon and Parks[12] in 1986 reported on a series of massively burned children. They compared one group, who had early total excision to fascia with application of expanded autograft and cadaver skin, to a second group treated by serial debridement or tangential debridement and subsequent meshed autografting on granulation tissue as it developed.

Mortality in these two groups was essentially the same, although survivors in the early excision group underwent fewer surgical procedures and had a significantly decreased hospital stay. The ultimate functional and aesthetic consequences of the two techniques are currently being evaluated, but the overall survival was significantly improved over

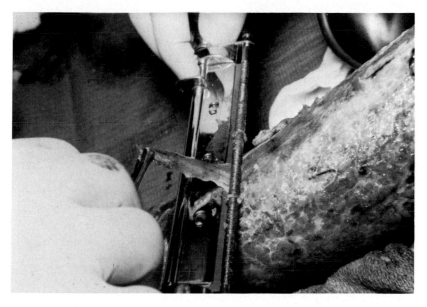

Fig. 24-9   Tangential debridement of deep third-degree burns to viable tissue. Procedure often performed under tourniquet and may be grafted immediately or more commonly dressed with antimicrobial drug or biologic dressings, including allograft or xenograft.

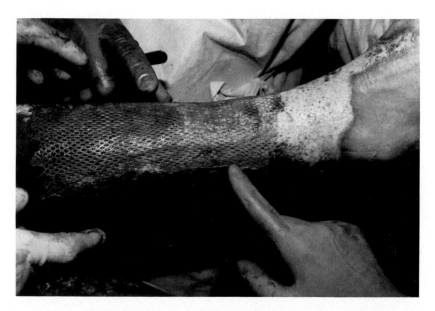

Fig. 24-10   1.5:1 meshed autograft applied to early, clean granulation tissue following tangential debridement and several days of hydrotherapy and topical antimicrobial agents.

much earlier reports. In support of the early massive excision, the search for suitable skin substitutes and other methods to resurface massive burns are being aggressively pursued to facilitate rapid wound coverage.[4]

Current research directed toward the use of autologous cultured epithelial cells is very promising, although further work is indicated.[10] Another promising development is a composite permanent skin substitute, in which a biologic "dermis" is allowed to integrate into the wound and then is covered by a very thin sheet of epidermal cells.[48]

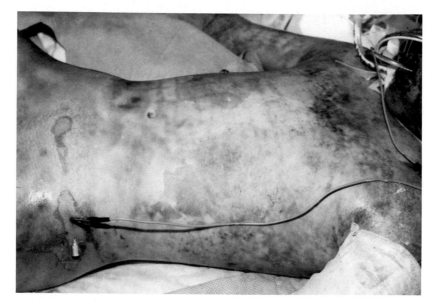

Fig. 24-11 Third-degree burn of anterior trunk in child with an 85% total body surface area flame burn. Prepared for surgical excision on the third day after the burn.

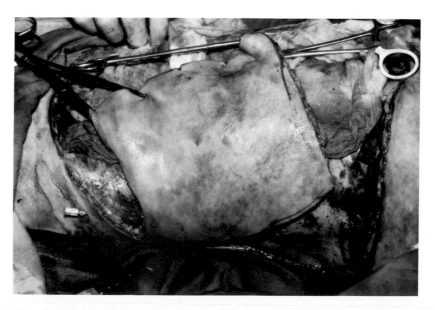

Fig. 24-12 Mass of eschar excised at fascial level preserving breast tissues. Excision achieved by electrocautery and scalpel with minimal blood loss.

The author's approach uses excision of a defined area of third-degree burn wound down to the fascia, with immediate split-thickness skin grafting using meshed autograft from all available donor sites as soon as practical, generally the postburn fifth day. The selected area of burned tissue is excised to the fascial plane over the anterior chest and abdomen if appropriate, after having first confirmed the third-degree nature of the wound with local tangential debridement. The exposed fascia is then covered with the available autograft, meshed 1.5 to 1 or greater (Figs. 24-11 to 24-14). Subse-

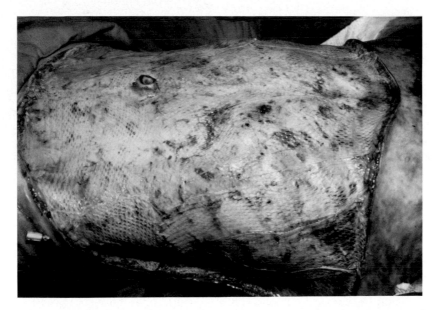

Fig. 24-13   All available autograft including scalp harvested at 7/1000 thickness, meshed 1.5:1, and immediately applied to exposed fascia.

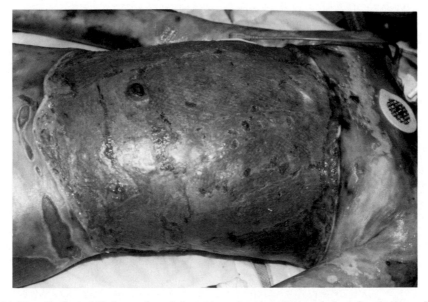

Fig. 24-14   Grafts stabilizing and mesh interstices closed on thirteenth day after the burn. Donor sites are ready for reharvesting.

quently, as the patient's condition allows, sequential tangential debridement of other areas is carried out, thereby rapidly reducing the bulk of dead tissue. As the debridement proceeds, the exposed tissues are maintained in an ideal environment using biologic dressings such as allograft, xenograft, synthetics, or often topical antimicrobial dressings until autograft is once again available. Our experience with graft acceptance on freshly exposed fascia has been excellent. Once donor sites have healed and are suitable for harvesting, a further localized excision to fascia or grafting on healthy granulation tissue, if present, is carried out.

In summary, a major therapeutic factor in the ultimate survival of the burned child seems related to the initial extensive excision of the bulk of necrotic tissue, with successful autografting to close a portion of the wound rapidly.

Excision in sepsis. Burn wound sepsis has been defined as existing when the burn wound is the site of microorganisms actively proliferating in numbers exceeding 10^5 per gram of burn wound tissue and actively invading subjacent unburned tissue.[41,42] The relatively poor blood supply to subcutaneous fat and an immunologically compromised host provide an excellent environment for the development of burn wound sepsis. Topical and systemic antimicrobial therapy is rarely successful in eradicating the septic focus; therefore radical surgical excision in the presence of burn wound sepsis may be a life-saving procedure for the burned child. Wounds are monitored by daily visual inspection as well as by systemic monitoring of the patient's progress. Suspicious changes in the wound prompt full-thickness tissue biopsies to be obtained from these areas and submitted for quantitative and qualitative microbiologic examination. If the biopsy proves to fulfill the criteria for burn wound sepsis, surgical excision of the affected areas may be urgently indicated. Other supportive methods for the management of sepsis are instituted.

Children have been particularly tolerant of surgical excision in the presence of burn wound sepsis. The feasibility and effectiveness of such intervention have been described by Parks, Linares, and Thomson[27] in a series of 22 burned children with biopsy-proved burn wound sepsis. Either tangential debridement of the involved area or excision to fascia locally may be indicated, and we prefer to dress the excised area with topical antimicrobial dressings. In some circumstances the exposed fas-

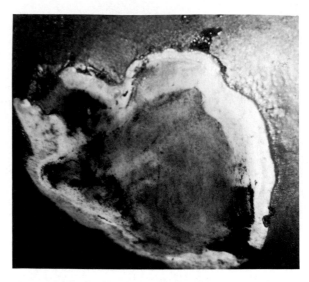

Fig. 24-15   Deep third-degree burn from muffler on chest of pedestrian trapped under vehicle.

cia may be grafted immediately with meshed skin, depending on the patient's condition and the ensured eradication of the septic focus by the surgeon. Alternatively, allograft and zenograft has been used as a temporary dressing.

The ultimate cosmetic appearance following excisions in facial areas with burn wound sepsis is less than ideal in most patients. However, the improved mortality figures outweigh the disadvantages.

Deep third-degree burns. Local deep third-degree burns in which gross evidence exists of primary major injury to the deep subcutaneous tissues provides a third definitive indication for excision to fascia. Hot muffler burns, hot press injuries, and similar burns can be appropriately managed by early excision to fascia and grafting as a primary procedure (Figs. 24-15 to 24-17). To wait for spontaneous debridement of such wounds is folly, and the presence of compromised subcutaneous fat may invite sepsis.

Skin Substitutes

Temporary biologic coverings with various synthetic and biologic materials are widely used in the management of the acutely burned child. In general, the indications include temporary wound closure in patients with massive burns while donor sites heal or cultured epidermal cells are grown in vitro. In patients with smaller superficial burns, skin substitutes are used for pain control, accel-

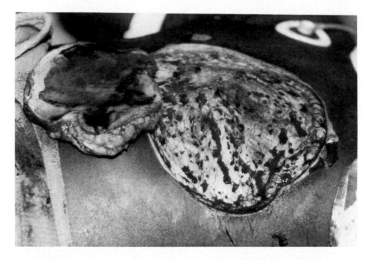

Fig. 24-16   Full-thickness excision of eschar, including involved pectoralis major muscle on second day, after the burn. Wound was immediately sheet autografted.

eration of healing, and minimization of wound manipulation. The ideal properties of these skin substitutes include[30,32,40]:

1. Adherence
2. Water vapor transport
3. Elasticity
4. Durability
5. Intact bacterial barrier
6. Nontoxic and nonantigenic
7. Antiseptic
8. Hemostatic
9. Easy to apply and remove
10. Inexpensive relative to alternatives

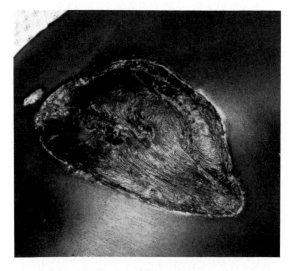

Fig. 24-17   Healed chest burn 14 days after injury.

Among the most widely used temporary skin substitutes are homografts, xenografts, amniotic membranes, and a variety of pure synthetics, including Biobrane. More recently a permanent substitute, specifically a two-layer composite membrane consisting of a collagen dermis under a layer of medical-grade silicon (Integra), has been developed.[48]

Biologic membranes

Allograft. Most allograft is used in the cadaver donor fresh form, although several facilities retain cadaver donor fresh, frozen, and lyophilized allograft for timely use. Allograft does vascularize, or "take," and fulfills many of the ideal characteristics of a skin substitute but is antigenic and thus will ultimately be rejected. It is generally not readily available and is very costly. Guidelines have been developed by the American Association of Tissue Banks Skin Council for the harvesting and storage of allograft, and physicians using allograft should be aware of the statutes regarding skin donation and removal.[39] Viruses and bacteria can be transmitted in allograft in some circumstances.

Xenograft. Xenografts, or porcine skin, are readily available commercially in many forms and may be used in situations similar to those for which allograft is used. Xenograft, however, does not "take," is antigenic, and often disintegrates on the wound, providing an increased risk of infection. We have used xenograft primarily to prepare and

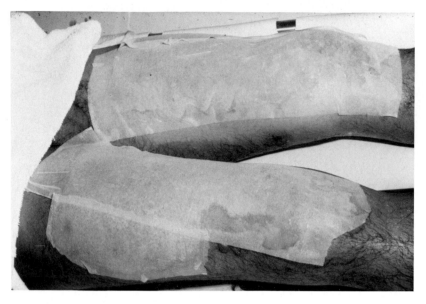

Fig. 24-18   Synthetic dressing (Biobrane) adherent to fresh second-degree burn.

test a granulating wound for subsequent autograft's acceptance and also to provide temporary coverage in large burns while awaiting donor site healing.

Amnion. Membranes collected from vaginal or cesarean deliveries have been prepared relatively inexpensively and used in fresh refrigerated, fresh frozen, and lyophilized forms. Excellent short-term use on a variety of burn wounds has been reported.[31,41,43] Amniotic membranes have been shown to promote angiogenesis in the burn wound, to decrease pain, and to control bacterial flora, but in our experience they tend to disintegrate in 4 to 5 days.[6,33]

Biosynthetic skin substitutes such as Biobrane have been used extensively primarily in the treatment of partial-thickness burns but also in situations where xenograft or allograft might be used (Fig. 24-18). Biobrane is a bilaminar membrane consisting of an outer silicone membrane over a collagen-derived layer. It possesses many of the properties of an ideal skin substitute, although it has little or no effect on wound bacterial counts and should be used on clean wounds.[32] Several other synthetic and biosynthetic skin substitutes are available in addition to other biologic ones.

Permanent skin substitutes. Much recent interest has been stimulated in the use of cultured autologous human epithelium used with a two-layer artificial skin consisting of a Silastic epidermal layer and a biodegradable, bovine collagen-glycosami-noglycan "dermis" that is incorporated into the body as a neodermis.[48] The neodermis becomes a permanent structure in approximately 4 weeks, whereas the Silastic layer is removed and replaced with autograft either directly harvested from the patient or cultured. A similar membrane seeded with autologous epidermal cells initially is being investigated.

A multicenter trial concluded that in patients with major burns, artificial dermis permitted early wound closure with acceptance as good as for allograft and a permanent cover at least as satisfactory as available skin-grafting techniques when covered with an epidermal graft.[11]

The development of permanent skin substitutes, probably using extracorporeal autologous epidermal cell culture methods, appears to hold great promise for the future coverage of burn wounds.[4]

REHABILITATION OF THE BURNED CHILD

Dramatic advances have occurred in the treatment of burn patients in recent years in terms of topical antimicrobial, nutritional, surgical, and other interventions, all directed toward improved survival. Although survival is the ultimate measure of successful therapy, functional, psychologic, and aesthetic considerations that lead to a quality life are a major part of the overall management program. Recently, burn care specialists have recognized that their rehabilitative efforts may not have kept pace with the improvements in mortality. Thus an increased effort in the understanding of scar, scar contractures, psychologic rehabilitation, surgical reconstruction, and other areas has been noted, particularly by such organizations as the American Burn Association.

Wound Healing in Burns

The processes of healing in burn wounds are conducive to the formation of hypertrophic scar and scar contracturing, as characterized by increased vascularity, fibroplasia, myofibroblast accumulation, collagen deposition, and the deposition of interstitial material, as well as scar edema.[19,21] Incised wounds heal in a reasonably satisfactory manner with similar characteristics, resulting in a decrease in wound size and facilitated wound healing by shortening the distance of marginal epithelial cell migration. Also, increased synthesis of structural collagen and cementing of mucopolysaccharide by the fibroblasts give strength to the wound. However, these same processes that are so beneficial in the incised wound can be devastating in the healing of the burn wound. Some of the factors in the healing of a burn wound that may potentiate hypertrophic scar formation and contracture deformities follow.

Collagen

The numerous fibroblasts in the healing burn wound synthesize large amounts of disorganized collagen. Burn scar, hypertrophic scar, and keloid are characterized by overabundant collagen deposition, which may result from alterations in the inflammatory and immune response, among other theoretic causes.[3]

The action of voluntary muscles contributes to positioning of the major joints in flexed positions of comfort. If maintained for a prolonged period, the young collagen fibers fuse into a solid shortened mass, ultimately producing fixed contractures, generally in a fetal posturing (Fig. 24-19). This process has been emphasized in burn care in that the "position of comfort is also the position of contracture" and must be prevented.

Ground substance

Fibroblasts found in granulations and early hypertrophic scar are characterized by having a rich array of dilated, rough endoplasmic reticulum, indicating a high degree of synthetic activity. Chondroitin sulfate B, the sulfate in mucopolysaccharide typically found in normal dermis, is largely replaced in the hypertrophic scar by a relative increase in chondroitin sulfate A, usually associated with firm tissues such as cartilage. An absolute increase occurs in mucopolysaccharide in the hypertrophic scar.

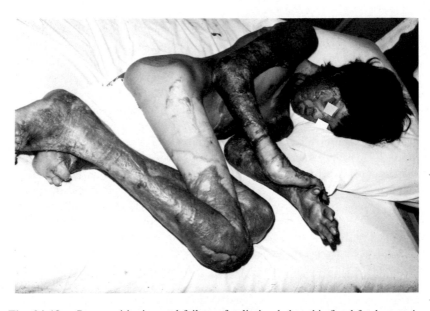

Fig. 24-19   Poor positioning and failure of splinting led to this fixed fetal posturing.

Myofibroblasts

Fibroblasts with contractile-like filaments, 40 to 80 angstroms in diameter, in the cytoplasmic matrix have been identified in early granulation tissue and ultimately result in hypertrophic scar formation.[19] Gabbiani et al.[9] first described fibroblasts with contractile properties in granulation tissues in animals and called them "myofibroblasts" because they had structural properties similar to smooth muscle cells. The myofibroblasts contract, and the resultant relief of stress on the adjacent collagen fibrils may allow the fibrils to form a wavy pattern with supracoils of collagen. Since the myofibroblasts are more frequently found in the reticular dermis, the compact collagen nodules are more frequently located in this area. It is postulated that contraction represented by whorls or nodules may provide the outward force producing the gross appearance of a hypertrophic scar.

In summary, the formation of hypertrophic scar and scar contractures in the burn wound of the child is conducive to discouraging results. Inappropriate positioning of the burned child during the recovery period may result in fixed contractures that may require surgical intervention for relief. The myofibroblasts' contribution to wound foreshortening may further promote contracture formation. The ultimate effect of all those processes in the burn wound results in two basic tenets: (1) the burn wound will shorten until it meets an equal opposing force, and (2) the position of comfort is the position of contracture.

Prevention of Musculoskeletal Deformities

Scar contractures and hypertrophic scar formation following thermal injury can be controlled by proper positioning of the patient, appropriate use of splints to maintain ideal position of all joints, and an intensive comprehensive exercise program in conjunction with the long-term use of splints and constant controlled pressure dressings after healing.[5] The prevention of musculoskeletal deformities is programmed according to the sequence of events in the healing process.

Prehealing Phase

Splints are developed within 24 to 48 hours of admission of the burned child, and strict patient positioning principles are outlined in an instructive diagram posted at the head of the bed. Splints are constructed of a thermoplastic material by the occupational therapist, allowing easy alteration and

replacement as appropriate. Splints are retained primarily by elastic wraps, but Velcro straps may also be useful. Most patients are maintained with the head of the bed elevated on blocks to enhance comfort and tolerance of the recumbent position and potentially to prevent cerebral edema and the features of burn encephalopathy.

Specific anatomic areas

Neck. The neck should be placed in mild hyperextension. Pillows should be avoided because they may produce neck flexion and promote contracture. Pillows are also contraindicated when burns to the ears are present and when bending and irritation may be predispose to chondritis. A neck-conforming splint is applied over the wound dressing, which usually consists of medicated fine-mesh gauze retained by elasticized fishnet dressing. The splint is worn virtually 24 hours a day but removed frequently for cleaning and drying. The splint's purpose is to prevent contracture by preventing flexion of the neck.

Axillae. Ideally the arms should be positioned at 80 to 90 degrees of abduction in a 15- to 20-degree forward plane. Axillary airplane splints may be helpful in the early stages of burn care.

Upper extremities and elbows. Flexion contractures of the antecubital fossae are prevented by the use of three-point splints or conformers constructed from thermoplastic material. These splints are worn continuously except during supervised exercise, mealtimes, and bathing.

Hand. Few greater challenges exist for the burn team than those presented by the burned hand. The deformity of the unsupported burned hand is extremely difficult to correct once established and is characterized by interphalangeal joint flexion, metacarpal phalangeal joint hyperextension, and thumb adduction and extension, all associated with wrist flexion. This position may be prevented by the use of a static splint providing 25 degrees of wrist extension and 45 degrees of metacarpal phalangeal flexion, interphalangeal joint extension, and thumb abduction and flexion. Throughout the postburn period, a carefully managed exercise program for the hand is supervised by therapists and nursing staff, but splinting should never be abandoned for any prolonged period.

Lower extremities. Ankles and feet are generally placed in a neutral position or at 90 degrees, either by using a footboard at the end of the bed or thermoplastic custom-made splints. It is quite unusual for children not to be ambulated early throughout the postburn period, however, since this is the most effective way for preventing foot contractures and particularly heel cord shortening.

Knees. Simple three-point splints or posterior conformers are worn while the patient is in bed. Lower extremities should be elevated at all times and extended while the children are out of bed and sitting. Supervised ambulation with appropriate range of motion exercise is usually indicated.

Hips. Hip contracturing may occur when burns extend over the inguinal area. The hips should be maintained in a neutral position with the leg abducted approximately 15 degrees from the midline to protect the hip joint from dislocation. Prolonged sitting should be avoided. We believe that no satisfactory splinting method for the hips is available.

In summary, contractures can be controlled during the prehealing phase by supervised positioning, splinting, and appropriate exercise programs. Children will generally tolerate ambulation early, particularly if the lower extremities are carefully wrapped with elasticized bandages from the base of the toes to midthighs. It has been our practice to ambulate children on the second postburn day.

Grafting Phase

The principles of proper positioning and splinting are followed during the grafting phase, but the presence of fresh grafts demand some modification of technique.

Specific anatomic areas

Neck. Extension of the neck can be maintained during grafting by using a short mattress with the head positioned on its end. Rarely do we use dressings other than a single layer of a membrane such as Nterface directly over the graft. Once acceptance has been ensured (for example, at 7 days), a conformer is prepared, and its subsequent use then is extremely critical to the eventual outcome.

Axillae. The use of an airplane splint fabricated before the surgical procedure has been used with good success in managing axillary grafts. These are usually made so that they are tolerated when the patient is supine.

Upper and lower extremities. Grafts are generally retained on the extremities with a layer of an interfacing material such as Nterface, a damp Kerlix gauze, and a splint incorporated over the dressing and retained with elastic wraps. Ambulation is usu-

ally discouraged for approximately 5 to 7 during grafting of the lower extremities.

Hand. Fresh sheet grafts are used to resurface the hand. Again, the procedure involves using an interfacing dressing to avoid sticking followed by carefully applying moist gauze individually to each digit and then incorporating the static hand splint, with retention by elasticized wraps. The dressing is left for approximately 3 to 5 days. We often prefer to apply the first dressing with children under general anesthesia and have the occupational therapist construct a custom thermoplastic splint at this dressing change.

Although all due respect should be given the fresh skin graft, the hidden threat of contractures developing, even during the grafting phase, cannot be forgotten. The methods described may hold back the forces leading to contracture while protecting the fragile grafts.

Postgrafting Phase

Hypertrophic scar and scar contracture are the most common sequelae of thermal injury. Many of the functional and cosmetic features of hypertrophic scar may be controlled by the use of constant pressure and conforming splints during the posthealing phase, in association with a specific exercise program and careful follow-up.

Investigators have shown that the application of constant controlled pressure of 25 to 30 mm Hg to scar during the hypertrophic phase, lasting from approximately 6 weeks to a year, induces scar flattening, scar softening, and decreased hyperemia, all features of the mature scar. Microscopically, collagen bundles obtain some degree of parallel orientation, and the nodules tend to disappear. The collagen maintains a loose pattern, and decreased vascularity and diminished tissue oxygen partial pressure under pressure has been described, along with decreased cellularity and mucopolysaccharide.

A program of conforming splints to oppose the forces of voluntary muscle action and myofibroblasts, in addition to constant controlled pressure, form the basis of successful management in the posthealing phase.

Methods of obtaining constant controlled pressure

Elastic bandages and woven fabric elastic (Ace) wraps are used in the early posthealing phase. When properly applied, these provide adequate constant pressure to the early scar and maintain hand or other splints in position. Each layer appears to provide 10 to 15 mm Hg pressure; therefore two to three layers suffice. The wraps are worn over all burn scar and donor sites 24 hours a day and may be augmented in certain areas such as the axillae with foam pads, although the use of a conforming airplane splint is most effective in the axillae.

Elasticized garments

Custom-made elasticized garments are available and provide a simple, effective method of applying constant controlled pressure to the healed burn wound 24 hours a day. Generally, patients are provided two sets of garments. Children usually have accepted the garments well, and the results have been gratifying. Garments are available for virtually all anatomic areas. We generally reserve the use of the garments until the scar has obtained some degree of durability at approximately 10 weeks, as a follow-up to the use of the bandage wraps.

Special Devices

Carefully fitted, high-topped laced shoes with a well-padded tongue, preferably a metatarsal bar,

are prescribed in the posthealing phase. The shoes are to be worn at all times, including at night in bed, by patients with burns of the feet and ankles.

Various methods of obtaining pressure on the face include a custom-made elasticized mask (Jobst) (Fig. 24-20), silicone sponge inserts used beneath the elasticized mask, and clear plastic (Uvex) used with elasticized straps, which is employed most frequently in our current practice with very good results. All devices usually must be worn 24 hours a day and removed only for bathing and during mealtime.

Elastomeres are being used more and more to facilitate pressure, particularly on difficult areas such as the presternum. These are custom-made devices worn beneath the elastic garments (Figs. 24-21 to 24-23). Various other devices, including mouth spreaders, nasal stents, and auricular stents, are available. All are essentially splinting devices and produce pressure on the developing hypertrophic scar.

Ongoing Research

Much research into the pathophysiology and prevention of hypertrophic scar and the closely related keloid is now underway. The lack of an animal

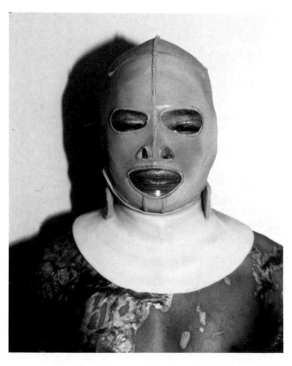

Fig. 24-20 Patient in Jobst hood and custom neck-conforming splint.

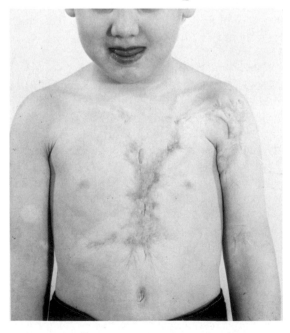

Fig. 24-21 Recently healed burn wound in difficult site to obtain pressure by garments alone.

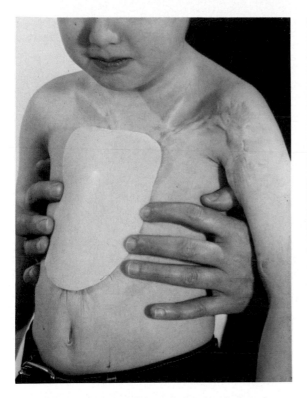

Fig. 24-22   Custom-fabricated elastomeric insert.

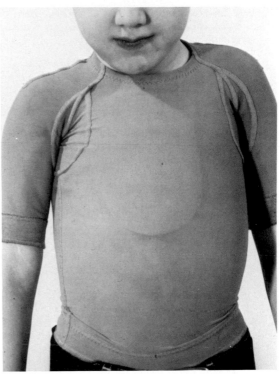

Fig. 24-23   Jobst garment over elastomere insert.

model that develops hypertrophic scar, however, among other problems, has made successful eradication of the problem elusive. Presently the most effective measures for the prevention and control of scar are mechanical and related to the use of pressure and splinting, as previously described. Numerous medications, both topical and systemic, have been evaluated, but until now none has been successful without also producing severe unacceptable side effects. Nevertheless the search continues in many laboratories throughout the United States and in the clinical sphere.

Psychosocial Rehabilitation

Although the scope of this chapter does not include the area of psychosocial rehabilitation, this is a multifaceted, extremely important, and mandatory component of the rehabilitative process.

During hospitalization, children should have a child-life therapy facility and therapist available. All involved in the care of the child must consider the family unit, and this can often be coordinated through the social workers.

REFERENCES

1. Asko-Seljavaara S, Sundell B, and Rytomaa T: The effect of early excision on bone marrow cell growth in burned mice, Burns Incl Therm Inj 2(3):140, 1976.
2. Bridges K and Lowbury JL: Drug resistance in relation to use of silver sulfadiazine cream in a burn unit, J Clin Pathol 30:160, 1977.
3. Cohen IK and McCoy BJ: The biology and control of surface overhealing, World J Surg 4:289, 1980.
4. Doherty D and Austin EV: Effective management of cultured epithelial cells—two case reports, J Burn Care Rehabil 7:33, 1986.
5. Evans EB and Parks DH: Burns. In Nichol VL, editor: Orthopedic rehabilitation, New York, 1982, Churchill Livingstone, Inc.
6. Faulk WP et al: Human amnion as an adjunct in wound healing, Lancet 1:1156, 1980.
7. Fodor PB: Scarlet red, Ann Plast Surg 4(1):45, 1980.
8. Fox CL: Silver sulfadiazine—a new topical therapy for *Pseudomonas* in burns, Arch Surg 96:184, 1968.
9. Gabbiani F et al: The presence of modified fibroblasts in granulation tissue and their possible role, Wound Exp 27:549, 1971.
10. Gallico GG III et al: Permanent coverage of large burn wounds with autologous cultured human epithelium, N Engl J Med 311:448, 1984.
11. Heinbach D et al: Artificial dermis for major burns, a multicenter randomized clinical trial, Ann Surg 208:313, 1988.

12. Herndon DN and Parks DH: Comparison of serial debridement and autografting and early massive excision with cadaver skin overlay in the treatment of large burns in children, J Trauma 26:2, 1986.

13. Hummel RP et al: The continuing problem of sepsis following enzymatic debridement of burns, J Trauma 14:572, 1974.

14. Jackson DM: Second thoughts on the burn wound, J Trauma 9:839, 1969.

15. Jackson DM and Stone PA: Tangential excision and grafting of burns: the method and a review of fifty consecutive cases, Br J Plast Surg 25:416, 1972.

16. Janzekovic Z: In Derganc M, editor: Present clinical aspects of burns. In Derganc M, editor: A symposium, Tisk, Yugoslavia, 1969, CP Mariborski.

17. Kiker RG et al: A controlled study of the effects of silver sulfadiazine on white blood cell counts in burned children, J Trauma 17:835, 1977.

18. Kozol RA, Gillies C, and Elgebaly SA: Effects of sodium hypochlorite (Dakin's solution) on cells of the wound module, Arch Surg 123:420, 1988.

19. Larson DL et al: Mechanisms of hypertrophic scar and contracture formation in burns, Burns Incl Therm Inj 1:2, 1975.

20. Larson SM: Anesthetic considerations. In Carvajal HF and Parks DH, editors: Burns in children: pediatric burn management, Chicago, 1988, Year Book Medical Publishers, Inc.

21. Linares HA: Hypertrophic healing: controversies and etiopathogenic review. In Carvajal HF and Parks DH, editors: Burns in children: pediatric burn management, Chicago, 1988, Year Book Medical Publishers, Inc.

22. Massiha H and Monafo WW: Dermal ischemia in thermal injury: the importance of venous occlusion, J Trauma 14:704, 1974.

23. Monafo WW and Moyer CA: The effectiveness of dilute aqueous silver nitrate in the treatment of burns, Arch Surg 91:200, 1965.

24. Moncrief JA: Topical antibacterial therapy of the burn wound. In Moncrief JA: Clinics in plastic surgery, Philadelphia, 1974, WB Saunders Co.

25. Munster AM and Winchurch RA: Infection and immunology. In Wachtel T: Crit Care Clin: Burns, 1:1, 1985.

26. Parks DH, Carvajal HF, and Larson DL: Management of burns, Surg Clin North Am 57:875, 1977.

27. Parks DH, Linares H, and Thomson PD: Surgical management of burn wound sepsis, Surg Gynecol Obstet 153:374, 1981.

28. Pennisi VR and Capozzi A: Travase: observations and controlled study of the effectiveness in burn debridement, Burns Incl Therm Inj 1(3):191, 1975.

29. Pruitt BA et al: Use of sulfamylon in burn patients. In Lynch JB and Lewis SR, editors: Symposium on the Treatment of Burns, St Louis, 1973, The CV Mosby Co.

30. Pruitt B and Levine N: Characteristics and uses of biologic dressings and skin substitutes, Arch Surg 119:312, 1984.

31. Quinby WC Jr et al: Clinical trials of amniotic membranes in burn wound care, Plast Reconstr Surg 70:711, 1982.

32. Robson M: Synthetic burn dressings: round table discussion, J Burn Care Rehabil 6:66, 1985.

33. Robson MC and Krizek T: The effect of human amniotic membranes on the bacterial population of infected rat burns, Ann Surg 177:144, 1973.

34. Robson MC and Kucan JO: The burn wound. In Current topics in burn care, Rockville, Md, 1983, Aspen Systems Corp.

35. Robson MC and Heggers JP: Pathophysiology of the burn wound. In Carvajal HF and Parks DH, editors: Burns in children: pediatric burn management, Chicago, 1988, Year Book Medical Publishers, Inc.

36. Schaner PJ et al: Succinyl choline–induced hyperkalemia in burned patients, Anesth Analg 48:764, 1969.

37. Silverstein P, Maxwell P, and Duckett L: Enzymatic debridement. In Boswick JA Jr, editor: The art and science of burn care, Rockville, Md, 1987, Aspen Systems Corp.

38. Smith CW and Goldman AS: Selective effects of thermal injury on mouse peritoneal macrophages, Infect Immun 5:938, 1977.

39. Standards Committee of the Skin Council of the American Association of Tissue Banks: Guidelines for the banking of skin tissues, Am Assoc Tissue Banks Newsletter 3:5, 1979.

40. Tavis MJ et al: Current status of skin substitutes, Surg Clin North Am 58:1233, 1978.

41. Teplitz C et al: Pseudomonas burn wound sepsis. I. Pathogenesis of experimental pseudomonas burn wound sepsis, J Surg Res 4:200, 1964.

42. Teplitz C et al: Pseudomonas burn wound sepsis. II. Hematogenous infection at the junction of the burn wound and the unburned hypodermis, J Surg Res 4:217, 1964.

43. Thomson PD and Parks DH: In Wise DL, editor: Burn wound coverings, Boca Raton, Fla, 1984, CRC Press, Inc.

44. Tompkins RG et al: Significant reductions in mortality for children with burn injuries through the use of prompt eschar excision, Ann Surg 208(5):577, 1988.

45. Wallace AB: The exposure treatment of burns, Lancet 1:501, 1985.

46. Wilson P, George R, and Raine PAM: Topical silver sulfadiazine and profound neutropenia in a burned child, Burns 12:295, 1986.

47. Winter G: Histological aspects of burn wound healing, Burns Incl Therm Inj 1(3):191, 1975.

48. Yannas IV et al: Wound tissue can utilize a polymeric template to synthesize a functional extension of skin, Science 215:174, 1982.

49. Zawacki BE: Reversal of capillary stasis and prevention of necrosis in burns, Ann Surg 180:98, 1974.

Index